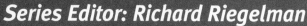

Series Editor: Richard Riegelman

ESSENTIAL PUBLIC HEALTH

Essentials of
Health Policy
and Law FOURTH EDITION

Sara E. Wilensky, JD, PhD
Department of Health Policy and Management, Milken Institute
School of Public Health, The George Washington University

Joel B. Teitelbaum, JD, LLM
Department of Health Policy and Management, Milken Institute
School of Public Health, The George Washington University

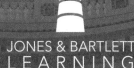

JONES & BARTLETT
LEARNING

World Headquarters
Jones & Bartlett Learning
5 Wall Street
Burlington, MA 01803
978-443-5000
info@jblearning.com
www.jblearning.com

Jones & Bartlett Learning books and products are available through most bookstores and online booksellers. To contact Jones & Bartlett Learning directly, call 800-832-0034, fax 978-443-8000, or visit our website, www.jblearning.com.

Substantial discounts on bulk quantities of Jones & Bartlett Learning publications are available to corporations, professional associations, and other qualified organizations. For details and specific discount information, contact the special sales department at Jones & Bartlett Learning via the above contact information or send an email to specialsales@jblearning.com.

15166-4

Production Credits

VP, Product Management: Amanda Martin
Director of Product Management: Cathy L. Esperti
Product Manager: Sophie Fleck Teague
Product Specialist: Carter McAlister
Product Assistant: Tess Sackmann
Project Specialist: Alex Schab
Digital Project Specialist: Rachel Reyes
Senior Marketing Manager: Susanne Walker
Production Services Manager: Colleen Lamy
Manufacturing and Inventory Control Supervisor: Amy Bacus

Composition: codeMantra U.S. LLC
Cover Design: Kristin E. Parker
Text Design: Kristin E. Parker
Director, Content Services and Licensing: Joanna Gallant
Rights & Media Manager: Shannon Sheehan
Rights & Media Specialist: Maria Leon Maimone
Cover Image (Title Page, Part Opener, Chapter Opener):
    © Mary Terriberry/Shutterstock
Printing and Binding: LSC Communications
Cover Printing: LSC Communications

Library of Congress Cataloging-in-Publication Data

Names: Teitelbaum, Joel Bern, author. | Wilensky, Sara E., author.
Title: Essentials of health policy and law / Sara E. Wilensky, Joel B. Teitelbaum.
Description: Fourth edition. | Burlington, Massachusetts: Jones & Bartlett Learning, [2020] |
Joel B. Teitelbaum's name appears first in previous edition. | Includes bibliographical references and index.
Identifiers: LCCN 2018058317 | ISBN 9781284151619
Subjects: | MESH: Health Policy—legislation & jurisprudence | Insurance,
Health—legislation & jurisprudence | Social Determinants of Health |
Health Care Reform | United States
Classification: LCC RA395.A3 | NLM WA 33 AA1 | DDC 362.10973—dc23
LC record available at https://lccn.loc.gov/2018058317

6048

Printed in the United States of America
23 22 21 20   10 9 8 7 6 5 4 3

Contents

Chapter 5 Public Health Institutions and Systems 81

PART II Essential Issues in Health Policy and Law   111

Chapter 6 Individual Rights in Health Care and Public Health 113

Chapter 7 Social Determinants of Health and the Role of Law in Optimizing Health 137

Chapter 8 Understanding Health Insurance 153

Chapter 12 Healthcare Quality Policy and Law 271

Chapter 13 Public Health Preparedness Policy 293

PART III Basic Skills in Health Policy Analysis   315

CHAPTER 14 The Art of Structuring and Writing a Health Policy Analysis 317

Prologue

The fourth edition of *Essentials of Health Policy and Law* is a textbook that describes and analyzes the transformations taking place across the healthcare delivery and public health systems in the United States. Building on the core content and engaging style of earlier editions, this edition is by necessity influenced by the shifts (both proposed and actual) occurring as a result of the 2016 election cycle, including of course the ways in which the Patient Protection and Affordable Care Act (commonly known as the ACA) is being interpreted and implemented.

Professors Sara Wilensky and Joel Teitelbaum are both experienced in analyzing and communicating about the ACA and many other aspects of health policy and law, and this edition benefits from their expertise. Beyond the issue of national and state health reform, *Essentials of Health Policy and Law, Fourth Edition* takes a broad approach to the study of health policy and law and provides a coherent framework for grappling with important healthcare, public health, and bioethical issues in the United States.

Health policies and laws are an inescapable and critical component of our everyday lives. The accessibility, cost, and quality of health care; the country's preparedness for natural and human-caused disasters; the safety of the food, water, and medications we consume; the right to make individual decisions about one's own health and well-being; and scores of other important issues are at the heart of health policy and law, and in turn at the heart of individual and community health and well-being. Health policies and laws have a strong and lasting effect on the quality of our lives as individuals and on our safety and health as a nation.

Professors Wilensky and Teitelbaum do a marvelous job of succinctly describing not only the nation's policy- and law-making machinery and the always-evolving healthcare and public health systems, but also the ways in which policy and law affect health care and public health, and vice versa. They have a unique ability to make complex issues accessible to various readers, including those without a background in health care or public health. Their training as policy analysts and lawyers shines through as they systematically describe and analyze the complex field of health policy and law and provide vivid examples to help make sense of it all.

Equally apparent is their wealth of experience teaching health policy and law at both the undergraduate and graduate levels. Between them, they have designed and taught many different health policy and/or law courses, supplemented the content of health policy and law by integrating writing and analytic skills into their courses, designed and directed a bachelor of science degree program in public health, and received teaching awards for their efforts. Readers of this textbook are the beneficiaries of their experience, enthusiasm, and commitment, as you will see in the pages that follow.

Essentials of Health Policy and Law, Fourth Edition stands on its own as a text. Even so, the accompanying *Essential Readings in Health Policy and Law* provides abundant illustrations of the development, influence, and consequences of health policies and laws. The carefully selected articles, legal opinions, and public policy documents in the supplemental reader allow students to delve deeper into the topics and issues explored in this book.

I am pleased that *Essentials of Health Policy and Law* is a part of the Essential Public Health series. From the earliest stages of the series' development, Professors Wilensky and Teitelbaum have played a central role. They have closely coordinated efforts with other series authors to ensure that the series provides a comprehensive approach with only intended overlap. This is well illustrated by the numerous additions and revisions that have taken place with the publication of this *Fourth Edition*, a description of which can be found in the Preface.

I am confident that you will enjoy reading and greatly benefit from *Essentials of Health Policy and Law*. Whether you are studying public health, public policy, healthcare administration, or a field within the clinical health professions, this textbook is a key component of your education.

—Richard Riegelman, MD, MPH, PhD
Editor, Essential Public Health Series

About the Editor

Richard K. Riegelman, MD, MPH, PhD, is professor of epidemiology-biostatistics, medicine, and health policy, and founding dean of the George Washington University Milken Institute School of Public Health in Washington, DC. He has taken a lead role in developing the Educated Citizen and Public Health initiative, which has brought together arts and sciences and public health education associations to implement the Health and Medicine Division of the National Academies' recommendation that "all undergraduates should have access to education in public health." Dr. Riegelman also led the development of the George Washington University's undergraduate major and minor and currently teaches Public Health 101 and Epidemiology 101 to undergraduate students.

Preface

In the context of health care and public health, the dozen years since the first edition of this textbook was published can be summed up in a well-worn phrase: change is the only constant. The first edition of *Essentials of Health Policy and Law* did not even include mention of the Patient Protection and Affordable Care Act—commonly known as the Affordable Care Act or ACA—because it was still 3 years from passage. Now hailed as the most important set of changes to health insurance since the 1965 enactment of Medicare and Medicaid, the ACA was signed into law by President Barack Obama in March of 2010. Since that time, the ACA itself has been on quite a journey, given the policy shifts and legal challenges it has undergone in a relatively short time. Broadly speaking, the ACA represents two landmark achievements in health policy: major reform of the private health insurance market and, relatedly, a redistribution of resources to groups and individuals who, by virtue of indigence and/or illness, have historically been excluded from the health insurance market and/or healthcare system. Additionally, the law includes dozens of other important reforms and programs unrelated to insurance. For example, more efficient and higher-quality health care, population health, healthcare access, long-term care, the health workforce, health disparities, community health centers, healthcare fraud and abuse, comparative effectiveness research, health information technology, and more all receive attention by the ACA. Indeed, it is fair to say that a fully implemented ACA would move the nation toward a more affordable, equitable, and stable insurance system, not only for the millions of individuals who have and are expected to gain insurance, but also for the tens of millions of people who no longer face the threat of a loss or lapse of coverage.

▶ Implementation of the ACA

Yet, full implementation of the ACA is still just a goal, as many federal and state policymakers and a substantial bloc of the voting public continue their efforts to undermine—if not totally destroy—the law. To understand these efforts, readers must understand

that many ACA reforms required a reordering of the relationships that lie at the heart of the nation's healthcare and public systems. Individuals, providers, insurers, employers, governments, and others were forced to alter once-normative behaviors in response to the policy and legal decisions underpinning the law. These types of major policy and legal shifts—such as, in the case of the ACA, the creation of the "individual insurance mandate," new prohibitions that prevent private insurers from using discriminatory enrollment practices, the creation of new health insurance "exchanges," and the expansion of Medicaid eligibility standards—are basically destined to create backlash, given the very nature of how people respond to change and the vast amounts of money that, for some industries, are at stake. Add to this the fact that (as described more fully in **Chapter 10**) the ACA bill that eventually became law passed in Congress by the slimmest of margins after months of rancorous debate, and fully half the states in the United States actively opposed the ACA's implementation after its passage. Even now, at the time of this writing, more than 8 years since the ACA became law, courts across the country have ACA-related cases on their dockets, the Trump administration has made a habit of slowing or reversing dozens of Obama-era ACA policy decisions, and the ACA continues to be used as a cudgel on the campaign trail. Needless to say, the outcomes of these lawsuits and policy debates will no doubt be discussed in both the national media and in the health policy and law courses in which you register, and they will be devoted space in the pages of this book in future editions.

▶ Other Changes in the Health Care and Public Health Landscape

Of course, the ACA is not the only significant shift in the healthcare/public health landscape since the first edition of this book. Just as that edition did not mention the ACA (for obvious reasons), neither did it include the term "social determinants of health," which is a growing focus of healthcare and public health systems nationwide and now has an entire chapter in this book to show for it. Furthermore, the 2007 edition included just a single reference to public health emergency preparedness, a topic that also is now rewarded with its own chapter. Back in 2005, when the first outline of the first draft of this book took shape, health informatics and health information technology were, relatively speaking, fringe topics in courses on medical care and public health. Not so today. And finally, of course, the country experienced a mainly unanticipated election at the very top of the ticket in 2016, a result that injected many new policies and legal interpretations into an already complex, costly, and oftentimes inequitable web of healthcare services and public health protections.

▶ Shifts in Public Health Education

Important shifts in public health education have taken place since 2007, as well. One particular change that is relevant to this textbook (and the entire Essentials of Public Health series) is the effort undertaken by the Association of American Colleges and Universities (AAC&U) and the Association of Schools and Programs of Public Health (ASPPH) to develop the Educated Citizen and Public Health Initiative. This initiative seeks to integrate public health perspectives into a comprehensive liberal education framework and to develop and organize publications, presentations, and resources to help faculty develop public health curricula in the nation's colleges and universities. As a result, public health perspectives generally, and health policy and law specifically, are increasingly being integrated into courses as diverse as political science, history, sociology, public policy, and a range of courses that prepare students for the health professions. We are proud that this textbook has played a role in shaping (and supplying) the market for health policy and law education as part of a liberal education framework, and we aim with this *Fourth Edition* to make the material as accessible to these diverse audiences as possible.

▶ Addressing Health Policy Challenges

On the topic of health system complexity, we offer four factors for your consideration as you delve into the

chapters that follow. First, like most challenging public policy problems, pressing health policy questions simultaneously implicate politics, law, ethics, and social mores, all of which come with their own set of competing interests and advocates. Second, health policy debates often involve deeply personal matters pertaining to one's quality—or very definition—of life, philosophical questions about whether health care should be a market commodity or a social good, or profound questions about how to appropriately balance population welfare with closely guarded individual freedoms and liberties. Third, it is often not abundantly clear how to begin tackling a particular health policy problem. For example, is it one best handled by the medical care system, the public health system, or both? Which level of government—federal or state—has the authority or ability to take action? Should the problem be handled legislatively or through regulatory channels? The final ingredient that makes health policy problems such a complex stew is the rapid developments often experienced in the areas of healthcare research, medical technology, and public health threats. Generally speaking, this kind of rapid evolution is a confounding problem for the usually slow-moving American policy- and law-making machinery.

Furthermore, the range of topics fairly included under the banner of "health policy and law" is breathtaking. For example, what effect is healthcare spending having on national and state economies? How should finite financial resources be allocated between health care and public health? How can we ensure that the trust funds established to account for Medicare's income and disbursements remain solvent in the future as an enormous group of baby boomers becomes eligible for program benefits? What kind of return (in terms of quality of individual care and the overall health of the population) should we expect from the staggering amount of money we collectively spend on health? Should individuals have a legal entitlement to health insurance? How should we attack extant health disparities based on race, ethnicity, and socioeconomic status? What policies will best protect the privacy of personal health information in an increasingly electronic medical system? Can advanced information technology systems improve the quality of individual and population health? Should the right to have an abortion continue to be protected under the federal Constitution? Should physician assistance in dying be promoted as a laudable social value? Will mapping the human genome lead to discrimination based on underlying health status? How prepared is the country for natural and man-made catastrophes, like pandemic influenza or bioterrorism attacks? What effect will chronic diseases, such as diabetes and obesity-related conditions, have on healthcare delivery and financing? How should we harness advancing scientific findings for the benefit of the public's health?

As seen from even this partial list of questions, the breadth of issues encountered in the study of health policy and law is virtually limitless, and we do not grapple with all of the preceding questions in this book. We do, however, introduce you to many of the policies and laws that give rise to them, provide an intellectual framework for thinking about how to address them going forward, and direct you to additional relevant readings. Given the prominent role played by policy and law in the health of all Americans, and the fact that the Health and Medicine Division of the National Academies recommends that students of public health and other interdisciplinary subjects (for example, public policy or medicine) receive health policy and law training, the aim of this book is to help you understand the broad context of American health policy and law, the essential issues impacting and flowing out of the healthcare and public health systems, and how health policies and laws are influenced and formulated. Broadly speaking, the goal of health policy is to promote and protect the health of individuals and of populations bound by common circumstances. Because the legal system provides the formal structure through which public policy—including health policy—is debated, effected, and interpreted, law is an indispensable component of the study of health policy. Indeed, law is inherent to the expression of public policy: major changes to policies often demand the creation, amendment, or rescission of laws. As such, students studying policy must learn about policymaking *and* the law, legal process, and legal concepts.

▶ About the Fourth Edition

As a result of the changes just described and also in response to comments we received from users of previous editions of the textbook, this edition of *Essentials of Health Policy and Law* has undergone updates to many chapters, including revised and expanded content; updated figures, tables, timelines, and discussion questions; and updated references and readings.

Part I

Part I of this textbook includes five preparatory chapters. **Chapter 1** describes the influential role of policy and law in health care and public health and introduces various conceptual frameworks through which the study of health policy and law can take place. The

chapter also illustrates why it is important to include policy and law in the study of health care and public health. However, an advanced exploration of health policy and law in individual and population health necessitates both a basic and practical comprehension of policy and law in general—including the policymaking process and the workings of the legal system—and an understanding of the nation's rather fragmented healthcare and public health systems. Thus, **Chapter 2** discusses both the meaning of policy and the policymaking process, including the basic functions, structures, and powers of the legislative and executive branches of government and the respective roles of the federal and state governments in policymaking. **Chapter 3** then describes the meaning and sources of law and several key features of the American legal system, including the separation of powers doctrine, federalism, the role of courts, and due process. **Chapter 4** provides an overview of the healthcare system, including basic information on healthcare finance, access, and quality, and examples of how the U.S. system differs from those in other developed nations. Part I closes with an overview, in **Chapter 5**, of the public health system, including its evolution and core functions.

Part II

Part II offers several chapters focusing on key substantive health policy and law issues. **Chapter 6** examines the ways in which the law creates, protects, and restricts individual rights in the contexts of health care and public health, including a discussion of laws (such as Medicaid and Medicare) that aim to level the playing field where access to health care is concerned. The chapter also introduces the "no-duty-to-treat" principle, which holds that there is no general legal duty on the part of healthcare providers to render care and that rests at the heart of the legal framework pertaining to healthcare rights and duties. **Chapter 7** describes how social factors play a critical role in the attainment (or not) of individual and population health, discusses the ways in which law can both exacerbate and ameliorate negative social determinants of health, and introduces readers to the concept of medical-legal partnership. **Chapters 8** and **9** cover the fundamentals of health insurance and health economics, respectively, and set up a subsequent thematic discussion in **Chapters 10** and **11**. Specifically, **Chapter 8** describes the function of risk and uncertainty in health insurance, defines the basic elements of health insurance, discusses important health policy issues relating to health insurance, and more; **Chapter 9** explains why it is important for health policymakers to be familiar with basic economic concepts; the basic tenets of supply, demand, and markets; and the way in which health insurance affects economic conditions.

The focus of **Chapter 10** is on health reform, including the ACA. The chapter discusses the reasons why for decades the United States failed to achieve national health reform prior to the ACA, how and why the ACA passed given this history, and what the ACA aims to achieve. **Chapter 11** explains how federal and state policymakers have created health insurance programs for individuals and populations who otherwise might go without health insurance coverage. The basic structure, administration, financing, and eligibility rules of the three main U.S. public health insurance programs—Medicaid, the Children's Health Insurance Program, and Medicare—are discussed, as are key health policy questions relating to each program. **Chapter 12** reflects on several important policy and legal aspects of healthcare quality, including the advent of provider licensure and accreditation of health facilities (both of which represent quality control through regulation), the evolution of the standard of care, tort liability for healthcare providers and insurers, preventable medical errors, and, with the ACA as the focal point, efforts to improve healthcare quality through quality improvement and provider incentive programs. Part II concludes with a chapter on public health preparedness policy, including discussions about how to define preparedness, the types of public health threats faced by the United States, policy responses to these threats, and an assessment of where the country stands in terms of preparedness.

Part III

The textbook concludes in Part III by teaching the basic skills of health policy analysis. The substance of health policy can be understood only as the product of an infinite number of policy choices regarding whether and how to intervene in many types of health policy problems. As such, **Chapter 14** explains how to structure and write a short health policy analysis, which is a tool frequently used by policy analysts when they assess policy options and discuss rationales for their health policy recommendations.

▶ New to this Edition

This *Fourth Edition* addresses the many changes related to health reform; the health care system; the ACA's effect on Medicaid, Medicare, and CHIP; as well as health care quality and private payer reform efforts.

The chapter on Public Health Preparedness Policy has been significantly revised, reflecting an increased focus on natural disasters, controlling infectious diseases, and military emergencies.

The chapter on writing a policy analysis has been updated with new detailed examples.

For instructors, we offer thoroughly updated PowerPoint lecture slides for classroom use, as well as an updated Test Bank for each chapter.

The resources in the accompanying Navigate 2 Advantage platform have also been thoroughly updated. These are available for either independent student study or for use in an instructor-led, online course. These materials include an interactive eBook with personalization tools such as highlighting, bookmarking, notes, and end-of-chapter quizzes to assess learning. Also included are Slides in PowerPoint format, an interactive glossary, practice quizzes, and more. These materials are available by redeeming the code found on the card inside this book.

Acknowledgments

We are grateful to the many people who generously contributed their guidance, assistance, and encouragement to us during the writing of this book. At the top of the list is Dr. Richard Riegelman, founding dean of the Milken Institute School of Public Health at the George Washington University (GW) and Professor of Epidemiology and Biostatistics, Medicine, and Health Policy. The Essential Public Health series was his brainchild, and his stewardship of the project as Series Editor made our involvement in it both enriching and enjoyable. We are indebted to him for his guidance and confidence.

We single out one other colleague for special thanks. Sara Rosenbaum, the Harold and Jane Hirsh Professor of Health Law and Policy and a past chair of GW's Department of Health Policy and Management, has been a wonderful mentor, colleague, and friend for decades. We are indebted to her for supporting our initial decision to undertake the writing of this textbook.

During the writing of the various editions of this book, we have been blessed by the help of several stellar research assistants. The *First Edition* could not have been completed without V. Nelligan Coogan, Mara B. McDermott, Sarah E. Mutinsky, Dana E. Thomas, and Ramona Whittington; Brittany Plavchak and Julia Roumm were essential to the completion of the *Second Edition*; Jacob Alexander's assistance was key to the *Third Edition*; and Joanna Theiss was instrumental in updating the current edition. To all of them we send our deep appreciation for their research assistance and steady supply of good cheer.

Our gratitude extends also to Mike Brown, publisher for Jones & Bartlett Learning, for his guidance and encouragement, and to his staff, for their patience and technical expertise.

Finally, we wish to thank those closest to us. Sara gives special thanks to Trish Manha—her wife, cheerleader, reviewer, and constant supporter—and to Sophia, and William, who make life fun, surprising, and ever-changing. Joel sends special thanks to his family: Laura Hoffman, Jared Teitelbaum, and Layna Teitelbaum, his favorite people and unending sources of joy and laughter.

About the Authors

Sara Wilensky, JD, PhD, is special services faculty for undergraduate education in the Department of Health Policy and Management at the Milken Institute School of Public Health at the George Washington University (GW) in Washington, DC. She is also the director of the Undergraduate Program in Public Health.

Dr. Wilensky has taught a health policy analysis course and health systems overview course required of all students in the Master of Public Health–Health Policy degree program, as well as the health policy course required of all undergraduate students majoring in public health. She has been the principal investigator or co-principal investigator on numerous health policy research projects relating to a variety of topics, such as Medicaid coverage, access and financing, community health centers, childhood obesity, HIV preventive services, financing of public hospitals, and data sharing barriers and opportunities between public health and Medicaid agencies.

As director of the Undergraduate Program in Public Health, Dr. Wilensky is responsible for the day-to-day management of the program, including implementation of the dual BS/MPH program. In addition, she is responsible for faculty oversight, course scheduling, new course development, and student satisfaction.

Dr. Wilensky is involved with several GW service activities: she has taught a service learning in public health course in the undergraduate program; she has been heavily involved in making GW's Writing in the Disciplines program part of the undergraduate major in public health; and she is the advisor to students receiving a master in public policy or a master in public administration with a focus on health policy from GW's School of Public Policy and Public Administration.

Prior to joining GW, Dr. Wilensky was a law clerk for federal Judge Harvey Bartle III in the Eastern District of Pennsylvania and worked as an associate at the law firm of Cutler and Stanfield, LLP, in Denver, Colorado.

Joel Teitelbaum, JD, LLM, is associate professor, director of the Hirsh Health Law and Policy Program, and co-director of the National Center for Medical-Legal Partnership at the George Washington University Milken Institute School of Public Health in Washington, DC. He also carries a faculty appointment in the GW School of Law, and for 11 years served as vice chair for academic affairs in the School of Public Health's Department of Health Policy and Management, a role in which he provided oversight of the Department's graduate degree programs, curriculum development, and faculty and student support services. As director of the Hirsh Health Law and Policy Program, he oversees a program designed to foster an interdisciplinary approach to the study of health law, health policy, health care, and public health through educational and research opportunities for law students, health professions students, and practicing lawyers. In his role at the National Center for Medical-Legal Partnership, he helps direct national efforts to embed civil legal services into healthcare delivery as a way of ameliorating social determinants that negatively affect individual and population health.

Professor Teitelbaum has taught law, graduate, or undergraduate courses on healthcare law, healthcare civil rights, public health law, minority health policy, and long-term care law and policy. In 2009 he became the first member of the School of Public Health faculty to receive the University-wide Bender Teaching Award. He is also a member of the GW Academy of Distinguished Teachers and a Fellow in the University's Cross-Disciplinary Cooperative; he has received the School's Excellence in Teaching Award and was an inaugural member of the School's Academy of Master Teachers; he was inducted in 2007 into the ASPPH/Pfizer Public Health Academy of Distinguished Teachers; and he has been named one of the "Stars" of undergraduate teaching at GW by an undergraduate leadership group. He is regularly invited to lecture at top universities and at national conferences and meetings.

In addition to *Essentials of Health Policy and Law*, Professor Teitelbaum is co-author of *Essentials of Health Justice* (2019), also published by Jones & Bartlett Learning. He has authored or co-authored dozens of peer-reviewed articles and reports in addition to many book chapters, policy briefs, and blogs on civil rights issues in health care, health reform and its implementation, medical-legal partnership, insurance law and policy, and behavioral healthcare quality, and he has directed many health law and policy research projects. In 2000, he was co-recipient of The Robert Wood Johnson Foundation Investigator Award in Health Policy Research, which he used to explore the creation of a new framework for applying Title VI of the 1964 Civil Rights Act to the modern healthcare system.

In 2016, during President Obama's second term, Professor Teitelbaum was named to the U.S. Department of Health and Human Services Secretary's Advisory Committee on National Health Promotion and Disease Prevention Objectives for 2030 (i.e., Healthy People 2030, the national agenda aimed at improving the health of all Americans over a 10-year span). He also serves as Special Advisor to the American Bar Association's Commission on Veterans' Legal Services and as a member of the Board of Advisors of PREPARE, a national advanced care planning organization.

Professor Teitelbaum is a member of Delta Omega, the national honor society recognizing excellence in the field of public health; the American Constitution Society for Law and Policy; the American Society of Law, Medicine, and Ethics; and the Society for American Law Teachers.

Contributors

▶ **Chapter 5: Public Health Institutions and Systems**

Richard Riegelman, MD, PhD, MPH
The George Washington University
Washington, DC

▶ **Chapter 13: Public Health Preparedness Policy**

Rebecca Katz, PhD, and Claire Standley, PhD
Georgetown University
Washington, DC

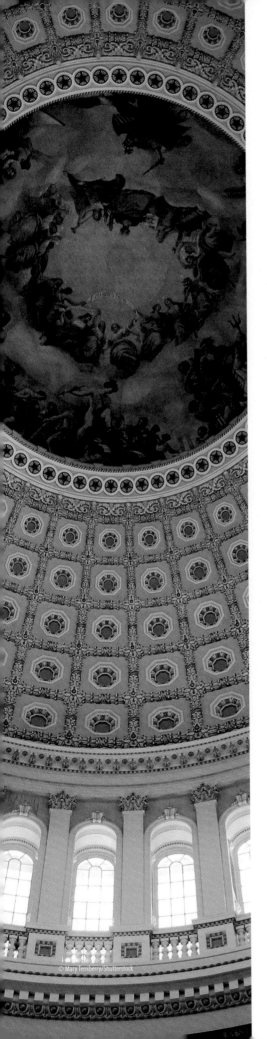

PART I

Setting the Stage: An Overview of Health Policy and Law

Part I of this textbook includes five contextual chapters aimed at preparing you for the substantive health policy and law discussions in Chapters 6–13 and for the skills-based discussion of policy analysis in Chapter 14. Chapter 1 describes generally the role of policy and law in health care and public health and introduces conceptual frameworks for studying health policy and law. Chapter 2 describes the meaning of policy and also the policymaking process itself. Chapter 3 provides an overview of the meaning and sources of law and of several important features of the legal system. Part I closes with overviews of the U.S. healthcare system (Chapter 4) and public health system (Chapter 5).

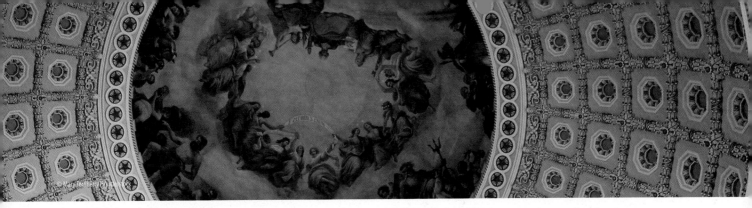

CHAPTER 1

Understanding the Role of and Conceptualizing Health Policy and Law

LEARNING OBJECTIVES

By the end of this chapter you will be able to:

- Describe generally the important role played by policy and law in the health of individuals and populations
- Describe three ways to conceptualize health policy and law

▶ Introduction

In this chapter, we introduce the role played by policy and law in the health of individuals and populations and describe various conceptual frameworks with which you can approach the study of health policy and law. In the chapters that follow, we build on this introduction to provide clarity in areas of health policy and law that are neither readily discernable—even to those who use and work in the healthcare and public health systems—nor easily reshaped by those who make, apply, and interpret policy and law.

The goals of this chapter are to describe why it is important to include policy and law in the study of health care and public health and how you might conceptualize health policy and law when undertaking your studies. To achieve these goals, we first briefly discuss the vast influence of policy and law in health care and public health. You will have a much better feel for how far policy and law reach into these areas as you proceed through this text, but we dedicate a few pages here to get you started. We then describe three ways to conceptualize health policy and law which, as you will discover, are interwoven, with no one framework dominating the discussion.

▶ Role of Policy and Law in Health Care and Public Health

The forceful influence of policy and law on the health and well-being of individuals and populations is undeniable. Policy and law have always been fundamental in shaping the behaviors of individuals and industries, the practice of health care, and the environments in which people live and work. They have also been vital in achieving both everyday and landmark public health improvements.

For example, centuries-old legal principles have, since this country's inception, provided the bedrock on which healthcare quality laws are built, and today the healthcare industry is regulated in many different ways. Indeed, federal and state policy and law shape virtually all aspects of the healthcare system, from structure and organization, to service delivery, to financing, to administrative and judicial oversight. Whether pertaining to the accreditation and certification of individual or institutional healthcare providers, requirements to provide care under certain circumstances, the creation of public insurance programs, the regulation of private insurance systems, or any other number of issues, policy and law drive the healthcare system to a degree unknown by most people.

In fact, professional digests that survey and report on the subjects of health policy and law typically include in their pages information on topics like the advertising and marketing of health services and products, the impact of health expenditures on federal and state budgets, antitrust concerns, healthcare contracting, employment issues, patents, taxation, healthcare discrimination and disparities, consumer protection, bioterrorism, health insurance, prescription drug regulation, physician-assisted suicide, biotechnology, human subject research, patient privacy and confidentiality, organ availability and donation, and more. Choices made by policymakers and decisions handed down through the judicial system influence how we approach, experience, analyze, and research all of these and other specific aspects of the healthcare system. Once you have read the next four preparatory chapters—one on policy and the policymaking process, one on law and the legal system, and one each covering the structure and organization of the healthcare and public health systems—and begin to digest the substantive chapters that follow them, the full force of policy and law in shaping the individual healthcare system will unfold. For now, simply keep in the back of your mind the fact that policy and law heavily influence the way in which overall health and well-being are achieved (or not), health care is accessed, medicine is practiced, treatments are paid for, and much more.

The role of policy and law in public health is no less important than in individual health care, but their influence in the field of public health is frequently less visible and articulated. In fact, policy and law have long played a seminal role in everyday public health activities. Think, for example, of food establishment inspections, occupational safety standards, policies related to health services for persons with chronic health conditions such as diabetes, and policies and laws affecting the extent to which public health agencies are able to gauge whether individuals in a community suffer from certain health conditions. Similarly, policy and law have been key in many historic public health accomplishments such as water and air purification, reduction in the spread of communicable diseases through compulsory immunization laws, reduction in the number of automobile-related deaths through seat belt and consumer safety laws, and several other achievements.[a] Public health professionals and students quickly learn to appreciate that combating public health threats requires both vigorous policymaking and adequate legal powers.

Additionally, in recent years, enhanced fears about bioterrorism and newly emerging infectious diseases have increased the public's belief that policy and law are important tools in creating an environment in which people can achieve optimal health and safety.

Of course, policies and laws do not always cut in favor of what many people believe to be in the best interests of public health and welfare. A policy or law might, for example, favor the economic interests of a private, for-profit company over the personal interests of residents of the community in which the company is located.[b] Such situations occur because one main focus of public health policy and law is on locating the appropriate balance between public regulation of private individuals and corporations and the ability of those same parties to exercise rights that allow them to function free of overly intrusive government intervention. Achieving this balance is not easy for policymakers, as stakeholders disagree on things like the extent to which car makers should alter their operations to reduce environmentally harmful vehicle emissions, or the degree to which companies should be limited in advertising cigarettes, or whether gun manufacturers should be held liable in cases where injuries or killings result from the negligent use of their products.

How do policymakers and the legal system reach a (hopefully) satisfactory balance of public health and private rights? The competing interests at the heart of public health are mainly addressed through two types of policies and laws: those that define the functions and powers of public health agencies and those that aim to directly protect and promote health.[c] State-level policymakers and public health officials create these types of policies and laws through what are known as their *police powers*. These powers represent the inherent authority of state and local governments to regulate individuals and private business in the name of public health promotion and protection. The importance of police powers cannot be overstated; it is fair to say that they are the most critical aspect of the sovereignty that states retained at the founding of the country, when the colonies agreed to a governmental structure consisting of a strong national government. Furthermore, the reach of police powers should not be underestimated: they give government officials the authority—in the name of public health and welfare—to coerce private parties to act (or refrain from acting) in certain ways. However, states do not necessarily need to exercise their police powers in order to affect or engage in public health–related policymaking. Because the public's health is impacted by many social, economic, and environmental factors, public health agencies also conduct policy-relevant research, disseminate information aimed at helping people engage in healthy behaviors, and establish collaborative relationships with healthcare providers and purchasers and with other government policymaking agencies.

Federal policy and law also play a role in public health. Although the word *health* does not appear in the U.S. Constitution, the document confers powers on the federal government—to tax and spend, for example—that allow it to engage in public health promotion and disease prevention activities. For example, the power to tax (or establish exemptions from taxation) allows Congress to incentivize healthy behaviors, as witnessed by the heavy taxes levied on packages of cigarettes; the power to spend enables Congress to establish executive branch public health agencies and to allocate public-health–specific funds to states and localities.

▸ Conceptualizing Health Policy and Law

You have just read about the importance of taking policy and law into account when studying health care and public health. The next step is to begin thinking about how you might conceptually approach the study of health policy and law.

There are multiple ways to conceptualize the many important topics that fall under the umbrella of health policy and law. We introduce three conceptual frameworks in this section: one premised on the broad topical domains of health policy and law, one based on prevailing historical factors, and one focused on the individuals and entities impacted by a particular policy or legal determination (**BOX 1-1**).

We draw on these frameworks to various degrees in this text. For example, the topical domain approach of Framework 1 is on display in the sections about individual rights in health care and public health and healthcare quality policy and law. Framework 2's focus

---

BOX 1-1 Three Conceptual Frameworks for Studying Health Policy and Law

Framework 1. Study based on the broad topical domains of:

a. Health care
b. Public health
c. Bioethics

Framework 2. Study based on historically dominant social, political, and economic perspectives:

a. Professional autonomy
b. Social contract
c. Free market

Framework 3. Study based on the perspectives of key stakeholders:

a. Individuals
b. The public
c. Healthcare professionals
d. Federal and state governments
e. Managed care and traditional insurance companies
f. Employers
g. Healthcare industries (e.g., the pharmaceutical industry)
h. The research community
i. Interest groups
j. Others

---

on historical perspectives is highlighted in the chapters on health reform and government health insurance programs. Finally, Framework 3, which approaches the study of health policy and law from the perspectives of key stakeholders, is discussed in the policy and policymaking process section and also in the chapter dedicated to the social determinants of health. We turn now to a description of each framework.

The Three Broad Topical Domains of Health Policy and Law

One way to conceptualize health policy and law is as consisting of three large topical domains. One domain is reserved for policy and law concerns in the area of *health care*, another for issues arising in the *public health* arena, and the last for controversies in the field of *bioethics*. As you contemplate these topical domains, bear in mind that they are not individual silos whose contents never spill over into the others. Indeed, spillage of one domain's contents into another domain is common (and, as noted, is one reason why fixing health policy problems can be terribly complicated). We briefly touch on each domain.

Healthcare Policy and Law

In the most general sense, this domain is concerned with an individual's access to care (e.g., What policies and laws impact an individual's ability to access needed care?), the quality of the care the person receives (e.g., Is it appropriate, cost-effective, and non-negligent?), and how the person's care will be financed (e.g., Is the person insured?). However, "access," "quality," and "financing" are themselves rather large subdomains, with their own sets of complex policy and legal issues; in fact, it is common for students to take semester-long policy and/or law courses focused on just one of these subdomains.

Public Health Policy and Law

The second large topical domain is that of public health policy and law. A central focus here is on why and how the government regulates private individuals and corporations in the name of protecting the health, safety, and welfare of the general public. Imagine, for example, that the federal government is considering a blanket policy decision to vaccinate individuals across the country against the deadly smallpox disease, believing that the decision is in the best interests of national security. Would this decision be desirable from a national policy perspective? Would it be legal? If the program's desirability and legality are not immediately clear, how would you go about analyzing and assessing them? These are the kinds of questions with which public health policy and law practitioners and scholars grapple.

Bioethics

Finally, there is the *bioethics* domain to health policy and law. Strictly speaking, the term *bioethics* is used to describe ethical issues raised in the context of medical practice or biomedical research. More comprehensively, bioethics can be thought of as the point at which public policy, law, individual morals, societal values, and medicine intersect. The bioethics domain houses some of the most explosive questions in health policy, including the morality and legality of abortion, conflicting values around the meaning of death and the rights of individuals nearing the end of life, and the policy and legal consequences of mapping the human genetic code.

Social, Political, and Economic Historical Context

Dividing the substance of health policy and law into broad topical categories is only one way to conceptualize them. A second way to consider health policy and law is in historical terms, based on the social, political, and economic views that dominate a particular era.[d] Considered this way, health policy and law have been influenced over time by three perspectives, all of which are technically active at any given time, but each of which has eclipsed the others during specific periods in terms of political, policy, and legal outcomes. These perspectives are termed *professional autonomy*, *social contract*, and *free market*.[e]

Professional Autonomy Perspective

The first perspective, grounded in the notion that the medical profession should have the authority to regulate itself, held sway from approximately 1880 to 1960, making it the most dominant of the three perspectives in terms of both the length of time it held favored status and its effect in the actual shaping of health policy and law. This model is premised on the idea that physicians' scientific expertise in medical matters should translate into legal authority to oversee essentially all aspects of delivering health care to individuals; in other words, according to proponents of the physician autonomy model, legal oversight of the practice of medicine should be delegated to the medical profession itself. During the period that this perspective remained dominant, policy- and lawmakers were generally willing to allow physicians to control the terms and amount of payments for rendered healthcare services, the standards under which medical licenses would be granted, the types of patients they would treat, the type and amount of information to disclose to patients, and the determination as to whether their colleagues in the medical profession were negligent in the treatment of their patients.

Social Contract Perspective

The second perspective that informs a historical conceptualization of health policy and law is that of the "modestly egalitarian social contract" (Rosenblatt, Law, & Rosenbaum, 1997, p. 2; the authors write that the American social contract lags behind those of other developed countries, and thus use the phrase "modestly egalitarian" in describing it). This paradigm overshadowed its competitors, and thus guided policymaking, from roughly 1960 to 1980, a time notable in U.S. history for social progressiveness, civil rights, and racial inclusion. At the center of this perspective is the belief that complete physician autonomy over the delivery and financing of health care is potentially dangerous in terms of patient care and healthcare expenditures, and that public policy and law can and sometimes should enforce a "social contract" at the expense of physician control. Put differently, this perspective sees physicians as just one of several stakeholders (including but not limited to patients, employers, and society more broadly) that lay claim to important rights and interests in the operation of the healthcare system. Health policies and laws borne of the social contract era centered on enhancing access to health care (e.g., through the Examination and Treatment for Emergency Medical Conditions and Women in Labor Act), creating new health insurance programs (Medicare and Medicaid were established in 1965), and passing antidiscrimination laws (one of the specific purposes of Title VI of the federal 1964 Civil Rights Act was wiping out healthcare discrimination based on race).

Free Market Perspective

The final historical perspective—grounded in the twin notions of the freedom of the marketplace and of market competition—became dominant in the 1990s and continues with force today (though one could argue that the Affordable Care Act evidences a curbing of the free market perspective and an elevation, again, of the social contract perspective). It contends that the markets for healthcare services and for health insurance operate best in a deregulated environment, and that commercial competition and consumer empowerment will lead to the most efficient healthcare system. Regardless of the validity of this claim, this perspective argues that the physician autonomy model is falsely premised on the idea of scientific expertise, when in fact most healthcare services deemed "necessary" by physicians have never been subjected to rigorous scientific validation (think of the typical treatments for the common cold or a broken leg). It further argues that even the modest version of the social contract theory that heavily influenced health policy and law during the civil rights generation is overly regulatory. Furthermore, market competition proponents claim that both other models are potentially inflationary: in the first case, self-interest will lead autonomous physicians to drive up the cost of their services, and in the second instance, public insurance programs like Medicare would lead individuals to seek unnecessary care.

To tie a couple of these historical perspectives together and examine (albeit in somewhat oversimplified fashion) how evolving social and economic mores have influenced health policy and law, consider the example of Medicaid, the joint federal–state health insurance program for low-income individuals. In 1965, Medicaid was born out of the prevailing societal mood that it was an important role of government to expand legal rights for the poor and needy. Its creation

exemplified a social contract perspective, which in the context of health promotes the view that individuals and society as a whole are important stakeholders in the healthcare and public health systems. Medicaid entitled eligible individuals to a set of benefits that, according to courts during the era under consideration, was the type of legal entitlement that could be enforced by beneficiaries when they believed their rights under the program were infringed.

These societal expectations and legal rights and protections withstood early challenges during the 1970s, as the costs associated with providing services under Medicaid resulted in state efforts to roll back program benefits. Then, in the 1980s, Medicaid costs soared higher, as eligibility reforms nearly doubled the program's enrollment and some providers (e.g., community health centers) were given higher payments for the Medicaid services they provided. Still, the social contract perspective held firm, and the program retained its essential egalitarian features.

As noted, however, the gravitational pull of the social contract theory weakened as the 1980s drew to a close. This, coupled with the fact that Medicaid spending continued to increase in the 1990s, led to an increase in the number of calls to terminate program members' legal entitlement to benefits.[f] Also in the 1990s, federal and state policymakers dramatically increased the role of private managed care companies in both Medicaid and Medicare, an example of the trend toward free market principles.

Key Stakeholders

A third way to conceptualize health policy and law issues is in terms of the stakeholders whose interests are impacted by certain policy choices or by the passage or interpretation of a law. For example, imagine that in the context of interpreting a state statute regulating physician licensing, your state's highest court ruled that it was permissible for a physician to not treat a patient who was in urgent need of care, even though the doctor had been serving as the patient's family physician. What stakeholders could be impacted by this result? Certainly the patient, as well as other patients whose treatment may be colored by the court's decision. Obviously the doctor and other doctors practicing in the same state could be impacted by the court's conclusion. What about the state legislature? Perhaps it unintentionally drafted the licensing statute in ambiguous fashion, which led the court to determine that the law conferred no legal responsibility on the physician to respond to a member of a family that was part of the doctor's patient load. Or maybe the legislature is implicated in another way—maybe it drafted the law with such clarity that no other outcome was likely to result, but the citizenry of the state was outraged because its elected officials have created public policy out of step with constituents' values. Note how this last example draws in the perspective of another key stakeholder—the broader public.

Of course, patients, healthcare providers, governments, and the public are not the only key stakeholders in important matters of health policy and law. Managed care and traditional insurance companies, employers, private healthcare industries, the research community, interest groups, and others all may have a strong interest in various policies or laws under debate.

▶ Conclusion

The preceding descriptions of the roles played by policy and law in the health of individuals and populations, and of the ways to conceptualize health policy and law, were cursory by design. But what we hope is apparent to you at this early stage is the fact that the study of policy and law is essential to the study of both health care and public health. Consider the short list of major problems with the U.S. health system as described in a book edited and written by a group of leading scholars: the coverage and financing of health care, healthcare quality, health disparities, and threats to population health (Mechanic, Rogut, Colby, & Knickman, 2005, p. 10). All of the responses and fixes to these problems—and to many other healthcare- and public health–related concerns—will invariably and necessarily involve creative policymaking and rigorous legal reform (and indeed, the Affordable Care Act, about which you will read in various sections, addressed each of these topics to one degree or another). This fact is neither surprising nor undesirable: policy and law have long been used to effect positive social change, and neither the healthcare nor public health field is immune to it. Thus, going forward, there is little reason to expect that policy and law will not be two of the primary drivers of health-related reform.

Policy and legal considerations are not relevant only in the context of major healthcare and public health transformations, however—they are critical to the daily functioning of the health system, and to the health and safety of individuals and communities across a range of everyday life events. Think about pregnancy and childbirth, for example. There are approximately 11,000 births each day in this country, and thus society views pregnancy and childbirth as more or less normal and unremarkable events. In fact, the process of becoming pregnant, accessing and receiving high-quality prenatal health care, and experiencing a successful delivery is crucial not only to the physical, mental, and emotional health and well-being of individuals and families, but to the long-term economic and social health of the nation. It also implicates a dizzying number of interesting and important policy questions. Consider the following:

- Should there be a legal right to health care in the context of pregnancy, and, if so, should that right begin at the point of planning to get pregnant, at the moment of conception, at the point of labor, or at some other point?

- Regardless of legal rights to care, how should the nation finance the cost of pregnancy care? Should individuals and families be expected to save enough money to pay out-of-pocket for what is a predictable event? Should the government help subsidize the cost of prenatal care? If so, in what way? Should care be subsidized at the same rate for everyone, or should subsidy levels be based on financial need?

- Regarding the quality of care, what is known about the type of obstetrical care women should receive, and how do we know they are getting that care? Given the importance of this type of care, what policy steps are taken to ensure that the care is sound? What should the law's response be when a newborn or pregnant woman is harmed through an act of negligence? When should clinician errors be considered preventable and their commission thus tied to a public policy response? And what should the response be?

- What should the legal and social response be to prospective parents who act in ways risky to the health of a fetus? Should there be no societal response because the prospective parents' actions are purely a matter of individual right? Does it depend on what the actions are?

- Is it important to track pregnancy and birth rates through public health surveillance systems? Why or why not? If it is an important function, should the data tracking be made compulsory or voluntary?

- How well does the public health system control known risks to pregnancies, both in communities and in the workplace?

- Finally, who should answer these questions? The federal government? States? Individuals? Should courts play a role in answering some or all of them, and, if so, which ones? Whose interests are implicated in each question, and how do these stakeholders affect the policymaking process?

There are scores of topics—pregnancy and child-birth among them, as you can see—that implicate a range of complex health policy questions, and these are the types of questions this text prepares you to ask and address. Before you turn your attention to the essential principles, components, and issues of health policy and law, however, you must understand something about policy and law generally, and about the organization and purposes of the healthcare and public health systems. The next two chapters provide a grounding in policy and law and supply the basic information needed to study policy and law in a health context. In those chapters, we define policy and law, discuss the political and legal systems, introduce the administrative agencies and functions at the heart of the government's role in health care and public health, and more. With this information at your disposal, you will be better equipped to think through some of the threshold questions common to many policy debates, including the following questions: Which sector—public, private, or not-for-profit (or some combination of them)—should respond to the policy problem? If government responds, at what level—federal or state—should the problem be addressed? What branch of government is best suited to address, or is more attuned to, the policy issue? When the government takes the lead in responding to a policy concern, what is the appropriate role of the private and not-for-profit sectors in also attacking the problem? What legal barriers might there be to the type of policy change being contemplated? Once you have the knowledge to critically assess these types of questions, you will be able to focus more specifically on how the healthcare and public health systems operate in the United States, and on the application of policy and law to critical issues in health care and public health.

References

Mechanic, D., Rogut, L. B., Colby D. C., & Knickman, J. R. (Eds.). (2005). *Policy challenges in modern health care.* New Brunswick, NY: Rutgers University Press.

Rosenblatt, R. E., Law, S. A., & Rosenbaum, S. (1997). *Law and the American health care system.* Westbury, CT: The Foundation Press.

▶ Endnotes

a. See, for example, Parmet W. E. (2006). Introduction: The interdependency of law and public health. In R. A. Goodman, R. E. Hoffman, W. Lopez, G. W. Matthews, M. A. Rothstein, & K. L. Foster (Eds.), *Law in public health practice* (2nd ed., pp. xxvii–xxvii). Oxford, England: Oxford University Press.

b. For a nonfictional and utterly engrossing example of the ways in which law and legal process might stand in the way of effective public health regulation, we recommend Harr, J. (1995). *A civil action.* New York, NY: Vintage Books.

c. See, for example, Gostin, L. O., Thompson, F. E., & Grad, F. P. (2006). The law and the public's health: The foundations. In R. A. Goodman, R. E. Hoffman, W. Lopez, G. W. Matthews, M. A. Rothstein, & K. L. Foster (Eds.), *Law in public health practice* (2nd ed., pp. 25–44). Oxford, England: Oxford University Press.

d. The particular historical framework described here was developed to apply to health care rather than to public health. We do not mean to imply, however, that it is impossible to consider public health from a historical, or evolutionary, vantage point. In fact, it is fair to say that public health practice may have just entered its third historical phase. Throughout the 1800s and most of the 1900s, protection of the public's health occurred mainly through direct regulation of private behavior. In the latter stages of the 20th century, strict reliance on regulation gave way to an approach that combined regulation with chronic disease management and public health promotion, an approach that necessitated a more active collaboration between public health agencies and healthcare providers and purchasers. Now, it appears that public health professionals are adding to this revised practice model another strategic initiative: building collaborative relationships with policymaking agencies whose responsibilities are not directly related to public health—for example, agencies whose primary fields are housing, transportation, or agriculture.

e. The discussion of these perspectives is guided by Rosenblatt, R. E., Law, S. A., & Rosenbaum, S. (1997). *Law and the American health care system* (pp. 24–35). Westbury, CT: The Foundation Press; Rosenblatt, R. E. (2004). The four ages of health law. *Health Matrix: Journal of Law-Medicine, 14*(1), 155–196.

f. By 2005, proponents of weakening Medicaid-enrolled persons' entitlement to program benefits had made significant strides: Congress passed a law called the Deficit Reduction Act that, among other things, granted states the ability to redefine the benefits and services to which Medicaid beneficiaries are entitled.

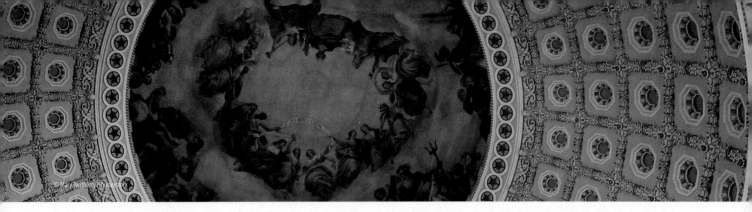

CHAPTER 2

Policy and the Policymaking Process

LEARNING OBJECTIVES

By the end of this chapter you will be able to:

- Describe the concepts of policy and policymaking
- Describe the basic function, structure, and powers of the legislative branch of government
- Describe the basic function, structure, and powers of the executive branch of government
- Explain the role of federal and state governments in the policymaking process
- Explain the role of interest groups in the policymaking process

▶ Introduction

The first steps for any student of health policy are to understand what policy is generally and to learn about the policymaking process. It is vital to consider policy questions in the particular context in which they arise, both in terms of the general politics of the issue and the values and powers of the policymaker. As you will discover, there is no single definition of policy. Even so, this chapter arms you with the information needed to know what issues to consider when thinking about a public policy problem, how to account for a variety of competing policy views, and what policy options are possible given the political process in the United States.

The chapter first defines what policy is and then moves to a discussion of the policymaking process by examining the roles and powers of two of the political branches of government—the legislative and executive branches. As part of this discussion, we intro-

duce you to federal and state agencies that make up the healthcare and public health bureaucracy. We conclude with a discussion about the roles of interest groups in policymaking and the influence they wield in the policymaking process.

▶ Defining Policy

In this section we consider various aspects of what we mean by the term *policy*. Before delving into the policymaking process, we identify which issues fall within the realm of a public policy decision and, generally, what kinds of decisions might be made by policymakers.

Identifying Public Problems

Scholars have defined policy in many different ways. Consider a few of them:

- Authoritative decisions made in the legislative, executive, or judicial branches of government that are intended to direct or influence the actions, behaviors, and decisions of others (Longest, 2016, p. 10).

- A course of action adopted and pursued by a government, party, statesman, or other individual or organization (Subcommittee on Health and Environment, 1976, p. 124).
- Authoritative decisions and guidelines that direct human behavior toward specific goals either in the private or the public sector (Hanley, 1999, p. 125).

The differences in these definitions raise several important issues. The first question to consider is whether private actors make policy or whether policymaking is an activity for the government only. The first definition refers only to governmental policymakers, the second definition allows for both public and private policymakers, and the third definition is unclear on this issue. Of course, the government is a key player in any policy field, and it is certainly true that decisions by government entities represent public policy. However, in this text we also focus on private actors who make policy, such as commercial insurance companies, private employers, influential individuals, and others who can all be part of health policy. For example, when a major health insurance company decides to cover obesity prevention measures, or when the Bill and Melinda Gates Foundation provides grants to develop crops that are high in essential vitamins and minerals to improve the nutrition of people in developing countries, they are making health policy decisions.

Regardless of whether the policymaker is a public or private figure, it is necessary that the decision being made is an *authoritative* decision. These are decisions made by an individual or group with the power to implement the decision, and there are a variety of levels where these kinds of decisions can take place. For example, within government, authoritative decisions may be made by the president, cabinet officials, agency heads, members of Congress, governors, state legislatures, public health commissioners, and many others.

But all decisions by public and private individuals or entities are not necessarily policy decisions. The key issue to determining whether a "decision" represents a "policy" is whether the question at hand is an individual concern or a public policy problem. A public policy problem goes beyond the individual sphere and affects the greater community. Whereas an individual might decide to take advantage of employer-sponsored health insurance, a public policy question is whether all employers should be required to offer health insurance to their employees. Whereas an individual might decide to purchase a generic (as opposed to a brand name) drug to save money, a public policy

question is whether patients should be induced to buy less expensive generic drugs. When deciding whether something is a public policy decision, the focus is not only on who is making a decision, but also on what kind of decision is being made.

Furthermore, just because a problem is identified as a public policy problem does not necessarily mean the only solution involves government intervention. For example, consider the problem of an influenza vaccine shortage. Although there are government-oriented solutions to this problem, such as expanding public research and development or creating production incentives (through tax cuts or subsidies) to encourage private manufacturers to produce more vaccine, other solutions may rely solely on private actors. Private companies may decide to invest in the research and development of new ways to produce vaccines, or to build new plants to increase production capacity, because they believe they can make a profit in the long run. Just as private individuals and entities can make policy decisions for their own benefit, they can also play a central role in solving public policy problems. A lengthier discussion about options for solving public policy problems and arguments for and against government intervention is found in a review of health economics.

Structuring Policy Options

Considered broadly, there are different ways to approach public policy problems. For example, some policy options are voluntary, whereas others are mandatory. It is important to recognize that authoritative decisions do not always *require* others to act or refrain from acting in a certain way. Some of the most important and effective policies are those that provide incentives to others to change their behavior. Indeed, the power of persuasion is very important to public officials, particularly those working for the federal government, which is limited in its ability to force states and individuals to take certain actions. This limitation stems from the fact that the 10th Amendment of the U.S. Constitution limits Congress and the executive branch to specific powers and reserves all other powers for the states. However, members of the federal government may use their enumerated powers, such as those to tax and spend, to persuade states and others to act in desired ways.

For example, the Constitution does not give the legislative or executive branches the power to protect the public's health, meaning that the area is primarily within the purview of states to regulate. As a result, Congress and the president cannot require states to create emergency preparedness plans. Yet, Congress may provide incentives to states to do so by offering them federal money in return for state preparedness plans that meet certain criteria established by the federal government.

In addition, it is important to remember that inaction can also be a policy decision. Deciding to do nothing may be a decision to keep a prior decision in place or not to engage in a new issue. For example, a governor could decide against trying to change a restrictive abortion law, or a state legislature could choose not to pass a law expanding the allowable scope of practice for nurse practitioners. Both of these inactions result in important policy decisions that will affect the choices and opportunities available to individuals, advocacy organizations, and others.

This brief discussion about policy has raised several important issues to consider when identifying policy options. The next section provides a detailed discussion of the policymaking process, providing you with the background knowledge necessary to identify and understand the roles and powers of various policymakers.

▶ Public Policymaking Structure and Process

The public policymaking structure refers to the various branches of government and the individuals and entities within each branch that play a role in making and implementing policy decisions. In this section, we review the structure, powers, and constituency of these branches, with a focus on the U.S. House of Representatives, the U.S. Senate, and various commissions and agencies that assist Congress, the president, White House staff, and federal executive branch administrative agencies. In addition to reviewing the policymaking structure, we discuss the processes used by these various individuals and entities for making public policy decisions.

State-Level Policymaking

The federal government does not have a monopoly on policymaking. Indeed, important policy decisions are regularly made at the state level as well, especially in the healthcare arena. However, because state governments are similar to the federal government in many ways, the policymaking duties and powers presented in the following discussion can often be applied to a state-level analysis. At the same time, there is a significant amount of variation in how states structure their legislative and executive branches, agencies, and offices, and it is not possible to review the differences

that exist among all 50 states. Accordingly, after a brief discussion of state-level policymaking, this chapter focuses primarily on the federal policymaking structure and process.

Like the federal government, each state has three branches of government. State legislatures pass laws, appropriate money within the state, and conduct oversight of state programs and agencies. States also have their own judiciary with trial and appellate courts. The governor is the head of the state executive branch and can set policy, appoint cabinet members, and use state administrative agencies to issue regulations that implement state laws. Although there are limits to a state's power to regulate healthcare issues, state regulation is an extremely important aspect of health policy. Just a few examples of the healthcare matters states can regulate include provider licensing, accreditation, some aspects of health insurance, and most public health concerns.

While state governments share these general characteristics, it is important to realize that all state governments are not exactly alike. The governor has more power in some states than in others, agencies are combined in different ways among the states, state legislatures may meet annually or biannually, state legislators may be full-time or part-time employees, and so on. Because these differences exist, it is essential for policy analysts to understand the specific structure of the state in which their client resides.

Furthermore, there are important differences between the federal government and the states. Unlike the federal government, almost all states are required to have a balanced budget, and most states cannot borrow money for operating expenses. These rules mean that states must act to raise revenue or cut programs if they project that their budget will be in deficit by the end of the fiscal year. In addition, in 2010, 30 states had at least one tax and expenditure limit rule that restricted the growth of government revenues or spending to a fixed numerical target, sometimes using changes in population level or the inflation rate as guideposts. Further, 15 states require a legislative supermajority or voter approval to raise taxes (a supermajority means that more than a simple majority—over 50%—is required; for example, a two-thirds majority vote could be required) (Waisanen, 2010). As a result, state officials may be more likely than federal officials to make the difficult choice to either limit programs or cut resources from one program to fund another.

As is evident from this brief discussion, state-level policymaking is both a rich area for discussion and a difficult area to make generalizations about because each state is unique. Having highlighted some of the key differences and similarities among the states and between the state and the federal governments, we now turn to the legislative and executive branches of the federal government.

The Federal Legislative Branch

Article I of the U.S. Constitution makes Congress the lawmaking body of the federal government by granting it "All legislative Powers" and the right to enact "necessary and proper laws" to effect its prerogatives (U.S. Const. art. I, § 1; U.S. Const. art. I, § 8). Congressional responsibilities are fulfilled by the two chambers of Congress, the Senate and the House of Representatives ("the House"). The Constitution grants specific powers to Congress, including but not limited to the power to levy taxes, collect revenue, pay debts, provide for the general welfare, regulate interstate and foreign commerce, establish federal courts inferior to the Supreme Court, and declare war (U.S. Const. art. I, § 1). The Senate has the specific power to ratify treaties and confirm nominations of public officials.

The Senate consists of 2 elected officials from each state, for a total of 100 senators.[a] Each senator is elected in a statewide vote for a 6-year term, whereas representatives in the House sit for 2-year terms. Due to the lengthy term of its members, the Senate is considered less volatile and more concerned with long-term issues than the House. A senator must be at least 30 years old, a U.S. citizen for at least 9 years, and a resident of the state he or she is seeking to represent (U.S. Const. art. I, § 3).

The House includes 435 members allocated proportionally based on the population of the 50 states, with each state guaranteed at least 1 representative.[b] For example, in 2018, California was allotted 53 representatives, while Vermont had only 1. Due to the proportionality rule, members from larger states dominate the House and often hold leadership positions. Members of the House are elected by voters in congressional districts and serve 2-year terms. They must be at least 25 years old, a U.S. citizen for at least 7 years, and a resident of the state where the election takes place (U.S. Const. art. I, § 2).

Leadership Positions

Leadership roles in Congress are determined by political party affiliation, with the party in the majority gaining many advantages. The vice president of the United States is also the president of the Senate and presides over its proceedings. In the vice president's absence, which is common given the other obligations of the office, the president pro tempore, a mostly ceremonial position, presides over the Senate. In most cases the vice president is not a major player in Senate voting, but with the power to break a tie vote, the vice president wields an important power. The Speaker of the House ("Speaker") presides over that chamber and has the authority to prioritize and schedule bills, refer bills to committees, and name members of joint and conference committees. Other than the vice president's senatorial role, leadership positions in Congress are not elected by the voters, but determined by the members from the party who have been elected to Congress. Other key Congressional leadership positions include the following:

- **Senate majority leader:** Speaks on behalf of the majority party, schedules floor action and bills, works on committees, directs strategy, and tries to keep the party united.
- **House majority leader:** Works with the Speaker to direct party strategy and set the legislative schedule.
- **House and senate minority leaders:** Speak on behalf of the minority party, direct strategy, and try to maintain party unity; as members of the minority, they do not have the legislative duties of the majority leader/Speaker.
- **House and senate majority and minority whips:** Track important legislation, mobilize members to support leadership positions, keep a count of how party members are planning to vote, and generally assist their leaders in managing their party's legislative priorities.

Committees

Committees have been referred to as the "workhorses" of Congress; they are where many key decisions are made and legislative drafting takes place. Given the vast array of issues that Congress contends with in any given legislative session, it is impossible for every member to develop expertise on every issue. Although members vote on bills that cover a wide range of issues, members often concentrate on the areas relevant to the committees on which they serve.

Committees have a variety of important roles, including drafting and amending legislation; educating members on key issues; shepherding the committee's legislation on the floor when it goes before a vote by all the members of one chamber; working with the president, his administration, and lobbyists to gain support for a bill; holding hearings; and conducting oversight of executive branch departments, agencies, commissions, and programs within their purview. Committee members often gain expertise in the areas covered by their committees, and other members often rely on their advice when making voting decisions.

Standing committees are generally permanent committees with specified duties and powers. There are 20 standing committees in the House and 16 in the Senate. House committees tend to be larger than those in the Senate, with about 40 members per committee. Some committees have *authorization* jurisdiction, allowing them to create programs and agencies. Other committees have *appropriation* authority, meaning they are responsible for funding various programs and agencies. Standing committees also have *oversight* authority, meaning they monitor how programs are run and funds are spent. Each chamber of Congress has established specific oversight committees for some programs and issues that cut across committee jurisdiction, as well as committees that review the efficiency and economy of government actions (Heitshusen, 2018).

Not surprisingly, some of the most powerful and popular committees are those that deal with appropriating money. These include the following:

■ **House Ways and Means and Senate Finance committees:** These committees have jurisdiction over legislation concerning taxes, tariffs, and other revenue-generating measures, and over entitlement programs such as Medicare and Social Security. The Constitution requires all taxation and appropriations bills to originate in the House, and House rules require all tax bills to go through the Ways and Means committee.

■ **House and Senate Appropriations committees:** These committees have responsibility for writing federal spending bills.

■ **House and Senate Budget committees:** These committees are tasked with creating the overall budget plan that helps guide tax and appropriation committee work.

■ **House Rules committee:** This committee has jurisdiction over the rules and order of business in the House, including rules for the floor debates, amendments, and voting procedures. Unlike in the Senate, all House bills must go to the House Rules committee before reaching the House floor for a vote by all representatives.

TABLE 2-1 identifies the key health committees and subcommittees and their health-related jurisdictions.

TABLE 2-1 Key Health Committees and Subcommittees	
Committee/Subcommittee	**Health-Related Jurisdiction**
Senate Finance Committee	
■ Subcommittee on Health Care	■ Department of Health and Human Services • Centers for Medicare and Medicaid Services (includes Children's Health Insurance Program [CHIP]) • Administration for Children and Families ■ Department of the Treasury • Group health plans under the Employee Retirement Income Security Act (ERISA)
Senate Appropriations Committee	
■ Subcommittee on Labor, Health, Human Services, Education, and Related Agencies	■ Department of Health and Human Services • All areas except Food and Drug Administration, Indian Health, and construction activities
■ Subcommittee on Agriculture, Rural Development, Food and Drug Administration, and Related Agencies	■ U.S. Agricultural Department (except Forest Service) • Includes child nutrition programs; food safety and inspections; nutrition program administration; special supplemental nutrition program for Women, Infants, Children (WIC); Supplemental Nutrition Assistance Program (SNAP) ■ Food and Drug Administration

(continues)

TABLE 2-1 Key Health Committees and Subcommittees   *(continued)*

Committee/Subcommittee	Health-Related Jurisdiction

▪ Subcommittee on Interior, Environment, and Related Agencies	▪ Department of Health and Human Services
	  • Indian Health Services
	  • Agency for Toxic Substances and Disease Registry

Senate Health, Education, Labor, and Pensions Committee	
▪ Subcommittee on Children and Families ▪ Subcommittee on Primary Health and Retirement Security	▪ Occupational safety and health, public health, Health Resources Services Act, substance abuse and mental health, oral health, healthcare disparities, ERISA
Senate Committee on Agriculture, Nutrition, and Forestry	
▪ Subcommittee on Nutrition, Specialty Crops, and Agricultural Research	▪ Food from fresh waters; SNAP; human nutrition; inspection of livestock, meat, and agricultural products; pests and pesticides; school nutrition programs; other matters related to food, nutrition, and hunger
Senate Committee on Environment and Public Works	
▪ Subcommittee on Clean Air and Nuclear Safety	▪ Air pollution, environmental policy, research and development, noise pollution, water pollution, nonmilitary control of nuclear energy, solid waste disposal and recycling
House Committee on Ways and Means	
▪ Subcommittee on Health	▪ Programs providing payments for health care, health delivery systems, and health research ▪ Social Security Act ▪ Maternal and Child Health Block Grant ▪ Medicare ▪ Medicaid ▪ Peer review of utilization and quality control of healthcare organizations ▪ Tax credit and deduction provisions of the Internal Revenue Service relating to health insurance premiums and healthcare costs

▪ Subcommittee on Human Resources	▪ Social Security Act
	  • Public assistance provisions
	  • Supplemental Security Income provisions
	  • Mental health grants to states

House Committee on Appropriations	

▪ Subcommittee on Labor, Health and Human Services, Education, and Related Agencies	▪ Department of Health and Human Services
	  • Administration for Children and Families
	  • Administration for Community Living
	  • Agency for Healthcare Research and Quality
	  • Centers for Disease Control and Prevention
	  • Centers for Medicare and Medicaid Services

	• Health Resources Services Administration • National Institutes of Health • Substance Abuse and Mental Health Services • Federal Mine Safety and Health Review Commission • Medicaid and CHIP Payment and Access Commission • Medicare Payment Advisory Committee • National Council on Disability • Occupational Safety and Health Review Commission • Social Security Administration
■ Subcommittee on Agriculture, Rural Development, Food and Drug Administration, and Related Agencies	■ Food and Drug Administration ■ Department of Agriculture (except Forestry)

■ Subcommittee on Energy, Water Development, and Related Agencies	■ Department of Energy
	  • National Nuclear Strategy Administration
	  • Federal Energy Regulatory Commission
	■ Department of Interior
	■ Bureau of Reclamation
	■ Defense Nuclear Facilities Safety Board
	■ Nuclear Regulatory Commission

■ Subcommittee on Interior, Environment, and Related Agencies	■ Department of Interior ■ Environmental Protection Agency ■ Indian Health Service ■ National Institute of Environmental Health Sciences ■ Chemical Safety and Hazards Investigation Board

House Committee on Agriculture

■ Subcommittee on Nutrition	■ Nutrition programs, including SNAP
■ Subcommittee on Biotechnology, Horticulture, and Research	■ Policies and statutes relating to horticulture, bees, organic agriculture, pest and disease management, bioterrorism, biotechnology
■ Subcommittee on Livestock and Foreign Agriculture	■ Policies and statutes relating to inspections of livestock, dairy, poultry, and seafood; aquaculture; animal welfare

Congressional Commissions and Staff Agencies

Although the committee system helps members of Congress focus on particular areas, members often need assistance with in-depth research and policy analysis. Commissions and staff agencies provide members with information they might not otherwise have the time to gather and analyze. There are too many commissions and agencies to list here, but a few key ones include the following:

■ **Congressional Budget Office:** An agency that provides Congress with cost estimates of bills and federal mandates to state and local governments, as well as forecasts economic trends and spending levels.

■ **Government Accountability Office:** An independent, nonpartisan agency that studies how federal tax dollars are spent and advises Congress and executive agencies about more efficient and effective ways to use federal resources.

■ **Congressional Research Service:** The public policy research service that conducts nonpartisan, objective research on legislative issues.

■ **Medicare Payment Advisory Commission:** An independent federal commission that gives Congress advice on issues relating to the Medicare program, including payment, access to care, and quality of care.

How Laws Are Made

One way that members of Congress indicate their policy preferences is by passing laws that embody their values and the values of their constituents. This is a lengthy process, with many steps along the way that could derail a bill (**FIGURE 2-1**).

Before a committee considers a bill, it must be introduced by a member of Congress. Once this occurs, the Speaker refers the bill to one or more committees in the House, and the majority leader does the same in the Senate. The bill may die in committee if there is not sufficient support for it, although there are rarely invoked procedures that allow a bill to be reported to the full chamber even without committee approval. While the bill is in committee, members may hold hearings on it or "mark up" the bill by changing or deleting language in the proposed bill or by adding amendments to it. If a majority of the committee members approves a bill, it

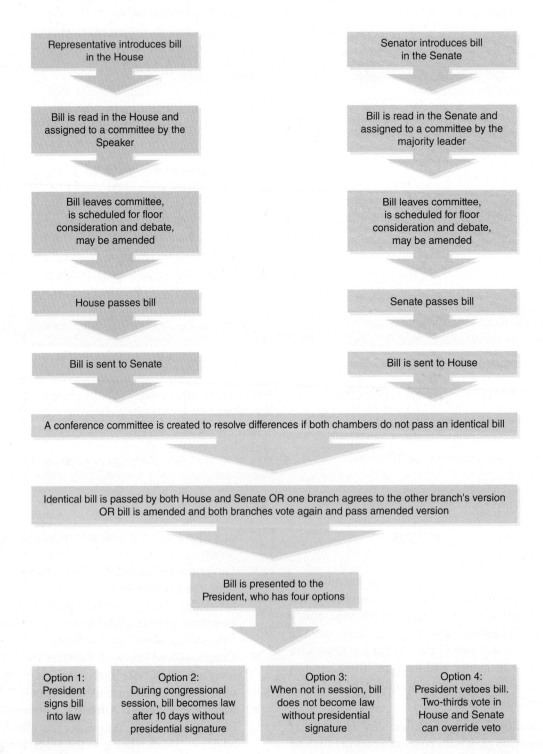

FIGURE 2-1 How a Bill Becomes a Law

goes to the full chamber (House or Senate, depending on where the bill originated).

The full House or Senate then debates the merits of the bill and puts it to a vote. If a majority does not support the bill, it dies on the chamber floor. If a majority supports the bill, it is sent to the other chamber for consideration. The second chamber may pass the exact same bill or a different version of the bill. If the second chamber does not pass any version of the bill, it dies on the chamber floor and no version of the bill moves forward. If the second chamber passes an identical bill, it goes directly to the president for consideration.

If there are differences in the bills passed by the House and Senate, the two chambers must reach a consensus through an exchange of amendments for the bill to have a chance of becoming law. Consensus building is facilitated by a "conference committee" made up of members from both chambers. If the committee cannot reach a consensus, the bill dies. If the committee reaches a consensus, the bill is sent back to each chamber for a vote on the new version of the bill. If either chamber does not approve it, the bill dies at that point. If both the House and the Senate pass the new version, it is sent to the president for consideration.

The president may choose to sign the bill into law, or the president may choose to veto the bill. If the president chooses not to sign the bill while Congress is in session, the bill becomes law after 10 days; if Congress is not in session and the bill goes unsigned, the bill dies (this is referred to as a "pocket veto"). If the president vetoes the bill, Congress may override the veto with approval of a two-thirds majority in each chamber.

Congressional Budget and Appropriations Process

Although the budget and appropriations process may sound dry, it is about much more than numbers and charts. If you take a close look at budget documents, they include narratives that discuss why certain programs are being funded and what the government hopes to achieve by doing so. In many ways, this process is a key policy tool for members of Congress and the president; they are able to show which programs and issues have their support through their funding decisions.

Given both the amount of money involved in running the United States ($4 trillion in 2017) and the various jurisdictions of congressional committees, it is not surprising that the federal budget process is fairly complex. The Congressional Budget and Impoundment Control Act of 1974 ("Budget Act") and subsequent amendments were passed by Congress to create a process that brings together the numerous committees involved in crafting an overall budget plan. The budget process works in concert with the appropriations process, which involves congressional passage of bills from each of the appropriations committees to distribute the funds provided for in the overall budget (House Committee on the Budget Majority Caucus, 2001; Senate Committee on the Budget, 1998).

The president is required to submit a budget proposal to Congress by the first Monday in February. This proposal is the administration's request; it is not binding on Congress. Each chamber then passes a *budget resolution*, identifying how the chamber would spend federal money delineated by different categories of spending (e.g., defense, agriculture, transportation). Members from each chamber then meet to develop a single *conference report* reflecting a consensus agreement on the overall budget. Congress then passes a *concurrent budget resolution*, which is binding upon the House and Senate as a blueprint for revenue collection and spending. However, it is not a law and the president is not bound by the budget resolution.

Over the 6 weeks subsequent to the passage of the concurrent budget resolution, the House and Senate budget committees hold hearings to discuss the budget, and other committees review the budget as it pertains to their jurisdiction. The latter committees provide the budget committees with their "views and estimates" of appropriate spending and/or revenue levels for the upcoming year. In addition, the Congressional Budget Office provides the budget committees with its budget and economic outlook reports and provides the budget and appropriations committees with its analysis of the president's proposal.

In March, the House and Senate budget committees each craft a budget plan during public meetings known as "markups." When the markups are complete, each committee sends a budget resolution to its respective chamber. The budget resolution contains a budget total, spending breakdown, reconciliation instructions, budget enforcement mechanisms, and statements of budget policy. Budget totals are provided as aggregates and as committee allocations.

The federal budget includes two types of spending: *discretionary* and *mandatory*. Discretionary spending refers to money that is set aside for programs that must be funded annually in order to continue. If the programs are not funded by Congress, they will not receive federal dollars to continue their operations. For example, the Head Start program, which provides early childhood education services, is a discretionary program that relies on annual appropriations. Mandatory spending refers to spending on entitlement and other programs that must be funded as a matter of law. For example, the Medicaid program is an entitlement that provides health insurance to eligible low-income individuals. The *authorizing legislation* (the law that created the program) for Medicaid includes eligibility rules and benefits. Because Medicaid is an entitlement program, Congress must provide enough money so the Medicaid agency can meet the obligations found in the authorizing legislation.

The appropriations committees write bills to cover discretionary spending. These committees make their decisions based on the amount of funds available and any *reconciliation instructions*, which direct the appropriate authorizing committee to make changes in the law for mandatory spending programs to meet budgetary goals. Appropriations bills and reconciliation instructions must be signed by the president to become law.

Members of the House and Senate have the opportunity to make changes to the work of the budget committees. Once the House and Senate pass their own versions of the budget resolution, they establish a conference committee to resolve any differences. Once the differences are resolved, each full chamber votes on the compromise budget.

Congress often does not meet Budget Act deadlines (shown in **TABLE 2-2**). If the appropriations bills are not passed by every October 1—the beginning of the fiscal year—Congress may pass a *continuing resolution* that allows the government to continue to spend money. If Congress does not pass a continuing resolution or if the president vetoes it, all nonessential activities of federal agencies must stop until additional funds are provided.

Constituents of Legislative Branch

With the wide array of issues they take on, members of Congress may have an equally wide array of constituents to be concerned about when making policy decisions. Clearly, members are concerned about pleasing the voters who elect them. Even though there may be a variety of policy views to consider, members often prioritize their home constituents. In addition to courting their home-state voters, members often try to court independents or voters from the opposing party in their home state to strengthen their appeal. High approval ratings deter challengers from trying to take an incumbent's congressional seat and allow members of Congress more leeway to pursue their goals and policies.

TABLE 2-2 Federal Budget Process Timeline

First Monday in February	President submits budget proposal to Congress.
March	House completes its budget resolution.
April	Senate completes its budget resolution.
April 15	House and Senate complete concurrent budget resolution.
May	Authorizing committees develop reconciliation language when necessary and report legislation to budget committees. House and Senate develop conference report on reconciliation, which is voted on by each chamber.
June 10	House concludes reporting annual House appropriations bills.
June 15	If necessary, Congress completes reconciliation legislation.
June 30	House completes its appropriations bills.
September 30	Senate completes its appropriations bills. House and Senate complete appropriations conference reports and vote separately on the final bills.
October 1	Fiscal year begins.

Modified from House Committee on the Budget Majority Caucus, *Basics of the Budget Process*, 107th Cong. Briefing Paper, 2001.

Although concern for their home-state base may be their first priority, representatives and senators often need to be concerned about supporting their party's position on issues. Today, elected federal politicians are usually affiliated with the Democratic or Republican Party, and voters may be influenced by the party's stance on issues. Also, if the balance of power between the two parties is close in Congress, the parties usually cannot afford to have members defect from their party's positions. Members' concern regarding keeping their party strong is magnified if they hold leadership positions in Congress or are considering running for national office.

Finally, the views of the president may be important for members to consider, depending on whether the member and the president share the same party, the particular issue involved, and the president's popularity. Members who are in the same party as the sitting president have incentive to help the president remain popular because they will likely advance many of the same policies. In addition, presidents are often prodigious fundraisers and campaigners who may be able to assist members during election season. Even when members disagree with the president, the president's power to affect their influence in Congress may be a deterrent to opposing the president. Of course, if the president is exceedingly popular, it is difficult for members of either party to oppose presidential policy goals.

The Federal Executive Branch

Article II of the U.S. Constitution establishes the executive branch and vests executive power in the most well-known member of the branch, the president (U.S. Const. art. II, § 1). Of course, the president does not act alone in running the executive branch. Presidents rely on Executive Office agencies and staff such as the Council of Economic Advisors and Office of Management and Budget, as well as policy development offices such as the National Security Council and Domestic Policy Council (see **BOX 2-1** for a description of one such office). In addition, there are 15 cabinet departments led by individuals selected by the president (subject to Senate confirmation) and additional non–cabinet-level agencies, all of which are responsible for, among other duties, interpreting and implementing the laws passed by Congress. All of these advisors identify issues to be addressed and formulate policy options for the president to consider. In theory, all of these parts of the executive branch work in furtherance of the goals set by the president.

BOX 2-1 Office of Management and Budget

The Office of Management and Budget (OMB) reports directly to the president and plays an important role in policy decisions. OMB is responsible for preparing the presidential budget proposal, which includes reviewing agency requests, coordinating agency requests with presidential priorities, working with Congress to draft appropriation and authorization bills, and working with agencies to make budget cuts when needed. In addition to these budgetary functions, OMB provides an estimate of the cost of regulations, approves agency requests to collect information, plays a role in coordinating domestic policy, and may act as a political intermediary on behalf of the president. OMB also has an oversight and evaluation function over select federal agencies as a result of the Government Performance and Results Act, which requires agencies to set performance goals and have their performance evaluated.

The Presidency

The president is the head of the federal executive branch. As powerful as that may sound, the country's founders created three distinct branches of government and limited the president's power in order to ensure that no single individual gained too much control over the nation. As you will see, in some ways the president is very powerful, and in other ways his power is quite limited.

Although there have been third-party candidates for president in the past, generally speaking the United States operates with a two-party system, with the Democratic and Republican parties as the major parties. Each party selects a candidate for president who represents the party in the election. Presidents (and their vice presidents) are elected through a nationwide vote to serve a 4-year term. An individual is limited to serving two 4-year terms as president, which may or may not be consecutive (U.S. Const. amend. XXII, § 1).[c] To be eligible for election, candidates must be at least 35 years old, a natural-born citizen of the United States, and a resident of the country for at least 14 years.

Presidents have many roles. As the unofficial *Chief of State*, the president is seen as the symbol of the country and its citizens (H.R. Doc. No. 106–216, 2000, p. 40). As the official *Chief Executive Officer*, the president manages the cabinet and executive branch. The president also holds the position of *Commander in Chief of the Armed Forces*, and as such is the top-ranking military official in the country. The U.S. Constitution vests the president with other powers, such as the ability to appoint judges to the federal courts, sign treaties with foreign nations, and appoint ambassadors as liaisons to other countries. These powers are all subject to the advice and consent of the Senate (H.R. Doc. No. 106–216, 2000, p. 41).

Agenda Setting. A key tool of the presidency is the ability to put issues on the national agenda and offer a recommended course of action: "Framing agendas is what the presidency is all about" (Davidson, 1984, p. 371). Presidents help set the national agenda because of the role of the president as the country's leader and the amount of media attention given to presidential actions, decisions, and policy recommendations. Unlike many other politicians or interest groups, the president does not have to work hard to receive media coverage. Whether it is the annual State of the Union address, release of the president's budget proposal, a major speech, a press conference, a photo shoot with a foreign leader, or the release of a report, the president's message is continually publicized. In addition, the president's message can be delivered by the vice president, cabinet officers, and party leaders in Congress.

The notion of appealing directly to the country's citizens to focus on a particular issue and to influence legislative debates is referred to as "going public." In going public, presidents try to use support from the American people to gain the attention of Congress and sway votes on policy decisions. Because members of Congress are highly concerned about pleasing their constituency to improve their chance for reelection, "the president seeks the aid of a third party—the public—to force other politicians to accept his preferences" (Kernell, 1997, p. 3).

Sometimes it may be advantageous for the president to place an item on the policy agenda in a less public manner. For example, if a policy is controversial with the general public or if members of the president's party disagree with a proposal, it may be more effective to promote a policy behind the scenes. The president, either directly or through intermediaries, can carefully let members of Congress know which policies are favored. Using combinations of promises of favors and threats to members' interests, the president may be able to influence the outcome of policy debates in Congress even without going public.

In addition to deciding whether to approach Congress publicly or behind the scenes, the president must choose whether to present a preferred policy decision with more or less detail. A policy can be presented broadly through principles or general guidelines, or specifically through proposed legislation that is presented to Congress. Each method for conveying the president's goals has pros and cons. If a policy choice is presented in a broad manner, Congress may interpret the policy in a way that the president dislikes. However, if the president presents Congress with a specific proposal or draft legislation, Congressional members may view the president as infringing upon their role as the legislative body and resist working with him.

Whether presidents are successful in placing policy issues on the national agenda and having them resolved in accordance with their preferences depends in part on how much "political capital" a president has available. Political capital is defined as the strength of the president's popularity and of his party, in Congress and in other contexts. Members of Congress are more likely to support a popular president who has the ability to mobilize the public's support, improve members' standing by association with the president and the president's party, and raise money for their campaigns.

Even the most popular president cannot always dictate what issues are on the national agenda, however. Events and decisions outside the president's control often influence what topics most concern the nation. The terrorist attacks of September 11, 2001, the subsequent anthrax scare, and the subway and bus bombings in London and Madrid all served to place combating terrorism at the top of the policy and political agenda during the George W. Bush administration. Concerns about an avian flu epidemic and numerous food recalls put public health and food safety issues on the national agenda. The devastation wrought by the BP oil spill in the Gulf of Mexico made improved responses to environmental disasters a high priority for a short time. Thus, even the most popular presidents must be responsive to national and international events that may be beyond their control.

Presidential Powers. As noted earlier, if Congress passes legislation the president dislikes, he has the power to veto it, thereby rejecting the bill. However, the president does not have to actually use the veto to shape policy. The president may be able to persuade Congress to change a piece of legislation simply by threatening to veto it, especially if it is a law that is expected to pass by only a slim majority. In general, vetoes are used infrequently, with presidents vetoing only 3% of all legislation since George Washington was president (H.R. Doc. No. 106–216, p. 43).

Presidents also have the power to issue executive orders. These are legally binding orders that the president gives to federal administrative agencies under the control of the Executive Office. In general, these orders are used to direct federal agencies and their officials in how they implement specific laws. Executive orders are controversial because under our system of government, Congress, not the executive, is tasked with making laws. In addition, significant policy decisions can be accomplished by using executive orders. For example, an executive order was used by President Truman to integrate the armed forces, by President Eisenhower to desegregate schools, by President Clinton to designate 1.7 million acres in southern Utah as a national monument, and by President George W. Bush to create the federal Office of Homeland Security (which subsequently became a cabinet-level department when Congress established it through legislation). As is discussed in the Health Reform in the United States chapter, President Trump issued several executive orders intended to undermine the Affordable Care Act after Congress was unable to pass a bill to repeal and replace it.

If Congress believes an executive order is contrary to congressional intent, it has two avenues of recourse. It can amend the law at issue to clarify its intent and effectively stamp out the executive order that is now clearly contrary to the law. (Bear in mind that because the president may veto any bill, in effect it takes a two-thirds majority of Congress to override an executive order.) As an alternative, Congress may challenge the executive order in court, claiming that the president's actions exceed his constitutional powers.

Constituents of the Executive Branch. From this description of the presidency, it is evident that presidents have several layers of constituents to consider when making policy choices. Certainly, the president represents every citizen and the country as a whole

as the only nationally elected official (along with the vice president) in the nation. However, the president is also a representative of a particular political party and therefore must consider the views of that party when making policies. The party's views may be evident from the party platform, policies supported by party leadership in Congress, and voters who identify themselves as party members. In addition, the president must keep in mind the foreign policy duties of the office. Depending on the issue, it may be important for the president to take into account the views of other nations or international organizations, such as the United Nations or the World Health Organization.

How does the president decide which policies to pursue? Presidents are driven by multiple goals. They want "their policies to be adopted, they want the policies they put in place to last, and they want to feel they helped solve the problems facing the country" (Weissert & Weissert, 2002, p. 82). In addition, presidents often speak of wanting to leave a legacy or ensure their place in history when they leave office.

Given the vast array of constituents that presidents must consider, the president's policy decision-making process involves several layers. As shown in **FIGURE 2-2**, presidents consult their agency staff to identify problems, decide which problems are priorities, determine what solutions are available to address those problems, and choose the policy option that is the preferred course of action. In addition, the president's staff interacts with members of Congress and other political

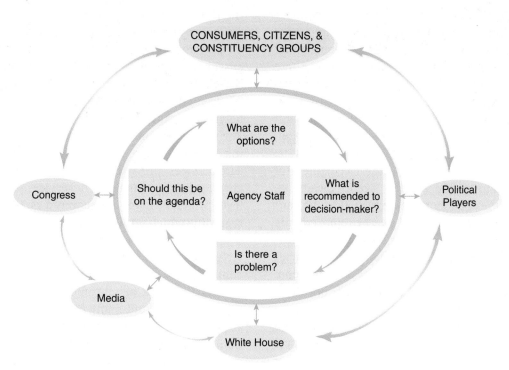

FIGURE 2-2 Executive Agency Policymaking

Source: Courtesy of Jeff Levi, Professor of Health Policy, George Washington University.

players to gauge their support for or opposition to various policies. Of course, how the media portrays both the problems and the potential solutions can be an important ingredient in whether politicians and the general public support the president's initiatives.

In addition, which policies presidents choose to promote may depend in part on when policy decisions are made. First-term presidents must satisfy their constituents if they hope to be reelected. Although all presidents want to see their favored policies implemented throughout their time in office, second-term presidents may be more willing to support more controversial goals because they cannot run for reelection. Yet, second-term presidents may also be constrained by the desire to keep their party in power, even though another individual will hold the presidential office.

Administrative Agencies

When studying the structure of our government, it is common to review Congress, the presidency, and the court system. Administrative agencies, however, are often overlooked despite the power they wield over the way our country is run.

Structurally, almost all administrative agencies are part of the executive branch and, thus, are under the power and control of the president. Practically, administrative agencies often work out of the public's eye to implement the laws passed by Congress and the executive orders signed by the president.

Federal agencies fall into two main categories: executive department agencies and independent agencies. Executive department agencies are under the direct control of the president, and department heads serve at the pleasure of the president. These departments include the 15 cabinet-level departments and their subunits; some of the more well-known executive departments are the Department of Health and Human Services, the Department of Education, the Treasury Department, the Department of State, the Department of Defense, and the Department of Homeland Security. Independent agency heads are appointed by the president and confirmed by the Senate. They serve a fixed term and may be removed only "for cause," meaning there must be a legitimate reason to fire them. Examples of independent agencies include the Securities and Exchange Commission, the U.S. Postal Service, and the National Labor Relations Board.

Overall, the president fills approximately 4,000 federal jobs (Yoder, 2016). In general, these political appointees have short tenures, lasting an average of 2 years (Weissert & Weissert, 2002, p. 161). When the

administration changes hands after an election, new appointees are usually selected to run the agencies. The daily operations of agencies are run by career civil servants, public employees who do not necessarily come and go with each administration but who often remain at an agency for years, gaining expertise and institutional knowledge about the agencies in which they work. Frequently, there may be tension between the goals of the political appointee and those of the career bureaucrat, who may have the advantage of familiarity with members of Congress and who knows that the political appointee is likely to be replaced in a few years.

Administrative agencies can be created by statute, internal department reorganization, or presidential directive (H.R. Doc. No. 106-216, 2000, p. 50). However they are initially created, agencies must have statutory authority in order to receive appropriations from Congress and act with the force of law. This statutory authority, or enabling statute, outlines the agency's responsibilities and powers.

Agency Powers. By necessity, statutes are usually written broadly. Congress does not have the time or expertise to include every detail about how a new program should operate or how a new department will be structured. It is up to the executive branch agency to fill in the details, and it does so by issuing policy statements, developing rules, and promulgating regulations.

The Affordable Care Act (ACA) is a classic example. Although the statute itself is lengthy (over 2,400 pages), the regulations needed to implement the law have been even more extensive—with some estimates putting the total page number at 20,000. To give just one example for now (a detailed discussion of the ACA occurs in the Health Reform in the United States chapter), the ACA includes a list of essential health benefits that must be provided by health insurance plans offered in state exchanges. The statute outlines numerous such services, including mental health services, maternity and newborn care services, prevention and wellness services, and chronic disease management services. Even with this level of detail, many unanswered questions remain regarding which services must be covered. Do mental health services include inpatient and outpatient services? Do prevention and wellness services include contraceptive coverage? Does chronic disease management include all chronic disease management models? These (and many other) questions must be answered through regulations. The ACA includes numerous provisions that require the relevant agencies to issue detailed regulations necessary to implementing the law.

TABLE 2-3 Summary of Public Policymaking Entities

	Congress	President	Administrative Agencies
Main function	Legislative body	Chief executive of the country	Implement statutes through rule making
Main tools/ powers	Support/oppose/pass legislation Appropriations Oversight	Agenda setting Persuasion Propose solutions Budget proposals Executive orders Sign legislation into law	Create regulations Provide information
Constituents	Voters in state or district Voters in nation if in leadership role or have national aspirations Party President	Nation (all voters) Public who voted for the president Party Other nations International organizations	President Congress Individuals and entities regulated or served by the agency

In addition, agencies must follow the requirements set forth in the Administrative Procedure Act of 1946 (APA). The APA contains detailed requirements compelling agencies to issue a notice of their intent to issue a new rule or change an existing rule, and provide for and respond to public comments on the proposed rule. Some agencies are also required to hold hearings and develop rules based on the evidence presented in those hearings (Weissert & Weissert, 2002, p. 172). It is important to know that the APA creates procedural standards that require an agency to follow a particular *process* when promulgating regulations, but that the APA does not relate to the *substance* of the regulations. As long as an agency follows the necessary notice and comment requirements of the APA, it has wide latitude to issue rules within its scope of power, even if many of the public comments opposed the proposed rules. If an agency does not follow the APA requirements, interested parties may sue the agency in court to force compliance with the law.

Constituents of Agencies. Agency heads, because they are not elected, do not have constituents in the same way that the president and members of Congress do. In theory, as members of the executive branch, agency heads should be concerned only with the wishes of the president. In reality, however, that is not always the case. Some presidents have firmer control of their departments than others. If the president gives the departments and agencies broad discretion to make policy decisions, the agencies may have few policy constraints. Practically, however, agency heads want their operation to run smoothly, which includes having a good working relationship with the individuals or entities regulated by that agency. If an agency antagonizes the people or groups being regulated, they might reach out to their congressional representatives to try to change or limit the agency's personnel or authority. In addition, because Congress appropriates funds to and maintains oversight of many agencies, agency heads are well served by taking Congress's interests into account.

TABLE 2-3 summarizes the general public policymaking machinery. We next turn our attention to the specific parts of the government bureaucracy that operate in the health arena.

▶ The Health Bureaucracy

The Federal Government

Although several federal agencies have healthcare-related responsibilities, three significant health agencies include the Department of Health and Human Services (HHS), the Department of Defense (DoD), and the Department of Veterans Affairs (VA). HHS houses many of the major public health insurance programs and health services that provide care, information, and more to millions of U.S. residents; the DoD and VA operate health insurance programs specifically for military personnel and their families.

Department of Health and Human Services

HHS includes hundreds of programs that cover activities as varied as medical and social science research, preschool education services, substance abuse and prevention services, and health insurance programs, just to name a few. As shown in **FIGURE 2-3**, the department

has 11 operating divisions. The main purpose of each agency is described in **TABLE 2-4**.

Each operating division has numerous bureaus or divisions that operate health programs. For example, the HIV/AIDS Bureau (HAB) is one of five bureaus in the Health Resources and Services Administration. The HIV/AIDs Bureau implements the Ryan White CARE Act of 1990, which provides health care to

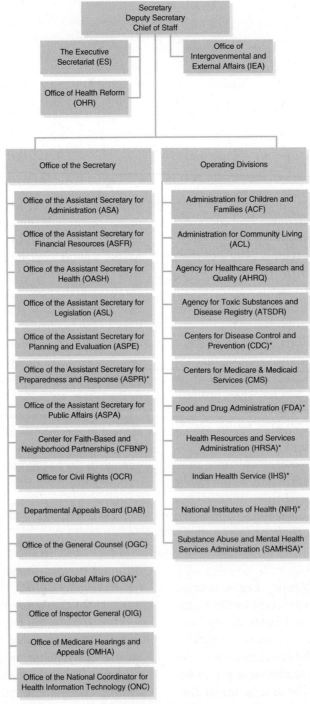

*denotes the components of the Public Health Service

FIGURE 2-3 Department of Health and Human Services Organizational Chart

Source: Reproduced from: the U.S. Department of Health and Human Services. HHS Organizational Chart. Retrieved from https://www.hhs.gov/about/agencies/orgchart/index.html#

TABLE 2-4 Department of Health and Human Services Agencies

Agency	Main Purpose of Agency
Administration for Children and Families (ACF)	To promote economic and social well-being of families, children, individuals, and communities through educational and supportive programs
Administration for Community Living (ACL)	To increase access to community support and resources for older adults and people with disabilities
Agency for Healthcare Research and Quality (AHRQ)	To produce evidence to make health care safer, high quality, more accessible, and affordable, and to work with HHS and other partners to make sure the evidence is understood and used
Agency for Toxic Substances and Disease Registry (ATSDR)	To prevent exposure to toxic substances and reduce the adverse health effects associated with such exposure
Centers for Disease Control and Prevention (CDC)	To protect the nation's health by providing leadership in the prevention and control of diseases and other preventable conditions, and to respond the public health emergencies
Center for Medicare and Medicaid Services (CMS)	To provide oversight of Medicare, the federal portions of Medicaid and CHIP, and the Health Insurance Marketplace, and to engage in quality assurance activities
Food and Drug Administration (FDA)	To assure the safety of human and veterinary drugs, biological products, and medical devices, and to ensure the safety and security of the nation's food supply and products that emit radiation
Health Resources and Services Administration (HRSA)	To provide health care to populations that are geographically isolated, or economically or medically vulnerable
Indian Health Services (IHS)	To provide American Indians and Alaska Natives with comprehensive health services
National Institutes of Health (NIH)	To support and conduct biomedical and behavioral research, to train promising young researchers, and to promote collecting and sharing knowledge
Substance Abuse and Mental Health Services Administration (SAMHSA)	To improve access to and reduce barriers to high-quality, effective programs for individuals who suffer from addictive or mental disorders, and for their families and communities

Department of Health and Human Services (2015).

Source: Department of Health and Human Services. (2015). *HHS agencies and offices.* Retrieved from https://www.hhs.gov/about/agencies/hhs-agencies-and-offices/index.html

individuals with HIV and AIDS. Similarly, the Food and Drug Administration has several offices or centers; the one whose job is perhaps best known to the general public is the Center for Drug Evaluation and Research, which is responsible for testing and approving new drugs before they can be sold to the public. These are just two examples of the many subagency units that perform vital functions in our federal healthcare bureaucracy.

HHS also includes numerous offices that assist the Secretary of HHS in running the department. The Office of the Assistant Secretary of Health (OASH) is the principal advisor to the HHS secretary on public health matters. Through the Office of the Surgeon General, OASH oversees the U.S. Public Health Service (PHS), the Commissioned Corps (health professionals used for both emergency responses and as health promoters), and the Office of Disease Prevention and

Health Promotion. The PHS employs both commissioned corps members and civilians to run its public health programs.

Nine of the offices and agencies within HHS are part of the PHS. In addition, the PHS employees also work in the Bureau of Prisons, U.S. Coast Guard, National Oceanic and Atmospheric Administration, Environmental Protection Agency (EPA), Division of Immigration Health Services, and U.S. Marshal Services. HHS also has divisions concerned with planning and evaluation, legislation, administration and management, budget and finance, program support, public affairs, and global health affairs. Offices concerned with the legality and efficiency of the department's activities include those of the General Counsel and Inspector General, and the Office of Civil Rights.

As a result of the focus on preventing terrorism, HHS includes an Assistant Secretary for Preparedness and Response. This individual is the principal advisor to the Secretary of HHS on matters relating to bioterrorism and other public health emergencies and helps coordinate efforts in these areas at all levels of government. Other federal departments also have a role in public health emergency preparedness. The Department of Homeland Security (DHS), which includes the Federal Emergency Management Agency (FEMA), is tasked with preparing for and coordinating the federal response to emergencies, whether due to natural or human-made disasters. The CDC houses the Strategic National Stockpile of emergency pharmaceutical supplies. Other agencies, such as the EPA, DoD, and VA, play significant roles in emergency preparedness and response.

Department of Veterans Affairs and Department of Defense

Any veteran who does not receive a dishonorable discharge is potentially eligible for healthcare services through the Veterans Health Administration (VHA). The VHA is the largest healthcare delivery system in the country, with hundreds of medical centers, nursing homes, and outpatient clinics that serve over 9 million patients each year (Department of Veterans Affairs, n.d.).

VHA-sponsored health plans offer a wide array of preventive, ambulatory, and hospital services as well as medications and medical and surgical supplies. VHA providers are organized into integrated networks aimed at providing cost-effective services based on local need. There are no premiums (monthly payments) for the plan, but veterans have to make co-payments (a charge per visit) unless they are exempt based on disability or income level. Unlike most healthcare plans, the VHA system is completely portable, meaning veterans can access VHA facilities anywhere in the country.

Veterans who wish to receive care through the VHA must enroll in the program. Because the VHA receives an annual appropriation from Congress, it may not have sufficient funds to pay for all of the care demanded by eligible veterans. For that reason, the VHA uses a priority system to ensure that veterans who are low-income or have service-related disabilities can be enrolled into a plan. Other veterans may have to wait to be enrolled if there are insufficient funds. In addition, priority in accessing care is given to enrolled veterans who need care for service-related disabilities or have a sufficiently severe service-related disability and need care for any health concern. Veterans not in a priority group may have to wait to see an appropriate provider once they are enrolled.

Although veterans may receive care through the VHA, they are not required to do so. If eligible, they may choose to obtain services through other public or private healthcare programs or health insurance plans. They may also choose to receive some services through the VHA and others from non-VHA programs or plans. As a result of scandals pertaining to excessive wait times and falsified patient logs, Congress passed several bills to improve the medical care veterans receive. For example, the bipartisan VA Mission Act of 2018 is intended to streamline various VA programs that allow veterans to access care in the private sector and improve payment systems for providers (Rein, 2018).

The VHA does not provide coverage to veterans' family members, but the DoD does through its TRICARE program. TRICARE provides healthcare services to current and retired military personnel and their families. TRICARE offers a variety of plans with various eligibility requirements and costs to the patient.

State and Local Governments

As discussed earlier, the Constitution gives states primary responsibility for protecting the public's health. States have health-related agencies that deal with health financing, aging, behavioral health, environmental health, children and family services, veterans, facility licensing and standards, provider credentialing, and more. Although all states have agencies that generally cover the same functions, their structure, responsibilities, and lines of authority vary greatly.

With the variation among state agencies, it is not surprising that there are significant differences across the states in terms of their approach to public health and health services needs. All states have agencies to run their Medicaid and CHIP programs, as well as other state-specific health services programs. Local health departments (LHDs) carry out the public health functions of the state. Most commonly, LHDs are formed by, managed by, and report to a local government, such as a county commission or local board of health. This structure provides LHDs with significant latitude to interpret and implement state statutes. In some states, the state and local governments jointly oversee the LHD. LHDs may provide services directly or, as is increasingly common, may contract or provide support to others who perform the services. The services provided by LHDs vary considerably, though there is an emphasis on addressing communicable diseases, environmental health, and children's health issues. LHDs often provide services such as immunizations; infectious disease investigations, epidemiology, and surveillance; food safety and inspections; nutrition services; and environmental health services. Some also provide diabetes care, glaucoma screening, substance abuse treatment, mental health services, and more (Turnock, 2016, pp. 235–239). (A more detailed discussion of various public health agencies is found in the Public Health Institutions and Systems chapter.)

Interest Groups

Before leaving the discussion of policy, the policy-making process, and the health bureaucracy, we must say a few words about interest groups. *Interest group* is a general term used for a wide variety of organizations that are created around a particular issue or population and have the goal of influencing policy and educating others about their views and concerns (Weissert & Weissert, 2002, p. 117). Interest groups are different from most of the other stakeholders that have been discussed because interest groups do not have the power to make policy. Although members of the executive and legislative branches of government have a key role in determining which policies are adopted, interest groups have the limited, but still significant, role of trying to influence the decisions of policymakers.

There are many types of interest groups, including trade associations, think tanks, advocacy groups, and lobbying firms. A few examples include the Pharmaceutical Research and Manufacturers of America (n.d), whose mission is to "conduct effective advocacy for public policies that encourage discovery of important new medicines for patients by pharmaceutical and biotechnology research companies" (Our Mission section, para. 1); America's Essential Hospitals (n.d), which "champions excellence in health care for all,

regardless of social or economic circumstance, and advances the work of hospitals and health systems committed to ensuring access to care and optimal health for America's most vulnerable people" (Mission and Service section, para. 2); the Center on Budget and Policy Priorities (n.d.), which conducts nonpartisan research and pursues "federal and state policies designed both to reduce poverty and inequality and to restore fiscal responsibility in equitable and effective ways" (About the Center section, para. 1); and the Heritage Foundation (n.d.), which strives to "formulate and promote conservative public policies based on the principles of free enterprise, limited government, individual freedom, traditional American values, and a strong national defense" (About Heritage section, para. 1).

Just as members of Congress do not have the time or ability to become experts in every issue that comes before them, the same is true for the average citizen. Many people do not have the time and ability to learn about all of the issues that are important to them, develop proposals, rally public support for their positions, monitor current activity, lobby to add or remove issues from the agenda, and reach out to politicians who make policy decisions. Instead, interest groups take on those duties: "Their job is to make the case for their constituents before government, plying the halls of Congress, the executive branch, the courts, and the offices of other interest groups to provide a linkage between citizens and government" (Weissert & Weissert, 2002, p. 119)

Interest Group Powers

Interest groups do not have the power to pass laws. However, they can influence policy in a variety of ways throughout the policymaking process. For example, recall all the steps it takes for a bill to become a law. Anywhere along that continuum is an opportunity for interest groups to make their case. The first step for interest groups is often to commission research that they use to support their position. This can be most important in the early stages of policy development, when politicians might have an open mind about various proposals (Weissert & Weissert, 2002, p. 131). However, it does not matter how much information a group has if it is not able to gain access to the decision makers. Even a few minutes with a politician may be a few more minutes than the opposition has to make its case directly to a decision maker (Weissert & Weissert, 2002, p. 131). Finally, interest groups need to develop a persuasive argument, a way to frame the issue that convinces politicians to agree with their view of a policy matter.

Interest groups have a variety of tools at their disposal when developing strategies for lobbying. They may initiate a *grassroots* campaign, asking their members to contact their representatives with a particular message. Because interest group members are the voters with the power to reelect public officials, strong grassroots campaigns can be quite effective. Or, they may try a *grasstops* strategy and harness the influence of community leaders and other prominent individuals (Weissert & Weissert, 2002, p. 1319), or, they may join with other interest groups to create coalitions and strengthen their influence through numbers. Interest groups may start a media campaign to align public sentiment with their goals. Of course, providing candidates with money, often through political action committees, is a time-honored way to try to influence the outcome of policy debates.

Whatever methodology they use, interest groups are an important part of the policymaking process. According to Lindbloom (1980), interest groups are an "indispensable" (p. 85) part of making policy decisions. They provide a way to give a voice to their members, who may not otherwise feel able to participate effectively in the policymaking process.

▶ Conclusion

This journey through the policymaking process in the United States was intended to provide you with an understanding of policy and a context for your discussions and analysis of health policy issues. It is vital that you become familiar with both the nature of policy and the institutions that make and influence policy. As you have seen, the definition of policy is subject to much debate, yet it is necessary to define what policy means before attempting to engage in policy analysis. We have also walked through the specific duties and powers of the executive and legislative branches of the federal government and included key points about state-level policymaking as well. Finally, all policy students must be aware of and understand the influence of interest groups. They have and use numerous opportunities to influence the policymaking process, and their strength and concerns must be accounted for when analyzing policy issues. As you move further into health policy study, use the information provided in this overview to help you think about and frame your own policy positions.

References

Administrative Procedure Act of 1946, 5 U.S.C. § 500 (2018).

America's Essential Hospitals. (n.d.). *Mission and service.* Retrieved from https://essentialhospitals.org/about-americas-essential-hospitals/mission-driven-and-ready-to-serve/

Center on Budget and Policy Priorities. (n.d.). *About the center.* Retrieved from https://www.cbpp.org/about/mission-history

Davidson, R. H. (1984). The presidency and the Congress. In M. Nelson (Ed.), *The presidency and the political system* (p. 371). Washington, DC: Congressional Quarterly Press.

Department of Veterans Affairs. (n.d.). *Veterans Health Administration.* Retrieved from https://www.va.gov/health/aboutVHA.asp

Hanley, B. E. (1999). Policy development and analysis. In J. K. Leavitt, D. J. Mason, & M. W. Chaffee (Eds.), *Policy and politics in nursing and health care* (3rd ed., pp. 125–138). Philadelphia, PA: W. B. Saunders.

Heitshusen, V. (2018). *Introduction to the legislative process in the U.S. Congress* (CRS Report No. R24843). Retrieved from https://fas.org/sgp/crs/misc/R42843.pdf

Heritage Foundation. (n.d.). *About Heritage.* Retrieved from https://www.heritage.org/about-heritage/mission

House Committee on the Budget Majority Caucus. (2001). *Basics of the budget process.* Washington, DC: U.S. Government Printing Office.

H.R. Doc. No. 106-216, at 40–50 (2000).

Kernell, S. (1997). *Going public: New strategies of presidential leadership* (3rd ed.). Washington, DC: CQ Press.

Lindbloom, C. (1980). *The policy-making process.* Englewood Cliffs, NJ: Prentice-Hall.

Longest, B. B., Jr. (2016). *Health policymaking in the United States* (6th ed.). Chicago, IL: Health Administration Press.

Pharmaceutical Research and Manufacturers of America. (n.d.). *Our mission.* Retrieved from https://www.phrma.org/about/our-mission

Rein, L. (2018, May 23). Congress sends massive veterans bill to Trump, opening door to more private care. *The Washington Post.* Retrieved from https://www.washingtonpost.com/politics/congress-sends-massive-veterans-bill-to-trump-opening-door-to-more-private-health-care/2018/05/23/48e91220-5ea8-11e8-a4a4-c070ef53f315_story.html?noredirect=on&utm_term=.6661a7a87de9

Ryan White Comprehensive AIDS Resources Emergency Act of 1990, 42 U.S.C. § 300ff (2000).

Senate Committee on the Budget. (1998). *The congressional budget process: An explanation.* Washington, DC: U.S. Government Printing Office.

Subcommittee on Health and Environment of the Committee on Interstate Commerce, U.S. House of Representatives. (1976). *A discursive dictionary of health care.* Washington, DC: U.S. Government Printing Office.

Turnock, B. J. (2016). *Public health: What it is and how it works* (6th ed.). Burlington, MA: Jones and Bartlett Learning.

Waisanen, B. (2010). *State tax and expenditure limits.* Retrieved from http://www.ncsl.org/research/fiscal-policy/state-tax-and-expenditure-limits-2010.aspx

Weissert, C. S., & Weissert, W. G. (2002). *Governing health: The politics of health policy* (2nd ed.). Baltimore, MD: Johns Hopkins University Press.

U.S. Const. amend. XXII, § 1.

U.S. Const. art. I, § 1.
U.S. Const. art. I, § 2.
U.S. Const. art. I, § 3.
U.S. Const. art. I, § 8.
U.S. Const. art. II, § 1.

Yoder, E. (2016, November 9). Trump and the federal workforce: Five key issues. *The Washington Post.* Retrieved from https://www.washingtonpost.com/news/powerpost/wp/2016/11/09/trump-and-the-federal-workforce-five-key-issues/?noredirect=on&utm_term=.4e8c427f5046

▶ Endnotes

a. Under Article 1 of the Constitution, Congress has jurisdiction over the District of Columbia. Both the Senate and the House have committees that oversee some governmental functions of the District. The District elects two "shadow senators" who are allowed to lobby Congress on issues but who do not have voting rights. In terms of representation, this places the District in a position similar to other political bodies administered by the United States, such as Puerto Rico, the U.S. Virgin Islands, and American Samoa. The District's shadow senators (and a shadow representative in the House) were created by the citizens of the District in anticipation of the passage of the 1978 District of Columbia Voting Rights amendment to the U.S. Constitution, which would have granted the District the same voting rights as the states. The amendment never passed, but the District government has maintained the shadow positions nonetheless.

b. In addition to the 435 representatives, Puerto Rico has a resident commissioner, and the District of Columbia, Guam, the U.S. Virgin Islands, and American Samoa each has a delegate who is allowed to sponsor legislation and vote in committees, but may not vote on the House floor. The citizens of the District of Columbia also elect a nonvoting shadow representative.

c. In circumstances where the president serves 2 years or less of the term of another president, that president may hold office for 10 years.

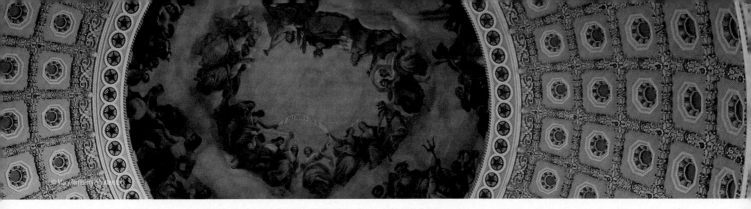

CHAPTER 3

Law and the Legal System

LEARNING OBJECTIVES

By the end of this chapter you will be able to:

- Describe the role of law in everyday life
- Define the term "law"
- Identify the various sources of law
- Describe key features of the legal system

"It is perfectly proper to regard and study the law simply as a great anthropological document."

—**Former U.S. Supreme Court Justice Oliver Wendell Holmes** (1899, p. 444).

▶ Introduction

The importance and complexity of law and the legal system in the United States cannot be overstated. Law's importance stems from its primary purpose: to function as the main tool with which we organize ourselves as an advanced, democratic society. The complexity of law and the legal process is a function of the multiple sources of law that may apply to any one of the millions of actions and interactions that occur daily in society, the division of legal authority between the federal and state governments and among the branches within them, the language the law and its players use to express themselves, and more. For all its complexity, however, there is also an undeniable pervasiveness and openness when it comes to law. We are not left to wonder where it comes from or how it is made. Generally speaking, we are privy to lawmakers' rationales for the laws they write and to judges' reasoning for their legal opinions, just as we are generally privy to the process by which law is made, and once made, laws are not hidden from us; to the contrary, they are discussed in the media and catalogued in books and online services available for public consumption. (Indeed, one is *expected* to know what the law is, since its violation can have potentially severe consequences.) If you want to know more about law than the average person, you can study it formally in law and other schools, or you can consult with one of the million or so lawyers in practice today. In other words, although law is complicated, it is equally accessible in a way that may not be clear at first blush.

Furthermore, beyond the law's sheer pervasiveness lies another simplicity: as the quotation at the outset of this chapter implies, the study of law is in essence the study of human beings, particularly their evolving customs, beliefs, and value systems. Because law is the key tool with which we regulate social behavior, it stands to reason that it also reflects our foremost values and normative standards. Indeed, law "takes an understanding, a norm, an attitude, and hardens it into muscle and bone" (Friedman, 2002, p. 29); however, this is subject to change, for as our society evolves, so too does our law. A relevant example of legal evolution can be seen in the updating of state public health laws, which before the tragic events of September 11, 2001, and the subsequent anthrax scare had not been updated in most states for over a century. Soon after the 2001 attacks, however, many states, concerned about new risks to the public's health, reviewed and overhauled these laws (Ziskin & Harris, 2007).

This chapter begins by briefly considering the role law plays in everyday life, and then turns to defining law and describing its multiple sources. It then discusses several key features of the legal system, including the separation of powers among branches of government, federalism (i.e., the separate sovereignty and authority of the federal and state governments), the role of courts, due process, and more.

For some, reading this chapter may bring to mind a course you have taken or a book you have read on civics or government. In this case, the chapter should serve as a helpful refresher. For those of you new to the study of law, consider the following pages a condensed but important introduction to one of the most critical and influential aspects of the society in which you live. In either event, this chapter is designed to better position you to understand the law's application to the specific fields of health care and public health and to digest the health policy and legal concepts discussed in this textbook.

▶ The Role of Law

The law reaches into nearly every corner of American life. Its impact is inescapable from the moment you wake up to the time you go back to sleep at night (and perhaps beyond, if your community has a curfew or other means of controlling activity and noise after dark). Have you ever stopped to think about the regulations pertaining to the flammability of the mattress you sleep on, or the safety of the water you shower with, cook with, and drink? How about the consumer protection laws regulating the quality of the food you eat throughout the day, and the quality of the establishments that serve it? Then there are the laws pertaining to the safety of the cars, buses, and subways you travel in each day, and the traffic laws that control their movement. You encounter laws daily pertaining to the environment, property ownership, the workplace, civil rights, copyright, energy, banking, and much more. And these are just the laws implicated by the relatively mundane actions of day-to-day life.

Steering into activities that are not as common—say, international travel, or adoption, or being admitted to a hospital—you encounter the law swiftly and noticeably. If you need final proof of the ubiquitous nature of law, pick up today's newspaper and count how many stories have some sort of legal angle to them. Then do it tomorrow and the next day. What you will almost certainly find is that a great majority of the stories concern law or legal process.

The law's pervasive nature is no surprise, given the important societal role we assign to it—namely, to serve as the tool with which we govern our relationships with one another, our government, and society at large. A society as sprawling and complex as ours needs formal, enforceable rules of law to provide a measure of control (for example, the need to regulate entities or actions that are potentially dangerous or invidious—a polluting power plant, or acts of discrimination based on race or gender). Furthermore, many people believe that law should be used not just to organize and control the society in which we live, but to achieve a more just society; in other words, according to this view, the country's key organizing principle should not simply be grounded in law, but rather grounded in a legal system designed to affirmatively produce outcomes based on fairness, justice, and equality (Smith, 1991).

The main way the law governs the many kinds of relationships in society is to recognize and establish enforceable legal rights and responsibilities that guide those relationships, and to create the institutions necessary to define and enforce them. Take constitutional law, for example. Constitutions are charters establishing governments and delineating certain individual and governmental rights and obligations. However, constitutional provisions are triggered only when one party to a relationship works for or on behalf of the government, whether federal or state. Thus, constitutional law governs the relationship between individuals and their government—not, for example, the relationship between two private parties, even when one party's actions are clearly discriminatory or wrongful. Thus, it takes affirmative action by a governmental actor to trigger constitutional protections. So, although it would be a violation of a public school student's First Amendment right to be forced by his principal to pray in class, forced prayer in private schools passes constitutional muster.

A legal right (constitutional or otherwise) denotes a power or privilege that has been guaranteed to an individual under the law, not merely something that is claimed as an interest or something that is a matter of governmental discretion. Conceptually, legal rights derive from the fact that the government sometimes creates what are called individual "property rights"—a generic term referring to an entitlement to personal or real property—for specified groups of persons (Reich, 1964). Importantly, legal rights also presuppose that their enforcement can be achieved through public institutions, including state and federal courts, because a person's ability to secure a remedy when a legal right is denied, reduced, or terminated goes to the very heart of what it means to be "entitled" to something. Indeed, whether particular healthcare benefits rise to the level of being a legal "right" and whether the healthcare right can be enforced in court are two of the most fundamental legal questions in the area of healthcare law. For example, the federal Medicare program for the aged and disabled confers on eligible individuals not only the right to healthcare services, but also the ability to enforce their right to benefits when program violations occur.

▶ The Definition and Sources of Law

Defining "Law"

Although many legal scholars agree on the general function of law in society, there is far less consensus on how to define "the law." As with many legal terms, there are several plausible interpretations of what is meant by the law, and thus there is no single way to correctly define it. For example, *Black's Law Dictionary* includes the following definitions in its primary entry:

> That which is laid down, ordained, or established. A rule or method according to which phenomena or actions co-exist or follow each other. Law, in its generic sense, is a body of rules of action or conduct prescribed by controlling authority, and having binding legal force. That which must be obeyed and followed by citizens subject to sanctions or legal consequences is a law. (Garner, 2014, p. 884)

However, even these commonly accepted definitions are not entirely satisfactory, because "a body of rules" that "must be obeyed" in the face of "sanctions or legal consequences" necessarily envisions a process by which the rules are created, disseminated, enforced, violated, disputed, interpreted, applied, revised, and so on. Considered in this way, "the law" essentially amounts to a "legal system"—and a system, by definition, entails regularly interacting or interdependent parts and subparts coming together to form a functional, unified whole. As you read this text, think of "the law" not just as words on a page (e.g., codified statutes or regulations), but as the many interacting

parts that are involved in drafting those words in the first place, and in bringing them to life once they have been enacted as laws. Note that this broad conceptualization of law as a system squares nicely with the primary purpose of law described previously, because there must, by necessity, be a sizeable system in place if law is going to carry out its role as the primary organizing tool in society. This broad definition of law also encompasses key legal doctrines, like separation of powers and federalism, described later in this chapter.

Sources of Law

Regardless of the breadth of the definition attached to the term *law*, at the core of the nation's expansive legal system lies a body of enforceable written rules meant to maintain order, define the outer limits of our interactions with one another and with our governments, and delineate legal rights and responsibilities. These rules derive from several sources, which collectively are called *primary* sources of law. The sources of primary legal authority include constitutions, statutes, regulations, and common (i.e., judge-made) law. There are also *secondary* sources of law, which are not laws in the technical sense, but rather are a collection of treatises, law review articles, reports, legal encyclopedias, and more that analyze, interpret, and critique primary laws. This section discusses each of the four types of primary sources of law.

Constitutions

A constitution is a charter that both establishes a government and delineates fundamental rights and obligations of that government and of individuals who fall within the territory covered by the constitution. In this country, there is a federal constitution and separate constitutions in each of the 50 states. The Constitution of the United States, completed in 1787 and subsequently ratified in each of the original 13 states, took effect in 1789. It provided for a federal union of sovereign states, and a federal government divided into three branches (legislative, executive, and judicial) to operate the union. This governmental structure was not easily agreed upon. Prior to the creation of the federal Constitution, the colonies of the American War of Independence first adopted, in 1777, the Articles of Confederation, which represented the first formal governing document of the United States and which were ratified in 1781. However, a defining feature of the Articles was a weak national government; fairly quickly, a movement for a stronger central government took hold, the colonies elected to throw out their original plan, and the Constitutional Convention—and with it the Constitution—was born.

The federal Constitution is rather short and, for the most part, quite general. One explanation for this is that the framers of the Constitution viewed it as a "document for the ages" that needed to include enduring principles to serve a growing, evolving society that has certainly proved to be more complex than it was at the time of the Constitution's ratification. In the words of former U.S. Supreme Court Justice Robert Jackson, the Constitution is a compilation of "majestic generalities" that collect meaning over a span of many years (*Fay v. New York*, 1947).

But the fact that some of the most important constitutional provisions are written in broad terms leads to many thorny legal controversies, because there are many competing approaches and theories as to how courts should interpret ambiguous constitutional phrases. Broadly speaking, the leading approaches to constitutional interpretation include the "living constitution," the "moral constitution," "originalism," and "strict constructionism." The living constitution model reflects a belief that the broadly written Constitution should be interpreted to reflect *current* moral, political, and cultural values in society, not the values that were predominant at the time of the Constitution's ratification. Under this view, the meaning of the Constitution is not fixed, but instead evolves along with society. Moral constitutionalists infuse their interpretation of constitutional law with principles of moral philosophy. Originalism, technically, is an umbrella term referring to a small group of constitutional interpretation theories, all of which share a common belief that constitutional provisions have a fixed and knowable meaning. For example, "original intent," one well-known theory under the originalism umbrella, adheres to the position that constitutional interpretation should be consistent with the intent of the Constitution's original drafters. Finally, strict constructionists limit their interpretation to the Constitution's actual words and phrases, and decline to consider contextual factors such as shifts in societal values or the commentaries or intent of the framers. The most well-known interpretational controversy in the area of health pertains to the breadth and reach of the due process clause of the federal Constitution's 14th Amendment, which prohibits states from depriving "any person of life, liberty, or property, without due process of law" (U.S. Const. amend. XIV, § 1). This provision rests at the heart of the Supreme Court's "right to privacy" jurisprudence, including the right to obtain an abortion. For readers interested in theories of constitutional interpretation, there is a vast body of literature at your disposal (Baker, 2004; Fallon, 1999).

One of the general principles underpinning the Constitution is that citizens should not be subjected to arbitrary and oppressive government. Given that the Constitution was drafted on the heels of the Revolutionary War, this is no surprise. But one consequence of the prevailing mood of the framers toward the reach of a national government is that they drafted the Constitution with an eye toward limiting federal government, as opposed to viewing the Constitution as a vehicle for extending benefits to the public—in other words, that "the men who wrote the Bill of Rights were not concerned that government might do too little for the people but that it might do too much to them" (*Jackson v. City of Joliet*, 1983). This logic helps explain why several key constitutional provisions were drafted in "negative" terms—the First Amendment prohibits government from abridging free speech, the Fourth Amendment makes unreasonable searches illegal—rather than as conferring positive rights, like a generalized right to receive healthcare services. At the same time, the First and Fourth Amendments, along with eight others, make up the Bill of Rights, a series of important, specifically guaranteed rights in the Constitution the framers believed to be inalienable.[b]

In addition to the federal Constitution, each state has its own constitution. All state constitutions are like the federal one in that they provide for the organizational structure of the particular state's government, and all contain some measure of a state bill of rights. Here the similarities can end, however. Although state constitutions cannot limit or take away rights conferred by the U.S. Constitution (or by federal statutes), some state constitutions go further than federal law in conferring rights or extending protections. For example, under current U.S. Supreme Court case law, the death penalty does not always violate the federal Constitution, but the Massachusetts Supreme Court has ruled that the death penalty is prohibited under the state's constitution in every instance. Maryland's constitution requires that a jury be unanimous in order to convict a person of a crime, a standard that differs from federal criminal law. Furthermore, state constitutions are amended much more easily and frequently than is their federal counterpart. While state constitutions have been amended, on average, 150 times per state (Dinan, 2018, p. 23), the language of the federal Constitution has not been dramatically altered since its inception; there have been just 27 amendments, and the 10 that make up the Bill of Rights were all added by 1791.

Statutes

Statutes are laws written by legislative bodies at all levels of government (federal, state, county, city) that, generally speaking, command or prohibit something.

It is the fact of their being legislatively created that sets them apart from other sources of law, because legislatures are understood as creating laws that are forward-looking and apply to large numbers of people. Indeed, the two hallmarks of statutes are their prospectivity and generality. These hallmarks result mainly from the fact that legislatures are in the "regulation business" across an enormous array of issues, and as a result, legislators often lack both the time and the substantive expertise to regulate other than in broad fashion.

Because statutes tend to be written as broad policy statements (and because words on a page can never communicate intent with absolute accuracy), there are few statutes that are utterly unambiguous. This, coupled with the fact that our evolving society continuously presents situations that may not have been foreseeable at the time a statute was written, results in the need for courts to interpret and apply general statutes to millions of specific legal cases or controversies. This practice is called "statutory construction." Although it is a tenet of the separation of powers doctrine (discussed later under Key Features of the Legal System) that legislatures represent the law-making branch of government and the judiciary's role is to interpret law, it is commonly understood that judges and courts "make" law as well through statutory construction, because the continual interpretation and application of broad policy statements (i.e., statutes) can put a "gloss" on the original product, potentially altering its meaning over time.

As discussed more fully later in the section on federalism, state legislatures have greater ability than does Congress to use statutes to regulate across a broad range of issues, pursuant to states' plenary authority under the Constitution. For instance, the number of state statutes regarding population health and safety (e.g., disease control and prevention, the creation of public health agencies, the ability of governors to classify public health emergencies) far exceeds congressional output on the same topic. Notwithstanding states' broader regulatory power, however, federal statutes have primacy over state statutes.

Administrative Regulations

The fact that statutes are written in broad generalities has another consequence beyond their need to be interpreted and applied in vast numbers of unique instances: specific regulations must be written to assist with the implementation of statutory directives and to promote statutes' underlying policy goals. This is where administrative agencies of the executive branch of government come in. Because these federal and state agencies—the U.S. Department of Health and Human Services, the U.S. Department of Labor, the California Department of Social Services, the Wisconsin Department of Commerce, and so on—are organized and created to deal with specific policy subject matters, they have more time and expertise than Congress or state legislatures have to enforce statutes and promulgate regulations, rules, and orders necessary to carry out statutory prerogatives. It is important to note that assuming the process for creating the regulations was itself legal, and provided that the regulations do not stray beyond the intent of the enacted statute, regulations have the full force of law.

Administrative law is crucial in the area of health policy and law.[c] For example, consider the Medicaid program, which functions primarily as a health insurance program for low-income individuals. The Medicaid statute embodies Congress's intentions in passing the law, including standards pertaining to program eligibility, benefits, and payments to participating healthcare providers. Yet there are literally thousands of administrative regulations and rules pertaining to Medicaid, which over the past 50 years have become the real battleground over the stability and scope of the program. In a very real sense, the Medicaid regulations passed by the federal Department of Health and Human Services and state-level agencies are what bring the program to life and give it vitality. This "operationalizing" function of administrative law can be seen across a wide spectrum of important health issues, including the reporting of infectious diseases, the development of sanitation standards, and the enforcement of environmental laws (Mensah et al., 2004). In order to be lawful, regulations must be proposed and established in a way that conforms to the requirements of the federal Administrative Procedure Act of 1946 (APA), which provides procedural restrictions for agency rule making and adjudication. Compared to state administrative procedure acts, which tend to be technical and detailed, the APA is broad and sweeping, thus relatively more ambiguous and open to various interpretations by federal courts.[d] Once Congress delegates rule-making authority to an executive branch agency via a statute (known as the "enabling statute"), the APA dictates how the agency must go about promulgating specific rules and regulations, unless the statute itself specifies the procedure an agency must follow. If the enabling statute dictates a formal rule-making process, the APA requires the agency to follow cumbersome procedures, and it can adopt rules only after a trial-like hearing on the proposed rule. If Congress does not specify in an enabling statute how an agency must adopt rules, the APA permits the agency to follow a more informal rule-making process. This requires the agency to publish the proposed rule in the *Federal Register* (the official daily publication for rules, proposed rules, and notices of federal agencies) and provide an opportunity for the public to comment on the proposed rule. The agency must take the comments under consideration (though it need not revise the proposed rule in response to them), and once it settles on a final rule, it must be published in the *Code of Federal Regulations* (which houses permanent federal regulations under 50 separate titles representing broad areas subject to federal oversight).

In delegating authority to an agency through an enabling statute, Congress must provide an "intelligible principle" that the agency can (and must) follow. That said, the amount of direction and discretion given to agencies varies widely. For example, the enabling statute for the Occupational Health and Safety Administration provides broad discretion by delegating the authority to create and enforce workplace safety standards (Occupational Health and Safety Act of 1970). Contrast this with the Americans With Disabilities Act, which has very specific provisions and does not allow agencies much discretion when implementing and enforcing the statutory language.

In addition to the power of rule making, Congress may also delegate adjudicatory and enforcement powers to administrative agencies. Adjudicatory power refers to claims of public rights, which are claims that involve private persons as one party and the government as the other party (excluding criminal cases). Congress may set up a court, known as an administrative court, within an agency to adjudicate these claims. Because these courts are located in the executive, rather than judicial, branch of government, they are not subject to the same rules and procedures as traditional courts, although they still must provide for the rights and protections prescribed by the Bill of Rights (e.g., the right to legal counsel). Administrative hearings are often much less formal than judicial trials: there are no juries, and although some evidence may be gathered through witness testimony, the majority of evidence derives from written reports. Decisions by administrative law judges (known as ALJs) often do not represent the final word on the matter being adjudicated, as these decisions are subject to approval or rejection by the agency's lead official or by a traditional (judicial branch) federal court. At the same time, federal courts generally apply a deferential standard of review to administrative decisions, reviewing only to see whether an agency has acted in an "arbitrary and capricious" manner.

The third type of authority granted to agencies by Congress is that of enforcement. As this authority already inherently resides in the executive branch

under the federal Constitution, Congress uses its power to specify which agencies have authority to enforce certain statutes and substantive areas of law.

Once Congress grants power to agencies to promulgate rules, adjudicate claims, and enforce statues, its ability to constrain agency action is limited. Because agencies are located in the executive branch and thus are under the control of the president, Congress is limited to passing a new statute overturning the questioned agency action or investigating agency action for impropriety.

Common Law

In each of the prior discussions about constitutions, statutes, and administrative regulations, we pointed out the generality and ambiguity of much of law, and the corresponding responsibility of courts to interpret and apply law to specific cases. It is via the common law—essay-like opinions written by appellate courts articulating the bases for their decisions in individual cases—that courts carry out this responsibility. Common law is also referred to as case law, judge-made law, or decisional law.

Common law is central to legal systems in many countries, particularly those that were territories or colonies of England, which is how the United States came to rely on common law as part of its legal system. Both historically and in modern times, case law is premised on the traditions and customs of society, the idea being that courts could continuously (and relatively efficiently, compared to the legislative process) interpret and apply law in such a way as to match the values of a society undergoing constant evolution. At the same time, the common law is heavily influenced by legal precedent and the doctrine of *stare decisis*, which refers to the legal principle that prior case law decisions should be accorded great deference and should not be frequently overturned. The importance and function of *stare decisis* in American law is discussed later in the section detailing the role courts play in maintaining stability in the law.

Although courts are expected to overturn their own prior decisions only in rare circumstances and lower courts can never overturn decisions by higher courts that have jurisdiction over them, legislatures can modify or even overturn common law decisions interpreting statutes and regulations. Imagine that the U.S. Supreme Court interpreted a federal civil rights statute as protecting individuals from intentional acts of race discrimination, but not from conduct that has the unintended effect of discriminating against racial minorities. If Congress disagreed with the court's interpretation of the statute, it could effectively

TABLE 3-1 Summary of the Primary Sources of American Law

Source of Law	Key Points
Constitutions	■ Establish governments and delineate fundamental rights and obligations of government and individuals.
	■ There is a federal constitution and separate constitutions in each state.
	■ The federal constitution restrains government more than it confers individual rights; however, the Bill of Rights specifically guarantees several important individual rights.
	■ The Supreme Court has the final word on the constitutionality of laws created by the political branches of government.
Statutes	■ Created by legislatures at all levels of government.
	■ Two hallmarks: prospectivity and generality.
	■ As broad policy statements, statutes are often ambiguous as applied to specific cases or controversies, requiring courts to interpret them through the practice of statutory construction.
	■ State legislatures can use statutes to regulate across a broader range of issues than can Congress; however, federal statutes have primacy over conflicting state statutes.
Regulations	■ Created by executive branch administrative agencies to implement statutes and clarify their ambiguities.
	■ Play a particularly critical role in health policy and law.
Common law	■ Court opinions interpreting and applying law to specific cases.
	■ Also referred to as case law, judge-made law, or decisional law.
	■ Based on the traditions and customs of society, yet heavily influenced by legal precedent and the doctrine of *stare decisis*.

overturn the court's decision by amending the statute to make it clear that the law was intended to prohibit intentional discrimination *and* presumably neutral acts that nonetheless resulted in unintended discrimination. However, because the judicial branch has final authority to determine whether statutes violate the federal Constitution, Congress would be powerless to overturn a federal court decision that ruled the same civil rights statute unconstitutional.

Notice the "checks and balances" at play in this example, with one branch of government acting as a restraint on another. In the next section, we discuss the separation of powers doctrine—including checks and balances—and other key features of the legal system. But first, see **TABLE 3-1**, which provides a summary of the sources of law.

▶ Key Features of the Legal System

Recall the earlier description of the law as something more than just words on a page, something more than statutes and constitutional provisions. Although the laws themselves are obviously critical, they are just one component of a complex, interacting legal system that creates the laws in the first instance and brings them to life after they hit the pages of legal code books, texts, and treatises.

All legal systems rest on unique principles, traditions, and customs. This section describes a handful of the most important features and principles of the U.S. legal system, including the separation of powers doctrine, federalism, the role and structure of federal and state courts, judicial review, due process, and constitutional standards of review.

Separation of Powers

This country's government, both federal and state, has an underpinning structure of three independent and equally powerful branches, a fact that sets it apart from parliamentary systems of government—such as those found in Canada, Germany, the United Kingdom, and many other countries—in which the legislature appoints the executive. The legal doctrine that supports the arrangement of shared governance among multiple branches is the *separation of powers* doctrine. This doctrine is considered one of the most important aspects of both federal and state constitutional design. The framers of the U.S. Constitution were well aware that nothing was more likely to foster tyrannical government than the concentration of governing powers in one person or political party. To guard against a concentration of political power, the framers did two related things: they divided governmental powers and responsibilities among separate, coequal branches, and they structured the elections of officials for the two political branches of government (legislative and executive) so that they would take place at different intervals and through different mechanisms (e.g., the president is elected through the electoral college system, whereas members of Congress are not).

Inherent in the separation of powers doctrine is the important concept of checks and balances. "Checks" refers to the ability and responsibility of one branch of government to closely monitor the actions of the other two, including when one branch grasps at an amount of power not envisioned by the Constitution. The "balance" at work in the separation of powers framework prevents one branch from exerting power in an area of responsibility that is the province of another branch.

The constitutional doctrine of separation of powers represents, in the words of one legal scholar, an "invitation to struggle for the privilege" of governing the country (Corwin, 1957, p. 171). Alexis de Tocqueville, a French philosopher and political theorist who studied American government in the 1830s, viewed the concept of checks and balances in much starker terms:

> The president, who exercises a limited power, may err without causing great mischief in the state. Congress may decide amiss without destroying the union, because the electoral body in which the Congress originates may cause it to retract its decision by changing its members. But if the Supreme Court is ever composed of imprudent or bad men, the union may be plunged into anarchy or civil war. (de Tocqueville, 1835, p. 152)

For example, a fairly common separation of powers debate between Congress and a president concerns the nation's soaring debt and the appropriateness of raising the debt ceiling. Some policymakers (and many presidents) maintain that the president can act unilaterally to raise the debt ceiling and allow the federal government to borrow more money, while others argue that such a move is solely within the purview of Congress and beyond the scope of presidential power.

Throughout this text, there are health policy and law questions that distinctly highlight our government's divided powers. For instance, how will the struggle between the executive branch and some members of Congress over implementation of the Affordable Care Act (ACA)—the former attempting to thwart implementation through fiscal, policy, and legal channels, while those in Congress who supported the ACA aim to keep the ACA functioning as fully and efficiently as possible—play out? And how has the Supreme Court applied its constitutional right to privacy jurisprudence to the matter of abortion in response to federal and state legislative enactments? As you consider these and other health policy and law questions from a separation of powers angle, consider the peculiar roles of each branch of government, taking into account their duties, powers, and limitations. Through this prism, continually reflect on which governmental body is best equipped to effectively respond to health policy problems.[e]

Federalism: Allocation of Federal and State Legal Authority

In the legal system, the powers to govern, make and apply law, and effect policy choices are not just apportioned among three governmental branches at both the federal and state levels; they are also divided *between* the federal government and the governments of the various states. This division of authority—which also plays a key role in the development of health policies and laws—is referred to as *federalism*. Like the separation of powers doctrine, federalism derives from the U.S. Constitution.

Under the Constitution, the federal government is one of limited powers, while the states more or less retain all powers not expressly given to the federal government. In essence, this was the deal consented to by the states at the time our federal republic was formed: they agreed to surrender certain enumerated powers (like foreign affairs) to the federal government in exchange for retaining many aspects of sovereignty.

The Constitution's 10th Amendment states that "the powers not delegated to the United States by the Constitution . . . are reserved to the States respectively." For example, because the Constitution does not explicitly define the protection and promotion of the public's health as a power of the federal government, public health powers are primarily held by the states. (In fact, compared to the federal government, the states handle the vast majority of *all* legal matters in this country. Consider just a sampling of typical legal affairs overseen by state government: marriages, divorces, and adoptions; law enforcement and criminal trials; schooling; driving, hunting, medical, and many other licenses; consumer protection; and much more [Adelson, 2003, pp. 481–488]. Furthermore, the vast majority of all litigation that takes place occurs in state, rather than federal, courts [Refo, 2004, p. 3].) As a result, all states regulate the area of public health through what are known as their "police powers," which allow state and local governments to (among other things) legislate to protect the common good. Examples of the kinds of laws passed under this authority include childhood immunization standards, infectious disease data collection mandates, and environmental hazard regulations. Moreover, under the 10th Amendment, states historically have had the power to regulate the practice of medicine and the licensing of hospitals and other healthcare institutions.

Recall, however, that the federal government also plays a role in regulating health care and public health. The national government's enumerated powers include the ability to tax, spend, and regulate interstate commerce, all of which have been utilized in ways to improve health care and promote public health. For example, Congress has used its taxing power to increase the cost of cigarettes (in the hopes of driving down the number of smokers) and to generate funds for programs such as Medicare, and congressional spending powers are the legal cornerstone for federal health programs like Medicaid. Furthermore, the sharing of power under the 10th Amendment notwithstanding, the Constitution's supremacy clause declares that federal laws—the Constitution, statutes, and treaties—are the "supreme" law of the land, and thus preempt state laws that conflict with them (U.S. Const. art. VI, para. 2).

While federalism is built solidly into the nation's political branches through separate federal and state legislatures and executives, it is also on display in the structure of U.S. courts. There are both federal and state court systems, and each has unique authority and jurisdiction: federal courts are limited to ruling only in certain kinds of cases, including those involving federal constitutional or statutory law, those in which the United States is a party to the lawsuit, and those specified by statutory law; state courts, by contrast, have jurisdiction to hear just about any case (unless explicitly precluded from doing so by federal statute), including those over which federal courts also have jurisdiction. State court jurisdiction includes cases implicating state statutory and regulatory law, the state constitution, and the U.S. Constitution.

Over the years, defining the boundaries of federalism (i.e., defining the federal government's sphere of authority and determining the scope of state sovereignty) has been a contentious legal and political issue. At the dawn of the country's independence, after the colonies scrapped the Articles of Confederation in favor of a stronger central government, the Supreme Court decided federalism cases with a nod toward expansive national powers (much to the dislike of some states). Two famous cases make the point. In the 1819 case of *McCulloch v. Maryland*, the Supreme Court enhanced the power of the U.S. government by establishing the principle that federal governmental powers are not strictly limited to those expressly provided for in the Constitution. At issue in the case was whether Congress had the power to charter a national bank to help the federal government shoulder wartime debt. In 1824, the court for the first time had the opportunity to review the Constitution's commerce clause (which grants Congress the authority to regulate interstate commerce) in the case of *Gibbons v. Ogden* (1824), which resulted from a decision by the state of New York to grant a monopoly to a steamboat operator for a ferry between New York and New Jersey. Again, the court ruled broadly in favor of the federal government, stating that the commerce clause reserved exclusively to Congress the power to regulate interstate navigation.

By the mid-1800s, however, this approach to defining the relative power of the federal and state governments gave way to one that was more deferential to states and more willing to balance their sovereign interests against the interests of the federal government. This approach, in turn, lost ground during the New Deal and civil rights eras, both of which were marked by an acceptance of federal authority to provide social services and regulate the economy. The arrival of Ronald Reagan's presidency in 1981 marked yet another turning point in the evolution of federalism. For 8 years, the Reagan administration acted to restrict national authority over the states, a process that took on even more force after the Republican Party took control of Congress in the mid-1990s. Indeed, since the early 1980s, a defining feature of federalism has been the purposeful devolution of authority and governance over social and economic policy from the federal government to state legislators and regulators.

The Role of Courts

Elsewhere, we have discussed the structure and powers of two of the political branches of government: the legislative and executive branches. The third branch is that of the judiciary, made up of justices, judges, magistrates, and other "adjudicators" in two separate court systems—one federal, one state. Although the federal and state court systems have critically distinctive authority, they do not look very different structurally. The federal court system has three tiers, with cases proceeding from the lowest-level court (a trial court) to two separate, higher-level courts (appellate courts). Federal trial courts are called district courts, and they exist in varying numbers in each state, with the size of the state determining the actual number of "districts," and thus the number of federal trial courts. In total, there are nearly 100 federal district courts. After a district court renders a decision, the losing party to a lawsuit is entitled to appeal the decision to a federal circuit court of appeals. There are 13 U.S. circuit courts of appeals—12 with jurisdiction over designated multistate geographic regions, or "circuits," and a court of appeals for the federal circuit (residing in Washington, DC), which has nationwide appellate jurisdiction over certain kinds of cases, such as patent and international trade disputes. For many individuals, losing a case in a federal circuit court represents the end of the line for their case, since litigants have no entitlement to have their case heard by the U.S. Supreme Court, the highest court in the country. Although parties have a right to *petition* the Supreme Court to hear their case, at least four of the nine justices on the court must agree to grant the petition. Although the Supreme Court is undeniably the most important court in the country in terms of its authority, it by no means renders the most decisions. Out of approximately 8,000 petitions annually, the Supreme Court typically accepts only 70 to 80, whereas the 13 circuit courts collectively decide approximately 61,000 cases each year. This fact is more than trivial; it effectively means that in the huge majority of federal cases, lower appellate courts, and not the Supreme Court, have final say over the scope and meaning of federal law.

As mentioned, each state also has its own court system, most of which are organized like the federal system: one trial court, followed by two separate appellate courts (generally termed "[name of state] court of appeals" and "[name of state] supreme court"). However, some state systems provide for only one appellate court. State systems also tend to include courts that are "inferior" even to their general trial courts; these handle relatively minor disputes (think of the small claims courts frequently shown on daytime television). Furthermore, state trial courts are sometimes divided by specialty, so that certain courts hear cases that involve only family matters, juvenile matters, and the like.

Within the federal and state court system hierarchy, appellate courts have two powers unavailable to trial courts: reviewing lower court decisions to determine whether there were errors of law made during the trial that necessitate a new one, and establishing legal precedents that lower courts are bound to follow. But appellate courts lack trial courts' powers to actually conduct trials, including empanelling juries, hearing testimony from witnesses, reviewing evidence, and the like. Instead, appellate reviews are generally limited to the written record created at trial by the lower court.

Adjudication refers to the legal process of resolving disputes. It is in the context of resolving specific legal disputes that the judiciary interprets and applies the law, and also indirectly "makes" law under its common law authority. The results of adjudication are the common law decisions described earlier. Because U.S. courts are generally not permitted to issue advisory opinions, courts in this country effectively only act in response to a specific "case or controversy" that is brought to them by parties to a lawsuit. (Where permitted, advisory opinions are released by courts not in response to a particular legal dispute, but in response to a request from another branch of government regarding the interpretation or permissibility of a particular law. Federal courts are bound from issuing advisory opinions because the Supreme Court has ruled that constitutional provisions establishing the federal courts prevent them from reviewing hypothetical or moot disputes. Although a couple exceptions exist, state courts are likewise prohibited from issuing advisory opinions.) This limitation essentially means that in order for a court to rule in a particular case, an individual initiating a lawsuit must assert an enforceable legal right, a measurable violation of that right, actual damage or harm, and a court-fashioned remedy that could appropriately respond to the lawsuit.

Courts play a vital role in the legal system. This role stems in large part from their responsibility to determine what, ultimately, the Constitution means, permits, and prohibits. In discharging this responsibility, courts are asked to protect and enforce individual legal rights, determine whether the political branches of government have acted in a way that violates the Constitution, and maintain stability in the law through the application of legal precedent. The judicial branch is viewed as uniquely able to fulfill these key responsibilities, at least at the federal level, because it is the branch of government most insulated (theoretically) from politics: federal judges are appointed, not elected, and granted life tenure under the Constitution to (theoretically) shield them from political influences that might otherwise interfere with their impartiality.[f] Most state judges, however, are now subject to popular election, either at the time of initial selection or subsequently, when it is determined whether they will be retained as judges (Brennan Center for Justice, 2015).[g]

Enforcing Legal Rights

As described earlier, two main functions of the legal system are to establish legal rights and to create institutions to enforce those rights. The primary enforcers of individual legal rights, and those in the best position to create remedies for their violation, are the courts. For example, the federal courts (and the Supreme Court in particular) were critical to the success of the civil rights movement, during which time federal judges expansively interpreted civil rights laws and maintained close oversight of the implementation of their rulings. At the same time, however, the Supreme Court has not often been at the forefront of advancing individual rights. Certainly, there have been times when the court has played an enormous role in advancing societal expectations with respect to individual equality—*Brown v. Board of Education* (1954) being the most obvious example—but this decision, and a few others, are actually quite anomalous, and the court has been more a follower of evolving attitudes and expectations.

Among the most important rights courts are expected to uphold and enforce is the constitutional right to *due process*, which protects individuals from arbitrary and unfair treatment at the hands of government. Both the 5th and 14th Amendments to the Constitution make clear that no person can be deprived of "life, liberty, or property, without due process of law," with the 5th Amendment applying to the federal government and the 14th applying to the states. An important component of due process is the principle that when government establishes a legal right or entitlement for individuals, it may not then decide to deny the right or entitlement unfairly.

When courts consider due process claims, they are often thought of as reviewing *how* laws operate and *why* laws have been established in the first place. This results from the fact that the due process clause has been interpreted by the Supreme Court as including *procedural* due process (the "how") and *substantive* due process (the "why"). Procedural due process requires that laws be enacted and applied fairly and equitably, including procedural fairness when individuals challenge government infringements on their life, liberty, or property. Thus, due process requirements might be triggered if a law is too vague or is applied unevenly, if government threatens to withdraw a previously granted license, or if an individual's public benefits are withheld. For example, before a physician can lose his state-granted license to practice medicine, the state must provide the physician advance notice of the termination and a formal hearing before an impartial examiner with all the usual legal trappings (right to legal representation, right to present evidence in one's defense, right to appeal the examiner's decision, etc.). Similarly, Medicaid beneficiaries must be given notice of, and an opportunity to challenge, benefit coverage denials made by a managed care company participating in the Medicaid program. And the courts' most well-known jurisprudence in the area of health-related due process rights concerns abortion, specifically whether federal and state laws impermissibly infringe on the right to terminate a pregnancy, which is part of the right to "liberty" under the due process clause.

But that clause has been interpreted by courts to require more than just procedural fairness when a law deprives an individual of life, liberty, or property; it also requires that government provide a sound reason for having invaded personal freedoms in the first place. This form of due process, which is termed *substantive due process*, serves as a proscription against arbitrary government activity. For instance, when states have been unable to adequately explain the reasoning behind statutes requiring involuntary confinement of mentally ill individuals who were not dangerous to themselves or others, courts ruled the laws unconstitutional on substantive due process grounds. Substantive due process is unquestionably more controversial than its procedural counterpart, because many critics argue that the former gives courts unrestrained power to invalidate, on constitutional grounds, government actions with which they simply disagree. In other words, some view this form of due process "as a potentially limitless warrant for judges to impose their personal values on the Constitution" (Lazarus, 1999, p. 474).

Reviewing the Actions of the Political Branches

An important piece of the separation of powers puzzle, and one that grants the courts wide authority to enforce individual legal rights in this country, is the doctrine of *judicial review*. Judicial review refers to the power of the courts to declare laws unconstitutional and to determine whether the actions of the legislative and executive branches of government are lawful. The theory behind judicial review is that, as the branch of government most independent of the political process, courts can pass judgment on the actions of the political branches free of partisanship.

Judicial review has its roots in the famous 1803 case of *Marbury v. Madison*, in which the Supreme Court ruled that it had the power to review acts of Congress and determine their constitutionality. The facts of the case are fascinating. In 1800, Thomas Jefferson won the presidential election, besting incumbent John Adams. In the final days of President Adams's term, the Federalist-controlled Congress passed, and Adams signed into law, a statute called the Judiciary Act of 1801. Among other things, the law created several new judgeships, and the idea was to fill the new judicial posts with Federalists before Jefferson assumed the presidency. Among the new judicial appointments made by Adams and approved by the Senate before Jefferson took office were 42 justices of the peace, including one for William Marbury. Prior to Jefferson's taking office, Marbury's commission was signed by Adams and by John Marshall—who at the time was Secretary of State under Adams—but not delivered. After his inauguration, Jefferson ruled that Marbury's commission (and those of several other Adams-appointed justices of the peace) were invalid because they had not been delivered during the Adams presidency, and therefore directed his new Secretary of State, James Madison, to withhold delivery. Marbury sued to force delivery of his commission, petitioning the Supreme Court directly to issue a *writ of mandamus*, which is an order by a court compelling a government officer to perform his duties. Marbury was able to ask the court directly for the writ because the recently enacted Judiciary Act also authorized the Supreme Court to issue writs of mandamus.

The Supreme Court's decision in *Marbury v. Madison*[h] first established the important principle that for every violation of a legal right, there must be a corresponding legal remedy. With this principle in place, the court ruled that Marbury was in fact entitled to his commission and to a legal remedy for Jefferson's decision to withhold it,

> since [Marbury's] commission was signed by the President, and sealed by the secretary of state ... and the law creating the office, gave the officer a right to hold for five years, independent of the executive, the appointment. ... To withhold his commission, therefore, is an act deemed by the court not warranted by law, but violative of a vested legal right.

The *Marbury* court then did something monumental: it established and justified the power of judicial review. This outcome flowed from the fact that Marbury had filed his legal petition directly with the Supreme Court, and the court needed to determine whether Congress acted constitutionally in granting the court power under the Judiciary Act to issue writs of mandamus as a matter of "original jurisdiction." (Original jurisdiction refers to cases on which a court rules before any other court does so, contrasted with situations in which a court reviews a decision of a lower court, which is called "appellate jurisdiction.")

It was not apparent that the mandamus component of the new Judiciary Act was constitutional because Article III of the Constitution—which established the judicial branch of the federal government, including the Supreme Court—says,

> In all Cases affecting Ambassadors, other public Ministers and Consuls, and those in which a State shall be a Party, the Supreme Court shall have original Jurisdiction. In all the other Cases [subject to Supreme Court jurisdiction], the Supreme Court shall have appellate Jurisdiction, both as to Law and Fact, with such Exceptions, and under such Regulations as the Congress shall make. (U.S. Const. art. III, § 2, clause 2)

Interpreting this clause, Chief Justice Marshall determined the court could issue a writ of mandamus under the Constitution only as an exercise of appellate—but not original—jurisdiction, and that Congress had no power to modify the court's original jurisdiction. As a result, the court held that the Judiciary Act of 1801 was in conflict with Article III, and thus unconstitutional.

Marbury represented the first time the Supreme Court exercised the power of judicial review and declared unconstitutional a law passed by Congress. Over the years, the court has exercised this power sparingly, explaining in 1867 that although it clearly had the authority to strike down congressional legislation repugnant to the Constitution, this "duty is one of great delicacy, and only to be performed where the repugnancy is clear, and the conflict unreconcilable" (*Mayor v. Cooper*, 1867).

For example, the Supreme Court invalidated few congressional acts in the first 50 years after *Marbury*, although the pace picked up somewhat after that, to an average of about one invalidation every 2 years. During William Rehnquist's term as chief justice (1986–2005), however, the court ruled unconstitutional more than 30 laws or statutory provisions, with most of these decisions occurring between 1995 and 2005. This uptick in the court's use of its most powerful judicial review tool has led to a discussion about the court's proper place in the separation of powers framework. As stated in one opinion piece,

Declaring an act of Congress unconstitutional is the boldest thing a judge can do. That's because Congress, as an elected legislative body representing the entire nation, makes decisions that can be presumed to possess a high degree of democratic legitimacy. (Gerwitz & Golder, 2005, p. A19)

When determining whether a statute violates the Constitution, courts necessarily take into account the subject of the regulation and Congress's purpose in regulating. Certain kinds of laws—say, affirmative action laws, or a law that classifies people on the basis of their gender—require a greater level of governmental justification and thus are held to a higher constitutional *standard of review*. In other words, these laws are scrutinized more closely by the court and thus stand a greater chance of failing the constitutionality test.

By way of example, the Supreme Court has developed a tiered standard of review framework for equal protection jurisprudence. Under the Constitution's equal protection clause, states are prohibited from denying "to any person within its jurisdiction the equal protection of the laws" (U.S. Const. amend. XIV, § 1).

The Court employs one of three standards when it reviews whether a particular law satisfies this constitutional mandate. The first, termed *rational basis* or *rational relations* review, is applied to everyday legislation pertaining to things like public safety, tax rates, and consumer protection and thus is the review standard most frequently used. It is nearly impossible for a law to run afoul of this standard, because as long as the challenged statute is *rationally* related to *any* legitimate government purpose in passing the law, it will be upheld as constitutional.

The second standard is that of *intermediate* review. This is the court's choice when the measure under review classifies individuals or groups on, for example, the basis of gender. The assumption here—and the point of the heightened review standard—is that when politicians legislate with gender (or another potentially baseless characteristic) in mind, there is a greater likelihood they are doing so for nefarious reasons. In order to pass constitutional muster under intermediate review, a statute must serve an *important* government objective and be *substantially* related to that objective. A good deal of legislation reviewed under this standard is found to be unconstitutional.

Finally, the court has at its disposal in equal protection lawsuits a review standard known as *strict scrutiny*. The court reserves this standard for laws that tread on fundamental constitutional rights (defined in part as those that are firmly established in American tradition), including an individual's right to be free of governmental discrimination on the basis of race. In theory, otherwise discriminatory laws that are *necessary* to achieve a *compelling* government interest—meaning that the law in question is the least discriminatory way to meet the legislature's compelling objective—can survive this intense form of scrutiny. However, of all the equal protection claims measured against this standard, only one survivor emerged—when the Supreme Court permitted the federal government to intern individuals of Japanese descent during World War II (*Korematsu v. United States*, 1944)—and this almost universally vilified decision was finally condemned (if not formally overruled) by the Supreme Court in 2018 (*Trump v. Hawaii*, 2018).[i]

Maintaining Stability in the Law

In addition to enforcing legal rights and passing on the constitutionality of actions of the two political branches of government, courts are expected to maintain a measure of stability, continuity, and predictability in the law. This expectation derives from the idea that those subject to the law should not have to contend with continuous swings in the direction law takes. In theory, the relatively nonpolitical judicial branch of government is in the best position to bring this expectation to fruition.

The way courts implement their responsibility to maintain legal stability is through application of *stare decisis*, a Latin legal term meaning "let it stand." *Stare decisis* is a policy of the courts to stand by existing legal precedent; that is, where rules of law have been established in prior judicial decisions, these decisions should be adhered to in subsequent cases where the questions of law and fact are substantially similar to those in the original case. Stability in the law is considered so important that *stare decisis* is usually applied, and the original judicial decision given deference, *even when the original decision is subsequently determined to be wrongly decided or not legally sound*. This is especially true where the original decision is an old one on which society has come to rest, as opposed to a relatively young decision with few deep roots in terms of societal expectations. The role of legal precedent has been described in this way:

Legal doctrines are shaped like family trees. Each generation of decisions is derived from ones that came before as, over time, each branch of the law grows and spreads or, occasionally, withers and dies away. The most recent decisions almost always draw their strength by tracing back through an ancestral line, choosing among parents, uncles, and cousins according to the aptness of their bloodlines. Rarely, a branch of doctrine is disowned, repudiated, and left vestigial until perhaps revived in another legal era. (Lazarus, 1999, p. 77)

At the same time, legal precedent is not completely sacred, and prior decisions are sometimes reconsidered and, on occasion, overturned. For instance, changes in societal values might outweigh strict application of *stare decisis*, as was the case with the Supreme Court's 1954 decision in *Brown v. Board of Education* to overturn the invidious idea of "separate but equal" from the court's 1896 decision in *Plessy v. Ferguson*. *Stare decisis* is, however, generally understood to trump mere changes in a court's makeup. In other words, courts are expected to remain anchored to precedential rules of law even when current individual members may not be.[j] Indeed, in a well-known Supreme Court case, former Justice John Marshall Harlan II wrote:

A basic change in the law upon a ground no firmer than a change in our membership invites the popular misconception that this institution is little different from the two political branches of the Government. No misconception could do more lasting injury to this Court and to the system which it is our abiding mission to serve. (*Mapp v. Ohio*, 1961)

▶ Conclusion

This chapter led you on a short journey through the complex world of the legal system. Along the way, you visited several of its essential elements and doctrines: legal rights, the various types of law, separation of powers, federalism, judicial review, and more. To be sure, the trip was abbreviated and in some cases concepts were oversimplified in an effort to concisely cover a complex and expansive topic.

As you encounter myriad health policy and law topics and concepts that are complex in their own right, bearing in mind a few important details about law might help you achieve a greater measure of clarity. First, law's primary purpose is to organize and control an ever-changing, ever-expanding, ever-more-complex society, and it does this in part by regulating a variety of relationships among parties with oftentimes competing interests (e.g., individual citizen and government; patient and physician; beneficiary and public program or private insurance company; physician and managed care organization; individual and her family). This function of law helps explain why in the context of a specific relationship, one party has a legal right and the other party has a legal responsibility to refrain from acting in a way that infringes that legal right. It also helps explain why an individual can justifiably claim a particular legal right in the context of one specific relationship, but not in others (for example, a patient who believes that he has been treated negligently might have a legitimate legal claim against the physician who provided his care, but not against the hospital where the care was provided).

A second detail worth reflecting on periodically is that law is established, enforced, interpreted, and applied by human beings, and thus one must accept that law and the legal process comprise a certain amount of imperfection. This characteristic of law helps explain why statutes and regulations are sometimes difficult to understand, why laws are sometimes enforced sporadically or not at all, why reasonable jurists can disagree about the intended meaning of statutory and constitutional provisions, and why law is too often applied unevenly or inequitably.

Finally, bear in mind the fact that laws and the broader legal system are reflective of the beliefs and values of the society from which they flow. This *fait accompli*, perhaps more than anything else, provides an object lesson in the role of law across a wide range of subjects, including matters related to health care and public health.

References

Adelson, R. G. (2003). The enumerated powers of states. *Nevada Law Journal, 3*, 469–494.

Administrative Procedure Act of 1946. 5 U.S.C. § 551 et seq.

Baker T. E. (2004). Constitutional theory in a nutshell. *William and Mary Bill of Rights Journal, 13*(1), 57–123.

Brennan Center for Justice. (2015). *Judicial selection: Significant figures*. Retrieved from https://www.brennancenter.org/rethinking-judicial-selection/significant-figures

Brown v. Board of Ed., 347 U.S. 483 (1954).

Corwin, E. S. (1957). *The president: Office and powers, 1787–1957*. New York, NY: New York University Press.

de Tocqueville, A. (1835). *Democracy in America* (H. Reeve, Trans.). New York, NY: Vintage Books; 1990.

Dinan, J. (2018). *State constitutional policies: Governing by amendment in the United States*. Chicago, IL: University of Chicago Press.

Fallon, R. H., Jr. (1999). How to choose a constitutional theory. *California Law Review, 87*(3), 535–579.

Fay v. New York, 332 U.S. 261 (1947).

Friedman, L. M. (1964). Law and its language. *George Washington University Law Review, 33*, 563–579.

Friedman, L. M. (2002). *Law in America: A short history*. New York, NY: The Modern Library.

Garner, B. (2014). *Black's law dictionary* (10th ed.). Eagan, MN: Thomson West.

Gewirtz, P., & Golder, C. (2005, July 6). So who are the activists? *The New York Times*. Retrieved from https://www.nytimes.com/2005/07/06/opinion/so-who-are-the-activists.html

Gibbons v. Ogden, 25 U.S. (9 Wheat.) 1 (1824).

Holmes, O. W. (1899). Law in science and science in law. *Harvard Law Review, 12*(7), 443–463.

Jackson v. City of Joliet, 715 F.2d 1203 (7th Cir. 1983).

Korematsu v. United States, 323 U.S. 214 (1944).

Lazarus, E. (1999). *Closed chambers: The rise, fall, and future of the modern Supreme Court*. New York, NY: Penguin Books.

Mapp v. Ohio, 367 U.S. 643 (1961).

Marbury v. Madison, 1 Cranch (5 U.S.) 137 (1803).

Mayor v. Cooper, 73 U.S. 247 (1867).

McCullough v. Maryland, 17 U.S. (4 Wheat.) 316 (1819).

Mensah, G. A., Goodman, R. A., Zaza, S., Moulton, A. D., Kocher, P. L., Dietz, W. H., . . . Marks, J. S. (2004). Law as a tool for preventing chronic diseases: Expanding the spectrum of effective public health strategies. *Preventing Chronic Disease: Public Health Research, Practice, and Policy, 1*(2), 1–6.

Occupational Health and Safety Act of 1970. 29 U.S.C. § 655.

Plessy v. Ferguson, 163 U.S. 537 (1896).

Refo, P. L. (2004). The vanishing trial. *Litigation Online, 30*(2), 1–4.

Reich, C. A. (1964). The new property. *The Yale Law Journal, 73*(5), 733–787.

Smith, S. D. (1991). Reductionism in legal thought. *Columbia Law Review, 91*(1), 68–109.

Trump v. Hawaii, 138 S. Ct. 923 (2018).

U.S. Const. amend. XIV, § 1.

U.S. Const. art. III, § 2, clause 2.

U.S. Const. art. VI, para. 2.

Ziskin, L. Z., & Harris, D. A. (2007). State health policy for terrorism preparedness. *American Journal of Public Health, 97*(9), 1583–1588.

▶ Endnotes

a. Although the important role that language plays in law is not a topic we delve into in this chapter, it is, particularly for students new to the study of law, one worth thinking about. Words are the basic and most important tool of the law and of lawyers. Without them, how could one draft a law, legal brief, contract, or judicial opinion? Or engage in oral advocacy on behalf of a client, or conduct a negotiation? Or make one's wishes known with respect to personal matters near the end of life? As one renowned legal scholar puts it, "law is primarily a verbal art, its skills verbal skills" (Friedman, 1964, p. 567).

   Of course, one problem with the language of law is that it is full of legal jargon, making it difficult sometimes for laypeople to understand and apply to their own particular situation. For example, if government regulation is to be effective, the language used to do the regulating must be understandable to those being regulated. Another problem relates to the interpretation of words and terms used in the law, because both ambiguity (where language is reasonably capable of being understood in two or more ways) and vagueness (where language is not fairly capable of being understood) are common to laws, leaving those subject to them and those responsible for applying them unsure about their true meaning. Furthermore, as the preface to *Black's Law Dictionary*, under the heading "A Final Word of Caution," states:

   The language of the law is ever-changing as the courts, Congress, state legislatures, and administrative agencies continue to define, redefine and expand legal words and terms. Furthermore, many legal terms are subject to variations from state to state and again can differ under federal laws. (Garner, 2014, p. iv)

b. For an overview of the Bill of Rights in a public health context, see Gostin, L. O. (2000). *Public health law: Power, duty, restraint* (pp. 62–65). Berkeley, CA: University of California Press.

c. For a full description of the intertwined nature of administrative and health law, see Jost, T. S. (2004). Health law and administrative law: A marriage most convenient. *Saint Louis University Law Journal, 49*, 1–34.

d. For an in-depth discussion of the relationship between the APA and state administrative procedures, see Bonfield, A. E. (1986). The federal APA and state administrative law. *Virginia Law Review, 72*(2), 297–336.

e. For a full discussion of each of the government branches' role in health policymaking, see Gostin, L. O. (1995). The formulation of health policy by the three branches of government. In R. E. Bulger, E. M. Bobby, & H. V. Fineberg (Eds.), *Society's choices: Social and ethical decision making in biomedicine* (pp. 335–357). Washington, DC: National Academy Press.

f.   However, since the 1980s, the selection (by the president) and approval (by the U.S. Senate) process for federal judges has become highly politicized. There is an extensive body of literature on this topic, as evidenced by a simple Internet search.

g.   The potential implications of increasingly injecting politics into the court system are very troubling, and there is likewise extensive literature on this topic.

h.   The decision was written, as it turned out, by Chief Justice John Marshall—the very same person who, as Secretary of State, signed Marbury's commission. Marshall was sworn in as Chief Justice of the United States just before Jefferson took office.

i.   For a fuller discussion of how the equal protection standards of review operate, see Lazarus, 2004, pp. 293–294.

j.   This understanding is often put to the test, however, as seen in the national discussion of the right to abortion that takes place each time a new U.S. Supreme Court nominee is announced whose political stripes seem to clash with the prevailing law that abortion is a constitutionally protected right.

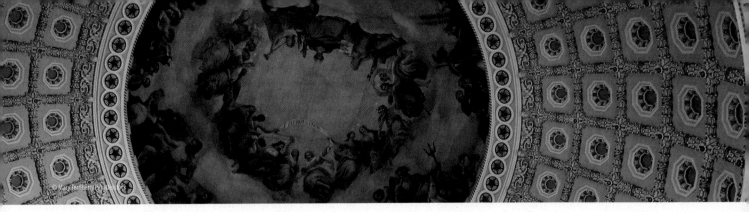
© Mary Terriberry/Shutterstock.

CHAPTER 4

Overview of the United States Healthcare System

LEARNING OBJECTIVES

By the end of this chapter you will be able to:

- Identify the key players who provide and finance health care in the United States
- Identify common characteristics of the uninsured
- Understand the effect of insurance on access to care and on health status
- Identify barriers to accessing health care
- Understand concerns regarding the quality of health care provided in the United States
- Describe differences in how health care is delivered in various countries

▶ Introduction

Coordinated. Efficient. Cost-effective. Goal oriented. These are words one might use to describe a well-functioning system. Unfortunately, they are not words that are often used when discussing how healthcare services are delivered in the United States. Unlike most other developed nations, the United States does not have a unified healthcare system. Even with the passage of the Patient Protection and Affordable Care Act of 2010 (ACA), the first major health reform law passed in this country in nearly 50 years, the United States will continue to provide healthcare services through a patchwork of public and private insurance plans; federal, state, and local governments; and institutions and individual providers who are often unconnected to one other.

The United States has never been accused of providing healthcare services in an efficient or cost-effective manner. On average, this country spends over twice as much on health care per person as other developed countries (Organization for Economic Cooperation and Development [OECD], 2017, p. 133). While the U.S. healthcare system does some things well, it ranks at or near the bottom on important health outcome measures such as life expectancy, infant mortality, and adult obesity rates (OECD, 2017, pp. 47–81). Even though the federal government establishes the nation's healthcare goals through initiatives such as *Healthy People 2020*, the lack of coordination within the healthcare system means that all parts of the system are not working together to achieve these goals (Office of Disease Prevention and Health Promotion, n.d.). The lack of a unified healthcare system makes it difficult to provide a straightforward overview of how healthcare services are delivered and financed. For example, the following are some of the various players in the provision and delivery of health care:

■ Educational institutions such as medical, dental, nursing, and physician assistant programs

■ Research organizations including private entities, public agencies, and nonprofit foundations

■ Private suppliers of goods and services such as hospital equipment manufacturers, home health agencies, and uniform suppliers

■ Private health insurance provided through employers, on the individual market, and through state health exchanges

■ Public health insurance programs such as Medicaid, Medicare, and TRICARE (the Department of Defense healthcare program for members of the uniformed services and their families)

■ Individual providers such as physicians, dentists, pharmacists, and physical therapists

■ Institutional providers such as hospitals, community health centers, and skilled nursing facilities

■ Private trade associations representing providers (e.g., the American Medical Association, which represents physicians), institutions (e.g., the National Association of Community Health Centers), and industries (e.g., PhRMA, which represents the pharmaceutical industry)

■ Private accreditation agencies that provide quality certifications to healthcare institutions

■ Consumers of healthcare goods and services

■ Local, state, and federal government agencies that have roles in delivering care, financing care, setting health policy, developing laws and regulations, and conducting and funding research

In the absence of a unified system or single government program to describe, it is easiest to understand the provision of U.S. health care through the concepts of finance (How do individuals pay for health care, and how are providers reimbursed for their services?), access (How do individuals access healthcare services, and what barriers to access exist?), and quality (What is the quality of healthcare services that are provided, and what can be done to improve the quality of care?). It is also helpful to consider the health system choices made by this country against those made by other developed countries. This chapter begins with a discussion of the concepts of finance, access, and quality and then turns to a comparative overview of how other countries have designed their healthcare systems.

▶ Healthcare Finance

In 2016, the United States spent $3.3 trillion on aggregate healthcare spending, the equivalent of $10,348 per person and 17.9% of the nation's gross domestic product (GDP) (**FIGURE 4-1**). This total represents a 4.3% increase over 2015 spending (Hartman, Martin, Espinosa, Catlin, & National Health Expenditures Accounts Team, 2018). Healthcare spending grew slowly during the Great Recession of 2007–2009 and the period

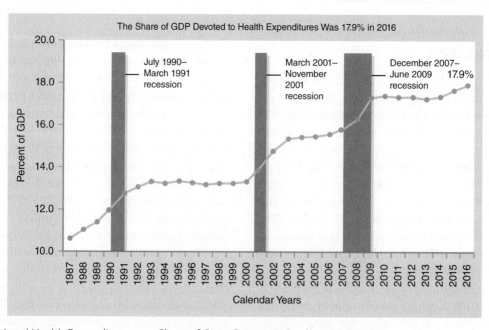

FIGURE 4-1 National Health Expenditures as a Share of Gross Domestic Product, 1987–2016

shortly thereafter. The implementation of the ACA led to 19 million newly insured individuals from 2014 to 2015. This reduction in the uninsured rate combined with strong prescription drug spending (due, in large part, to increased spending on a new drug for hepatitis C) resulted in robust spending growth in 2014 and 2015, though growth slowed in 2016. As shown in **FIGURE 4-2**, spending growth was due to higher medical prices and increased use of health services by newly insured individuals (Hartman et al., 2018).

National health expenditures are expected to average 5.6% growth from 2017 to 2026 and reach 19.7% of the GDP by 2026 (Cuckler et al., 2018). This growth is expected to be driven by an increase in prices for medical goods and services, and increases in Medicare and Medicaid spending due to the aging Baby Boomer population (Cuckler et al., 2018). Put differently, come 2026, one-fifth of the nation's economy will be consumed by healthcare spending. This is nothing short of staggering. As shown in **FIGURE 4-3**, the largest portion of national healthcare spending in 2016 was on hospital services, followed by physician and clinical services.

Health Insurance

Having health insurance reduces the risk of financial ruin when expensive health services are needed and often provides coverage for preventive services at low or no cost. As discussed in the upcoming section on healthcare access, individuals without health insurance must pay for services themselves, find services provided at no cost, or go without care. While most people in the United States have health insurance, one of the main goals of the ACA is to decrease the number of uninsured people.

The ACA includes a number of provisions designed to reduce the uninsured rate in this country. While these provisions, as well as the changes that have taken place since the ACA was signed into law, will be discussed in detail in the chapter on health reform, a brief overview is useful here. The ACA attempts to reduce the number of uninsured through three main strategies. First, the law includes mandates on individuals to purchase insurance and on (many) employers to provide insurance. Second, the law expands Medicaid, the federal–state program for the poor, to the poorest uninsured individuals across the country. Third, the ACA created state health insurance exchanges, which are aimed at individuals and small businesses that are not able to obtain affordable health insurance through other means.

When President Obama signed the ACA into law in 2010, the uninsured rate was 16.3%, or 49.9 million individuals (U.S. Census Bureau, 2011, pp. 22–23). The ACA was effective in reducing the uninsured rate; by 2016 it had dropped to 8.8%, or 28.1 million individuals (U.S. Census Bureau, 2017). A number of legal and policy developments since the

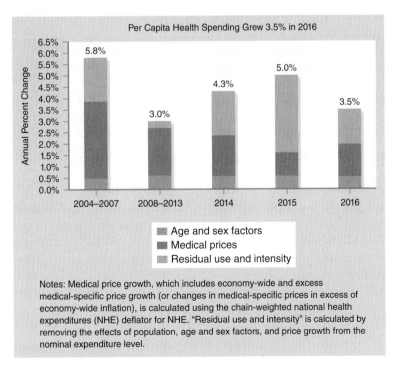

FIGURE 4-2 Factors Accounting for Growth in per Capita National Health Expenditures, Selected Calendar Years, 2004–2016

Source: Reproduced from: Centers for Medicare and Medicaid Services, Office of the Actuary. (n.d.). National Health Care Spending in 2016. Retrieved from https://www.cms.gov/Research-Statistics-Data-and-Systems/Statistics-Trends-and-Reports/NationalHealthExpendData/Downloads/NHE-Presentation-Slides.pdf

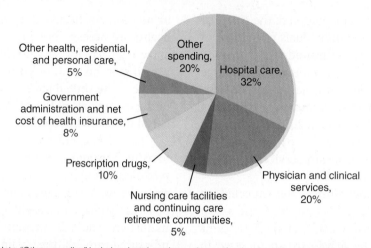

FIGURE 4-3 The Nation's Health Dollar, Calendar Year 2016: Where it Went

Note: "Other spending" includes dental services, other professional services, home health care, durable medical equipment, other nondurable medical products, government public health activities, and investment.

Source: Reproduced from: Centers for Medicare and Medicaid Services, Office of the Actuary. (n.d.). National Health Care Spending in 2016. Retrieved from https://www.cms.gov/Research-Statistics-Data-and-Systems/Statistics-Trends-and-Reports /NationalHealthExpendData/Downloads/NHE-Presentation-Slides.pdf

2016 election have reduced the ACA's effectiveness. As a result, the Congressional Budget Office (CBO) estimates that the number of individuals younger than 65 years without insurance will increase to 35 million (13%) by 2028 (CBO, 2018). According to the CBO, one of the main reasons for this increase is the 2018 repeal of the penalty associated with the individual mandate. The elimination of this penalty is projected to increase the uninsured rate by 4 million in 2019 and another 3 million by 2021. This is a result of individuals choosing not to purchase health insurance while they remain in good health, do not face a penalty for going without coverage, or cannot afford the higher premiums that are expected due to the repeal of the individual mandate penalty (CBO, 2018).

As shown in **FIGURE 4-4**, most people in the United States are privately insured and obtain their health insurance through their employer. Employer-sponsored insurance plans may be self-funded (meaning employers set aside funds to pay for their employees' health insurance claims instead of paying a premium to a health insurance carrier) or fully insured (meaning employers pay a premium to a private health insurance company to administer employees' plans and pay the healthcare claims of the employees). Another significant portion of the population is publicly insured through Medicaid, the Children's Health Insurance Program (CHIP), Medicare, the Veteran's Administration, and the Department of Defense. Public programs are funded and run by federal and/or state government agencies, depending on the program.

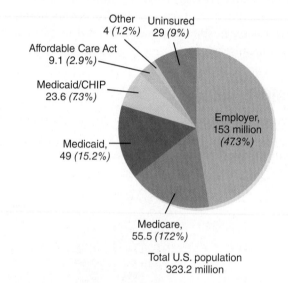

FIGURE 4-4 Healthcare Coverage in the United States, March 2016

Source: Hiltzik, M. (2016, March 29). Where America gets its health coverage: Everything you wanted to know in one handy chart. *L.A. Times.* Retrieved June 11, 2018 from http://www.latimes.com/business/hiltzik/la-fi-hiltzik-gaba-20160329-snap-htmlstory.html

FIGURE 4-5 illustrates how health insurers act as an intermediary between consumers (sometimes referred to as "insureds") and providers (which refers to both individual providers, such as physicians or nurses, and institutions, such as hospitals and community health centers). The specifics regarding eligibility for a particular insurance plan, choice of plans, how much a plan costs to enroll in or use, what benefits are covered, and how much providers are reimbursed vary by plan or government program. In some circumstances, providers may accept insurance from only a single plan, but often providers will accept patients from a variety of plans.

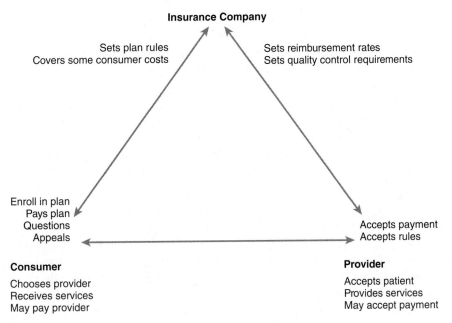

Insurance Company

Sets plan rules
Covers some consumer costs

Sets reimbursement rates
Sets quality control requirements

Enroll in plan
Pays plan
Questions
Appeals

Accepts payment
Accepts rules

Consumer

Chooses provider
Receives services
May pay provider

Provider

Accepts patient
Provides services
May accept payment

FIGURE 4-5 Insurance Company–Consumer–Provider Interaction

Consumers interact with health insurance companies or government programs by enrolling into an insurance plan by which they are accepted (in the case of private plans) or for which they are eligible (in the case of public programs), providing payments to the insurance plan for being enrolled (either directly or through a payroll deduction), choosing which provider to see based on plan restrictions or incentives, and working with the plan if they have questions or complaints. Providers that agree to be part of a plan's "network" (i.e., the group of providers who will see patients insured by the plan) are reimbursed a contractually agreed-upon amount from the insurance company and/or the patient for providing services covered under the plan, may accept consumers who are enrolled in the plan, may be subject to plan quality-control measures, and will participate as necessary in plan appeals processes.

Direct Services Programs

In addition to providing publicly funded health insurance to certain populations through programs such as Medicare and Medicaid, federal, state, and local governments also fund numerous programs that directly provide healthcare services to vulnerable populations. Many of these programs also receive private funding and donations to support their operations. Direct service programs generally exist to fill gaps in the private healthcare delivery system. Examples of these types of programs include the following:

- **Federally qualified health centers (FQHCs):** These centers are located in medically underserved areas and provide primary care services to individuals on a sliding fee scale (meaning that how much one pays for services depends on the individual's income level). While anyone may use an FQHC, the health center patient population is made up of mostly uninsured and publicly insured patients. Funding for health centers usually comes from the federal and state governments, and sometimes from local governments and private donations.

- **HIV/AIDS services:** The Ryan White HIV/AIDS Program works with states, cities, and local organizations to provide services to patients with human immunodeficiency virus (HIV) or acquired immunodeficiency syndrome (AIDS) who do not have health insurance coverage or the financial resources to pay for needed care. The program is federally funded and provides grants to state agencies that deliver care to patients. The Ryan White program includes the state AIDS Drug Assistance Program (ADAP), which provides medications to low-income individuals with HIV. A supplementary ADAP for high-need states includes federal funding and a state matching requirement. States often supplement federal funding with state-funded HIV prevention and treatment programs. Some local public health departments provide HIV testing and counseling services and help individuals access treatment. Many programs also accept private donations.

■ **Family planning services:** Title X of the Public Health Service Act provides federal funding for family planning services offered to women who do not qualify for Medicaid, maintains family planning centers, and establishes standards for providing family planning services (although federal dollars may not be used to support abortion services except in the case of rape, incest, or danger to the life of the pregnant woman). In addition, states also fund family planning services. Services provided vary by state but may include contraception, cervical cancer screening, tubal sterilization, sexually transmitted disease screening, HIV testing, and abstinence counseling. State laws vary on the use of state funds for abortion services. Local health departments may also offer some of these services as well as help people access family planning services from private providers. Private donations provide revenue to many family planning clinics.

▶ Healthcare Access

Access to care refers to the ability to obtain needed health services. There are a variety of factors that can hinder access to care. Barriers may exist if individuals are underinsured and cannot afford the cost sharing required by their health insurance policy, if needed services are not covered by health insurance, if providers will not take a particular insurance plan, or if providers are not available in certain geographic areas. Access problems are exacerbated by provider shortages, especially in primary care fields (e.g., internal medicine and pediatrics). Many areas of the country already experience workforce shortages, and the influx of newly insured individuals as a result of health reform will make this problem even more pronounced in the years to come.

Of course, one important factor relating to access is lack of health insurance. Individuals without health insurance have to pay more for comparable services because they do not have the advantage of sharing costs as part of a pool of consumers. Because many individuals without health insurance are low-income, they may be unable to pay for the cost of needed care, and providers are often unwilling to accept uninsured patients because of the risk of not being paid for their services. Some providers, referred to as "safety net" providers, focus on providing care to uninsured patients, but gaining access to needed care remains a significant issue for this population.

As noted previously, many changes that took place in 2014 as part of ACA implementation are intended to reduce the number of uninsured people. Even so, it is important to understand the healthcare problems faced by the uninsured due to the uncertainty surrounding the ACA's future. Furthermore, millions would remain uninsured even with a fully implemented ACA. The ACA did not help almost half the uninsured in 2017 because their state did not expand Medicaid, their income was too high to allow them to obtain subsidies, or they were ineligible for insurance or assistance due to immigration restrictions (Foutz, Damico, Squires, & Garfield, 2017). Many of those who could be assisted by the ACA's provisions also remain uninsured. A 2016 survey conducted by the Commonwealth Fund found that only about half (52%) of the uninsured knew they could look for coverage in a state marketplace, and two-thirds of uninsured adults who knew about state exchanges did not think they could find affordable coverage (Commonwealth Fund, n.d.).

The Uninsured

Characteristics of the Uninsured

There are many myths relating to the uninsured. It is often assumed that the uninsured do not work or simply choose not to purchase health insurance even though it is available and affordable. Although this assumption may be true in some cases, in most instances it is not. Furthermore, many people believe that all employers offer insurance or that those individuals without private insurance are always eligible for public programs. As you will see, these and other assumptions are also false.

Income Level While the poor saw significant gains in insurance coverage under the ACA, the primary reason people do not have health insurance is still financial—available coverage is simply too expensive (**FIGURES 4-6** and **4-7**). There was an increase of 17 million Medicaid and CHIP enrollees from September 2013 to June 2017, accounting for much of the decrease in the uninsured rate among the poor. Not surprisingly, between 2013 and 2016, the uninsured rate for nonelderly adults dropped more significantly in states that expanded Medicaid (9.2% decrease) than in states that did not (4.8% decrease) (Foutz et al., 2017). In addition, another 10 million individuals received premium subsidies to purchase health insurance in a state exchange. These subsidies are available to individuals whose income is between 100% and 400% of the federal poverty level (FPL) ($20,160 to $80,640 for a family of three in 2016) (Foutz et al., 2017).

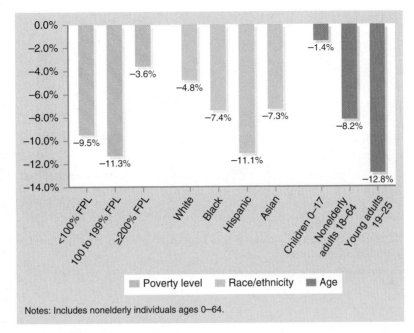

FIGURE 4-6 Percentage Point Change in Uninsured Rate Among the Nonelderly Population by Selected Characteristics, 2013–2016

Source: Foutz et al., 2017, Figure 4; Kaiser Family Foundation analysis of the 2013 and 2016 National Health Interview Survey.

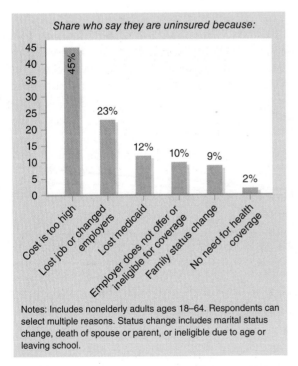

FIGURE 4-7 Reasons for Being Uninsured Among Uninsured Nonelderly Adults, 2016

Source: Kaiser Family Foundation. (n.d.). Key facts about the uninsured population. Retrieved from https://www.kff.org /uninsured/fact-sheet/key-facts-about-the-uninsured-population/

Race, Ethnicity, and Immigrant Status

Prior to the ACA, the uninsured rate was much higher for Hispanics (30.7%) and Blacks (20.8%) than for non-Hispanic Whites (11.7%) (U.S. Census Bureau, 2011, pp. 22–23). As shown in Figure 4-6 and **FIGURE 4-8**, minority populations experienced significant coverage gains in the early years of the ACA, although Whites continued to have the lowest uninsured rate (U.S. Census Bureau, 2017). These differences are due to a variety of factors, such as language barriers, income level, work status, state of residence, and immigration status (Foutz et al., 2017).

In 2016, noncitizens were three times as likely to be uninsured as were citizens (Foutz et al., 2017). Restrictive eligibility rules pertaining to immigrants in public programs make it difficult for non-natives to obtain public coverage. While legal immigrants may obtain subsidies to assist with purchasing health insurance through the state exchanges under the ACA, undocumented immigrants are not eligible for federal subsidies and are prohibited from purchasing insurance through an exchange, even at full cost.

Employment Status While over half (57%) of employers offered health insurance coverage in 2013, this number has declined significantly since 66% of employers provided this benefit in 1999 (Foutz et al., 2017). Most of the decrease is due to small businesses dropping coverage. As shown in **FIGURE 4-9**, premium costs nearly doubled while wages and inflation grew at a much slower pace, meaning coverage became less affordable even for those employees who were offered coverage (Foutz et al., 2017). While the ACA includes an employer mandate that requires medium and large employers

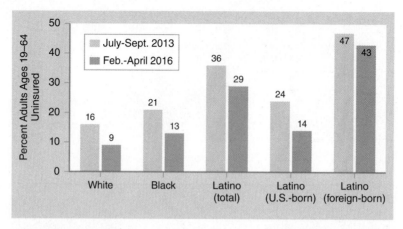

FIGURE 4-8 After 3 Years of the ACA, Uninsured Rates for Blacks, Latinos, and Whites Have Declined Significantly, but Large Numbers of Immigrant Latinos Remain Uninsured

Source: Reproduced from Foutz et al., 2017; The Commonwealth Fund Affordable Care Act Tracking Surveys. July–September 2015 and February–April 2016.

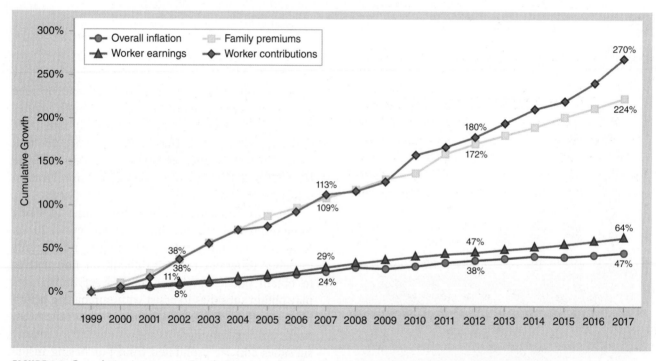

FIGURE 4-9 Cumulative Increase in Family Premiums, Worker Contribution to Premiums, and Worker Earnings, 1999–2017

Source: Kaiser/HRET Survey of Employer-Sponsored Health Benefits, 1999-2017; Bureau of Labor Statistics, Consumer Price Index, U.S. City Average of Annual Inflation (April to April), 1999-2017; Bureau of Labor Statistics, Seasonally Adjusted Data from the Current Employment Statistics Survey, 1999-2017 (April to April).

(those with over 50 full-time-equivalent employees) to provide coverage, the percentage of employers offering health insurance coverage, the number of employees eligible for coverage, and the take-up rate by employees choosing to purchase coverage did not change significantly after the ACA was implemented (Foutz et al., 2017). This is not surprising since medium and large businesses were the most likely to offer coverage before the ACA and concerns about affordability remain the primary obstacle for individuals obtaining insurance.

As shown in **FIGURE 4-10**, most of the uninsured work or are in families with at least one full-time worker, and many more have part-time workers in the family. In 2017, 74% of nonelderly uninsured workers were not offered health insurance by their employer, and over 40% of uninsured workers were employed by small businesses who were not subject to the ACA's employer mandate (Foutz et al., 2017). Most uninsured workers are low-income and/or work in blue-collar fields such as agriculture, construction, and the service industry.

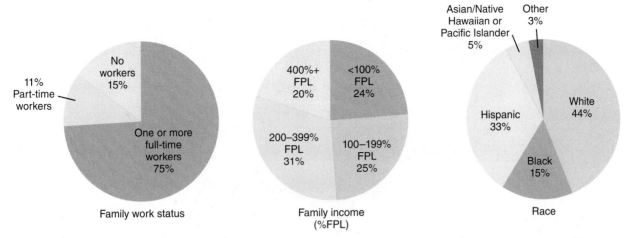

Total = 27.5 Million Nonelderly Uninsured

FIGURE 4-10 Characteristics of the Nonelderly Uninsured, 2016

Notes: Includes nonelderly individuals ages 0–64. The U.S. Census Bureau's poverty threshold for a family with two adults and one child was $19,318 in 2016. Data may not total 100% due to rounding. Persons of Hispanic origin may be of any race; all other race/ethnicity groups are non-Hispanic.

Source: Kaiser Family Foundation analysis of the March 2017 Current Population Survey, Annual Social and Economic Supplement.

Age Because Medicaid and CHIP provide extensive coverage to low-income children and Medicare covers older adults, working-age adults between 19 and 64 years are the age group most likely to be uninsured. In 2016, 98.8% of adults older than 65 years and 94.6% of children younger than 19 years were insured, compared to 87.9% of working-age adults (U.S. Census Bureau, 2017). Even though many young adults (ages 26–34 years) gained insurance under the ACA, 15.7% of them were still uninsured in 2016.

As young adults transition from school to the workforce, they may become ineligible for their family's coverage for the first time, may have entry-level jobs earning too little income to afford a policy, or may work for an employer that does not offer health insurance. The ACA addresses part of this problem by requiring insurers to cover dependents (someone who relies on the primary insured for support) until age 26 years. Although some young adults do not consider health insurance a priority expense because they are relatively healthy, studies have shown that cost is the primary determinant of whether people in this age bracket obtain coverage (Institute of Medicine [IOM], 2001a, pp. 73–74). While adults 55 to 64 years of age are more likely to be insured than are younger adults, the uninsured who fall into this age group are a cause for concern because they are medically high risk and often have declining incomes (IOM, 2001a, p. 72). The disability provisions of Medicaid and Medicare and the availability of employer-based insurance keep the number of uninsured in this group relatively small, which is important because it is very expensive for individuals in this demographic to purchase individual insurance policies in the private market.

Education Level Education level is also an important factor in insurance status because it is easier, for example, for college graduates to earn higher incomes and obtain jobs that provide affordable employment-based insurance as compared to less-educated individuals (IOM, 2001a, p. 74). The higher the education level, the more likely one is to be insured. In 2016, the uninsured rate was 6.8% for working adults with a bachelor's degree, compared to 15.2% for high school graduates and 27.3% for those without a high school diploma (U.S. Census Bureau, 2017).

Geography As shown in **FIGURE 4-11**, residents of the South and West are more likely to be uninsured than are residents of the North and Midwest. There are variations in the uninsured rate from state to state. These differences are based on numerous factors, including racial/ethnic composition, other population characteristics, public program eligibility, and employment rates and sectors (Kaiser Family Foundation (KFF) 2017). This trend is likely to continue, at least in the short run, with many states in the South opting not to expand Medicaid coverage under the ACA.

Uninsurance is a particular problem among the 16% of the population who live in rural areas. They are more likely to be poorer, unemployed, or employed in blue-collar jobs and are less likely to have access to employer coverage than are their urban counterparts (Newkirk & Damico, 2014). In addition, rural residents have relatively high healthcare needs—they tend to be older, poorer, and less healthy than urban residents—and there is often a provider shortage in these areas. Because many rural residents live in states that have not chosen to expand Medicaid and also have incomes

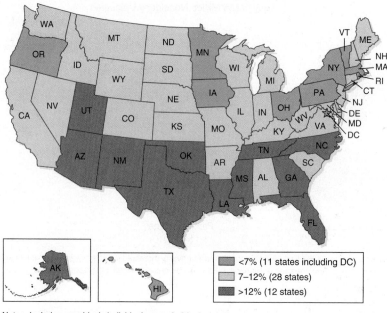

Notes: Includes nonelduals individuals ages 0–64.

FIGURE 4-11 Uninsured Rates Among the Nonelderly by State, 2016

Source: Kaiser Family Foundation analysis of the March 2017 Current Population Survey, Annual Social and Economic Supplement.

BOX 4-1 Discussion Questions

From a policy perspective, are the characteristics just described interrelated, or should they be addressed separately? If you are trying to reduce the number of uninsured, do you believe the focus should be on altering insurance programs or changing the effect of having one or more of these characteristics? Whose responsibility is it to reduce the number of uninsured? Government? The private sector? Individuals?

BOX 4-2 Discussion Questions

The ACA made it a priority to reduce the number of uninsured. At what point, if any, should the government step in to provide individuals with assistance to purchase insurance coverage? Do you think such assistance should be a federal or a state responsibility?

Source: Reproduced from Centers for Disease Control and Prevention, *MMWR* 1996;45: 526–528.

---

too low to qualify for premium subsidies, insurance is more likely to be unaffordable for them than for urban residents (Newkirk & Damico, 2014).

The Importance of Health Insurance Coverage to Health Status

Having health insurance provides tangible health benefits. For a variety of reasons discussed in this section,

having health insurance increases access to care and positively affects health outcomes. Conversely, the uninsured, who do not enjoy the benefits of health insurance, are more likely to experience adverse health events and a diminished health-related quality of life and are less likely to receive care in appropriate settings or receive the professionally accepted standard of care (Foutz et al., 2017).

Health insurance is an important factor in whether someone has a "medical home," or consistent source of care. Having a consistent source of care is positively associated with better and timelier access to care, better chronic disease management, fewer emergency department (ED) visits, fewer lawsuits against EDs, and increased cancer screenings for women (Foutz et al., 2017; Lambrew, DeFriese, Carey, Ricketts, & Biddle, 1996; Starfield & Shi, 2004). Unfortunately, the uninsured are much less likely to have a usual source of care than are insured individuals (**FIGURE 4-12**).

The uninsured are also less likely to follow treatment recommendations and more likely to forgo care due to concerns about cost (Foutz et al., 2017). In addition, the uninsured are less likely to receive preventive care and appropriate routine care for chronic conditions (Foutz et al., 2017). One result of these conditions is that children without insurance are more likely to have developmental delays, often leading to difficulties in education and employment. Also, quality of life may be lower for the uninsured due to their lower health status and anxiety about both monetary and medical problems.

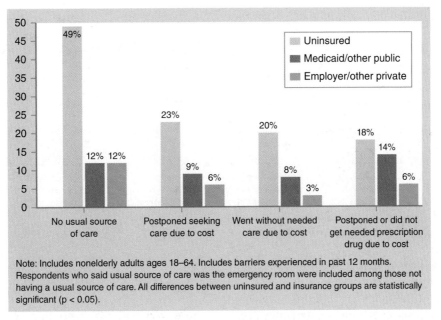

FIGURE 4-12 Barriers to Health Care Among Nonelderly Adults by Insurance Status, 2016

Source: Foutz et al., 2017; Kaiser Family Foundation analysis of the 2016 National Health Interview Survey.

Because the uninsured are less likely to obtain preventive care or treatment for specific conditions, they have a higher mortality rate overall, have a higher in-hospital mortality rate, and are more likely to be hospitalized for avoidable health problems (Foutz et al., 2017). Of course, without regular access to care, it is less likely that a disease will be detected early when treatment may be cheaper and more effective. For example, uninsured cancer patients are diagnosed at later stages of the disease and die earlier than insured cancer patients.

Ways to Assess the Cost of Being Uninsured

There are several ways to think about the costs of being uninsured. These costs include the health status costs to the uninsured individual, as discussed previously; financial cost to the uninsured individual; financial cost to state and federal governments and to private insurers; financial cost to providers; productivity costs from lost work time due to illness; costs to other public priorities that cannot be funded because of the resources spent on providing care to the uninsured; and costs to the health status and patient satisfaction of *insured* individuals.

The financial burden of being uninsured is significant. Although on average the uninsured spend fewer dollars on health care than the insured, those without insurance spend a greater proportion of their overall income on medical needs. Furthermore, when the uninsured receive care, it is often more expensive because the uninsured are not receiving care as

part of an insurance pool with leverage to negotiate lower rates from providers. In fact, the uninsured are charged rates two to four times higher than the rates paid by insurance companies or public programs (Foutz et al., 2017). The uninsured are less likely to be able to pay for healthcare needs because the average uninsured household does not have net assets and half of the uninsured living under the 200% poverty level have no savings (Foutz et al., 2017). Not surprisingly, the uninsured are much more likely to be concerned about being able to pay their medical bills than are their insured counterparts (**FIGURE 4-13**).

Costs of medical care provided by, but not fully reimbursed to, health professionals are referred to as uncompensated care costs. In 2013, it was estimated that uncompensated care costs surpassed $84 billion in the United States, with federal, state, and local spending covering most of the tab, primarily through "disproportionate share" (DSH) payments to hospitals that serve many uninsured individuals and Medicaid beneficiaries (Foutz et al., 2017). Under the ACA, however, DSH payments are set to be reduced drastically—a $43 billion reduction between 2018 and 2025 (Foutz et al., 2017). Although hospitals provide about 60% of all uncompensated care services and receive significant government assistance, most of the uncompensated care provided by nonhospital physicians is not subsidized (Foutz et al., 2017). Every dollar spent by providers, governments, and communities to cover uncompensated care costs is a dollar that is not spent on another public need. There are a variety of high-cost public health needs, such as battling infectious

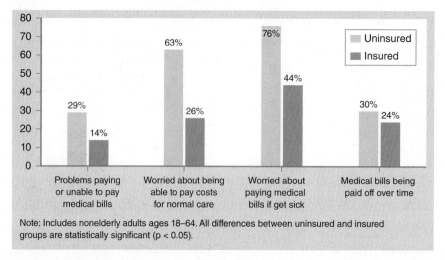

FIGURE 4-13 Problems Paying Medical Bills by Insurance Status, 2016

Source: Foutz et al., 2017; Kaiser Family Foundation analysis of the 2016 National Health Interview Survey.

diseases like tuberculosis, engaging in emergency preparedness planning, and promoting healthy behaviors. Public and private funds used to cover uncompensated care, especially when the care is more expensive than necessary because of the lack of preventive care or early interventions, are resources that are no longer available to meet the country's other health needs.

An additional cost associated with the uninsured is the cost of lower productivity. This cost refers to the reduced productivity in the workforce stemming from the lower health status associated with being uninsured. Productivity may be reduced when workers are absent or when they are not functioning at their highest level due to illness. In addition, several studies show that providing health insurance helps employers recruit better employees and that workers with health insurance are less likely to change jobs, reducing the costs of hiring and training new employees (Families USA, 2005).

Finally, there is a "spillover" effect of uninsurance for insured individuals. In communities with high rates of uninsured, even *insured* individuals are less likely to have a usual source of care, schedule an office visit, be satisfied with the quality of care they receive, and obtain needed care (Gresenz & Escarce, 2011; Pauly & Pagán, 2007). This spillover occurs because providers in communities with high uninsured rates may earn less revenue relative to costs. Insured individuals may suffer if subsidies are not available to providers to allow for higher revenue or if government spending on subsidies for the uninsured crowd out spending on services that might benefit the insured (Pauly & Pagán, 2007). In addition, physicians in communities with high uninsurance rates may choose to provide fewer types of services or fewer office hours due to profitability concerns. Finally, the insured may suffer if their provider treats them the same as

uninsured patients, who may demand and receive fewer services or lower-quality services from their providers (Gresenz & Escarce, 2011).

The Underinsured

While there are disagreements about how to measure the underinsured, in general being underinsured means individuals do not have the financial means to cover the gap between what their insurance coverage pays for and the total cost of their medical bills. As a result, they spend a high proportion of their income on healthcare services. A July 2014 survey found that 23% (31 million) of adults ages 19 to 64 years were underinsured (Collins, Rasmussen, Beutel, & Doty, 2015). Of particular concern are the 45% of underinsured adults younger than 65 years who are on Medicare, because they were the sickest population in the survey. Ninety-one percent of them are in fair or poor health or are disabled, and they are the second-poorest population after Medicaid beneficiaries (Collins et al., 2015).

The underinsured problem is exacerbated during a recession when more individuals cannot afford to pay their deductibles and co-payments. Insurance status is clearly linked to the decision to delay care due to cost. In the 2014 survey, 57% of uninsured individuals and 44% of underinsured respondents reported avoiding care due to cost, compared to 23% of insured individuals (Collins et al., 2015). In addition, over half (51%) of underinsured adults indicated they had problems paying medical bills or were currently paying off medical debt, which is twice the rate of other insured adults who are not underinsured (Collins et al., 2015). As a result, everyone ends up paying for the underinsured. Providers attempt to shift the cost associated with the underinsured and uninsured to others who can afford to pay, including the government and insured individuals. Institutions such as hospitals may try to negotiate higher reimbursement for their services, which leads insurers to charge higher premiums to their clients to cover the additional costs.

Insurance Coverage Limitations

Even individuals with insurance coverage may face healthcare access problems due to coverage limitations. These limitations could include high levels of cost sharing, reimbursement and visit caps for specific services, and service exclusions. (Another problem—annual and lifetime dollar limits on coverage—was eliminated by the ACA.)

Cost Sharing

A typical insurance plan includes premiums, deductibles, and co-payments (the latter can also be designed as co-insurance). A premium is an annual cost, typically charged monthly, for enrolling in a plan. For those with health insurance through their employer, the premium is often split between employer and employee. The average annual premium for a single coverage was $6,690 in 2017, although individuals in high-deductible plans averaged somewhat less in premiums ($6,024) (KFF & Health Research Educational Trust [HRET], 2017). Figure 4-9 and **FIGURE 4-14** show the increase in monthly premiums over the last decade and also how much faster premiums have

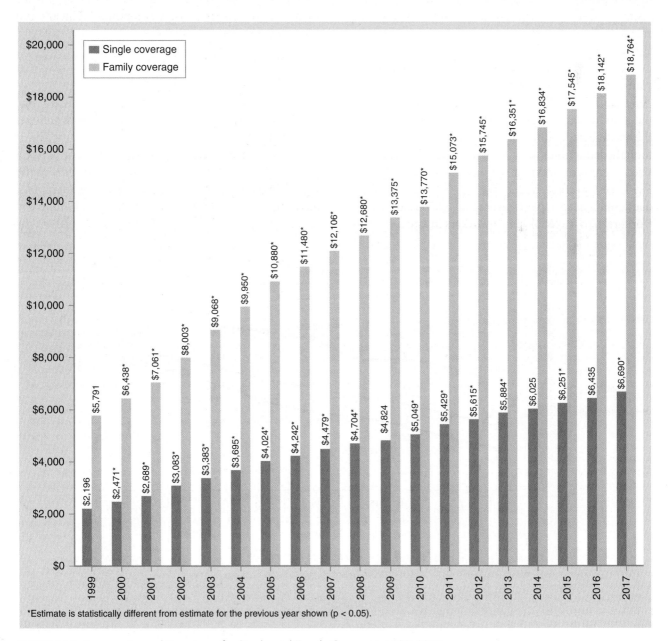

*Estimate is statistically different from estimate for the previous year shown ($p < 0.05$).

FIGURE 4-14 Average Annual Premiums for Single and Family Coverage, 1999–2017

Source: Kaiser/HRET Survey of Employer-Sponsored Health Benefits, 1999–2017.

risen relative to wages and inflation. A deductible is an amount the insured pays out-of-pocket before the insurance plan assists with the costs of healthcare services. There may be an annual deductible for the plan overall or separate deductibles for different types of services covered by the plan, such as inpatient care, outpatient care, and prescription drug coverage. Co-payments refer to a specific dollar amount that patients pay when they receive services or drugs. For example, one might have a $15 co-payment to see a primary care provider for an office visit. Co-insurance refers to a percentage of service cost that patients pay when they receive services or drugs. For example, an insured might have a 20% co-insurance requirement to see a primary care provider for an office visit. If the visit cost $150, a 20% co-insurance requirement would cost $30. Co-payment and co-insurance amounts may vary depending on the service received.

Cost-sharing requirements can vary widely by plan and plan type. Some plans do not have general deductibles, and for those with general deductibles, the amount varies significantly. For example, in 2017 the average deductible for a single worker was $1,505, though deductibles vary by plan type and employer size. Preferred provider organizations (PPOs) had the lowest average deductible ($1,046), while high-deductible health plans averaged $2,304 for single workers. Coverage for single workers in small firms is much higher ($1,594) than it is for those in large firms ($856) (KFF & HRET, 2017). A significant number of plans have deductibles of $1,000 or more (**FIGURE 4-15**).

Variation also exists for service-specific costs. It is rare for private plans to have separate deductibles for hospital admissions, outpatient surgery, or ED visits, but patients generally have cost-sharing arrangements for these services. For example, in private plans the average co-payment for ED visits is $180 and the average co-payment for outpatient surgery is $231 (KFF & HRET, 2017). Medicare, on the other hand, charged a $1,340 deductible for the first 60 days of hospitalization in 2018. Medicare beneficiaries do not pay a per diem for the first 60 days in a hospital, but they then pay $335 per day for the next 3 months. This fee increases for longer stays (Centers for Medicare and Medicaid Services, 2017).

Reimbursement and Visit Caps

Insurance plans may limit the amount they will reimburse for a specific service during the year, with patients responsible for costs that exceed dollar amount limits. In addition, plans may limit the number of times a patient may see a certain type of provider during the year. Visit caps vary by insurance plan. For example, a plan might limit a member to 90 physical therapy visits per year per injury, or to 20 visits per calendar year

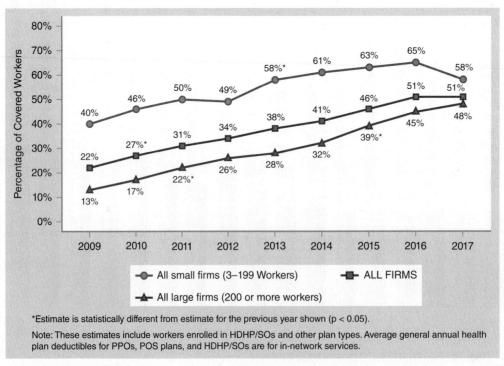

FIGURE 4-15 Percentage of Covered Workers Enrolled in a Plan With a General Annual Deductible of $1,000 or More for Single Coverage, by Firm Size, 2009–2017

Source: "2017 Employer Health Benefits Survey," 2017.

for acupuncture. Once a patient reaches these limits, the insurance plan will not cover additional visits and the patient would have to pay the entire cost of a visit out-of-pocket.

Service Exclusions

Health insurance plans may also partially or fully exclude certain types of services from coverage altogether. For example, a plan might cover high-dose chemotherapy associated with bone marrow transplants for only specified organ and tissue transplants and home health services only if certain conditions are met. Examples of services not covered at all by a plan include nonrigid orthopedic or prosthetic devices such as wigs or elastic stockings, eyeglasses, hearing aids, exercise programs, assisted reproductive technology, or physical exams for obtaining or continuing employment.

Coverage for abortion and family planning services is also limited in many instances. Federal funds may be used for abortion services only in cases of rape or incest or to save the life of the pregnant woman. The ACA does not include abortion services as part of its essential health benefits package, and any coverage of abortion services must be paid with private dollars, not with federal subsidies. As of June 2018, 11 states have enacted laws that restrict abortion coverage in all private plans in the state, 25 states restrict abortion coverage in private plans offered through their exchange, and 21 states restrict abortion coverage in public employee plans (Guttmacher Institute, n.d., 2018a).

Regarding contraceptive coverage, the ACA requires most health insurance plans to cover all contraceptive methods approved by the Food and Drug Administration and related counseling services without cost-sharing. Federal regulations exempt religious organizations from having to provide contraceptive coverage and make an accommodation for certain other employers with religious objections to avoid paying for or arranging contraceptive coverage, while still allowing employees to obtain coverage through their health insurance plan (Guttmacher Institute, 2018b). In October 2017, the Trump administration issued regulations that expand the ability of organizations to refuse to provide contraceptive coverage due to religious or moral objections, but these regulations are, at the time of this writing, blocked by court rulings. Due to concerns that federal guarantees for contraceptive coverage may be limited in the future, many states have passed laws protecting coverage. As of June 2018, 29 states require insurance plans to cover the full range of contraceptive drugs, 9 states prohibit cost-sharing for contraceptives, and 5 states prohibit other restrictions and delays by insurers. At the same time, 21 states exempt select employers and insurers from providing contraceptive coverage based on religious objections (Guttmacher Institute, 2018b). Given the litigation relating to contraceptive coverage requirements and exemptions/accommodations, it is not yet clear what requirements, if any, plans will have to follow regarding contraceptive coverage in the future.

Safety Net Providers

Securing access to care can be difficult for those without comprehensive private insurance. For the uninsured, the high cost of care is often a deterrent to seeking care. For those with public coverage, it is often difficult to find a provider willing to accept their insurance due to the low reimbursement rates and administrative burdens associated with participating in these programs. For these patients and the underinsured, the "healthcare safety net" exists.

The healthcare safety net refers to providers who serve disproportionately high numbers of uninsured, underinsured, and publicly insured patients. Although there is no formal designation indicating that one is a safety net provider, the Health and Medicine Division (HMD) of the National Academy of Sciences (formerly the Institute of Medicine [IOM]) defines the healthcare safety net as "those providers that organize and deliver a significant level of health care and other related services to uninsured, Medicaid, and other vulnerable populations" (IOM, 2000a, p. 21). "Core" safety net providers are those who serve vulnerable populations and have a policy of providing services regardless of patients' ability to pay. Some safety net providers have a legal requirement to provide care to the underserved, while others do so as a matter of principle (IOM, 2000a, p. 21).

Who are safety net providers? It is a difficult question to answer because there is no true safety net "system." Safety net providers can be anyone or any entity providing health care to the uninsured and other vulnerable populations, whether community or teaching hospitals, private health professionals, school-based health clinics, or others. Those providers that fit the narrower definition of "core" safety net providers include some public and private hospitals, community health centers, family planning clinics, and public health agencies that have a mission to provide access to care for vulnerable populations. Safety net provider patient loads are mostly composed of people who are poor, on Medicaid, or uninsured, and are members of racial and ethnic minority groups. For example, in 2016, 92% of federally qualified community health center (FQHC) patients had incomes at or below 200% FPL, 72% were on Medicaid or uninsured, 23% were African American, and 35% were Hispanic/Latino (National Association of Community Health Centers [NACHC], 2018a). Of the America's Essential Hospitals (formerly National Association of Public Hospitals and Health Systems) member hospital inpatient discharges, in 2016, about 46% were covered by Medicaid or uninsured, and 68% were racial or ethnic minorities (America's Essential Hospitals, 2018).

FQHCs provide comprehensive primary medical care services, culturally sensitive care, and enabling services such as transportation, outreach, and translation that make it easier for patients to access services. Many health centers also provide dental, mental health, and pharmacy services. Because health centers are not focused on specialty care, public hospitals are often the sole source of specialty care for uninsured and underserved populations (Makaroun et al., 2017). In addition, public hospitals provide traditional healthcare services, diagnostic services, outpatient pharmacies, and highly specialized trauma care, burn care, and emergency services (America's Essential Hospitals, 2018). Although not all local government health departments provide direct care, many do. Local health departments often specialize in caring for specific populations, such as individuals with HIV or drug dependency, as compared to public hospitals and health centers, which provide a wider range of services (IOM, 2000a, pp. 63–65).

Safety net providers receive funding from a variety of sources, but they often struggle financially. Medicaid is the single largest funding stream for health centers, accounting for 43% of their revenue (NACHC, 2018b). Due to low Medicaid reimbursement, Medicaid revenue accounts for only 80% of the cost of providing care to Medicaid patients served by health centers (NACHC, 2018a). Federal grants to health centers are intended to cover the cost of caring for the uninsured; however, this grant funding has not kept pace with the cost of provided care. Due to low federal reimbursement, health centers incurred a $1 billion gap in the cost of care for treating the uninsured in 2016 (NACHC, 2018a). In addition, payment from private insurance is unreliable due to the high-cost-sharing plans held by many privately insured, low-income individuals. Furthermore, Medicare payments to health centers are capped under federal law at an amount that does not match the growth in healthcare spending.

Public hospitals face a similarly difficult economic picture. Many public hospital services are not fully reimbursed because payments made by individuals or insurers do not match the cost of care. In 2016, Essential Hospitals members provided almost $5.5 billion in uncompensated care, which equals almost 14% of all the uncompensated care provided nationally (America's Essential Hospitals, 2018). Like health centers, public hospitals receive funds to cover low-income patients, including Medicaid DSH payments, state and local subsidies, and other revenues such as sales tax and tobacco settlement funds. In 2016, Essential Hospitals had an average aggregate operating margin of 4%, compared to 7.8% for all U.S. hospitals. Without DSH payments, Essential Hospitals' aggregate operating margin would dip to –1.4% (America's Essential Hospitals, 2018). Thus, the reduction in DSH payments that occurred as part of health reform is particularly concerning for safety net hospitals.

For all the positive work accomplished by safety net providers, they cannot solve all healthcare problems for vulnerable populations. Safety net patients may lack continuity of care, whether because they cannot see the same provider at each visit or because they have to go to numerous sites or through various programs to receive all the care they need. Even though safety net providers serve millions of patients every year, there are not enough providers in enough places to satisfy the need for their services. While the ACA included an infusion of funds to safety net providers, they also will serve an influx of newly insured patients. Health centers received $11 billion under the ACA and increased their patient population by 10% over 2 years, to serve 24 million patients in 2015 (Rosenbaum et al., 2017). And, as noted earlier, many safety net providers are underfunded and constantly struggling to meet the complex needs of their patient population.

The problems facing the uninsured and the stressors on the healthcare safety net highlight the inadequacies of the current "system" of providing health care, and many of these problems will remain even after the ACA is implemented. Given the country's patchwork of programs and plans, decisions made in one area can significantly affect another. For example, if Medicaid reimbursement rates are cut or program eligibility is reduced, safety net providers will have a difficult time keeping their doors open while, simultaneously, more patients will become uninsured and seek care from safety net providers. If more people choose high-deductible private insurance plans that they cannot easily afford, individuals may go without needed services or safety net providers will end up providing an increasing amount of uncompensated care. If employers decide to reduce or end coverage or increase employee cost sharing, previously insured people may fall into the ranks of the uninsured. As a result, safety net providers and their patients

BOX 4-3 Discussion Questions

Safety net providers mostly serve uninsured and publicly insured low-income patients. Many of the safety net provider features you just read about are in place to assist these patients in accessing health care. Instead of pursuing universal coverage, would it be an equally good strategy to expand the number of safety net providers? Are there reasons for both safety net providers and health insurance to exist? How does having insurance relate to accessing care?

are affected by many policies that are not directed at them, but still greatly impact their ability to provide or access care.

Workforce Issues

Problems accessing care may also occur due to provider shortages and an uneven distribution of providers throughout the country. This problem affects both the uninsured and the insured alike. If a provider is not available to take you as a patient, it matters little if you have an insurance plan that would cover the cost of your care. Of course, if a provider shortage is so great that those with insurance are turned away, the uninsured will have an even harder time accessing care.

There are a variety of estimates regarding a future healthcare workforce shortage. For example, the Association of American Medical Colleges estimates a physician shortfall between 42,600 and 121,300 by 2030 (Dall, West, Chakrabarti, Reynolds, & Iacobucci, 2018). On the other hand, if healthcare delivery approaches that rely heavily on nonphysician providers are used more often in the future, the estimates for physician shortages decline significantly. Two such models are the patient-centered medical home (PCMH), which relies on a team of providers to supply and coordinate care, and the nurse-managed health center (NMHC), which is a clinic with nurse practitioners (NPs) as the primary caregiver (Auerbach et al., 2013). One study estimated that increased use of PCMHs or NMHCs alone would reduce a primary care physician shortage from 45,000 to 35,000. Used together, the combination of approaches could cut the physician shortage in half (Auerbach et al., 2013).

One of the main concerns with the healthcare workforce is a shortage of primary care providers. It is expected that there will be between 14,800 and 49,300 fewer primary care physicians than are needed to meet demand by 2030 (Dall et al., 2018). More providers are choosing specialty care over primary care. About 30%

of physicians practice primary care today, as opposed to 70% 50 years ago (Mitra, 2016). Midlevel provider career choices have followed a similar pattern. From 1974 to 2012, the percentage of physician assistants (PAs) working in primary care declined from 70% to 34% (Dunker, Krofah, & Isasi, 2014). NPs and PAs are more likely to work in hospitals or specialty care offices than to provide services in office-based primary care (Colwill, Cultice, & Kruse, 2008). The long work hours, increased demands (particularly administrative demands associated with insurance companies), lack of respect, and comparatively low pay for primary care providers are sending future practitioners to other fields (Castellucci, 2016). For example, one study showed that, over a lifetime, a cardiologist will make $2.7 million more than a primary care physician (Vaughn, DeVrieze, Reed, & Schulman, 2010).

While fewer graduates are turning to primary care, demand for primary care services is expected to increase in the next several years. Most of the increased demand will be due to population growth and aging, with the remaining uptick in demand based on the increase of insured individuals under the ACA (Dall et al., 2018). The U.S. population is aging, with individuals older than 65 years projected to increase from 15% in 2017 to 21% in 2030 (U.S. Census Bureau, 2018). These older patients are heavy users of healthcare services. Even though older patients made up about 12% of the population in 2008, they accounted for over 45% of all primary care office visits that year (Centers for Disease Control and Prevention [CDC], 2010). Furthermore, geriatric training is lacking among primary care providers. An IOM report on aging and the healthcare workforce found medical school curricula on geriatric medicine to be "inadequate" (IOM, 2008, p. 129). Physicians agree: in a 2002 survey, only half of all responding physicians thought their colleagues could adequately treat a geriatric condition (IOM, 2008, pp. 128–129), and in a 2007 study, only 23% of medical school graduates indicated they received expert geriatric training (Association of American Medical Colleges, 2012).

In addition to provider shortages, access problems may exist because providers are not distributed as needed throughout the country (**FIGURES 4-16** through **4-18**). In 2013, 29 states had a primary care physician shortage, with Texas and Florida experiencing the greatest deficits (over 1,000 full-time-equivalent [FTE] providers). By 2025, it is estimated that 37 states will have a primary care physician shortage, with 12 states experiencing a deficit of 1,000 FTE providers or more (Health Resources Services Administration [HRSA], 2016). In contrast, Massachusetts has a primary care physician surplus that it

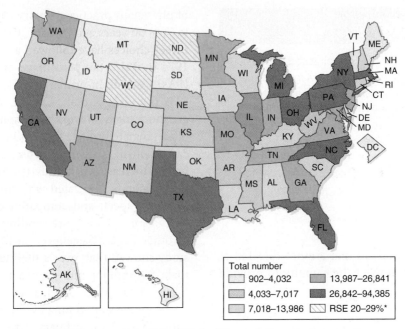

*Note: Estimates in states with an RSE > 20% should be used with caution because of large sampling error.

FIGURE 4-16 Number of Physicians by State, 2008–2010

Source: See Figure 2 from *The US Health Workforce Chartbook*, HRSA, 2013, retrieved from https://bhw.hrsa.gov/sites/default/files/bhw/nchwa/chartbookpart1.pdf

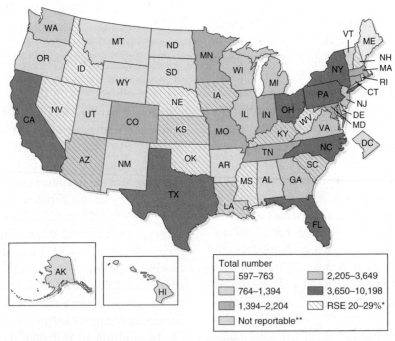

*Note: Estimates in states with an RSE > 20% should be used with caution because of large sampling error.
**Data are not reported at the state level, because the RSE ≥ 30%; estimate does not meet standards of reliability.

FIGURE 4-17 Number of Physician Assistants by State, 2008–2010

Source: See Figure 7 from *The US Health Workforce Chartbook*, HRSA, 2013, retrieved from https://bhw.hrsa.gov/sites/default/files/bhw/nchwa/chartbookpart1.pdf

expects to maintain through 2025. Similarly, primary care NP and PA shortages vary across the country. In 2013, 23 states had a primary care NP shortage, but no states are projected to have a shortfall by 2025 (HRSA, 2016). Regarding primary care PAs, 22 states had a shortage in 2013. In 2025, 9 states are expected to have a PA shortage, while 5 states (New York, North Carolina, Texas, California, and Colorado) are projected to have a surplus of more than 1,000 FTE (HRSA, 2016).

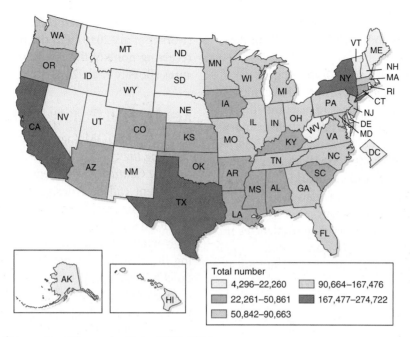

FIGURE 4-18 Number of Nurse Practitioners by State, 2008–2010

Source: See Figure 21 from *The US Health Workforce Chartbook*, HRSA, 2013, retrieved from https://bhw.hrsa.gov/sites/default/files/bhw/nchwa/chartbookpart1.pdf

Rural areas are particularly susceptible to provider shortages. This is an especially pressing problem because individuals who live in rural areas are more likely to be sicker, older, and poorer than their urban counterparts. Compared to urban dwellers, rural residents are more likely to lack access to a primary care physician, have higher rates of chronic diseases and teen pregnancies, and engage in more unhealthy behaviors such as smoking (National Conference of State Legislatures, 2017).

In 2017, 59% of designated Health Professional Shortage Areas were in rural areas (National Conference of State Legislatures, 2017). The number of specialists in rural areas is only 30 per 100,000 people, compared to 263 per 100,000 in urban areas (National Rural Health Association [NRHA], n.d.). While the gap is not as prominent for primary care physicians, they also prefer urban locations. The patient–primary care physician ratio in rural areas is 39.8 per 100,000, compared to 53.3 per 100,000 in urban areas (NRHA, n.d.). Primary care providers are vital to the healthcare workforce in rural areas. While family physicians comprise only 15% of outpatient physicians in the country, they provide 42% of services in rural areas (NRHA, n.d.).

Rural areas are more likely to attract NPs and PAs than physicians, suggesting that alternative care models that focus on nonphysician providers may be particularly useful in addressing access issues in rural areas (Graves et al., 2016). FQHCs have already embraced this model, hiring NPs, PAs, and nurse–midwives at a faster rate than physicians (Proser, Bysshe, Weaver, & Yee, 2015).

Shortages also exist within the public health workforce. The public health workforce has been defined to include anyone who is providing 1 of the 10 essential public health functions (discussed in the Public Health Institutions and Systems chapter), regardless of whether their employer is a government agency, not-for-profit organization, private for-profit entity, or some other type of organization (Center of Excellence, 2013). The public health workforce includes professions such as public health physicians and nurses, epidemiologists, health educators, and administrators. It is difficult to count everyone involved in the public health workforce, given the wide array of jobs and the numerous data sources needed to compile the information. In 2012, the public health field was estimated to include between 310,000 and 342,000 workers. This represents a worker-to-population ratio of 99 to 110 per 100,000 people, which is substantially lower than the earlier estimates in 1980 (220 per 100,000 people) and 2000 (158 per 100,000 people) (Center of Excellence, 2013).

The ACA contains a number of provisions, intended to address some of the more pressing healthcare and public health workforce issues, which could accomplish the following goals:

- Increase funding for community health centers
- Increase funding for the National Health Service Corps, which provides scholarships and loan

repayments to students who agree to become primary care providers and work in medically underserved communities

- Increase funding for PA and NP training
- Provide new funding to establish NP-led clinics
- Provide new funding for states to plan and implement innovative strategies to boost their primary care workforce
- Establish a National Health Care Workforce Commission to coordinate federal workforce efforts and bolster data collection and analysis
- Establish teaching health centers
- Provide payments for primary care residencies in community-based ambulatory care centers
- Increase the number of Graduate Medical Education slots available to primary providers by redistributing unused slots
- Promote residency training in outpatient settings
- Provide grants to training institutions to promote careers in the healthcare sector
- Increase reimbursement for primary care providers under Medicare and Medicaid

Given the uncertain political future of the ACA, it remains to be seen whether these provisions will be implemented or funded in the years to come.

▶ Healthcare Quality

As noted earlier in this chapter, the United States spends more on health care than most other developed countries, yet frequently the care provided does not result in good health outcomes. Researchers and policymakers have highlighted the need to improve the quality of care provided in this country. A 2003 landmark study raised many quality concerns, including findings that patients received the appropriate medical care only 55% of the time and that patients were much more likely not to receive appropriate services than to receive potentially harmful care (McGlynn, Asch, & Adams, 2003). The lack of appropriate care was seen across medical conditions, similarly affecting treatments relating to preventive care, acute care, and chronic diseases (McGlynn et al., 2003, p. 2641). The degree to which patients received appropriate care varied greatly. For example, only 10% of patients with alcohol dependence received the standard of care, as opposed to 78% of those with senile cataracts (McGlynn et al., 2003, p. 2641). In addition, many adults do not receive all of the recommended preventive measures. A 2015 study found that only 8% of respondents age 35 years and older reported receiving all of the recommended preventive measures,

and only 20% reported receiving most (75%) of them (Borsky et al., 2018). On the other hand, 5% reported receiving none of the recommended preventive measures (Borsky et al., 2018).

Key Areas of Quality Improvement

In 2001, the IOM (again, now the HMD) released *Crossing the Quality Chasm: A New Health System for the 21st Century*, which represented nothing less than an urgent call to redesign the healthcare system to improve the quality of care provided (IOM, 2001b). The IOM attributes our inability to provide consistent, high-quality health care to a number of factors, including the growing complexity of health care, including quickly developing technological advancements; an inability to meet rapid changes; shortcomings in safely using new technology and applying new knowledge to practice; increased longevity among the population, which carries concerns relating to treating chronic conditions in a system better designed to address episodic, acute care needs; and a fragmented delivery system that lacks coordination, leading to poor use of information and gaps in care (IOM, 2001b, pp. 2–4). In its call to redesign the healthcare system to improve quality, the IOM focuses on six areas of improvement: safety, efficacy, patient-centeredness, timeliness, efficiency, and equity (IOM, 2001b, p. 43).

Safety

In a safe healthcare system, patients should not be endangered when receiving care that is intended to help them, and healthcare workers should not be harmed by their chosen profession (IOM, 2001b, p. 44). In an earlier report, *To Err Is Human*, the IOM found that deaths due to medical errors in hospitals could be as high as 98,000 annually and cost up to $29 billion, over half of which is attributable to healthcare costs (IOM, 2000b, pp. 1–2). A safe healthcare system also means that standards of care should not decline at different times of the day or week or when a patient is transferred from one provider to another. In addition, safety requires that patients and their families are fully informed and participate in their care to the extent they wish to do so (IOM, 2001b, p. 45).

Efficacy

While scientific evidence regarding a particular treatment's effectiveness is not always available, an effective healthcare system should use evidence-based treatments whenever possible. This effort includes avoiding the underuse of effective care and the overuse of ineffective care (IOM, 2001b, p. 47). Evidence-based medicine is not limited to findings from randomized clinical trials, but may use results from a variety of research designs. To promote the use of evidenced-based medicine, healthcare providers and institutions should improve their data collection and analysis capabilities so it is possible to monitor results of care provided (IOM, 2001b, p. 48).

Patient-Centeredness

A patient-centered healthcare system is sensitive to the needs, values, and preferences of each patient, includes smooth transitions and close coordination among providers, provides complete information and education at a level and in a language patients can understand, involves the patient's family and friends according to the patient's wishes, and, to the extent possible, reduces physical discomfort experienced by patients during care (IOM, 2001b, pp. 49–50). A language or cultural barrier may be a significant hurdle to receiving high-quality and patient-centered care. In 2013, one in five Americans spoke a language other than English at home (Camarota & Zeigler, 2014). Individuals with language barriers are less likely to adhere to medication regimens, have a usual source of care, and understand their diagnosis and treatment, and are more likely to leave a hospital against a provider's advice and miss follow-up appointments (Speaking Together, 2007). While use of interpreters can improve a patient's quality of care, when friends or family members serve as interpreters, there is greater risk that the interpreter will misunderstand or omit a provider's questions and that the patient will not disclose embarrassing symptoms (Speaking Together, 2007). Similarly, cultural differences between provider and patient can result in patients receiving less than optimal care. Cultural differences can define how healthcare information is received, whether a problem is perceived as a healthcare issue, how patients express symptoms and concerns, and what type of treatment is most appropriate. As a result, healthcare organizations should ensure that patients receive care that is both linguistically and culturally appropriate (Office of Minority Health, n.d.).

Timeliness

A high-quality healthcare system will provide care in a timely manner. Currently, U.S. patients experience long waits when making appointments, sitting in doctors' offices, standing in hallways before receiving procedures, waiting for test results, seeking care at EDs, and appealing billing errors (IOM, 2001b, p. 51).

These delays can take an emotional as well as physical toll if medical problems would have been caught earlier with more timely care. Timeliness problems also affect providers because of difficulties in obtaining vital information and delays that result when consulting specialists. In addition, lengthy waits are the result of a system that is not efficient and does not respect the needs of its consumers (IOM, 2001b, p. 51).

Efficiency

An efficient healthcare system makes the best use of its resources and obtains the most value per dollar spent on healthcare goods and services. The uncoordinated and fragmented U.S. system is wasteful when it provides low-quality care and creates higher than necessary administrative and production costs (IOM, 2001b, p. 52). As indicated previously, the high level of spending and poor outcomes relating to preventable conditions, the number of patients who do not receive appropriate care, and the high number of medical errors make it clear that the quality of healthcare services provided can be improved.

In addition, significant geographic variations in the provision of healthcare services suggest a lack of efficiency in the system; however, this is a complicated issue to understand and solve. For example, the Dartmouth Atlas Project has studied regional variations in healthcare practices and spending for several decades. Even after controlling for level of illness and prices paid for services, researchers have found a two-fold difference in Medicare spending in the country.

Furthermore, higher spending areas are not associated with better quality of care, more patient satisfaction, better access to care, more effective care, or improved outcomes (Fisher, Goodman, Skinner, &

BOX 4-4 Discussion Questions

Unfortunately, evidence is not available to support the effectiveness or cost–benefit of every procedure or drug. How should policymakers and providers make decisions when faced with a dearth of evidence? Do you prefer a more cautious approach that does not approve procedures or drugs until evidence is available or a more aggressive approach that encourages experimentation and use of treatments that appear to be effective? What about medical care for children, who are generally excluded from clinical and research trials for ethical reasons? When, if ever, is it appropriate for insurers to cover or the government to pay for treatments that are not proven effective?

Bronner, 2009). Instead, both health system capacity and local practice styles appear to be key factors in geographic variations in cost. An IOM report addressing this issue also found that health status, demographics, insurance plan coverage, and market factors did not explain the variation (IOM, 2013). The report highlighted the use of post-acute care and acute care services as a key concern and noted that other factors, such as patient preference and provider discretion, are not included in the data analyzed. In the end, the IOM concluded, "an overall explanation for geographic variation remains elusive" (IOM, 2013). As policymakers try to improve quality of care in the United States, they will have to continue to untangle difficult questions of why some parts of the country spend more on services than others.

The nation also spends close to one-quarter of healthcare expenditures on administration, which is more than twice what the country spends on cardiovascular disease and three times the amount it spends on cancer (Cutler, 2018). As shown in **FIGURE 4-19**, this high level of administrative spending dwarfs that of other countries (Bodenheimer, 2005, p. 934; Papanicolas, Woskie, & Jha, 2018). Extensive use of private insurers, who often have high administrative costs relative to public insurance programs, as well as the use of multiple insurers instead of a single-payer system, result in high administrative costs in the United States.

Equity

An equitable healthcare system provides essential health benefits to all people and includes universal access to care. Equity can be considered on an individual level and on a population level (IOM, 2001b, p. 53). While the ACA should improve individual access to services by reducing the number of uninsured, insurance alone is not sufficient to ensure access to care. The care itself still must be accessible (providers are willing to accept you as a patient), affordable, and available (sufficient providers are available).

Population-level equity refers to reducing healthcare disparities among subgroups. In the United States, racial and ethnic minority groups often receive lower-quality care and fewer routine preventive procedures than White people. A 2003 IOM report found that African Americans were less likely than Whites to receive appropriate cardiac medication, undergo necessary artery bypass surgery, and use dialysis or receive a kidney transplant even when controlling for factors such as age, insurance status, income level, and comorbidities. Not surprisingly, African Americans also had higher mortality rates than their White counterparts (IOM, 2003, pp. 2–3).

These trends continue. In 2014, African Americans were still more likely than Whites to have asthma, diabetes, cardiovascular disease and AIDS. African American men have the shortest life expectancy

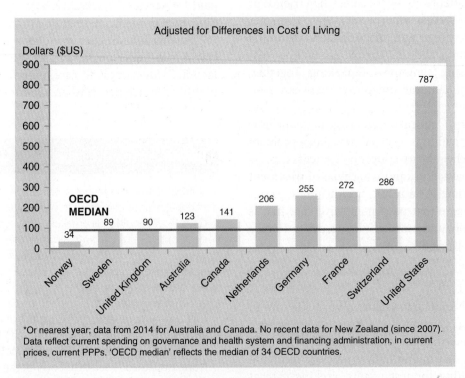

FIGURE 4-19 Spending on Health Insurance Administration per Capita, 2015

Source: Retrieved from https://www.commonwealthfund.org/publications/publication/2017/nov/multinational-comparisons-health-systems-data-2017

(Orgera & Artiga, 2016). As compared to Whites, Hispanics were more likely to be diabetic, experience periodontitis, be HIV positive, and be uninsured, and less likely to be screened for colorectal cancer or receive the flu vaccine as an infant (CDC, 2013). Hispanics are more likely than Whites to have asthma, liver disease, tuberculosis, and diabetes, and to die from cervical cancer, HIV, and end-stage renal disease (Families USA, 2014). In 2016, the Agency for Healthcare Quality and Research (AHQR) found access to care was worse for African Americans on 50% of their measures and for Hispanics on 75% of their measures (AHQR, 2016).

While this country continues to struggle with health disparities, the ACA has made a positive difference. From 2013 to 2015, racial disparities narrowed in terms of percentage of working adults who were uninsured, who skipped care due to cost, and who lacked a usual source of care (Hayes, Riley, Radley, & McCarthy, 2017).

Assessment of Efforts to Improve Quality

The IOM has called for sweeping changes to the healthcare system to address the numerous ways in which the quality of care could be improved. In 2015, the Department of Health and Human Services (HHS) issued a progress report on its Action Plan to Reduce Racial and Ethnic Health Disparities, which included a number of activities HHS had already taken and goals for future activities (HHS, 2015). While the ACA makes significant changes to the healthcare system, the law is focused more on improving access than improving quality or the delivery system. Many of the law's quality improvement provisions are pilot programs and demonstration projects that may eventually result in significant changes—or fall to the wayside once they expire.

None of the quality improvement tasks the IOM calls for will be simple to achieve, and, at times, they seem to have conflicting goals. For example, making the healthcare system patient-centered may not always result in enhanced efficiency. Furthermore, the IOM's proposed changes would require increased resources at a time when the United States is facing record deficits and unsustainable healthcare spending levels. Improving the quality of the healthcare system is an enormous challenge and one that is likely to remain on the nation's agenda for years to come.

▶ Comparative Health Systems

A review of the U.S. healthcare system and a discussion of its flaws often leads one to ask, how do other countries deliver health care, and do they do a better job? Because the United States spends more overall and more per person on health care comparatively speaking and yet often lags in many quality and outcome indicators, perhaps there are lessons to learn from other countries (**FIGURE 4-20**). While there are many problems with healthcare delivery in the United States, it is also true that each type of healthcare system has its advantages and drawbacks.

There are three types of healthcare systems often found in other countries: (1) a national health insurance system that is publicly financed, but in which care is provided by private practitioners (e.g., Canada); (2) a national health system that is publicly financed and where care is provided by government employees or contractors (e.g., Great Britain); and (3) a socialized insurance system that is financed through mandatory contributions by employers and employees and in which care is delivered by private practitioners (e.g., Germany) (Shi & Singh, 2019, p. 22). Of course, variations exist within these types of systems in terms of the role of the central government, the presence of private insurance, the way the healthcare system is financed, and how care is administered by providers and accessed by patients. While comparing the systems in the three countries used as examples does not cover all possible permutations of how healthcare systems are designed, it provides an overview of the choices made by policymakers in different countries (**TABLE 4-1**).

A National Health Insurance System: Canada

Canada's healthcare system is called Medicare. Prior to establishing the Medicare program in 1966, Canada provided insurance in a manner that was similar to the U.S. method, with private plans offering coverage to many, even while millions remained uninsured. Incremental changes were made to the Canadian healthcare system until the Medical Care Act of 1966 established Medicare's framework; it was later modified through the Canadian Health Act of 1984. The Canadian Health Act established five principles for health care delivery: (1) public administration, (2) comprehensive coverage, (3) universality, (4) portability across Canada, and (5) uniform and reasonable access to care (Johnson, Stoskopf, & Shi, 2018).

Canada's healthcare system is largely decentralized, with Canada's provinces and territories responsible for setting up their own delivery system. As such, Canada's Medicare system is a collection of single-payer systems governed by the provinces and territories, with the central government taking a more limited role. The provinces and territories set their own policies regarding

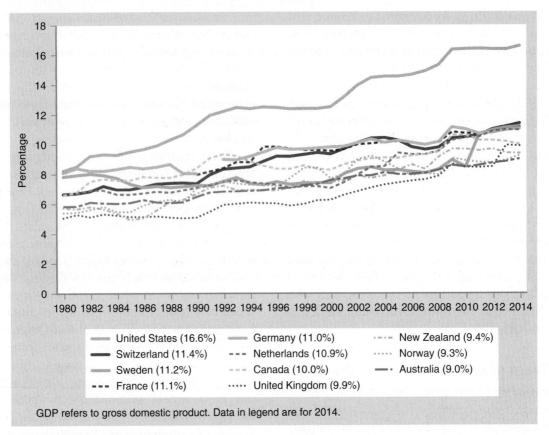

FIGURE 4-20 Healthcare Spending as a Percentage of Gross Domestic Product, 1980–2014

Source: Retrieved from https://www.commonwealthfund.org/chart/2017/health-care-spending-percentage-gdp-1980-2014

TABLE 4-1 Comparison of Health Systems Across Four Countries

	United States	Canada	Great Britain	Germany
System type	No unified system	National health insurance	National health system	Socialized health insurance
Universal coverage	Near universal if ACA fully implemented	Yes	Yes	Yes
Role of private insurance	Significant	Supplemental to Medicare, two-thirds purchase	Minimal	Minimal
Financing	Private payments and tax revenue	Mostly tax revenue (federal, provincial, territorial)	All federal income tax revenue	Mandatory employer and employee contributions to national health fund
Hospital reimbursement	Varies by payer (DRG[a], FFS[b], capitation, per diem)	Global budget	Global budget	DRG[a]
Physician reimbursement	Fee schedule or capitation	Negotiated fees with provinces/ territories	Salary or capitation	Negotiated fees with funds

DRG[a] = diagnostic-related group (payment based on bundle of services needed for diagnosis). FFS[b] = fee for service (payment per service rendered).

many healthcare and other social issues, administer their own individual single-payer systems, reimburse hospitals directly or through regional health authorities, and negotiate physician fees schedules with provincial medical associations. Provinces and territories use regional health authorities as their primary payer of healthcare services. While funding methods vary by location, regional health authorities have the ability to tailor funds in a way that best serves the needs of their population. In addition to paying for care, regional health authorities also organize the delivery of care. They hire staff at most acute care facilities and contract for some ambulatory care services. General practitioners and specialists mostly work on a fee-for-service arrangement and in private practice (Allin & Rudoler, n.d.). The federal government has responsibility for specific health areas such as prescription drugs, public health, and health research, as well as for providing care to certain populations (e.g., veterans, indigenous peoples) (Allin & Rudoler, n.d.).

Financing for health benefits varies by benefit type. Hospital services, physician services, and public health services are financed through public taxation. Hospitals mostly operate under global budgets they negotiate with a ministry of health or regional health authority, although a few provinces are considering activity-based funding (Allin & Rudoler, n.d.). Certain services, including prescription drugs, home care, and institutional care, are financed through a combination of public taxation and private insurance coverage. Other goods and services, such as dental and vision care, over-the-counter drugs, and alternative medicines are covered only through private insurance. Approximately two-thirds of Canadians purchase private insurance, which is used to cover goods and services not provided by Medicare (Allin & Rudoler, n.d.).

Tax revenue from the provincial, territorial, and federal governments pays for 70% of total Medicare expenditures, while private insurance reimbursement accounts for 12% of costs, patient out-of-pocket payments cover 14%, and various sources account for the remaining amount (Allin & Rudoler, n.d.). Healthcare spending is expected to reach C\$242 billion in 2017 (Canadian Institute for Health Information [CIHI], "How much," n.d.). Healthcare spending varies considerably across the country. For example, Alberta spends C\$7,329 per person, compared to Yukon's C\$11,222 per-person costs (CIHI, "How does," n.d.).

A National Health System: Great Britain

Great Britain's healthcare system was designed by Sir William Beveridge as part of a social reconstruction plan after World War II. The National Health Services Act of 1946 created the National Health Service (NHS), a centrally run healthcare system that provides universal insurance coverage to all residents of Great Britain. It was designed based on the principle that the government is responsible for providing equal access to comprehensive health care that is generally free at the point of service (Johnson et al., 2018, pp. 174–176).

The Health and Social Care Act of 2012 introduced significant changes to the NHS system. In the prior system, health care was delivered through a variety of trusts that covered services such as primary care, mental health care, acute care, and ambulance services (Johnson et al., pp. 178–179). In the new system, Primary Care Trusts were replaced with Clinical Commissioning Groups (CCGs), which are led by clinicians. CCGs are bodies that consist of general practitioners in their service area, and they are responsible for providing urgent and emergency care, elective hospital care, community health services that go beyond general practitioner services, maternity and newborn services, and mental health and learning disability services. The 2012 legislation also created an independent organization called NHS England to focus on improving health outcomes and quality of care. NHS England provides national leadership, supervises CCGs, allocates resources to CCGs, and commissions primary care, certain specialty care, military care, and offender care (Thorlby, Arora, & Nuffield Trust, n.d.).

The NHS is the largest publicly financed national health system in the world. The 2017–2018 budget is £124.7 billion, with only a 1.2% growth rate projected from 2010 to 2021. This is far below the needed growth rate, which is expected to exceed 4% (King's Fund, 2018). Due to this discrepancy, NHS projects a \$6 billion deficit by 2021 (Thorlby et al., n.d.). NHS is using a number of cost containment strategies to address its budgetary concerns, including freezing wages, increasing use of generic drugs, reducing hospital payments, lowering administrative costs, and improving hospital management (Thorlby et al., n.d.).

The NHS is financed primarily through general tax revenues. It is NHS England's responsibility to identify necessary healthcare services and Monitor's (England's regulatory body for health care) role to set prices for those services. While most residents receive their care through the NHS, private insurance is also available. Approximately 10.5% of residents have private health insurance, which provides the same benefits as the NHS but allows for reduced waiting times, more convenient care, and greater access to specialists (Johnson et al., 2018, p. 182; Thorlby et al., n.d.).

NHS services are provided by provider organizations that are classified as NHS foundation trusts or

NHS trusts. NHS foundation trusts are not directed by the government and are free to make financial decisions based on a framework established by law and regulation. NHS trusts are directed by the government and are financially accountable to the government (Johnson et al., 2018, p. 181; Thorlby et al., n.d.). Most general practice physicians and nurses are private practitioners who work for the NHS as independent contractors, not salaried employees, while the NHS owns the hospitals and the hospital staff are salaried employees. Patients select a general practitioner in their service area, and this provider is the gateway to NHS services. Almost everyone has a registered general practitioner, and most patient contact is with this provider (Thorlby et al., n.d.). Services are provided free of charge, except for specific services designated by law.

The Health and Social Care Act also renewed focus on public health needs. Public Health England was created in 2013 as an autonomous executive agency of the Department of Health. Its role is to protect the public's health, reduce health disparities, promote health knowledge and information, and ensure that high-quality healthcare services are delivered to the public. In addition, local Health and Wellbeing Boards were created to improve the public's health and reduce disparities through local government action (Public Health England, n.d.).

In 2014, NHS unveiled the Five Year Forward plan to address challenges to the healthcare system, with a focus on improving early identification of high-risk patients and exploring new payment models. Based on the plan, 50 "vanguards," or pilot programs, have been established to test ideas such as "scaled-up primary care, enhanced health care in long-term care homes, vertically integrated hospital and community care, and networks to improve emergency care" (Thorlby et al., n.d.). In addition, the plan includes a diabetes initiative, a commitment to 7-day workweeks by 2020, and "footprints" that bring together purchasers and providers in a local community to provide services under a consolidated budget (Thorlby et al., n.d.).

A Socialized Insurance System: Germany

In 1883, Germany's Otto von Bismarck created the first healthcare system in the world. He viewed a strong health and pension system as a way to build a superior nation, earn support from Germany's working class, and undermine any attempts by Germany's socialist party to gain power. The central government is responsible for setting health policy and regulating the Social Health Insurance System (SHIS). German healthcare

policy emphasizes solidarity, the idea that all should have equal access to health care regardless of ability to pay (Johnson et al., 2018, pp. 217–223). Germany's legislature passed several major health reform bills in recent years. These reforms include integration of inpatient and ambulatory care, premium payment changes, an insurance mandate, and revised long-term care policies (Johnson et al., 2018, pp. 230–31).

SHIS is composed of a collection of nonprofit regional sickness funds with a standard benefit package that includes inpatient services, outpatient services, medications, rehabilitation therapy, and dental benefits. The funds are organized around industry or geography and are responsible for managing healthcare services. Germans must enroll in sickness funds or obtain coverage through private insurance (Blümel & Busse, n.d.). Some populations are required to be under SHIS, including individuals who earn less than $60,000 per year or are pensioners, students, unemployed, disabled, poor, or homeless. Funds may not refuse to cover these individuals, and physicians may not refuse to treat them. Germans who earn more than $60,000 per year for 3 consecutive years or who are self-employed may choose to opt out of SHIS and purchase private coverage. Exempt citizens and individuals choosing to opt out of SHIS may purchase private substitutive private health insurance (PHI). In 2015, almost 9 million people—often young, wealthy workers who could secure a low-premium plan—enrolled in substitutive PHI (Blümel & Busse, n.d.).

Health care is provided in the public and private sectors. SHIS ambulatory care physicians generally work in private practice and are members of regional associations that negotiate a fee schedule with sickness funds. Fee schedules are also used by private insurers, but often at a higher rate than the SHIS fee schedule. Hospitals are split between public, private nonprofit, and private for-profit institutions, with the latter increasing its share of the market in recent years. Hospitals are staffed by salaried providers and reimbursed based on a diagnostic-related group methodology (Blümel & Busse, n.d.; Johnson et al., 2018, p. 235).

Sickness funds are financed through employer and employee contributions. As of 2016, employer and employees split the 14.6% of gross wage contribution. In addition, there is a supplementary contribution based on income that is set by each sickness fund. The sickness fund contributions are pooled and then reallocated to individuals based on a risk-adjusted formula that accounts for age, sex, and morbidity (Blümel & Busse, n.d.). In 2014, Germany spent $492 billion in health expenditures, mostly through SHIS (Johnson et al., 2018, p. 234).

The Importance of Health Insurance Design

Reviewing the healthcare systems of four countries—the United States, Canada, Great Britain, and Germany—shows how varied healthcare systems are around the world. Differences exist regarding the role of government, the ability to purchase private insurance, cost-sharing requirements, and how the system is financed. Even countries that share the same general type of system have variations based on their specific culture, politics, and needs. How a system is designed matters in terms of access to care, financing, and patient satisfaction. A 2016 survey in 11 countries asked residents about their experience with their country's healthcare system (Obsorne, Squires, Doty, Sarnak, & Schneider, 2016). What issues were primary concerns and how different residents fared within a system varied by country (**FIGURES 4-21** through **4-25**).

While affordability was a key concern in the United States, Americans reported fewer access problems than residents in many other countries. Of those surveyed, a third of U.S. residents went without care due to cost, as compared to 7% of respondents in England and Germany (Osborne et al., 2016). Cost barriers to accessing dental care were a much bigger concern for American and Canadian respondents than for those living in England or Germany. Low-income adults reported worse health and more cost concerns than wealthier individuals across all of the countries surveyed, with the United States having the highest rate of low-income respondents indicating that cost was a barrier to care. England was the only country where low-income adults did not report greater access problems due to cost (Osborne et al., 2016). In terms of same-day or next-day appointments, Canadians (53%) and Germans (47%) reported more problems than American (42%) and British (41%) respondents (Osborne et al., 2016). In addition, about 30% of Canadian adults and 19% of British adults reported having to wait at least 2 months for a specialty appointment, compared to less than 10% of adults in Germany and the United States. Germans obtained care through EDs at a much lower rate (11%) than residents of other countries, with Canadians (41%) and Americans (35%) reporting much higher use of emergency care.

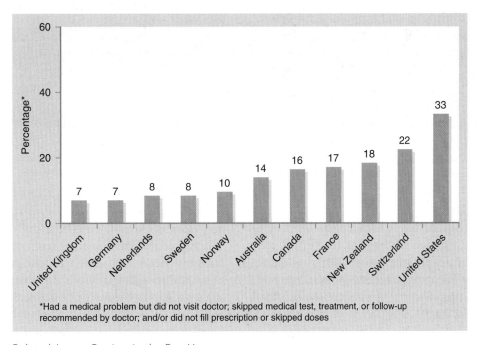

*Had a medical problem but did not visit doctor; skipped medical test, treatment, or follow-up recommended by doctor; and/or did not fill prescription or skipped doses

FIGURE 4-21 Cost-Related Access Barriers in the Past Year

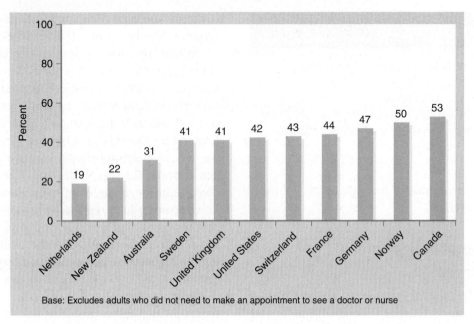

FIGURE 4-22 Did Not Get Same or Next-Day Appointment Last Time You Needed Care

Source: Retrieved from https://www.commonwealthfund.org/publications/surveys/2016/nov/2016-commonwealth-fund-international-health-policy-survey-adults

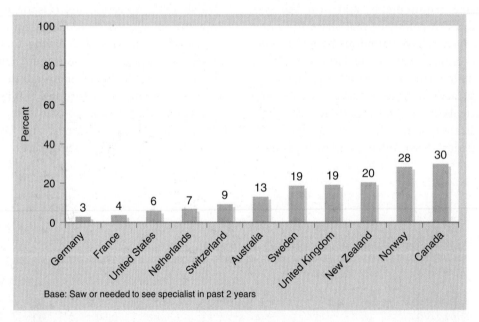

FIGURE 4-23 Waited 2 Months or Longer for a Specialist Appointment

Source: Retrieved from https://www.commonwealthfund.org/publications/surveys/2016/nov/2016-commonwealth-fund-international-health-policy-survey-adults

▶ Conclusion

This wide-ranging review of the U.S. healthcare system was intended to provide readers with a general sense of how health care is accessed, financed, and administered in this country. Understanding the various players in the healthcare system, from providers to researchers to policymakers, is crucial to being able to participate in debates over current issues in health policy and law. While the U.S. system excels on many fronts, it falls short in many areas relating to access, quality, and efficiency. Perhaps policymakers in this country could learn lessons from successes abroad, but the United States has a unique political environment and it is clear there is no silver bullet that will solve all the problems we face. Specific health policy and law concerns will be described in much greater detail elsewhere, providing a foundation to tackle the many problems that will confront the country in the years ahead.

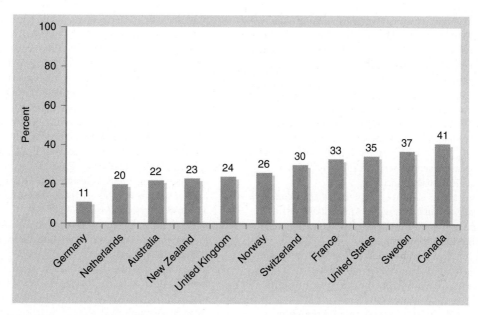

FIGURE 4-24 Used the ED in the Last 2 Years

Source: Retrieved from https://www.commonwealthfund.org/publications/surveys/2016/nov/2016-commonwealth-fund-international-health-policy-survey-adults

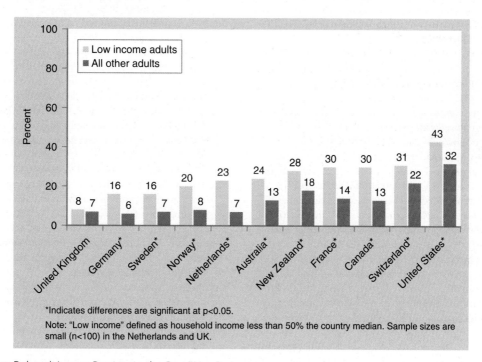

FIGURE 4-25 Cost-Related Access Barriers in the Past Year, By Income

Source: Retrieved from https://www.commonwealthfund.org/publications/surveys/2016/nov/2016-commonwealth-fund-international-health-policy-survey-adults

References

Agency for Healthcare Quality and Research. (2018). *2016 national healthcare quality and disparities report.* Retrieved from https://www.ahrq.gov/research/findings/nhqrdr/nhqdr16/index.html

Allin, S., & Rudoler, D. (n.d.). *The Canadian health care system.* Retrieved from https://international.commonwealthfund.org/countries/canada/

America's Essential Hospitals. (2018, June). *Essential data: Our hospitals, our patients.* Retrieved from https://essentialhospitals.org/wp-content/uploads/2018/06/AEH_Essential Data_2018Web.pdf

Association of American Medical Colleges. (2012). *Recent studies and reports on physician shortages in the U.S.* Retrieved from https://www.aamc.org/download/100598/data/

Auerbach, D. I., Chen, P. G., Friedberg, M. W., Reid, R., Lau, C., Buerhaus, P. I., & Mehrotra, A. (2013). Nurse-managed health centers and patient centered medical homes could mitigate expected primary care physician shortage. *Health Affairs, 32*(11), 1933–1941. doi:10.1377/hlthaff.2013.0596

Blümel, M., & Busse, R. (n.d.). *The German health care system.* Retrieved from https://international.commonwealthfund.org /countries/germany/

Bodenheimer, T. (2005). High and rising health care costs, part 2: Technological innovation. *Annals of Internal Medicine, 142*(11), 932–937. doi:10.7326/0003-4819-142-11-200506070-00012

Borsky, A., Zhan, C., Miller, T., Ngo-Metzger, Q., Bierman, A. S., & Myers, D. (2018). Few Americans receive all high-priority, appropriate clinical preventive services. *Health Affairs, 37*(6), 925–928. doi:0.1377/hlthaff.2017.1248

Camarota, S. A., & Zeigler, K. (2014). *One in five U.S. residents speaks foreign language at home, record 61.8 million.* Retrieved from https://cis.org/One-Five-US-Residents-Speaks-Foreign -Language-Home-Record-618-million

Canadian Institute for Health Information. (n.d.). *How does health spending differ across provinces and territories?* Retrieved from https://www.cihi.ca/en/how-does-health-spending-differ -across-provinces-and-territories-2017

Canadian Institute for Health Information. (n.d.). *How much does Canada spend on health care?* Retrieved from https://www.cihi .ca/en/how-much-does-canada-spend-on-health-care-2017

Castellucci, M. (2016, November 5). Medical schools tackle primary-care shortages. *Modern Healthcare.* Retrieved from http://www.modernhealthcare.com/article/20161105 /MAGAZINE/311059982

Center of Excellence in Public Health Workforce Studies. (2013). *Public health workforce enumeration, 2012.* Retrieved from http://www.phf.org/resourcestools/Documents/UM_CEPHS _Enumeration2012_Revised_July_2013.pdf

Centers for Disease Control and Prevention. (2010). *Population aging the use of office-based physician services.* Retrieved from https://www.cdc.gov/nchs/data/databriefs/db41.pdf

Centers for Disease Control and Prevention. (2013). *Health disparities and inequalities report.* Retrieved from https://www.cdc.gov /mmwr/preview/ind2013_su.html#HealthDisparities2013

Centers for Medicare and Medicaid Services. (2017, November 17). *2018 Medicare parts A and B premiums and deductibles.* Retrieved from https://www.cms.gov/Newsroom/MediaReleaseDatabase/ Fact-sheets/2017-Fact-Sheet-items/2017-11-17.html

Collins, S. R., Rasmussen, P. W., Beutel, S., & Doty, M. M. (2015, May 20). *The problem of underinsurance and how rising deductibles will make it worse.* Retrieved from https://www .commonwealthfund.org/publications/issue-briefs/2015/may /problem-underinsurance-and-how-rising-deductibles-will -make-it

Colwill, J. M., Cultice, J. M., & Kruse, R. L. (2008). Will generalist physician supply meet demands of an increasing and aging population? *Health Affairs, 27*(3), w232. doi:10.1377 /hlthaff.27.3.w232

Commonwealth Fund. (n.d.). *Why do millions of U.S. adults remain uninsured?* Retrieved from http://www.commonwealthfund .org/publications/lists/2016/remaining-uninsured

Congressional Budget Office. (2018). *Federal subsidies for health insurance coverage for people under age 65: 2018 to 2028.* Retrieved from https://www.cbo.gov/system/files/115th -congress-2017-2018/reports/53826-healthinsurance coverage.pdf

Cuckler, G. A., Sisko, A. M., Poisal, J. A., Keehan, S. P., Smith, S. D., Madison, A. J., . . . Hardesty, J. C. (2018). National health expenditure projections, 2017–2026: Despite uncertainty, fundamentals primarily drive spending growth. *Health Affairs, 37*(3), 482–492. doi:10.1377/hlthaff.2017.1655

Cutler, D. (2018). What is the US health spending problem? *Health Affairs, 37*(3). doi:10.1377/hlthaff.2017.1626

Dall, T., West, T., Chakrabarti, R., Reynolds, R., & Iacobucci, W. (2018). *The complexities of physician supply and demand: Projections from 2016 to 2030.* Retrieved from https://aamc -black.global.ssl.fastly.net/production/media/filer_public/85 /d7/85d7b689-f417-4ef0-97fb-ecc129836829/aamc_2018 _workforce_projections_update_april_11_2018.pdf

Dunker, A., Krofah, E., & Isasi, F. (2014, September 22). *The role of physician assistants in health care delivery.* Retrieved from https://www.nga.org/files/live/sites/NGA/files/pdf/2014/1409 TheRoleOfPhysicianAssistants.pdf

Families USA. (2005). *Paying a premium: The added cost of care for the uninsured.* Retrieved from http://www.policyarchive.org /handle/10207/6261

Families USA. (2014). *Latino health disparities compared to non-Hispanic Whites.* Retrieved from https://familiesusa. org/product/latino-health-disparities-compared-non -hispanic-whites

Fisher, E., Goodman, D., Skinner, J., & Bronner, K. (2009). *Health care spending, quality, and outcomes: More isn't always better.* Retrieved from http://www.dartmouthatlas.org/downloads /reports/Spending_Brief_022709.pdf

Foutz, F., Damico, A., Squires E., & Garfield R. (2017, December 14). *The uninsured: A primer—key facts about health insurance and the uninsured under the Affordable Care Act.* Retrieved from https://www.kff.org/uninsured/report/the-uninsured -a-primer-key-facts-about-health-insurance-and-the -uninsured-under-the-affordable-care-act/

Graves, J. A., Pranita, M., Dittus, R. S., Parikh, R., Perloff, J., Buerhaus, P. I. (2016). Role of geography and nurse-practitioner scope of practice in efforts to expand primary care system capacity: Health reform and the primary care workforce. *Medical Care, 54*(1), 81–89. doi:10.1097/MLR.0000000000000454

Gresenz, C. R., & Escarce, J. J. (2011). Spillover effects of community uninsurance on working age adults and seniors: An instrumental variable analysis. *Medical Care, 49*(9), e14–e21. doi:10.1097/MLR.0b013e31822dc7f4

Guttmacher Institute. (n.d.). *Abortion—Insurance coverage.* Retrieved from https://www.guttmacher.org/united-states /abortion/insurance-coverage

Guttmacher Institute. (2018a, June 1). *An overview of abortion laws.* Retrieved from https://www.guttmacher.org/state-policy /explore/overview-abortion-laws

Guttmacher Institute. (2018b, June 11). *Insurance coverage of contraceptives.* Retrieved from https://www.guttmacher.org /state-policy/explore/insurance-coverage-contraceptives

Hartman, M., Martin, A. B., Espinosa N., Catlin, A., & National Expenditures Accounts Team. (2018). National health care spending in 2016: Spending and enrollment growth slow after initial coverage expansions. *Health Affairs, 37*(1), 150–160. doi:10.1377/hlthaff.2017.1299

Hayes, S. L., Riley, P., Radley, D., & McCarthy, D. (2017). *Reducing racial and ethnic disparities in access to care: Has the Affordable Care Act made a difference?* Retrieved from https://www .commonwealthfund.org/publications/issue-briefs/2017/aug /reducing-racial-and-ethnic-disparities-access-care-has

Health Resources Services Administration. (2016). *State- level projections of supply and demand for primary care practitioners: 2013–2025.* Retrieved from https://

bhw.hrsa.gov/sites/default/files/bhw/health-workforce -analysis/research/projections/primary-care-state -projections2013-2025.pdf

Institute of Medicine. (2000a). *America's health care safety net: Intact but endangered.* Washington, DC: National Academy Press.

Institute of Medicine. (2000b). *To err is human: Building a safer health care system.* Washington, DC: National Academy Press.

Institute of Medicine. (2001a). *Coverage matters: Insurance and health care.* Washington, DC: National Academy Press.

Institute of Medicine. (2001b). *Crossing the Quality Chasm: A New Health System for the 21st Century.* Washington, DC: National Academy Press.

Institute of Medicine. (2003). *Unequal treatment: Confronting racial and ethnic disparities in health care.* Washington, DC: National Academy Press.

Institute of Medicine. (2008). *Retooling for an aging America: Building the health care workforce.* Washington, DC: National Academy Press.

Institute of Medicine. (2013). *Variation in health care spending: Target decision making, not geography.* Washington, DC: National Academy Press.

Kaiser Family Foundation. (2017). *Key facts about the uninsured.* Retrieved from https://www.kff.org/uninsured/fact-sheet /key-facts-about-the-uninsured-population/

Kaiser Family Foundation & Health Research Educational Trust. (2017, September 19). *2017 Employer health benefits survey.* Retrieved from https://www.kff.org/health-costs /report/2017-employer-health-benefits-survey/

King's Fund. (2018). *The NHS budget and how it has changed.* Retrieved from https://www.kingsfund.org.uk/projects /nhs-in-a-nutshell/nhs-budget

Johnson, J., Stoskopf, C., & Shi, L. (2018). *Comparative health systems: A global perspective* (2nd ed.). Burlington, MA: Jones and Bartlett Learning.

Lambrew, J. M., DeFriese, G. H., Carey, T. S., Ricketts, T. C., & Biddle, A. K. (1996). The effects of having a regular doctor on access to primary care. *Medical Care, 34*(2), 138–151.

Makaroun, L. K., Bowman, C., Duan, K., Handley, N., Wheeler, D. J., Pierluissi, E., & Chen, A. H. (2017). Specialty care access in the safety net—The role of public hospitals and health systems. *Journal of Health Care for the Poor and Underserved, 28(1),* 566–681. doi:10.1353/hpi.2017.0040

McGlynn, E. A., Asch, S. M., & Adams, J. (2003). The quality of health care delivered to adults in the United States. *New England Journal of Medicine, 348,* 2635–2645.

Mitra, A. (2016, June 24). *Why don't young doctors want to work in primary care?* Retrieved from http://sideeffectspublicmedia .org/post/why-dont-young-doctors-want-work-primary-care

National Association of Community Health Centers. (2018a, June). *Community health center chartbook.* Retrieved from http:// www.nachc.org/wp-content/uploads/2018/06/Chartbook _FINAL_6.20.18.pdf

National Association of Community Health Centers. (2018b, May). *Health centers and Medicaid.* Retrieved from http:// www.nachc.org/wp-content/uploads/2018/05/Medicaid _FS_5.15.18.pdf

National Conference of State Legislatures. (2017). *Improving access to care in rural and underserved communities: State workforce strategies.* Retrieved from http://www.ncsl.org/research /health/improving-access-to-care-in-rural-and-underserved -communities-state-workforce-strategies.aspx

National Rural Health Association. (n.d.). *About rural health care.* Retrieved from https://www.ruralhealthweb.org/about-nrha /about-rural-health-care

Newkirk, V., & Damico, A. (2014). *The Affordable Care Act and insurance coverage in rural areas.* Retrieved from https://www .kff.org/uninsured/issue-brief/the-affordable-care-act-and -insurance-coverage-in-rural-areas/

Office of Disease Prevention and Health Promotion. (n.d.). Healthy People 2020 homepage. Retrieved from https://www .healthypeople.gov/

Office of Minority Health. (n.d.). *The national CLAS standards.* Retrieved from https://minorityhealth.hhs.gov/omh/browse .aspx?lvl=2&lvlid=53

Organization for Economic Cooperation and Development. (2017). *Health at a glance 2017: OECD indicators.* Retrieved from http://dx.doi.org/10.1787/health_glance-2017-en

Orgera, K., & Artiga, S. (2018). *Disparities in health and health care: Five key questions and answers.* Retrieved from https:// www.kff.org/disparities-policy/issue-brief/disparities -in-health-and-health-care-five-key-questions-and-answers/

Osborne, R., Squires, D., Doty, M. M., Sarnak, D. O., & Schneider, E. C. (2016). In new survey of eleven countries, US adults still struggle with access to and affordability of health care. *Health Affairs, 35*(12). doi:10.1377/hlthaff.2016.1088

Papanicolas, I., Woskie, L. R., & Jha, A. K. (2018). Health care spending in the United States and other high-income countries. *New England Journal of Medicine, 319*(10), 1024 –1039. doi:10.1001/jama.2018.1150

Patient Protection and Affordable Care Act of 2010, 42 U.S.C. § 18001 (2010).

Pauly, M. V., & Pagán, J. A. (2007). Spillovers and vulnerability: The case of community uninsurance. *Health Affairs, 5,* 1304–1314. doi:10.1377/hlthaff.26.5.1304

Proser, M., Byshhe, T., Weaver, D., & Yee, R. (2015). Community health centers at the crossroads: Growth and staffing needs. *Journal of the American Academy of PAs, 28*(4), 49–53. doi:10.1097/01.JAA.0000460929.99918.e6

Public Health England. (n.d.). *About us.* Retrieved from https://www.gov.uk/government/organisations/public -health-england/about

Rosenbaum, S., Paradise, J., Markus, A., Sharac, J., Tran, C., Reynolds, D., & Shin, P. (2017). *Community health centers: Recent growth and the role of the ACA.* Retrieved from http:// files.kff.org/attachment/Issue-Brief-Community-Health -Centers-Recent-Growth-and-the-Role-of-the-ACA

Shi, L., & Singh, D. A. (2019). *Delivering health care in America: A systems approach* (7th ed.). Burlington, MA: Jones and Bartlett Learning.

Speaking Together. (2007). *Addressing language barriers in health care: What's at stake.* Retrieved from https://www .rwjf.org/content/dam/farm/reports/issue_briefs/2007 /rwjf30140

Starfield, B., & Shi, L. (2004). The medical home, access to care, and insurance: A review of evidence. *Pediatrics, 113,* 1493– 1498. doi:10.1542/peds.113.5.S1.1493

Thorlby, R., Arora, S., & Nuffield Trust. (n.d.). *The English health care system.* Retrieved from https://international .commonwealthfund.org/countries/england/

U.S. Census Bureau. (2011). *Income, poverty, and health insurance coverage in the United States: 2010* (Current Population Reports, P60-239). Washington, DC: U.S. Government Printing Office.

U.S. Census Bureau. (2017). *Health insurance coverage in the United States: 2016* (Current Population Reports, P60-260). Washington, DC: U.S. Government Printing Office.

U.S. Census Bureau. (2018). *Demographic turning points for the United States: Population projections from 2020 to 2016* (Current Population Reports, P25-1144). Washington, DC: U.S. Government Printing Office.

U.S. Department of Health and Human Services. (2015). *HHS action plan to reduce racial and ethnic health disparities: Implementation progress report 2011–2014.* Retrieved from https://aspe.hhs.gov/basic-report/hhs-action-plan-reduce-racial-and-ethnic-health-disparities-implementation-progress-report-2011-2014

Vaughn, B. T., DeVrieze, S. R., Reed, S. D., & Schulman, K. A. (2010). Can we close the income and wealth gap between specialists and primary care physicians? *Health Affairs, 29*(5), 933–940. doi:10.1377/hlthaff.2009.0675

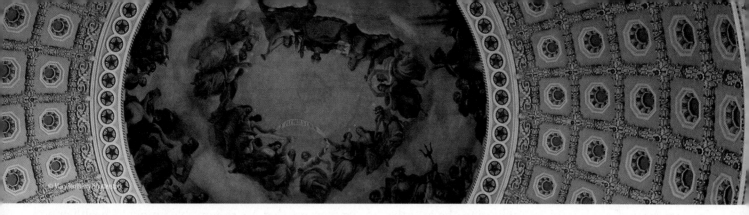

CHAPTER 5

Public Health Institutions and Systems

Richard Riegelman

LEARNING OBJECTIVES

By the end of this chapter you will be able to:

- Identify goals of governmental public health
- Identify the 10 essential services of public health
- Describe basic features of local, state, and federal public health agencies in the United States
- Identify global public health organizations and agencies and describe their basic roles
- Identify roles in public health for federal agencies not identified as health agencies
- Illustrate the need for collaboration by governmental public health agencies with other governmental and nongovernmental organizations
- Describe approaches to connecting public health and the healthcare system

▶ Introduction

The cases in **BOX 5-1** all reflect the responsibilities of public health agencies at the local, federal, and global levels. While they illustrate public health working the way it is supposed to work, this is of course not always the case. Let us start by taking a look at the goals and roles of public health agencies.

▶ What Are the Goals and Roles of Governmental Public Health Agencies?

Public health is often equated with the work of governmental agencies. The role of government is only a portion of what we mean by "public health," but it is an important component. It is so important, in fact, that we often define the roles of other components in terms of how they relate to the work of governmental public health agencies. That is, we may refer to them as nongovernmental public health.

In 1994, the U.S. Public Health Service put forth the Public Health in America statement, which provided the framework that continues to define the goals and services of governmental public health agencies (Centers for Disease Control and Prevention [CDC], 2018):

- To prevent epidemics and the spread of disease
- To protect against environmental hazards
- To prevent injuries
- To promote and encourage healthy behaviors

- To respond to disasters and assist communities in recovery
- To ensure the quality and accessibility of health services

These are ambitious and complicated goals to achieve. To achieve them, it is important to further define the roles that governmental public health agencies themselves play and, by implication, the roles that other governmental agencies and NGOs need to play.

The Public Health in America statement built upon a 1988 report by the Institute of Medicine (IOM; now called the Health and Medicine Division [HMD]) called *The Future of Public Health*. The IOM defined three core public health functions that governmental public health agencies need to perform. The concept of "core function" implies that the job cannot be delegated to other agencies or to NGOs. It also implies that the governmental public health agencies will work together to accomplish these functions, because as a group, they are responsible for public health as a whole; that is, no one agency at the local, state, or federal level is specifically or exclusively responsible for accomplishing the essential public health services.[a]

BOX 5-1 Vignette

A young man in your dormitory is diagnosed with tuberculosis. The health department works with the student health service to test everyone in the dorm, as well as in his classes, with a tuberculosis skin test. Those who are positive for the first time are advised to take a course of a medicine called INH. You ask, is this standard operating procedure?

You go to a public health meeting and learn that many of the speakers are not from public health agencies, but from the Departments of Labor, Commerce, Housing, and Education. You ask, what do these departments have to do with health?

You hear that a new childhood vaccine was developed by the National Institutes of Health (NIH), approved by the Food and Drug Administration (FDA), endorsed for federal payment by the Centers for Disease Control and Prevention (CDC), and recommended for use by the American Academy of Pediatrics. You ask, do all these agencies and organizations always work so well together?

A major flood in Asia leads to disease and starvation. Some say it is due to global warming, others to bad luck. Coordinated efforts by global health agencies, assisted by nongovernmental organizations (NGOs) and individual donors, help get the country back on its feet. You ask, what types of cooperation are needed to make all of this happen?

A local community health center identifies childhood obesity as a problem in the community. The center collects data demonstrating that the problem begins as early as elementary school. They develop a plan that includes clinical interventions at the health center and also at the elementary school. They ask the health department to help them organize an educational campaign and assist in evaluating the results. Working together, they are able to reduce the obesity rate among elementary school children by 50%. This seems like a new way to practice public health, you conclude. What type of approach is this?

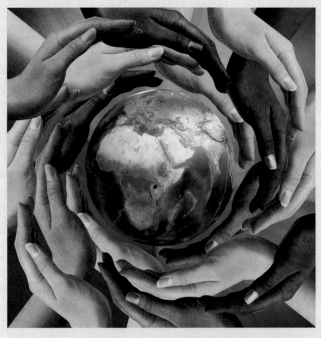

Source: © maxstockphoto/ShutterStock, Inc.

The core functions defined by the IOM are (1) assessment, (2) policy development, and (3) assurance (Institute of Medicine [IOM], 1988).

- Assessment includes obtaining data that define the health of the overall population and specific groups within the population, including defining the nature of new and persisting health problems.
- Policy development includes developing evidence-based recommendations and other analyses of options, such as health policy analysis, to guide implementation, including efforts to educate and mobilize community partnerships.
- Assurance includes governmental public health's oversight responsibility for ensuring that key components of an effective health system, including health care and public health, are in place even though the implementation will often be performed by others.

The three core functions, while useful in providing a delineation of responsibilities and an intellectual framework for the work of governmental public health agencies, were not tangible enough to provide a clear understanding or definition of the work of public health agencies. Thus, in addition to the goals of public health, the Public Health in America statement defined a series of 10 essential public health services that build upon the IOM's core functions, guide day-to-day responsibilities, and provide a mechanism for evaluating whether the core functions are fulfilled. These 10 services have come to define the responsibilities of the combined local, state, and federal governmental public health system.

▶ What Are the 10 Essential Public Health Services?

TABLE 5-1 outlines the 10 essential public health services and organizes them according to which IOM core function they aim to fulfill (CDC, 2018). A description of each service is presented in column 2, and examples of these essential services are listed in column 3.

TABLE 5-1 10 Essential Public Health Services

Essential Service	Meaning of Essential Service	Examples
Core function: assessment		
1. Monitor health status to identify and solve community health problems	This service includes accurate diagnosis of the community's health status; identification of threats to health and assessment of health service needs; timely collection, analysis, and publication of information on access, utilization, costs, and outcomes of personal health services; attention to the vital statistics and health status of specific groups that are at a higher risk than the total population; and collaboration to manage integrated information systems with private providers and health benefit plans.	Vital statistics Health surveys Surveillance, including reportable diseases
2. Diagnose and investigate health problems and health hazards in the community	This service includes epidemiologic identification of emerging health threats; public health laboratory capability using modern technology to conduct rapid screening and high-volume testing; active communicable disease epidemiology programs; and technical capacity for epidemiologic investigation of disease outbreaks and patterns of chronic disease and injury.	Epidemic investigations CDC–Epidemic Intelligence Service State public health laboratories
Core function: policy development		
3. Inform, educate, and empower people about health issues	This service includes social marketing and media communications; providing accessible health information resources at community levels; active collaboration with personal healthcare providers to reinforce health promotion messages and programs; and joint health education programs with schools, churches, and worksites.	Health education campaigns, such as comprehensive state tobacco programs

(continues)

TABLE 5-1 10 Essential Public Health Services   *(continued)*

Essential Service	Meaning of Essential Service	Examples
4. Mobilize community partnerships and action to identify and solve health problems	This service includes convening and facilitating community groups and associations, including those not typically considered to be health-related, in undertaking defined preventive, screening, rehabilitation, and support programs; and skilled coalition-building to draw upon the full range of potential human and material resources in the cause of community health.	Lead control programs: testing and follow-up of children, reduction of lead exposure, educational follow-up, and addressing underlying causes
5. Develop policies and plans that support individual and community health efforts	This service requires leadership development at all levels of public health; systematic community and state-level planning for health improvement in all jurisdictions; tracking of measurable health objectives as a part of continuous quality improvement strategies; joint evaluation with the medical/healthcare system to define consistent policy regarding prevention and treatment services; and development of codes, regulations, and legislation to guide public health practice.	Newborn screening and follow-up programs for PKU and other genetic and congenital diseases

Core function: assurance

6. Enforce laws and regulations that protect health and ensure safety	This service involves full enforcement of sanitary codes, especially in the food industry; full protection of drinking water supplies; enforcement of clean air standards; timely follow-up of hazards, preventable injuries, and exposure-related diseases identified in occupational and community settings; monitoring quality of medical services (e.g., laboratory, nursing home, home health care); and timely review of new drug, biologic, and medical device applications.	Local: Fluoridation and chlorination of water State: Regulation of nursing homes Federal: FDA drug approval and food safety
7. Link people to needed personal health services and ensure the provision of health care when otherwise unavailable	This service (often referred to as "outreach" or "enabling" services) includes ensuring effective entry for socially disadvantaged people into a coordinated system of clinical care; culturally and linguistically appropriate materials and staff to ensure linkage to services for special population groups; ongoing "care management"; and transportation.	Community health centers
8. Ensure the provision of a competent public and personal healthcare workforce	This service includes education and training for personnel to meet the needs of public and personal health services; efficient processes for licensure of professionals and certification of facilities with regular verification and inspection follow-up; adoption of continuous quality improvement and lifelong learning within all licensure and certification programs; active partnerships with professional training programs to ensure community-relevant learning experiences for all students; and continuing education in management and leadership development programs for those charged with administrative/executive roles.	Licensure of physicians, nurses, and other health professionals

9. Evaluate effectiveness, accessibility, and quality of personal and population-based health services	This service calls for ongoing evaluation of health programs, based on analysis of health status and service utilization data, to assess program effectiveness and to provide information necessary for allocating resources and reshaping programs.	Development of evidence-based recommendations
All three IOM core functions		
10. Research for new insights and innovative solutions to health problems	This service includes continuous linkage with appropriate institutions of higher learning and research and an internal capacity to mount timely epidemiologic and economic analyses and conduct needed health services research.	NIH, CDC, AHRQ, other federal agencies

Abbreviations: Agency for Healthcare Research and Quality = AHRQ; Centers for Disease Control and Prevention = CDC; Food and Drug Administration = FDA; National Institutes of Health = NIH; phenylketonuria = PKU.

Source: Data from Public Health in America. Essential public health services. Retrieved from http://www.cdc.gov/nphpsp/ essentialservices.html. Accessed October 26, 2015.

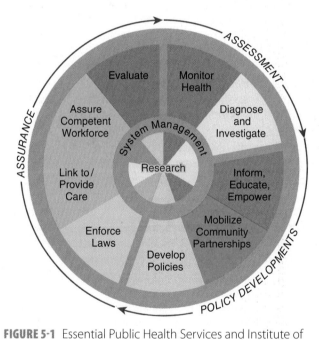

FIGURE 5-1 Essential Public Health Services and Institute of Medicine's Core Functions

Source: Centers for Disease Control and Prevention. (2017). The public health system & the 10 essential public health services. Retrieved from https://www.cdc.gov/stltpublichealth/publichealthservices/essentialhealthservices.html

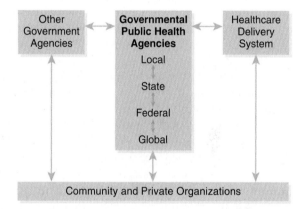

FIGURE 5-2 Framework for Viewing Governmental Public Health Agencies and Their Complicated Connections

FIGURE 5-1 then combines the core functions of public health with the essential services of public health agencies so that you can see the connections.

Public health services are delivered through a complex web of local and federal agencies, as well as through increasing involvement from global organizations. What follows is a description of the work of public health agencies at each of these levels.

FIGURE 5-2 provides a framework to guide our review of the delivery of public health services.

It diagrams the central role of governmental public health agencies and the complicated connections required to accomplish their responsibilities. We begin by taking a look at the structure and function of governmental public health agencies at the local/ state, federal, and global levels. We then examine the key connections with other governmental agencies, community organizations, and private organizations, and finally the connections with the healthcare delivery system.

▶ What Are the Roles of Local and State Public Health Agencies?

The U.S. Constitution does not mention public health. Because public health is not a delineated federal responsibility, it is an authority retained by the states. States may retain their authority, voluntarily request or accept help from the federal government, or delegate their responsibility and/or authority to local agencies at the city, county, or other local levels.[b]

BOX 5-2 briefly describes the history of public health agencies in the United States. It is a complex history and has resulted in more structures than there are states—more because large cities often have their own public health systems (Turnock, 2009). In addition, the District of Columbia and several U.S. territories have their own systems and often have the authority to make public health system decisions as if they were states.

To understand the role of local health departments, it is useful to think of two models (Turnock, 2007). In the first model, which we will call the "home rule" or "local autonomy" model, authority is delegated from the state to the local health department. The local health department, or the local government, has a great deal of autonomy in setting its own structure and function and often raising its own funding.

BOX 5-2 Brief History of Public Health Agencies in the United States

An understanding of the history of U.S. public health institutions requires an understanding of the response of local, state, and federal governments to public health crises and the complex interactions among these levels of government.

The colonial period in the United States saw repeated epidemics of smallpox, cholera, and yellow fever, primarily focused in the port cities. These epidemics brought fear and disruption of commerce, along with accompanying disease and death. One epidemic in 1793 in Philadelphia, which was then the nation's capital, nearly shut down the federal government. These early public health crises brought about the first municipal boards of health, made up of respected citizens authorized to act in the community's interest to implement quarantine, evacuation, and other public health interventions of the day. The federal government's early role in combating epidemics led to the establishment in 1798 of what later became known as the U.S. Public Health Service.

Major changes in public health occurred in the last half of the 1800s, with the great expansion of the understanding of disease and the ability to control it through community actions. The Shattuck Commission in Massachusetts in 1850 outlined the roles of state health departments as responsible for sanitary inspections, communicable disease control, food sanitation, vital statistics, and services for infants and children. Over the next 50 years, the states gradually took the lead in developing public health institutions based on delivery of these services.

Local health departments did not exist outside of the largest cities until the 1900s. The Rockefeller Foundation stimulated and helped fund early local health departments and campaigns, in part to combat specific diseases, such as hookworm. There was no standard model for local health departments; they developed in different ways in the various states and were chronically underfunded.

The federal government played a very small role in public health throughout the 1800s and well into the 20th century. However, an occasional public health crisis stimulated federal action, often as a result of media attention. The founding of the FDA in 1906 resulted in large part from the journalistic activity known as "muckraking," which exposed the status of food and drug safety. The early years of the 1900s set the stage for expansion of the federal government's role in public health through the passage of the 16th Amendment to the Constitution, which authorized federal income tax as a major source of federal government funding.

The Great Depression, in general, and the Social Security Act of 1935, in particular, brought about a new era in which federal funding became a major source of financial resources for state and local public health departments and NGOs. The founding of the CDC (which at that time stood for Communicable Disease Center) in 1946 led to a national (and eventually international) leadership role for the CDC, which attempts to connect and hold together the complex local, state, and federal public health efforts and integrate them into global public health efforts.

The Johnson administration's War on Poverty, as well as the Medicare and Medicaid programs, brought about greatly expanded funding for healthcare services and led many health departments to provide direct healthcare services, especially for those without other sources of care. The late 1980s and 1990s saw a redefinition of the roles of governmental public health, including the IOM definition of core functions and the development of the 10 essential public health services. These documents have guided the development of a broad population focus for public health and a move away from the direct provision of healthcare services by health departments.

The terrorism of September 11, 2001, and the subsequent anthrax scare moved public health institutions to the center of efforts to protect the public's health through emergency response and disaster preparedness. The development of flexible efforts to respond to expected and unexpected hazards is now a central feature of public health institutions' roles and funding. The success of these efforts has led to new levels of coordination of local, state, federal, and global public health agencies using state-of-the-art surveillance, laboratory technology, and communications systems.

In the second model, which we will call the "branch office" model, the local health department can be viewed as a branch office of the state agency, with little or no independent authority or funding. There are several thousand local health departments across the country. The majority of these lie somewhere in between these two extreme models; however, these models provide a framework for understanding the many varieties of department structures. Thus, when we speak of local public health, we may be speaking of a state agency with branch offices or a relatively independent local agency. Regardless of which model a state uses, many public health responsibilities of local public health departments are quite similar, and they usually have authority and responsibility for at least the following (Turnock, 2007):

- Immunizations for those individuals not covered by the private health insurance system
- Communicable disease surveillance and initial investigation of outbreaks
- Communicable disease control, often including at a minimum tuberculosis and syphilis case finding and treatment
- Inspection and licensing of restaurants
- Environmental health surveillance
- Coordination of public health screening programs, including newborn and lead screenings
- Tobacco control programs
- Public health preparedness and response to disasters

Health departments in many parts of the United States also serve as the healthcare provider for those without other sources of health care. This function is generally referred to as the healthcare safety net. In recent years, many health departments have reduced or discontinued these services, often transferring them to the healthcare system or integrating their efforts into community health centers. The concept of core functions holds that while these activities can be performed by other organizations or agencies, the public health agencies retain responsibility for ensuring access to and the quality of these services.

The work of local public health agencies cannot be viewed in isolation. The state health department usually retains important roles even in those states where the local departments have home rule authority. These responsibilities often include collecting vital statistics, running a public health laboratory, licensing health professionals, administering nutrition programs, and regulating health facilities, such as nursing homes. In addition, drinking water regulation, administration of the state Medicaid program, and the office of the medical examiner may also fall under the authority of the state health department.

The 2003 IOM report *The Future of the Public's Health in the 21st Century*, in conjunction with the Futures Initiative of the CDC, initiated the establishment of a voluntary national accreditation program for state and local health departments to advance quality and performance in health departments. Through these efforts, the Public Health Accreditation Board was formed, and in early 2013, the first set of health departments achieved national accreditation. The accreditation standards and measures address each of the 10 essential public health services to evaluate health department processes and services and their outcomes (Public Health Accreditation Board, 2013).

Today, the federal government has a great deal of involvement in national and global issues of public health and often works closely with local agencies. We now turn to a discussion of the structure and role of the federal government in public health.

▶ What Are the Roles of Federal Public Health Agencies?

The federal government's role in public health does not explicitly appear in the U.S. Constitution. It has been justified largely by that document's Interstate Commerce clause, which provides federal government authority to regulate commerce between the states. Federal public health authority often rests on the voluntary acceptance by the states of funding provided by the federal government. The federal government may require that states take certain actions to qualify for the funding.

The Department of Health and Human Services (HHS) is the central public health agency of the federal government. It includes operating agencies, each of which reports directly to the cabinet-level secretary of HHS. **TABLE 5-2** outlines most of these agencies, their roles and authority, and their basic public health structure and activities (U.S. Department of Health and Human Services, 2017).

The NIH, one of the larger agencies within HHS, is devoted to basic science research and the translation of research into clinical practice. Some of the other federal health agencies, such as the Health Resources and Services Administration, the Substance Abuse and Mental Health Services Administration, and the Indian Health Service, provide or fund individually oriented health services in addition to population-oriented preventive services. The Indian Health Service is unique because it is responsible for both public health and healthcare services for a defined population.

TABLE 5-2 Key Federal Health Agencies of the Department of Health and Human Services

Agency	Roles/Authority	Examples of Structures/Activities
Centers for Disease Control and Prevention (CDC) and the Agency for Toxic Substances and Disease Registry (ATSDR)	The CDC is the lead agency for prevention, health data, epidemic investigation, and public health measures aimed at disease control and prevention. The CDC administers the ATSDR, which works with the Environmental Protection Agency to provide guidance on health hazards of toxic exposures.	The CDC and ATSDR work extensively with state and local health departments. The CDC's Epidemic Intelligence Service functions domestically and internationally at the request of governments.
National Institutes of Health (NIH)	Serves as lead research agency; also funds training programs and communication of health information to the professional community and the public.	NIH comprises 17 institutes in all—the largest being the National Cancer Institute. The National Library of Medicine is part of NIH Centers, which also include the John E. Fogarty International Center for Advanced Study in the Health Sciences. NIH is the world's largest biomedical research enterprise, with intramural research at NIH and extramural research grants throughout the world.
Food and Drug Administration (FDA)	Acts as consumer protection agency with authority for safety of foods and safety and efficacy of drugs, vaccines, and other medical and public health interventions.	Divisions of FDA are responsible for food safety, medical devices, drug efficacy, and safety pre- and post-approval.
Health Resources and Services Administration (HRSA)	Seeks to ensure equitable access to comprehensive quality health care.	HRSA funds community health centers, HIV/AIDS services, and scholarships for health professional students.
Agency for Healthcare Research and Quality (AHRQ)	Sets research agenda to improve the outcomes and quality of health care, including patient safety and access to services.	AHRQ supports U.S. Preventive Services Task Force, evidence-based medicine research, and Guidelines Clearinghouse.
Substance Abuse and Mental Health Services Administration (SAMHSA)	Works to improve quality and availability of prevention, treatment, and rehabilitation for substance abuse and mental illness.	SAMHSA provides research, data collection, and funding of local services.
Indian Health Service (IHS)	Provides direct health care and public health services to federally recognized tribes.	IHS provides services to approximately 550 federally recognized tribes in 35 states. It is the only comprehensive federal agency responsibility for health care plus public health services.

The CDC is perhaps the agency most closely identified with public health at the federal level. **BOX 5-3** describes its first 50 years, from 1946 to 1996, in a reprint of its official history first published in the *Morbidity and Mortality Weekly Report* (*MMWR*), a weekly publication of the agency (CDC, 1996). Today, the CDC is a global partner in conducting research and epidemiologic investigations in addition to working closely with states to monitor and prevent disease through health surveillance, taking an

BOX 5-3 History of the CDC

The following is reprinted as it originally appeared in 1996 in the Morbidity and Mortality Weekly Report *(CDC, 1996):*

The Communicable Disease Center was organized in Atlanta, Georgia, on July 1, 1946; its founder, Dr. Joseph W. Mountin, was a visionary public health leader who had high hopes for this small and comparatively insignificant branch of the Public Health Service (PHS). It occupied only one floor of the Volunteer Building on Peachtree Street and had fewer than 400 employees, most of whom were engineers and entomologists. Until the previous day, they had worked for Malaria Control in War Areas, the predecessor of CDC, which had successfully kept the southeastern states malaria-free during World War II and, for approximately 1 year, from murine typhus fever. The new institution would expand its interests to include all communicable diseases and would be the servant of the states, providing practical help whenever called.

Distinguished scientists soon filled CDC's laboratories, and many states and foreign countries sent their public health staffs to Atlanta for training. Medical epidemiologists were scarce, and it was not until 1949 that Dr. Alexander Langmuir arrived to head the epidemiology branch. Within months, he launched the first-ever disease surveillance program, which confirmed his suspicion that malaria, on which CDC spent the largest portion of its budget, had long since disappeared. Subsequently, disease surveillance became the cornerstone on which CDC's mission of service to the states was built and, in time, changed the practice of public health.

The outbreak of the Korean War in 1950 was the impetus for creating CDC's Epidemic Intelligence Service (EIS). The threat of biological warfare loomed, and Dr. Langmuir, the most knowledgeable person in PHS about this then-arcane subject, saw an opportunity to train epidemiologists who would guard against ordinary threats to public health while watching out for alien germs. The first class of EIS officers arrived in Atlanta for training in 1951 and pledged to go wherever they were called for the next 2 years. These "disease detectives" quickly gained fame for "shoe-leather epidemiology," through which they ferreted out the cause of disease outbreaks.

The survival of CDC as an institution was not at all certain in the 1950s. In 1947, Emory University gave land on Clifton Road for a headquarters, but construction did not begin for more than a decade. PHS was so intent on research and the rapid growth of the National Institutes of Health that it showed little interest in what happened in Atlanta. Congress, despite the long delay in appropriating money for new buildings, was much more receptive to CDC's pleas for support than either PHS or the Bureau of the Budget.

Two major health crises in the mid-1950s established CDC's credibility and ensured its survival. In 1955, when poliomyelitis appeared in children who had received the recently approved Salk vaccine, the national inoculation program was stopped. The cases were traced to contaminated vaccine from a laboratory in California; the problem was corrected, and the inoculation program, at least for first and second graders, was resumed. The resistance of these 6- and 7-year-olds to polio, compared with that of older children, proved the effectiveness of the vaccine. Two years later, surveillance was used again to trace the course of a massive influenza epidemic. From the data gathered in 1957 and subsequent years, the national guidelines for influenza vaccine were developed.

CDC grew by acquisition. When CDC joined the international malaria-eradication program and accepted responsibility for protecting the earth from moon germs and vice versa, CDC's mission stretched overseas and into space.

CDC then played a key role in one of the greatest triumphs of public health: the eradication of smallpox. In 1962 it established a smallpox surveillance unit, and a year later tested a newly developed jet gun and vaccine in the Pacific island nation of Tonga. CDC also achieved notable success at home tracking new and mysterious disease outbreaks. In the mid-1970s and early 1980s, it found the cause of Legionnaires disease and toxic-shock syndrome. A fatal disease, subsequently named acquired immunodeficiency syndrome (AIDS), was first mentioned in the June 5, 1981, issue of *MMWR*.

Although CDC succeeded more often than it failed, it did not escape criticism. For example, television and press reports about the Tuskegee study on long-term effects of untreated syphilis in black men created a storm of protest in 1972. This study had been initiated by PHS and other organizations in 1932 and was transferred to CDC in 1957. Although the effectiveness of penicillin as a therapy for syphilis had been established during the late 1940s, participants in this study remained untreated until the study was brought to public attention. CDC was also criticized because of the 1976 effort to vaccinate the U.S. population against swine flu, the infamous killer of 1918–1919. When some recipients of the vaccines developed Guillain-Barre syndrome, the campaign was stopped immediately; the epidemic never occurred.

As the scope of CDC's activities expanded far beyond communicable diseases, its name had to be changed. In 1970 it became the Center for Disease Control and in 1981, after extensive reorganization, Center became Centers. The words "and Prevention" were added in 1992 but, by law, the well-known three-letter acronym was retained. In health emergencies, CDC means an answer to SOS calls from anywhere in the world, such as the recent one from Zaire where Ebola fever raged.

Fifty years ago, CDC's agenda was non-controversial (hardly anyone objected to the pursuit of germs), and Atlanta was a backwater. In 1996, CDC's programs are often tied to economic, political, and social issues, and Atlanta is as near to Washington as the tap of a keyboard.

Source: Reproduced from Centers for Disease Control and Prevention, *MMWR* 1996;45: 526–528.

action-oriented approach to disease prevention, and maintaining health statistics through the National Center for Health Statistics, which has been a part of the CDC since 1987.

The CDC's role in connecting federal, state, and local governmental public health efforts is central to the success of the system. Approximately half of the CDC's over $10 billion total budget is channeled to state and local health departments. A key function of the CDC is to provide national leadership and to coordinate the efforts of local/state and federal public health agencies.

To understand the local/state and federal public health system, it is important to appreciate that less than 5% of all health-related expenditures in the United States goes to governmental public health agencies, and of that, less than half goes to population-based prevention (as opposed to providing safety net healthcare services to individuals). In addition, the role of governmental public health is limited by social attitudes toward government. For instance, there are constitutional limitations on the authority of public health and other government agencies to impose actions on individuals. These may limit public health agencies' abilities to address issues ranging from tuberculosis and HIV control to responses to emergencies.

The social attitudes of Americans may also limit the authority and resources provided to public health agencies. Americans often favor individual or private efforts over governmental interventions when they believe that individuals and private organizations are capable of success. For instance, some Americans resist active efforts in schools to provide information and access to contraceptives, while others resist the type of case-finding efforts for HIV/AIDS that have been used successfully in investigating and controlling other communicable diseases.

Today, governmental public health is a global enterprise. As a result, we now turn to a discussion of the roles of global health organizations and agencies.

▶ What Are the Roles of Global Health Organizations and Agencies?

Public health is increasingly becoming a global undertaking. Global governmental efforts have grown dramatically in recent years. The World Health Organization (WHO), created in 1948, has become decidedly more prominent in the 2000s with the increasing importance of global health issues. WHO is a part of the United Nations organizations, which also include the United Nations International Children's Emergency Fund (UNICEF) and the Joint United Nations Programme on HIV/AIDS (UNAIDS).

Today, the World Bank and other multilateral financial institutions are the largest funding source for global health efforts (World Bank, 2018). National governmental aid programs, including the U.S. Agency for International Development (USAID), also play an important role in public health. **TABLE 5-3** outlines the

TABLE 5-3 Global Public Health Organizations

Type of Agency	Structure/Governance	Role(s)	Limitations
World Health Organization	United Nations Organization Seven "regional" semi-independent components (e.g., Pan American Health Organization covers North and South America)	Policy development (e.g., tobacco treaty, epidemic control policies) Coordination of services (e.g., SARS control) Vaccine development Data collection and standardization (e.g., measures of healthcare quality, measures of health status)	Limited ability to enforce global recommendations, limited funding, and complex international administration
Other UN agencies with focused agenda	UNICEF UNAIDS	Focus on childhood vaccinations Focus on AIDS	Limited agendas and limited financing

International financing organizations	The World Bank Other multilateral regional banks (e.g., InterAmerican and Asian Development Banks)	World Bank is largest international funder. Increasingly supports "human capital" projects and reform of healthcare delivery systems and population and nutrition efforts Provides funding and technical assistance, primarily as loans	Criticized for standardized approach with few local modifications
Bilateral governmental aid organizations	USAID Many other developed countries have their own organizations and contribute a higher percentage of their gross domestic product to those agencies than does the United States	Often focused on specific countries and specific types of programs (e.g., the focus on HIV/AIDS in the United States), and maternal and child health	May be tied to domestic politics and global economic, political, or military agendas

Abbreviations: AIDS = acquired immunodeficiency syndrome; HIV = human immunodeficiency virus; SARS = severe acute respiratory syndrome; UN = United Nations; UNAIDS = Joint United Nations Programme on HIV/AIDS; UNICEF = United Nations International Children's Emergency Fund; USAID = U.S. Agency for International Development.

structure/governance, roles, and limitations of global public health agencies.

The complexity of local, state, federal, and global public health agencies raises the question of whether these agencies can and do work together. It should not surprise you that close collaboration, while the goal, is often difficult to achieve with so many organizations involved. Thus, it is important to ask: How can public health agencies work together?

▶ How Can Public Health Agencies Work Together?

Coordination among just local, state, and federal public health agencies has been a major challenge. Increasingly, coordination also requires a global aspect. Efforts toward efficient collaboration, on all levels, have a long way to go. There are signs of hope with progress in such fields as tobacco control, food safety, and the response to severe acute respiratory syndrome (SARS). **BOX 5-4** discusses the dramatic events of the 2003 SARS epidemic, providing an example of what can be done and what needs to be done to address future public health emergencies (Duffin & Sweetman, 2006).

Collaboration needs to be an everyday effort, not just a requirement for emergencies or epidemics. Let us look at the relationships and needed collaboration among governmental public health and other governmental agencies, NGOs, and the healthcare delivery system.

▶ What Other Government Agencies Are Involved in Health Issues?

To address the full range of issues that affect population health, it is important to recognize the important roles that government agencies not designated as health agencies play in public health. Such agencies exist at the local/state, federal, and global levels. To illustrate the involvement of these agencies in health issues, let us begin with the roles of non-health agencies at the federal level.

A number of federal agencies serve public health functions even though they are not defined as health agencies. The roles they play are important, especially when we take the population health perspective, which includes the totality of efforts to promote and protect health and prevent disease, disability, and death.

Environmental health issues are an important part of the role of the Environmental Protection Agency. Reducing injury and hazardous exposures in the workplace are key goals of the Occupational Safety and Health Administration, which is part of the Department of Labor.

Protecting health as part of preparation and response to disasters and terrorism is central to the role of the Department of Homeland Security. The Department of Agriculture shares with the FDA the role of protecting the nation's food supply. The Department of Housing and Urban Development influences the built environment and its impacts on health. The Department of Energy plays important roles in setting

---

BOX 5-4   SARS and the Public Health Response

The SARS epidemic of 2003 began with little notice, most likely somewhere in the heartland of China, and then spread to other areas of Asia. The world took notice following televised reports of public health researchers who were sent to Asia to investigate the illness subsequently contracting and dying from the disease. Not an easily transmissible disease except for between those in very close contact, such as investigators, family members, and healthcare providers, the disease spread slowly but steadily through areas of China. Among those infected, the case-fatality rate was very high, especially without the benefits of modern intensive care facilities.

The disease did not respond to antibiotics and was thought to be a viral disease by its epidemiologic pattern of spread and transmission, but at first, no cause was known. The outside world soon felt the impact of the brewing epidemic when cases appeared in Hong Kong that could be traced to a traveler from mainland China. Fear spread when cases were recognized that could not be explained by close personal contact with a SARS victim.

The epidemic continued to spread, jumping thousands of miles to Toronto, Canada, where the second-greatest concentration of disease appeared. Soon, the whole world was on high alert, if not quite on the verge of panic. At least 8,000 people worldwide became sick, and nearly 10% of them died. Fortunately, progress came quite quickly. Researchers coordinated by WHO were able to put together the epidemiologic information and laboratory data and establish a presumed cause—a new form of the coronavirus never before seen in humans—leading to the rapid introduction of testing.

WHO and the CDC put forth recommendations for isolation, travel restrictions, and intensive monitoring that rapidly controlled the disease, even in the absence of an effective treatment aimed at a cure. SARS disappeared as rapidly as it emerged, especially after systematic efforts to control spread were put in place in China. Not eliminated, but no longer a worldwide threat, SARS left a lasting global impact. WHO established new approaches for reporting and responding to epidemics, which now have the widespread formal acceptance of most governments.

Once the world could step back and evaluate what happened, it was recognized that the potential burden of disease posed by the SARS epidemic had worldwide implications and raised the threat of interruption of travel and trade. Local, national, and global public health agencies collaborated quickly and effectively. Infection control recommendations made at the global level were rapidly translated into efforts to identify disease at the local level and manage individual patients in hospitals throughout the world. It is a model of communicable disease control that will be needed in the future.

---

radiation safety standards for nuclear power plants and other sources of energy.

When multiple federal agencies are involved in health-related matters, coordination and collaboration are required across agencies. This interaction is certainly important when it comes to food safety and disaster planning and response. It is also key for efforts to address problems that cut across agencies, such as childhood lead exposure or efforts to reduce the environmental causes of asthma.

The collaboration needed to address complex public health issues lends itself to a "health in all policies" approach, which acknowledges that the variety of influences impacting population health are outside the control of the health sector. Collaborative efforts are not restricted to governmental agencies. We will now explore the roles of NGOs in public health.

▶ What Roles Do NGOs Play in Public Health?

Nongovernmental Organizations

NGOs play increasingly important roles in public health in the United States and around the world. In the United States, there is a long tradition of private

groups organizing to advocate for public health causes, delivering public health services, and providing funding to support public health efforts. In recent years, these efforts have been expanding globally as well.

The American Red Cross and its network of international affiliates represent a major international effort to provide public health services. The organization plays a central role in obtaining volunteers for blood donations and ensuring the safety and effectiveness of the U.S. and world supply of blood products in collaboration with the FDA. The ability of the Red Cross to obtain donations, mobilize volunteers, and publicize the need for disaster assistance has allowed it to play a central role in providing lifesaving public health services.

Many private organizations provide public health education, support research, develop evidence-based recommendations, and provide other public health services. Many of these organizations are organized around specific diseases or types of disease, such as the American Cancer Association, the American Heart Association, the American Lung Association, and the March of Dimes, which today focuses on birth defects. Other private organizations focus primarily on advocacy for individuals with specific diseases, but these organizations also may advocate for specific public health interventions. For instance, Mothers Against Drunk Driving has had a major impact on the passage and enforcement of drunk-driving laws. HIV/AIDS advocacy groups have influenced policies on confidentiality, funding, and public education.

Globally, NGOs increasingly play a key role in providing services and advocating for public health policies. CARE and Oxfam International are examples of the types of organizations involved in global health-related crises. Physician groups, including Physicians for Social Responsibility and Doctors Without Borders, have been active in advocating for public health efforts, seeking funding for public health needs, and addressing the ethical implementation of public health programs.

New combinations of governmental and NGOs are increasingly developing to fill in the gaps. At the global level, the Global Fund to Fight AIDS, Tuberculosis, and Malaria, which is a public–private effort, provides funding for evidence-based interventions to address these diseases. It is funded not only by governments, but also by private foundations, such as the Bill and Melinda Gates Foundation.

Private foundations have long played major roles in both funding public health efforts and stimulating governmental funding. The Rockefeller Foundation's efforts were instrumental in developing local health departments and initiating schools of public health in the United States during the early years of the 1900s. The Kellogg Foundation, the Robert Wood Johnson Foundation, and most recently the Gates Foundation have all played key roles in advancing public health efforts in areas ranging from nutrition to tobacco control to the advancement of new public health technologies.

Foundation funding has been the catalyst in initiating new funding efforts and sustaining those that are not adequately funded by governments. They cannot be expected, however, to provide long-term support for basic public health services. Thus, additional strategies are required. One key strategy is to link public health efforts with the efforts of healthcare professionals and the healthcare system.

▶ How Can Public Health Agencies Partner With Health Care to Improve the Response to Health Problems?

Clinicians and public health professionals increasingly share a common commitment to evidence-based thinking, cost-effective delivery of services, and computerized and confidential data systems. They also increasingly share a commitment to provide quality services to the entire population and eliminate health disparities. The potential for successful collaboration between public health and health care is illustrated by the National Vaccine Plan, which is discussed in **BOX 5-5** (IOM, 2008).

BOX 5-5 National Vaccine Plan

In 1994, a National Vaccine Plan was developed as part of a coordinated effort to accomplish the following goals:

1. Develop new and improved vaccines.
2. Ensure the optimal safety and effectiveness of vaccines and immunizations.
3. Better educate the public and members of the health profession on the benefits and risks of immunizations.

A recent IOM report evaluated progress since 1994 on achieving these goals and made recommendations for the development of a revised National Vaccine Plan (IOM, 2008). The IOM highlighted a number of successes since 1994 in achieving each of the goals of the plan. These successes illustrate the potential for improved collaboration between public health systems and healthcare systems.

In terms of the development of new and improved vaccines since 1994, over 20 new vaccine products resulting from the collaborative efforts of the NIH, academicians, and industry researchers were approved by the FDA. Novel vaccines introduced include vaccines against pediatric pneumococcal disease, meningococcal disease, and the human papillomavirus—a cause of cervical cancer.

In terms of safety, vaccines and vaccination approaches with improved safety have been developed since 1994, including those directed against rotavirus, pertussis (whooping cough), and polio. The FDA Center for Biologics Evaluation and Research, which regulates vaccines, now has an expanded array of regulatory tools to facilitate the review and approval of safe and efficacious vaccines. The FDA and the CDC have collaborated on surveillance for and evaluation of adverse events. Efforts have also been made to increase collaboration with the Centers for Medicare and Medicaid Services, the Department of Defense, and the Department of Veterans Affairs to improve surveillance and reporting of adverse events following immunization in the adult populations these agencies serve.

In terms of better education of health professionals and the public, progress has also been made. The American Academy of Pediatrics collaborates with the CDC for its childhood immunization support. The American Medical

(continues)

BOX 5-5 National Vaccine Plan *(continued)*

Association cosponsors the annual National Influenza Vaccine Summit, a group that represents 100 public and private organizations interested in preventing influenza.

Despite the growing collaboration and success in vaccine development and use, new issues have appeared in recent years. Vaccines are now correctly viewed by health professionals and the broader public as having both benefits and harms. In recent years, the public has grown more concerned about the safety of vaccines, including the issue of the use of large numbers of vaccines in children. The limitations of vaccines to address problems, such as HIV/AIDS, have also been increasingly recognized. Hopefully, the continued efforts to develop and implement national vaccine plans will build upon these recent successes and address the new realities and opportunities.

BOX 5-6 Community-Oriented Primary Care

Community-oriented primary care (COPC) is a structured effort to expand the delivery of health services from a focus on the individual to include an additional focus on the needs of communities. Serving the needs of communities brings healthcare and public health efforts together. COPC can be seen as an effort on the part of healthcare delivery sites, such as community health centers, to reach out to their community and to governmental public health institutions.

TABLE 5-4 outlines the six steps in the COPC process and presents a question to ask when addressing each of these steps. Notice the parallels between COPC and the evidence-based approach.

A series of principles underlies COPC:

- Healthcare needs are defined by examining the community as a whole, not just those who seek care.
- Needed healthcare services are provided to everyone within a defined population or community.
- Preventive, curative, and rehabilitative care are integrated within a coordinated delivery system.
- Members of the community directly participate in all stages of the COPC process.

The concept of COPC, if not the specific structure, has been widely accepted as an approach for connecting the organized delivery of primary health care with public health. It implies that public health issues can and should be addressed, when possible, at the level of the community with the involvement of healthcare providers and the community members themselves.

TABLE 5-4 The Six Sequential Steps of Community-Oriented Primary Care

Steps in the COPC Process	Questions to Ask
1. Community definition	How is the community defined based on geography, institutional affiliation, or other common characteristics (e.g., use of an Internet site)?
2. Community characterization	What are the demographic and health characteristics of the community, and what are its health issues?
3. Prioritization	What are the most important health issues facing the community, and how should they be prioritized based on objective data and perceived need?
4. Detailed assessment of the selected health problem	What are the most effective and efficient interventions for addressing the selected health problem based on an evidence-based assessment?
5. Intervention	What strategies will be used to implement the intervention?
6. Evaluation	How can the success of the intervention be evaluated?

Data from Mullan, F., & Epstein, L. (2002). Community-oriented primary care: New relevance in a changing world. *American Journal of Public Health*, 92(11), 1748–1755.

In the mid-1990s, the Medicine–Public Health Initiative was implemented to investigate better ways to connect public health with medicine, in particular, and health care, in general. Connecting these two fields has not always been easy or yielded successful results. Additional structures are needed to formalize effective and efficient bonds. Models do exist and new ideas are being put forth to connect clinical care and public health. **BOX 5-6** discusses one such model, called community-oriented primary care (COPC) (Gofin & Gofin, 2011).

Despite efforts in the healthcare system to reach out to the community and address public health issues (such as COPC), it remains the primary responsibility of governmental public health to organize and mobilize community-based efforts. Working with NGOs and healthcare professionals and organizations is imperative to effectively and efficiently accomplish the goals of public health. But how exactly can public health agencies accomplish these goals?

▶ How Can Public Health Take the Lead in Mobilizing Community Partnerships to Identify and Solve Health Problems?

An essential service of public health is the mobilization of community partnerships and action to identify and solve health problems. These efforts by public health agencies are critical to putting the pieces of the health system together to protect and promote health and prevent disability and death.

Increasingly, community members themselves are becoming active participants in addressing health and disease in their communities. One approach to engage community members in the process is through community-based participatory research (CBPR). Through CBPR, community members are involved in all phases of the research process, contributing their expertise while sharing ownership and responsibility over the research, and assisting to build trust, knowledge, and skill to facilitate the research and development and implementation of interventions.

Examples of successful collaboration include state tobacco control programs that have been led by public health agencies but rely heavily on NGOs, healthcare professionals, and other governmental agencies. These efforts have substantially reduced statewide cigarette smoking rates.

Efforts to organize coordinated programs for lead control have also been met with success. Collaborative efforts between public health and health care have identified and treated children with elevated lead levels. Cooperation with other agencies has provided for the removal of lead paint from homes and testing and control of lead in playgrounds, water, and, most recently, toys.

It is possible to view the coordinated mobilization of public and private efforts as community-oriented public health (COPH). We can see this as a parallel to COPC. In COPC, healthcare efforts are expanded to take on additional public health roles. In COPH, public health efforts are expanded to collaborate with healthcare delivery institutions, as well as other community and other governmental efforts. Child oral health, an example of COPH, is illustrated in **BOX 5-7**.

Developing community partnerships is a time-consuming and highly political process that requires great leadership and diplomatic skills. Central authority and command and control approaches are generally not effective in the complex organizational structures of the United States. New approaches and new strategies are needed to bring together the organizations and individuals who can get the job done.

BOX 5-7 Child Oral Health and Community-Oriented Public Health

The problem of childhood dental disease illustrates the potential for COPH. A lack of regular dental care remains a major problem for children in developed, as well as developing, countries. Oral health is often high on the agenda of parents, teachers, and even the children themselves.

The history of public health interventions in childhood oral health is a story of great hope and partial success. Public health efforts to improve oral health go back to the late 1800s and early 1900s, when toothbrushes and toothpaste were new and improved technologies. The public health campaigns of the early 1900s were very instrumental in making

(continues)

BOX 5-7 Child Oral Health and Community-Oriented Public Health   *(continued)*

toothbrushing a routine part of life in the United States. Unfortunately, the fluoridization of drinking water, despite the well-grounded evidence of its benefits, has not been so readily accepted. The American Dental Association and the American Medical Association have supported this intervention for over half a century. Resistance from those who view it as an intrusion of governmental authority, however, has prevented universal use of fluoridation in this country. After over a half century of effort, fluoridation has reached less than 66% of Americans through the water supply.

Today, new technologies, from dental sealants to more cost-effective methods for treating cavities, have again made oral health a public health priority. However, the number of dentists has not grown in recent years to keep up with the growing population. In addition, dental care for those without the resources to pay for it is often inadequate and inaccessible. Thus, a new approach is needed to bring dental care to those in need. Perhaps a new strategy using a COPH approach can make this happen.

COPH can reach beyond the institutional and geographical constraints that COPC faces when based in a community health center or other institutions serving a geographically defined population or community. COPH as a government-led effort allows a greater range of options for intervention, including those that require changes in laws, incentives, and governmental procedures. Interventions may include authorizing new types of clinicians, providing services in nontraditional settings such as schools, funding innovations to put new technologies into practice, and addressing the regulatory barriers to rapid and cost-effective delivery of services.

▶ Conclusion

In summary, the chapter offered a look at the organization of the public health system and the challenges it faces in accomplishing its core functions and providing its essential services. The role of public health will continue to evolve as current and emerging issues impact the health of the population.

References

Centers for Disease Control and Prevention. (1996). History of CDC. *Morbidity and Mortality Weekly Report, 45*(25), 526–530.

Centers for Disease Control and Prevention & Centers for State, Tribal, Local, and Territorial Support. (2018). *Public health professionals gateway: The public health system and the 10 essential public health services.* Retrieved from https://www.cdc.gov/stltpublichealth/publichealthservices/essentialhealthservices.html

Duffin, J., & Sweetman, A. (2006). *SARS in context: Memory, history, policy.* Montreal, Canada: McGill-Queen's University Press.

Gofin, J., & Gofin, R. (2011). *Essentials of global community health.* Sudbury, MA: Jones and Bartlett Learning.

Institute of Medicine. (1988). *The future of public health.* Washington, DC: National Academies Press.

Institute of Medicine. (2008). *Initial guidance for an update of the National Vaccine Plan: A letter report to the national vaccine program office.* Washington, DC: National Academies Press.

Public Health Accreditation Board. (2013). *Standards and measures.* Retrieved from http://www.phaboard.org/accreditation-process/public-health-department-standards-and-measures

Turnock, B. J. (2007). *Essentials of public health.* Burlington, MA: Jones and Bartlett Learning.

Turnock, B. J. (2009). *Public health: What it is and how it works* (4th ed.). Burlington, MA: Jones and Bartlett Learning.

U.S. Department of Health and Human Services. (2017). *HHS organizational chart.* Retrieved from http://www.hhs.gov/about/orgchart

World Bank. (2018). *Health.* Retrieved from http://www.worldbank.org/en/topic/health

▶ Endnotes

a. This does not imply that components of the work cannot be contracted to nongovernmental organizations. This activity is increasingly occurring. The concept of core function, however, implies that public health agencies remain responsible for these functions even when the day-to-day work is conducted through contracts with an outside organization.

b. This delegation may occur at the discretion of the state government or it may be included in the state's constitution, providing what is called home rule authority to local jurisdictions. In general, jurisdictions with home rule authority exercise substantially more autonomy.

PART I ADDENDUM: TIMELINE

	Pre-1800	1800s	1820s
Political Party in Power—Federal Government			
President	Federalist (1789–1801)	Dem-Rep (1801–1829)	
	George Washington (1789–1797); John Adams (1797–1801)	Thomas Jefferson (1801–1809); James Madison (1809–1817); James Monroe (1817–1825); John Quincy Adams (1825–1829)	
U.S. House of Representatives	Pro-Administration (1789–1793); Anti-Administration (1793–1795); Jeffersonian Republican (1795–1797); Federalist (1797–1801)	Jeffersonian Republican (1801–1823)	Adams–Clay Republican (1823–1825); Adams (1825–1827); Jacksons (1827–1829)
U.S. Senate	Pro-Administration (1789–1795); Federalist (1795–1801)	Republican (1801–1823)	Jackson–Crawford Republican (1823–1825); Jacksonian (1825–1833)
Major Social and Political Events		**Industrial Revolution (~1790–1860)** and increased urbanization	
		War of 1812 (1812–1814) and post-war economic growth	
Key Federal Legislative Proposals/Laws and Key Legal Decisions	**1798** U.S. Public Health Service Act: Creates the **Marine Hospital Service,** predecessor to the Public Health Service, to provide medical care to merchant seamen.	*Marbury v. Madison,* 5 U.S. 137 (1803): Established the Supreme Court's power of judicial review; **1818 Office of the Surgeon General** established.	
Important Developments in Health and Medicine	State Poor Laws require communities to care for residents who are physically or mentally incapable of caring for themselves; States begin building dispensaries in the late 1700s to provide medication to the poor; Almshouses serve as primitive hospitals, providing limited care to the indigent; Public health focuses on fighting plague, cholera, and smallpox epidemics, often through quarantine.		

	1830s	1840s	1850s
Political Party in Power— Federal Government President	Democrat (1829–1841)	Whig (1841–1845); Democrat (1845–1849)	Whig (1849–1853); Democrat (1853–1861)
	Andrew Jackson (1829–1837); Martin Van Buren (1837–1841)	William Henry Harrison (1841); John Tyler (1841–1845); James K. Polk (1845–1849); Zachary Taylor (1849–1850)	Millard Fillmore (1850–1853); Franklin Pierce (1853–1857); James Buchanan (1857–1861)
U.S. House of Representatives	Jacksons (1829–1837); Democrat (1837–1841)		
U.S. Senate	Anti-Jacksonian (1833–1835); Jacksonian (1835–1837); Democrat (1837–1841)	Whig (1841–1845) (27th–28th); Democrat (1845–1861) (29th–36th)	
Major Social and Political Events	**Industrial Revolution (~1790–1860)** and increased urbanization	**U.S.–Mexican War** (1846–1848)	**Crimean War** (1853–1856)
Key Federal Legislative Proposals/Laws and Key Legal Decisions		**1848 Import Drug Act:** Initiates drug regulation; U.S. Customs Service is required to enforce purity standards for imported medications.	
Important Developments in Health and Medicine		**1846** First publicized use of general anesthetic; Use of anesthetics increases the number of surgeries performed; **1847** American Medical Association (AMA) is founded.	Studies by Edwin Chadwick in England, Lemuel Shattuck in Massachusetts, and others reveal that overcrowded and unsanitary conditions breed disease, and advocate establishment of local health boards; By the end of the 1800s, 40 states and several localities establish health departments.

	1860s	1870s	1880s
Political Party in Power—Federal Government			
President	Republican; Democrat Abraham Lincoln (1861–1865); Andrew Johnson (1865–1869)	Republican Ulysses S. Grant (1869–1877); Rutherford B. Hayes (1877–1881)	Republican (1881–1885); Democrat (1885–1889) James A. Garfield (1881); Chester A. Arthur (1881–1885); Grover Cleveland (1885–1889)
U.S. House of Representatives	Republican (1859–1875)	Democrat (1875–1881)	Republican (1881–1883); Democrat (1883–1889)
U.S. Senate	Republican (1861–1879) (37th–45th)	Democrat (1879–1881) (46th)	Republican (1881–1893) (47th–52nd)
Major Social and Political Events	**Industrial Revolution (~1790–1860)** and increased urbanization **U.S. Civil War** (1861–1865) and post-war expansion in interstate commerce	**U.S.–Mexican War** (1846–1848)	**Crimean War** (1853–1856)
Key Federal Legislative Proposals/Laws and Key Legal Decisions	**1862 Bureau of Chemistry** (forerunner of the Food and Drug Administration [FDA]) is established as a scientific laboratory in the Department of Agriculture.	**1870s Medical Practice Acts:** Establish state regulation of physician licensing; **1870 Marine Hospital Service** is centralized as a separate bureau of the Treasury Department; **1878 National Quarantine Act:** Grants the Marine Hospital Service quarantine authority due to its assistance with yellow fever outbreak.	**1887** National Hygienic Laboratory, predecessor lab to the National Institutes of Health, is established in Staten Island, New York, by the National Marine Health Service.
Important Developments in Health and Medicine	**1861** First nursing school is founded and the important role of nursing is established during the Civil War; **1860s** Louis Pasteur develops the germ theory of disease; **1865 antiseptic surgery** is introduced by Joseph Lister, decreasing death rates from surgical operations; With the advent of licensing, the practice of medicine begins to become a more exclusive realm.	**1877** Louis Pasteur discovers that anthrax is caused by bacteria; Scientists find bacteriologic agents causing tuberculosis, diphtheria, typhoid, and yellow fever; Immunizations and water purification interventions follow recent discoveries; State and local health departments create laboratories; States begin passing laws requiring disease reporting and establishing disease registries.	**1880s** First hospitals established and the importance of hospitals in the provision of medical care increases; **1882** first major employee-sponsored mutual benefit association was created by Northern Pacific Railway, includes healthcare benefit; Social Insurance movement results in the creation of "sickness" insurance throughout many countries in Europe; **1895** X-rays discovered.

	1890s	1900s
Political Party in Power—Federal Government		
President	Republican (1889–1893); Democrat (1893–1897); Republican (1897–1901) Benjamin Harrison (1889–1893); Grover Cleveland (1893–1897); William McKinley (1897–1901)	Republican/Progressive Theodore Roosevelt (1901–1909)
U.S. House of Representatives	Republican (1889–1891); Democrat (1891–1895); Republican (1895–1911)	
U.S. Senate	Democrat (1893–1895) (53rd); Republican (1895–1913) (54th–62nd)	Republican
Major Social and Political Events		**Progressive Era** (1900–1920): Characterized by popular support for social reform, part of which included compulsory health insurance; Roosevelt campaigned on a social insurance platform in 1912.
Key Federal Legislative Proposals/ Laws and Key Legal Decisions	**1890 Sherman Antitrust Act:** Prohibits interstate trusts so economic power would not be concentrated in a few corporations.	*Hurley v. Eddingfield,* 59 N.E. 1058 (Ind. 1901): Physicians are under no duty to treat, and a physician is not liable for arbitrarily refusing to render medical assistance; **1902 Marine Health Service** renamed the **Public Health and Marine Hospital Service (PHMHS)** as its role in disease control activities expands; **1902 Biologics Control Act:** Regulates safety and effectiveness of vaccines, serums, etc.; *Jacobson v. Massachusetts,* 197 U.S. 11 (1905): State statute requiring compulsory vaccination against smallpox is a constitutional exercise of police power; **1906 Food and Drug Act** (Wiley Act): Gives regulatory power to monitor food manufacturing, labeling, and sales to FDA predecessor; **1908** Federal Employers Liability Act: Creates workers compensation program for select federal employees.
Important Developments in Health and Medicine		**1901** AMA reorganizes at local/state level and gains strength, beginning era of "organized medicine" as physicians as a group become a more cohesive and increasingly professional authority.

	1910s	**1920s**
Political Party in Power— Federal Government		
President	Republican — William H. Taft (1909–1913); Democrat — Woodrow Wilson (1913–1921)	Republican — Warren G. Harding (1921–1923); Republican — Calvin Coolidge (1923–1929)
U.S. House of Representatives	Democrat (1911–1919) (62nd–65th)	Democrat (1913–1919) (63rd–65th); Republican (1919–1933) (66th–72nd); Republican (1919–1931) (66th–71st)
U.S. Senate	Republican	Democrat (1913–1919) (63rd–65th); Republican (1919–1933) (66th–72nd); Republican; Republican
Major Social and Political Events		**World War I** (1914–1919; United States enters in 1917)
Key Federal Legislative Proposals/Laws and Key Legal Decisions	**1912 Children's Bureau of Health** established in Department of Commerce (later moved to Department of Labor); **1912 Public Health and Marine Hospital Service** is renamed the **Public Health Service** and is authorized to investigate human disease and sanitation; **1914 Clayton Antitrust Act:** Clarifies the Sherman Antitrust Act and includes additional prohibitions.	**1911:** First state workers compensation law enacted; **1918 Chamberlain-Kahn Act:** Provides first federal grants to states for public health services; **1921 Sweet Act:** Establishes the Veterans Administration; **1922 Shepherd-Towner Act:** Provides grants for the Children's Bureau and state maternal and child health programs, and is the first direct federal funding of health services for individuals.
Important Developments in Health and Medicine	**1910** Flexner Report on Medical Education creates medical school standards; "sickness" insurance established by Britain in 1911 and Russia in 1912; Socialist and Progressive parties in the United States support similar "sickness" insurance.	**1913 American College of Surgeons (ACS)** is founded; **1918** ACS begins accreditation of hospitals; **1918–1919 pandemic flu** kills over 600,000 people in the United States; **1920** AMA passes resolution against compulsory health insurance; AMA opposition combined with entry into World War I (and the anti-German sentiments aroused), undermines support for national health reform and government insurance; **1929 Blue Cross** established its first hospital insurance plan at Baylor University; Chronic illnesses begin to replace infectious diseases as most significant health threat; With innovations in medical care, healthcare costs begin to rise.

	1930s	1940s
Political Party in Power—Federal Government	Republican	Democrat
President	Herbert Hoover (1929–1933)	Franklin D. Roosevelt (1933–1945)
U.S. House of Representatives	Democrat (1931–1947) (72nd–79th)	Democrat
U.S. Senate	Democrat (1933–1947) (73rd–79th)	Democrat
Major Social and Political Events	**Great Depression** (1929 through 1930s); **New Deal** (1933–1939)	**World War II** (1939–1945), Pearl Harbor 1941)
Key Federal Legislative Proposals/Laws and Key Legal Decisions	**1930 National Institutes of Health** established; **1933 Federal Emergency Relief Administration** provides limited medical services for the medically indigent; **1935 Social Security Act:** Provides federal grant-in-aid funding for states to create and maintain public health services and training, expands responsibilities for the Children's Health Bureau, and establishes Aid to Families with Dependent Children (AFDC) welfare program; **1935 Works Project Administration** is created, including projects to build and improve hospitals; **1938 Food, Drug and Cosmetic Act:** Expands regulatory scope of FDA to require premarket approval (in response to deaths from an untested product); **1939** Public Health Service is transferred from the Treasury Department to the new Federal Security Agency.	**1941 Manham Act:** Funds wartime emergency building of hospitals; **1942 National War Labor Board** rules that the provision of benefits, including health insurance, does not violate wage freeze; **1944 Public Health Service Act:** Consolidates the laws related to the functions of the PHS; **1946 Hill-Burton Act:** Funds hospital construction to improve access to hospital-based medical care; **1946 The Communicable Disease Center (CDC)** opens as part of the Public Health Service; **1949** Truman's national health insurance proposal is defeated.
Important Developments in Health and Medicine	The Great Depression threatens financial security of physicians, hospitals, and individuals; Commercial insurance industry rises in the absence of government-sponsored insurance plans; In the **late 1930s** the Blue Cross (hospital services) and Blue Shield (physician services) health insurance plan created; Prepaid group health plans/medical cooperatives gain popularity with some providers and consumers, but are opposed by AMA.	**(1932–1972) Tuskegee Syphilis Study** **1945** Nobel Prize in Medicine awarded for development of penicillin treatment for humans, which is used extensively in the war; **1945** Kaiser Permanente, a large prepaid, integrated health plan is opened to the public; 1946 the Emerson Report released proposing overall plan for public health in the United States; **1948** AMA opposes Truman's plan for national health insurance and sentiments against national health reform also fueled by the Cold War; Employer-based health insurance grows rapidly with no national health insurance program and as employers compete for a short supply of employees due to the war and because health benefits are exempted from the wage freeze; After WWII, labor unions gained the right to bargain collectively, leading to another expansion in employee health plans; Commercial insurance has taken over 40% of the market from Blue Cross.

	1950s		1960s	
Political Party in Power—Federal Government				
President	Democrat Harry S. Truman (1945–1953)	Republican Dwight D. Eisenhower (1953–1961)	Democrat John F. Kennedy (1961–1963)	Democrat Lyndon B. Johnson (1963–1969)
U.S. House of Representatives	Republican (1947–1949) (80th); Democrat (1949–1953) (81st–82d)	Republican (1952–1955) (83rd); Democrat (1955–1994) (84th–103rd)	Democrat	Democrat
U.S. Senate	Republican (1947–1949) (80th); Democrat (1949–1953) (81st–82nd)	Republican (1953–1955) (83rd); Democrat (1955–1981) (84th–96th)	Democrat	Democrat
Major Social and Political Events	Cold War ideology and McCarthyism (1950–1954); **Korean War** (1950–1953)		Economic downturn	
Key Federal Legislative Proposals/Laws and Key Legal Decisions	**1953 Department of Health, Education, and Welfare (HEW)** is created from the Federal Security Agency, and the Public Health Service is transferred to HEW; **1954** Internal Revenue Service declares that employers can pay health insurance premiums for their employees with pre-tax dollars; *Brown v. Board of Education,* 347 U.S. 483 (1954): Racial segregation in public education violates the Equal Protection Clause of 14th Amendment; **1956 Dependents Medical Care Act:** Creates government medical care program for military and dependents outside the Veterans Affairs system; **1956 Social Security Act** is amended to provide Social Security Disability Insurance.		**1962 Amendments to Food, Drug and Cosmetic Acts** require that new drugs be "effective."	**1960 Kerr-Mills program** provides federal funding through vendor payments to states for medically indigent elderly; *Simpkins v. Moses H. Cone Memorial Hospital,* 323 F.2d 959 (4th Cir. 1963): Racial segregation in private hospitals receiving federal Hill-Burton funds violates the Equal Protection Clause of the 14th Amendment; **1964: Civil Rights Act** passed; **1965 Medicare and Medicaid** programs created through Social Security Amendments; *Griswold v. Connecticut,* 381 U.S. 479 (1965): The Constitution protects a right to privacy, state law forbidding the use of contraceptives or provision of them to married couples violates a constitutional right to marital privacy; **1966 Civilian Health and Medical Program for the Uniformed Services** (CHAMPUS) created.
Important Developments in Health and Medicine	**1951 Joint Commission on Accreditation of Hospitals (JCAH)** is created to provide voluntary accreditation; **1953** Salk creates polio vaccine; **1954** first organ transplant is performed; Continued progression in medical science and technology leads to increased costs; Political focus turns to Korean War and away from medical care reform.		**1965:** Medicare and Medicaid created; **1967** first human heart transplant.	

	1970s		1980s	
Political Party in Power—Federal Government				
President	Republican — Richard M. Nixon (1969–1974)	Republican — Gerald R. Ford (1974–1977)	Democrat — Jimmy Carter (1977–1981)	Republican — Ronald Reagan (1981–1989)
U.S. House of Representatives	Democrat	Democrat	Democrat	Democrat
U.S. Senate	Democrat	Democrat	Democrat	Republican (1981–1987) (97th–99th); Democrat (1987–1995) (100th–103rd)
Major Social and Political Events				1989 "New Federalism" of the Reagan administration; Berlin Wall falls
Key Federal Legislative Proposals/Laws and Key Legal Decisions	President Nixon's proposed comprehensive health insurance plan fails; **1971** proposed Health Security Act from Senator Edward Kennedy (D-MA) fails; **1970** Communicable Disease Center is renamed the **Centers for Disease Control; 1972 Social Security Amendments** extend Medicare eligibility and create Supplemental Security Income (SSI) program; *Canterbury v. Spence,* 464 F.2d 772 (D.C. Cir. 1972): Established modern law of informed consent based on a reasonable patient standard; *Roe v. Wade,* 410 U.S. 113 (1973): Constitutional right to privacy encompasses a woman's decision to terminate her pregnancy; **1973 Health Maintenance Organization Act:** Supports growth of health maintenance organizations; **1974 Employment Retirement Income Security Act (ERISA)** passed; **1977 Health Care Financing Administration (HCFA)** is created to administer the Medicare and Medicaid programs.		**1979** Carter introduces a National Health Plan to Congress; **1979 Department of Health and Human Services (HHS)** is created from a reorganized HEW.	**1983** Medicare implements prospective payment system for reimbursing hospitals; **1986 Emergency Medical Treatment and Active Labor Act (EMTALA):** Ensures access to emergency services in Medicare-participating hospitals regardless of ability to pay; **1986 Health Care Quality Improvement Act:** Creates the National Practitioner Databank; **1986 Consolidated Omnibus Budget Reconciliation Act (COBRA):** Includes health benefit provisions that establish continuation of employer-sponsored group health coverage; **1989 Medicare Catastrophic Coverage Act of 1988:** Includes outpatient prescription drug benefit and other changes in Medicare (repealed 1989).
Important Developments in Health and Medicine	Healthcare costs continue to rise dramatically, due to advances in medical technology, high-tech hospital care, the new pool of paying patients from Medicaid and Medicare, increased utilization of services, and increased physician specialization; **1972** computed tomography (CT) scan first used; **1978** first baby conceived through in vitro fertilization is born.			**1980** World Health Assembly declares smallpox eradicated; **1981** Scientists identify AIDS; **1987** the Joint Commission on Accreditation of Hospitals changes name to the Joint Commission on Accreditation of Healthcare Organizations (JCAHO); Shift away from traditional fee-for-service insurance plans and toward managed care.

	1990s	
Political Party in Power—Federal Government		
President	Republican	Democrat
	George Bush (1989–1993)	William J. Clinton (1993–2001)
U.S. House of Representatives	Democrat	*First time since 1955 that both houses are Republican;* Republican (1995–2005) (104th–108th)
U.S. Senate	Democrat	Republican (1995–2005) (104th–108th [Jan. 3–20, 2001, and June 6, 2001–Nov. 12, 2002 Democrat])
Major Social and Political Events	**1990–1991** Gulf War	Foreign crises in Haiti and Bosnia; **1993** North American Free Trade Agreement (NAFTA); Whitewater investigation; **1995** Oklahoma City bombing; **1998** President Clinton impeached
Key Federal Legislative Proposals/Laws and Key Legal Decisions	**1989 Agency for Healthcare Policy and Research** created; **1990 Americans With Disabilities Act (ADA):** Provides protection against disability discrimination; **1990 Ryan White CARE Act:** Creates federal support for AIDS-related services; ***Cruzan v. Director, Missouri. Dep't of Health,*** 497 U.S. 261 (1990): First "right to die" case before Supreme Court, in which the Court held that a competent person has a constitutionally protected liberty interest in refusing medical treatment.	**1993** President Clinton's proposed **Health Security Act** is defeated; **1995** PHS reorganized to report directly to the Secretary of HHS; **1996 Health Insurance Portability & Accountability Act (HIPAA):** Includes privacy rules to protect personal health information, attempts to simplify coding for health bills, makes it difficult to exclude patients from insurance plans due to preexisting conditions; **Personal Responsibility and Work Opportunity Reconciliation Act of 1996** replaces AFDC with the Temporary Assistance for Needy Families (TANF) program; **1996 Mental Health Parity Act:** Requires insurance carriers that offer mental health benefits to provide the same annual and lifetime dollar limits for mental and physical health benefits; **1997 Food and Drug Administration Modernization Act:** Relaxes restrictions on direct-to-consumer advertisements of prescription drugs; **1997 Balanced Budget Act:** Adds Medicare part C, the Medicare managed care program, and creates the State Health Insurance Program, which allows states to extend health insurance coverage to additional low-income children; **The Ticket to Work and Work Incentives Improvement Act of 1999:** Creates a new state option to help individuals with disabilities stay enrolled in Medicaid or Medicare coverage while returning to work.
Important Developments in Health and Medicine		Enrollment in managed care doubles; Greater use of outpatient services; Rate of health spending is relatively stable at roughly 12% to 13% of gross domestic product; Direct-to-consumer advertising of pharmaceuticals increases dramatically and the Internet is used as a source of medical information; **1994** Oregon Health Plan rations Medicaid services through a prioritized list of medical treatments and conditions; **1997** Ian Wilmut clones a sheep from adult human cells.

	2000s	
Political Party in Power—Federal Government		
President	Republican	Democrat
	George W. Bush (2001–2009)	Barack Obama (2009–2017)
U.S. House of Representatives	Republican (2005–2007) (109th); Democrat (2007–2009) (110th)	Democrat (2009–2011) (111th); Republican 2011– (112th)
U.S. Senate	Republican (2005–2007) (109th); Democrat (2007–2009) (110th)	Democrat (2009–2015) (111th–113th)
Major Social and Political Events	**September 11, 2001,** terrorist attacks on World Trade Center in New York and the Pentagon; **2001** U.S. military action in Afghanistan; **2003** Iraq War begins	Great Recession (began in December 2007), including financial crisis and collapse of housing market; Passage of the 2010 Patient Protection and Affordable Care Act
Key Federal Legislative Proposals/Laws and Key Legal Decisions	Congressional attention and spending turns to international and security concerns, little discussion of health reform; **2002 Homeland Security Act** transfers some HHS functions, including the Strategic National Stockpile of emergency pharmaceutical supplies and the National Disaster Medical Service, to the new Department of Homeland Security; **2003 Medicare Modernization Act:** Adds a prescription drug benefit to Medicare beginning in 2006; **2004 Project BioShield Act:** Provides funding for vaccines and medications for biodefense and allows expedited FDA review of treatments in response to attacks; **2005 Deficit Reduction Act:** Makes changes to Medicaid cost sharing, premiums, benefits, and asset transfers; **2006 Medicare Part D Prescription Drug Plan** goes into effect; **2008 Mental Health Parity Act** amended to require insurers to treat mental health conditions on the same basis as physical conditions.	Congressional focus on health reform, spending cuts; President Obama establishes the **Office of Health Reform: 2009 American Reinvestment and Recovery Act (ARRA)** creates incentives to help develop health information technology and expand the primary care workforce, among other things; **2009 Children's Health Insurance Program Reauthorization Act** extending (for 4.5 years) and expanding the program; **2010 Patient Protection and Affordable Care Act (ACA):** Comprehensive health reform including an "individual mandate" to purchase insurance coverage, Medicaid expansion, creation of state health insurance exchanges, and much more.
Important Developments in Health and Medicine	After the September 11, 2001, attacks, public health becomes focused on emergency preparedness; **2003** Sequencing of human genome completed; **2003** SARS epidemic and 2004 flu vaccine shortage raises concerns about public health readiness; Worldwide concern about a possible Avian flu epidemic; High level of concern in the United States about the rising rate of obesity; **2006** Gardasil vaccine protecting against two strains of the human papillomavirus, which is associated with cervical cancer, approved by the FDA; **2007** International Health Regulations, passed by the World Health Organization in 2005, are implemented by member states.	Rate of health spending continues to skyrocket, accounting in 2009 for 17% of the gross domestic product; **2009** H1N1 swine flu virus pandemic.

	2010s	
Political Party in Power—Federal Government	Democrat	Republican
President	Barack Obama (2009–2017)	Donald Trump (2017–)
U.S. House of Representatives	Republican 2011–Present (112th–115th)	
U.S. Senate	Republican 2015 (114th–115th)	
Major Social and Political Events	Great Recession ended but many not prospering during the recovery; **Continued political debate regarding the ACA,** including debates in nearly half the states concerning whether to adopt the ACA's Medicaid expansion; Several states continue to experience financial and/or technical issues in the establishment and operation of ACA insurance exchanges; Increasing political and legal acceptance of same-sex marriage likely to impact use and cost of health insurance and public health programs; Growth of ISIS as a terrorist threat; **U.S. Supreme Court Justice Antonin Scalia dies** suddenly in February 2016, after which the U.S. Senate, under Republican power, refuses to consider President Obama's replacement nomination until after the 2016 election.	Mainly **unanticipated outcome in 2016** national election results in abrupt shift in federal policymaking, views about entitlement and welfare programs, and revised immigration policies, among other key national political and social issues; **Racial tensions escalate: Robert Mueller appointed as Special Counsel** in 2017 to investigate the alleged role of Russian interference in the 2016 national election; **Neil Gorsuch confirmed** to take Justice Scalia's seat on the U.S. Supreme Court; **U.S. Supreme Court Justice Anthony Kennedy retires** at the end of the 2017–2018 term, is replaced by **Brett Kavanaugh** by the smallest margin for a Supreme Court Justice since 1881 and after a deeply troubling and polarizing nomination process; National economy mainly recovers from Great Recession, **yet income inequality continues to grow.**
Key Federal Legislative Proposals/Laws and Key Legal Decisions	Congressional focus continues to be on debating the ACA as well as international security issues; **Don't Ask Don't Tell Repeal Act of 2010** ended the discriminatory military policy regarding gay service members; **2012 *NFIB v. Sebelius*,** Supreme Court held that the ACA's individual insurance requirement was constitutional but also ruled that the ACA's requirement that all states expand Medicaid was unduly coercive; **2014 *Burwell v. Hobby Lobby*,** the Supreme Court held that one provision of the ACA violated federal law by requiring closely held corporations to pay for insurance coverage for certain types of contraception; **Medicare and CHIP Reauthorization Act of 2015** replaced the Sustainable Growth Rate formula used for physician payment and funded CHIP through 2017; **2015 *Obergefell v. Hodges*,** the Supreme Court held that the fundamental right to marriage is guaranteed to same-sex couples; In **2015 in *Burwell v. King*** the Supreme Court upheld the ACA's statutory and regulatory scheme permitting federal subsidies to flow through both state-run and federally facilitated insurance exchanges; The **Global Food Security Act of 2016** authorized a comprehensive, strategic approach for U.S. foreign assistance to developing countries to reduce global poverty and hunger, achieve food security, promote sustainable agricultural-led economic growth, and improve nutritional outcomes, particularly for women and children; The **21st Century Cures Act** became law in 2016 and was designed to help accelerate medical product development and bring new innovations and advances to patients who need them faster and more efficiently; In Whole ***Woman's Health v. Hellerstedt*** (2016), the Supreme Court struck down strict Texas abortion regulations, ruling that abortion provider regulations must be based on convincing medical evidence and cannot unduly burden a woman's right to abortion.	After President Trump's inauguration, multiple Republican **efforts to repeal and replace the Affordable Care Act fail** (though several executive/regulatory actions halt or limit the reach of the ACA); **CHIP reauthorized** and funded through 2027; The **Tax Cuts and Jobs Act of 2017** represents the biggest federal tax overhaul in 30 years—among other things, it cut the maximum corporate income tax rate to 21%, eliminated the tax on people who do not obtain adequate health insurance coverage, and increased the standard deduction and the estate tax exemption, which together will reduce federal revenues by significant amounts and likely make the distribution of after-tax income more unequal. In ***Cooper v. Harris*** (2017), the Supreme Court ruled that racial gerrymandering violated the rights of voters to equal protection of the laws; The Supreme Court ruled 5–4 that President Trump had the legal authority to restrict travel from several mostly Muslim countries in the 2018 case of ***Trump v. Hawaii***; In ***Masterpiece Cakeshop v. Colorado Civil Rights Commission*** (2018), the Supreme Court ruled in favor of a Colorado baker who refused to create a wedding cake for a gay couple, determining that the baker had been mistreated by the state civil rights commission based on remarks of one of its members indicating hostility to religion; In 2018, the Supreme Court ruled 5–4 that foreign corporations may not be sued in American courts for complicity in human rights abuses abroad (***Jesner v. Arab Bank***).

	2010s
Important Developments in Health and Medicine	**2010** cholera outbreak in Haiti, one of the worst outbreaks in recent history; **2012** emergence of MERS-CoV, a viral respiratory illness that is new to humans, first reported in the Middle East but later spread to several countries including the United States; **2013** healthcare spending reached almost $3 trillion and accounted for 17.4% of the gross domestic product; **2014** Ebola outbreak was the largest in history and first Ebola epidemic; **2015** Ebola research advances quickly, scientists discovered a new class of antibiotics, and doctors performed the world's first rib cage transplant using a three-dimensional-printed chest prosthetic; **2015** represents the start of a worldwide Zika virus epidemic; **2016** marks the point at which the nation's opioid crisis finally becomes front-page news; **2016** the U.S. Drug Enforcement Agency permits the first-ever clinical trial in which patients will be smoking marijuana, in order to establish whether pot-smoking can have positive medical benefits for patients with post-traumatic stress disorder; **2016** witnesses both Hurricane Matthew, which kills nearly 50 people and causes more than $15 billion in damage in Florida, Georgia, and the Carolinas, and also the Great Smoky Mountain wildfires in Tennessee, which destroyed nearly 2,000 structures and burned nearly 18,000 acres of land. **2017** scientists successfully cut out the HIV virus from mouse cells using gene editing therapy; **2017** healthcare spending accounted for 18% of the gross domestic product; **2017** Hurricanes Harvey, Irma, and Maria, result in thousands of deaths and hundreds of billions of dollars in damages in Texas, Louisiana, Alabama, Florida, South Carolina, Georgia, Puerto Rico, and multiple islands in the eastern Caribbean Sea.

Further Reading

For more on these and other related historical timeline details and trends, see the following:

Day, J. G. (1997). Managed care and the medical profession: Old issues and old tensions the building blocks of tomorrow's health care delivery and financing system. *Connecticut Insurance Law Journal, 3*(1), 60–78.

Hall, M. A. (1999). *Health care corporate law: Formation and regulation.* New York, NY: Aspen Law & Business.

Public Broadcasting System. (n.d.). *Healthcare crisis: Healthcare timeline.* Retrieved from http://www.pbs.org/healthcarecrisis/history.htm

Wing, K. R., Jacobs, M. S., & Kuszler, P. C. (1998). *The law and American health care.* New York: Aspen Law & Business.

References

Birn, A. (2003). Struggles for national health reform in the United States. *American Journal of Public Health, 93*(1), 86–94.

Institute of Medicine. (2002). *The future of the public's health in the 21st century* (pp. 96–177). Washington, DC: National Academies Press (Ch. 3).

Shi, L., & Singh, D. A. (2004). *Delivering health care services in America: A systems approach.* Sudbury, MA: Jones and Bartlett Learning.

Sultz, H., & Young, K. (2003). *Health care USA: Understanding its organization and delivery* (4th ed.). Sudbury, MA: Jones and Bartlett Learning.

Other Sources Consulted

American Medical Association. (n.d.). *Chronology of AMA history.* Retrieved from https://www.ama-assn.org/ama-history

U.S. Food and Drug Administration. (n.d.). *A history of the FDA and drug regulation in the United States.* Retrieved from https://www.fda.gov/downloads/drugs/resourcesforyou/consumers/buyingusingmedicinesafely/understandingover-the-countermedicines/ucm093550.pdf

U.S. National Library of Medicine. (2012). *History of medicine.* Retrieved from http://www.nlm.nih.gov/exhibition/phs_history/contents.html

Source for Political Affiliation of Senate

U.S. Senate. (n.d.). *Party division.* Retrieved from http://www.senate.gov/pagelayout/history/one_item_and_teasers/partydiv.htm

Source for Political Affiliation of the House of Representatives

U.S. House of Representatives. (n.d.). *House history timeline.* Retrieved from http://history.house.gov/Education/Timeline/Timeline/

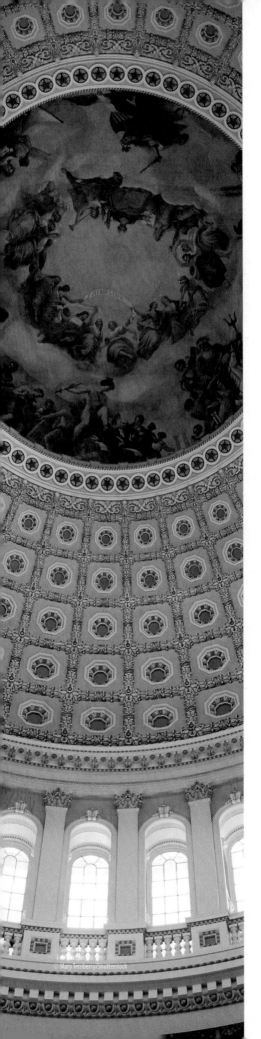

PART II

Essential Issues in Health Policy and Law

Part I of this book introduced frameworks for conceptualizing health policy and law and described basic aspects of policy, the policymaking process, law, the legal system, and the healthcare and public health systems. Part II covers many of the essential issues in health policy and law. Chapter 6 addresses individual rights in health care and public health, Chapter 7 describes how law itself is a determinant of health and how law relates to other social determinants of health, and Chapters 8 and 9 cover the fundamentals of health insurance and health economics, respectively. Chapter 10 provides an overview of national health reform. Chapters 11 through 13 cover government insurance programs, healthcare quality, and public health preparedness, respectively. After completing Part II, among other things you will understand how social factors influence individual and population health, how health insurance functions, why private employer-based coverage dominates the health insurance market, why gaps in health insurance coverage remain, the importance of health economics to health policymaking, key provisions in the Affordable Care Act, various policy and legal dimensions to healthcare quality, and the role of public health in preparing for and responding to national and global emergencies.

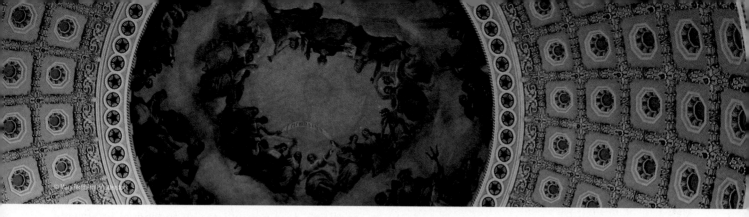

CHAPTER 6

Individual Rights in Health Care and Public Health

LEARNING OBJECTIVES

By the end of this chapter you will be able to:

- Describe the meaning and importance of the "no-duty to treat" principle
- Explain generally how the U.S. approach to health rights differs from that of other developed countries
- Describe the types and limitations of individual legal rights associated with health care
- Describe the balancing approach taken when weighing individual rights against the public's health

▶ Introduction

The real-life scenarios in **BOX 6-1** touch upon the key issues you will confront in this chapter: namely, the ways in which the law creates, protects, and restricts individual rights in the contexts of health care and public health. Individuals are deeply impacted by law on a daily basis, and this fact is no less true when they navigate the healthcare system, or when an individual's actions are measured against the broader interests of the public's health. Over many decades, legal principles have been rejected, developed, and refined as the law continually struggles to define the appropriate relationship between individuals and the physicians, hospitals, managed care companies, and others they encounter in the healthcare delivery system, and between individuals and government agencies charged with protecting public health and welfare. These balancing acts are made all the more difficult as the legal system bumps up against the quick pace of technological

advancements in medicine and against amorphous, potentially deadly risks to the public's health, such as bioterrorism and fast-spreading influenzas.

After a background section, this chapter considers individual legal rights in health care, beginning with a brief overview of health rights under international and foreign law. This sets up a much lengthier discussion of healthcare rights in the United States, which for purposes of this chapter are classified according to an important distinction: legal rights *to* health care and rights that individuals can claim only *within* the context of the healthcare system—that is, only once they have found a way to access needed care.[a] Examples of the latter type of rights include the right to refuse unwanted treatment, the right to autonomy in making personal healthcare decisions, and the right to be free from wrongful discrimination when receiving care. Finally, the chapter turns to a discussion of individual rights in the context of government-initiated public health efforts. This topic

BOX 6-1 Vignette

At the turn of the 20th century, an Indiana physician named George Eddingfield repeatedly refused to come to the aid of Charlotte Burk, who was in labor, even though he was Mrs. Burk's family physician. Doctor Eddingfield conceded at trial that he made this decision for no particular reason and despite the facts that he had been offered monetary compensation in advance of his performing any medical services and that he was aware that no other physician was available to provide care to Mrs. Burk. Unattended by any medical providers, Mrs. Burk eventually fell gravely ill, and both she and her unborn child died. It was determined upon trial and subsequent appeals that Dr. Eddingfield did not wrongfully cause either death.

Around the same time as the scenario just described, the Cambridge, Massachusetts, Board of Health ordered everyone within city limits to be vaccinated against the smallpox disease under a state law granting local boards of health the power, under certain circumstances, to require the vaccination of individuals. After refusing to abide by the Cambridge Board's order, Henning Jacobson was convicted by a state trial court and sentenced to pay a $5 fine. Remarkably, Mr. Jacobson's case not only made its way to the U.S. Supreme Court, it resulted in one of the court's most important public health rulings and a sweeping statement about limitations to fundamental individual rights in the face of threats to the public's health.

is dominated by the role and scope of government "police powers," which permit governments, when acting to promote or protect public health, to curtail individual freedoms and liberties.

▶ Background

Lurking behind any discussion of individual rights in a health context is one of the most basic principles in U.S. health law: generally speaking, individuals have no legal right to healthcare services (or to public health insurance), and, correspondingly, there exists on the part of healthcare providers no general legal duty to provide care. This is referred to as the "no-duty" or "no-duty-to-treat" principle, which is aptly described by the Indiana Supreme Court in the well-known 1901 case of *Hurley v. Eddingfield*, the facts of which were referred to in the first vignette in Box 6-1. In its decision, the court wrote that the state law permitting the granting of a medical license

provides for…standards of qualification… and penalties for practicing without a license. The [state licensing] act is preventive, not a

compulsive, measure. In obtaining the state's license (permission) to practice medicine, the state does not require, and the licensee does not engage, that he will practice at all or on other terms than he may choose to accept. (*Hurley v. Eddingfield*, 1901)

In other words, obtaining a license to practice medicine does not obligate an individual to actually practice, or to practice in a particular fashion or with a particular clientele; the licensure requirement exists instead to filter out individuals who may not have the requisite knowledge or skills to practice medicine. The same can be said for obtaining a law license, or even a driver's license: the former does not obligate a lawyer to practice, or to choose certain types of clients or cases; the latter does not require that a person actually drive, or drive a certain make of car. As with a medical license, the point of a law or driver's license is to guarantee that should the licensee *choose* to practice law or operate a motor vehicle, he or she is qualified to do so. Furthermore, you will recall from the facts provided in the vignette that Dr. Eddingfield was Mrs. Burk's family physician, and many students believe that this fact is enough to establish a sufficient legal relationship between the two to hold Dr. Eddingfield accountable for the death of Mrs. Burk. However, the general legal rule is that physician–patient relationships are specific to "spells of illness" and that past treatment is not tantamount to an *existing* physician–patient relationship. Put another way, under the law a physician–patient relationship does not exist as a general, continuous matter—even with one's family physician, internist, primary care physician, and so on—but rather it exists for a specific period of time and must be established (or renewed) accordingly.

Note that this basic premise—that there is no fundamental right to healthcare services in the United States—was not altered by the passage in 2010 of the Affordable Care Act (ACA). While it is arguable that the ACA moves the country in a direction that makes a legal right to health care more plausible down the road (Friedman & Adashi, 2010), and while there can be no arguing that it makes health care more accessible to millions of people by virtue of its health insurance reforms (as discussed later in this chapter and in greater detail elsewhere), the ACA does not create a right to care.

As you begin to think through the significance and implications of the no-duty principle, it is important to understand that there are many other legal principles and health laws that define the relationship between an individual and another health system stakeholder (e.g., a physician, hospital, or government program). In fact, there are several federal and state laws that narrow the scope of the no-duty principle. For example, a federal law called the Examination and Treatment for Emergency Medical Conditions and Women in Labor Act enables all individuals to access some hospital care in medical emergencies, irrespective of the individual's ability to pay for that care or a hospital's willingness to treat the individual. Also, both federal and state laws that generally prohibit certain forms of discrimination (say, based on race or disability) apply in the context of health care and might thus result in access to health services that otherwise would not be forthcoming. Furthermore, some public health insurance programs—Medicaid and Medicare, most prominently—create entitlements (a legal concept denoting a legal claim to something) to services for individuals who meet the programs' eligibility criteria (Jost, 2003), and some health insurance products obligate physicians participating in the plan's networks to extend care to plan members. Finally, some states implemented universal healthcare coverage programs, such as Maine's Dirigo Health Reform Act, which was designed to provide access to health coverage to every person in Maine (and which ended at the end of 2014 as residents of the state were transitioned into the health insurance exchanges created by the ACA).

When thinking about the law's no-duty principle, you must also take into account the role of medical ethics, which might require more of a healthcare professional than does the law. For example, no law mandates that licensed physicians aid a stranger in medical distress, but many believe an ethical obligation exists in this instance. And although legally the no-duty principle would dictate otherwise, many healthcare providers consider themselves ethically obligated to furnish at least some level of care to those who cannot pay for it. In short, although there is no universal legal right to health care in the United States, certain situations give rise to healthcare rights, and specific populations may be entitled to health care or receive it purely through the magnanimity of ethics-conscious providers.

Perhaps because of the federal and state laws that chip away at the no-duty-to-treat principle, many students new to the study of health law erroneously assume that the principle is a legal anomaly, borne solely of the incredible historical power and autonomy of the medical profession and without modern precedent. In this case, it is instructive to place the principle in a broader "welfare rights" context. During the 1960s, public-interest lawyers, social reform activists, and others pressed for an interpretation of the federal Constitution that would have created an individual right to welfare. Under this view, the government must provide individuals with minimally adequate levels of education, food, housing,

health care, and so on (Davis, 1993). But in a series of cases, the Supreme Court rejected the notion of a constitutional right to welfare.

Consider the right to education. Even though every state provides free public schools and makes education for minors compulsory, there is no national, generalized legal right to education. In the case of *San Antonio Independent School District v. Rodriguez* (1973), the Supreme Court ruled that education is not a fundamental right under the federal Constitution's Equal Protection Clause. The plaintiffs in the *Rodriguez* case were Mexican-American parents whose children attended elementary and secondary schools in an urban San Antonio school district. They had attacked as unconstitutional Texas's system of financing public education and filed the suit on behalf of school children throughout the state who were members of minority groups or who resided in relatively poor school districts. But the court turned the plaintiffs' argument away, noting that although education is one of the most important services states perform,

> it is not among the rights afforded explicit protection under our Federal Constitution. Nor do we find any basis for saying it is implicitly so protected. . . . [T]he undisputed importance of education will not alone cause this Court to depart from the usual standard for reviewing a State's social and economic legislation. (*San Antonio Indep. School Dist. v. Rodriguez*, 1973)

In the wake of the *Rodriguez* decision, several states interpreted their own constitutions as prohibiting inequitable methods of financing public education, thereby recognizing on some level a right to a minimally "meaningful" education. Subsequently, lawyers and social activists seeking to promote equal access to all manner of critical services seized on these state determinations, arguing that an egalitarian approach to constitutional interpretation should not be limited to education (Stacy, 1993). Note, for example, how one author's writings about the right to education could just as well have been written with respect to health care:

> Requiring an adequate education will help to fulfill our nation's promise, articulated in *Brown* [*v. Board of Education*], that an individual be free to achieve her full potential. Ensuring educational adequacy will promote children's emotional and intellectual development, their career path and earning potential and thus their success throughout life. A meaningful education offers the hope that children can escape the degradation of

poverty and its lack of opportunity, and attain pride, participation in this country's economic and political life, and financial and emotional success. (Smith, 1997, p. 825)

However, efforts around ensuring adequate education have not been emulated in other social policy areas, such as health care. In fact, health care is treated not as a right, but as a commodity (like televisions or vacuum cleaners) subject to private market forces and socioeconomic status. During the public debate in 1993 over President Bill Clinton's failed attempt at national health reform, U.S. Representative Dick Armey (R-TX) stated that "health care is just a commodity, just like bread, and just like housing and everything else" (Reinhardt, 1996, p. 102). But why should this be the case, particularly when the private health insurance market has presumably found equilibrium at a point that continually leaves tens of millions of Americans uninsured, and particularly because health care (like education) is different from vacuum cleaners and other everyday goods in that it has "a fundamental bearing on the range of one's opportunities to realize one's life plans"? (Stacy, 1993, p. 80).

There is no single answer to the question of why health care is generally treated in this country as something less than an individual legal right. Many factors beyond the scope of this chapter are implicated: the nature and interpretation of the federal Constitution, politics, a weak labor movement, powerful interest groups, the nation's free market philosophies, the public's often negative view of the government, and more (Blum et al., 2003; Rich, 2000; Vladeck, 2003). In this chapter, we limit the discussion to describing the kinds of health rights that do exist, and how they operate in the context of the healthcare delivery system and when considered against government-initiated public health efforts. Before we explore in depth the scope of individual health-related rights under U.S. law, however, we briefly describe these same types of rights under international law and under the law of other countries. Through this examination, we provide a backdrop for understanding this country's approach to legal rights in the context of health.

▶ Individual Rights and Health Care: A Global Perspective

Despite being the world leader in terms of the development of medical technologies and the quantity of medical services, the United States is one of the only high-income nations that does not guarantee health care as a fundamental right, and it is the only developed nation that has not implemented a system for insuring at least all but the wealthiest segment of its population against healthcare costs (Jost, 2003, p. 3). In essence, other high-income nations with social democracies treat the provision of health care as a social good[b] (i.e., something that could be supported through private enterprise but is instead supported by the government and financed from public funds). Furthermore, it is worth noting that nations that provide universal healthcare entitlements have not been bankrupted as a result. In fact, according to Professor Timothy Jost, "all of the other developed nations spend less on health care than does the U.S., in terms of both dollars per capita and proportion of gross domestic product" (Jost, 2003, p. 3).

A foreign nation's universal healthcare rights—whether an unlimited right to health, a right to medical care generally or to a basic package of services, a right to healthcare insurance, or something else—exist as the result of either a commitment to human rights principles generally or fidelity to the particular country's own constitution. When recognized by governments, human rights accrue to all individuals because the rights are based on the dignity and worth of the human being; thus, technically, a human right exists regardless of whether positive law (a constitution or statute) has given it expression (Barnes & McChrystal, 1998). Examples of positive expressions of health as a human right include Article 25 of the 1948 Universal Declaration of Human Rights, which states that "everyone has the right to a standard of living adequate for the health and well-being of himself and of his family, including…medical care…and the right to security in the event of…sickness [or] disability" (Claiming Human Rights, 2010), and the Constitution of the World Health Organization, which says that "the enjoyment of the highest attainable standard of health is one of the fundamental rights of every human being without distinction of race, religion, political belief, economic or social condition" (World Health Organization, 2006).

In terms of national constitutions, some two-thirds of constitutions worldwide specifically address health or health care, and almost all of them do so in universal terms, rather than being limited to certain populations (Kinney & Clark, 2004). For example, consider the health-related aspects of the constitutions of four politically and culturally diverse countries—Italy, the Netherlands, South Africa, and Poland—that have some type of "right to health": Italy's Constitution guarantees a right to health; under the Dutch Constitution, the government is mandated "to promote the

Depending on one's personal experience in obtaining health care, or one's view of the role of physicians in society, of law as a tool for social change, of the scope of medical ethics, or of the United States' place in the broader global community, the no-duty principle might seem appropriate, irresponsible, or downright wrong. Imagine you are traveling in a country where socialized medicine is the legal norm, and your discussion with a citizen of that country turns to the topic of your countries' respective health systems. When asked, how will you account for the fact that health care is far from being a fundamental right rooted in American law?

health of the population"; the Constitution of South Africa imposes on government the obligation to provide access to health services; and under Polish constitutional law, citizens are guaranteed "the right to health protection" and access to publicly financed healthcare services (Littell, 2002).

Of course, including language respecting health rights in a legal document—even one as profound as a national constitution—does not guarantee that the right will be recognized or enforced. As in the United States, multiple factors might lead a foreign court or other tribunal to construe rights-creating language narrowly or to refuse to force implementation of what is properly considered a right. Examples of these factors include the relative strength of a country's judicial branch vis-a-vis other branches in its national governance structure and a foreign court's view of its country's ability to provide services and benefits inherent in the health right.

▶ Individual Rights and the Healthcare System

The "global perspective" you just read was brief for two reasons. First, a full treatment of international and foreign health rights is well beyond the scope of this chapter, and second, historically speaking, international law has played a limited role in influencing this nation's domestic legal principles. As one author commented, "historically the United States has been uniquely averse to accepting international human rights standards and conforming national laws to meet them" (Yamin, 2005, p. 1156). This fact is no less true in the area of health rights than in any

other major area of law. As described earlier in this chapter, universal rights to health care are virtually nonexistent in this country, even though this stance renders it almost solitary among the world's developed nations.

This is not to say that the United States has not contemplated health care as a universal, basic right. For instance, in 1952, a presidential commission stated that "access to the means for attainment and preservation of health is a basic human right" (President's Commission, 1983, p. 4). Medicaid and Medicare were the fruits of a nationwide debate about universal healthcare coverage. And during the 1960s and 1970s, the claim that health care was not a matter of privilege, but rather of right, was "so widely acknowledged as almost to be uncontroversial" (Starr, 1982, p. 389). Nor is it to say that certain populations do not enjoy healthcare rights beyond those of the general public. Prisoners and others under the control of state governments have a right to minimal health care (Wing, 1993), some state constitutions expressly recognize a right to health or healthcare benefits (for example, Montana includes an affirmative right to health in its constitution's section on inalienable rights), and individuals covered by Medicaid have unique legal entitlements. Finally, it would be inaccurate in describing healthcare rights to cover only rights to obtain health care in the first instance, because many important healthcare rights attach to individuals once they manage to access needed healthcare services.

The remainder of this section describes more fully the various types of individual rights associated with the healthcare system. We categorize these rights as follows:

1. Rights related to receiving services explicitly provided under healthcare, health financing, or health insurance laws—for example, the Examination and Treatment for Emergency Medical Conditions and Women in Labor Act, Medicaid, and the ACA
2. Rights concerning freedom of choice and freedom from government interference when making healthcare decisions—for example, choosing to have an abortion
3. The right to be free from unlawful discrimination when accessing or receiving health care—for example, Title VI of the federal Civil Rights Act of 1964, which prohibits discrimination on the basis of race, color, or national origin by entities that receive federal funding (Annas, 2004; Barnes & McChrystal, 1998, p. 12)

Rights Under Healthcare and Health Financing Laws

We begin this discussion of rights-creating health laws with the Examination and Treatment for Emergency Medical Conditions and Women in Labor Act (also referred to as EMTALA, which is the acronym for the law's original name—the Emergency Medical Treatment and Active Labor Act—or, for reasons soon to become clear, the "patient anti-dumping statute"). We then briefly discuss the federal Medicaid program in a rights-creating context and wrap up this section with a brief discussion of the ACA.

Rights Under Healthcare Laws: EMTALA

Because EMTALA represents the only truly universal legal right to health care in this country—the right to access emergency hospital services—it is often described as one of the building blocks of health rights. EMTALA was enacted by Congress in 1986 to prevent the practice of "patient dumping"—that is, the turning away of poor or uninsured persons in need of hospital care. Patient dumping was a common strategy among private hospitals aiming to shield themselves from the potentially uncompensated costs associated with treating poor and/or uninsured patients. By refusing to treat these individuals and instead "dumping" them on public hospitals, private institutions were effectively limiting their patients to those whose treatment costs would likely be covered out-of-pocket or by insurers. Note that the no-duty principle made this type of strategy possible.

EMTALA was a conscious effort on the part of elected federal officials to chip away at the no-duty principle: by creating legally enforceable rights to emergency hospital care for all individuals regardless of their income or health insurance status, Congress created a corresponding legal *duty* of care on the part of hospitals. At its core, EMTALA includes two related duties, which technically attach only to hospitals that participate in the Medicare program (but then again, nearly every hospital in the country participates). The first duty requires covered hospitals to provide an "appropriate" screening examination to all individuals who present at a hospital's emergency department seeking care for an "emergency medical condition." Under the law, an appropriate medical screening is one that is nondiscriminatory and that adheres to a hospital's established emergency care guidelines. EMTALA defines an emergency medical condition as a

medical condition manifesting itself by acute symptoms of sufficient severity (including severe pain) such that the absence of immediate medical attention could reasonably be expected to result in (i) placing the health of the individual (or, with respect to a pregnant woman, the health of the woman or her unborn child) in serious jeopardy, (ii) serious impairment to bodily functions, or (iii) serious dysfunction of any bodily organ or part; or with respect to a pregnant woman who is having contractions, that there is inadequate time to effect a safe transfer to another hospital before delivery, or that transfer may pose a threat to the health or safety of the woman or the unborn child. (Examination and Treatment, 2011)

The second key duty required of hospitals under EMTALA is to either stabilize any condition that meets the preceding definition or, in the case of a hospital without the capability to treat the emergency condition, undertake to transfer the patient to another facility in a medically appropriate fashion. A proper transfer is effected when, among other things, the transferring hospital minimizes the risks to the patient's health by providing as much treatment as is within its capability, a receiving medical facility has agreed to accept the transferred patient, and the transferring hospital provides the receiving facility all relevant medical records.

The legal rights established under EMTALA are accompanied by heavy penalties for their violation. The federal government, individual patients, and "dumped-on" hospitals can all initiate actions against a hospital alleged to have violated EMTALA, and the federal government can also file a claim for civil money penalties against individual physicians who negligently violate an EMTALA requirement.

Rights Under Healthcare Financing Laws: Medicaid

Many laws fund programs that aim to expand access to health care, such as state laws authorizing the establishment of public hospitals or health agencies, and the federal law establishing the vast network of community health clinics that serve medically underserved communities and populations. However, the legal obligations created by these financing laws are generally enforceable only by public agencies, not by individuals.

The Medicaid program is different in this respect. (Medicaid is covered elsewhere in greater depth, but because of its importance in the area of individual healthcare rights, we mention it also in this context.) Although most certainly a law concerning healthcare financing, Medicaid is unlike most other health financing laws in that it confers the right to individually enforce program obligations through the courts (Rosenblatt, Law, & Rosenbaum, 1997, pp. 419–424). This right of individual enforcement is one of the reasons why Medicaid, 50 years after its creation, remains a hotly debated public program. This is because the legal entitlements to benefits under Medicaid are viewed as a key contributor to the program's high cost. Yet whether Medicaid's legal entitlements are any more of a factor in the program's overall costs than, say, the generally high cost of health care, is not clearly established.

Rights Under Health Insurance Laws: The ACA

As you will learn in subsequent chapters, the ACA is far more than a law that concerns only health insurance; it is a sweeping set of reforms that touch on healthcare quality, public health practice, health disparities, community health centers, healthcare fraud and abuse, comparative effectiveness research, the health workforce, health information technology, long-term care, and more. However, for purposes of this chapter, we mention it briefly in terms of its impact on the rights of individuals to access health insurance and to equitable treatment by their insurer. Details concerning the ACA's effect on the public and private insurance markets are discussed elsewhere.

Through a series of major reforms to existing policies, the ACA reshapes the private health insurance market, transforming private health insurance from a commodity that regularly classified (and rejected) individuals based on their health status, age, disability status, and more into a social good whose availability is essential to individual and population health (Rosenbaum, 2011). The key elements of this shift include a ban on exclusion and discrimination based on health status or preexisting health conditions; new protections that ensure that, once covered by insurance, individuals will have access to necessary care without regard to artificial annual or lifetime expenditure caps; a guarantee that once insurance coverage is in place, it cannot be rescinded except in cases of applicant fraud; a ban on additional fees for out-of-network emergency services; the provision of financial subsidies to help low- and moderate-income individuals and small businesses purchase insurance coverage; the inclusion, in the individual and small group insurance markets, of a package of "essential health benefits" that must be covered; and the creation of state health insurance "exchanges" through which individuals and small employer groups can purchase high-quality health insurance in a virtual marketplace that is substantially regulated and that simplifies the job of learning about, selecting, and enrolling in insurance plans.

The ACA also reforms the public health insurance market, primarily through an expansion of Medicaid eligibility to cover all non-elderly low-income persons who are legal residents or citizens (this expansion is now voluntary on the part of states, as the result of a Supreme Court decision described in a subsequent chapter). If fully implemented, this reform would substantially close one of Medicaid's last remaining coverage gaps for the poor—namely, the program's historical denial of coverage for nonpregnant, working-age adults without minor children—and in so doing would provide insurance coverage (and the resulting access to health care that often follows coverage) to many millions of people.

Rights Related to Freedom of Choice and Freedom From Government Interference

EMTALA and Medicaid are remarkable in terms of the rights *to* health care that they each provide, though as mentioned earlier in this chapter, individual rights that attach *within* the context of healthcare provision can be equally important. Important individual rights within health care include the right to make informed healthcare decisions and the right to personal privacy and autonomy.

The Right to Make Informed Healthcare Decisions

One of the most important healthcare rights is the right of individual patients to make informed decisions about the scope and course of their own care. This includes the right to *refuse* treatment, regardless of the treatment's nature or urgency. That is, the right to refuse treatment exists whether the patient is considering ingesting prescribed medication for minor pain, undergoing a minimally invasive test or procedure, or consenting to a major, potentially life-sustaining operation like the removal of a brain tumor. However, the right pertaining to informed decision making does not come without qualifiers and exceptions, as described here.

Modern notions of informed consent have their roots in the Nuremberg Code, which derived from the Nuremberg trials in the late 1940s of German physicians who performed horrendous experiments on prisoners in Nazi concentration camps during the Second World War. The code spells out principles of research ethics, including the need to secure in advance the voluntary consent of the research subject. These principles have been codified and expanded in American federal statutory and regulatory law concerning federally funded biomedical research (Protection of Human Subjects, 2009). But if the Nuremberg Code can be thought of as the roots of U.S. informed consent law, then the decision in *Canterbury v. Spence* (1972) can be thought of as the trunk.

In 1959, Jerry Canterbury was a 19-year-old suffering from severe back pain. His neurosurgeon, Dr. William Spence, informed him that he would need a laminectomy—a surgical procedure in which the roofs of spinal vertebrae are removed or trimmed to relieve pressure on the spinal cord—to correct what the doctor believed was a herniated disc. However, Dr. Spence did not inform Canterbury of any risks associated with the surgery. The day after the operation, while appearing to recuperate normally, Canterbury fell from his hospital bed while no attendant was on hand and a few hours later began suffering paralysis from the waist down. This led to a second spinal surgery, but Canterbury never fully recovered; years later, he needed crutches to walk and he suffered from paralysis of the bowels.

Canterbury sued Dr. Spence, alleging negligence in both the performance of the laminectomy and the doctor's failure to disclose risks inherent in the operation. The federal trial judge ruled in Dr. Spence's favor and Canterbury appealed, setting the stage for the now-famous decision in 1972 by the federal Court of Appeals for the District of Columbia Circuit (considered second in national importance to the Supreme Court).[c] The decision includes two important determinations pertinent to this chapter. The first is that "as a part of the physician's overall obligation to the patient, [there exists a] duty of reasonable disclosure of the choices with respect to proposed therapy and the dangers inherently and potentially involved." The court viewed this duty as a logical and modest extension of a physician's existing general duty to his patients. Importantly, the court discarded the notion that "the patient should ask for information before the physician is required to disclose." In other words, the duty to disclose requires more than just answering patient questions; it demands voluntary disclosure on the part of the physician of pertinent medical information.

The *Canterbury* court's second key determination concerns the actual scope of the disclosure required—in other words, once the physician's duty to disclose is triggered, what information satisfies the legal requirement? On this matter the court made several observations: that the patient's right of "self-decision" is paramount, that the right to consent can be properly exercised only if the patient has sufficient information to make an "intelligent choice," that the sufficiency test is met when all information "material to the decision" is disclosed, and that the disclosure's legality should be measured objectively, not subjectively from the perspective of a particular physician or patient. From these observations, the court settled on three required pieces of disclosed information: a proposed treatment's inherent and potential risks, any alternatives to a proposed treatment, and the likely outcome of not being treated at all. Applying these criteria, the court ruled that Dr. Spence's failure to disclose even the tiniest risk of paralysis resulting from the laminectomy entitled Canterbury to a new trial.

As mentioned earlier, the right to make informed healthcare decisions is not boundless. For example, the court in *Canterbury* wrote that where disclosure of a treatment's risks would pose a threat of harm to the patient (for example, because it would severely complicate treatment or psychologically damage the patient) as to become "unfeasible or contraindicated from a medical point of view," the physician's duty to disclose could be set aside. Furthermore, a patient's competency from a legal vantage point plays a major role in his or her ability to consent to treatment.

The *Canterbury* decision and its progeny have over the years been interpreted expansively, and today the right to make informed healthcare decisions has many facets beyond a clear explanation of proposed treatments, potential risks and complications, and the like. For example, patients have the right to know whether outside factors, such as research interests or financial considerations, are coloring a physician's thinking about a proposed course of treatment; patients whose first language is not English have the right to an interpreter; and patients have the right to designate in advance their treatment wishes, whether through written advance directives or another individual.

The Right to Personal Privacy

Another right related to freedom of choice and freedom from government interference is the constitutional right to personal privacy. Although the federal Constitution makes no explicit mention of the right to privacy, the Supreme Court has recognized some form of it since the 1890s.[d] The court has taken a more or less two-pronged approach to the right. The first approach defines the protected personal interest as

Go back to the first legal principle drawn from the *Canterbury* decision: namely, that physicians have a duty of reasonable disclosure to include therapy options and the dangers potentially involved with each. Do you agree with the court that this duty is both a logical and modest extension of physicians' "traditional" obligation to their patients? Why or why not? Depending on your answer, are you surprised to learn that some states have opted not to follow the *Canterbury* court's patient-oriented standard of informed consent, relying instead on the more conventional approach of measuring the legality of physician disclosure based on what a reasonable physician would have disclosed?

"informational privacy," meaning the limiting of others' access to and use of an individual's private information.[e] The second approach—the focus of this section—is concerned with individual autonomy and freedom from governmental interference in making basic personal decisions. This right is one of the most debated in law, both because of its implicit nature (constitutionally speaking) and because it has served as the legal underpinning of several divisive social issues, including abortion, intimate associations, and the decisions as to whether, when, and how to end one's life.

The right to privacy achieved prominence beginning with the Supreme Court's landmark 1965 decision in *Griswold v. Connecticut* (1965), in which the court considered the constitutionality of a state law criminalizing the provision of contraception to married couples. In the early 1960s, Estelle Griswold, the Executive Director of the Planned Parenthood League of Connecticut, and one of her colleagues were convicted of aiding and abetting "the use of a drug, medicinal article, or instrument for the purpose of preventing conception" by providing contraceptives to a married couple in violation of Connecticut law. The court determined that although the Constitution does not explicitly protect a general right to privacy, certain provisions in the Bill of Rights create "penumbras," or zones, of guaranteed privacy, and that Connecticut's law constituted an undue intrusion into one of these zones (i.e., marriage).

After the *Griswold* decision, advocates of the constitutional right to privacy flooded the federal courts with cases designed to expand the scope of the right. Quickly, laws banning interracial marriage were struck down (*Loving v. Virginia*, 1967), as were laws

prohibiting unmarried individuals from using contraception (*Eisenstadt v. Baird*, 1972). At the same time, federal courts were confronted with cases asking them to determine how the right to privacy applied in the context of abortion. The remainder of this section analyzes the courts' response to this particular issue. We selected the constitutional right to abortion as the focal point of the right to privacy discussion because it is not only one of the most contested rights in a health context, but also one of the most contested areas of public policy generally.

The *Roe v. Wade* Decision. Few judicial decisions have affected this country's legal, political, and social landscape as much as *Roe v. Wade* (1973).[f] In 1970, an unmarried pregnant woman filed a lawsuit under the pseudonym "Roe" challenging the constitutionality of a Texas criminal law that prohibited procuring or attempting an abortion at any stage of pregnancy, except for the purpose of saving the pregnant woman's life. Roe was joined in the lawsuit by a doctor who performed abortions in violation of the law. They argued that the constitutional right to privacy articulated in *Griswold* and its progeny included a woman's right to choose to obtain an abortion. Texas, through district attorney Henry Wade, claimed that the law was permissible because the state had a compelling interest in protecting women from an unsafe medical procedure and in protecting prenatal life. The federal trial court agreed with Roe and declared the law unconstitutional, and Texas immediately appealed to the U.S. Supreme Court, which agreed to hear the case (in rare circumstances, the Supreme Court will hear a case without an intermediate appellate court ruling).

At the Supreme Court, the work of drafting the majority opinion in *Roe v. Wade* fell to Justice Harry Blackmun, who earlier in his legal career had been counsel to a well-known and highly regarded medical clinic. By a 7–2 margin, the court ruled that the constitutional right to privacy, which in its view most strongly emanates from the 14th Amendment's due process protections, is broad enough to encompass a woman's decision to terminate her pregnancy.

Once the court established that a woman has a constitutional right to obtain an abortion, it went on to discuss the limits of that right. Roe had argued that the right to obtain an abortion is absolute and that no state or federal law abridging the right could be enacted. The court did not agree. Justice Blackmun wrote that states have both an interest in protecting the welfare of its citizens and a duty to protect them and that the duty extends to the unborn. According to the court, "a State may properly assert important interests in safeguarding health, in maintaining medical standards, and in protecting potential life. At some point in pregnancy, these respective interests become sufficiently compelling to sustain regulation of the factors that govern the abortion decision" (*Roe v. Wade*, 1973). The court then linked both a woman's "right to choose" and states' interest in protecting potential life to the viability of the fetus, setting forth the following "trimester framework" that enhances state power to regulate the abortion decision and restricts a pregnant woman's right as the fetus grows older:

a. For the stage prior to approximately the end of the first trimester, the abortion decision and its effectuation must be left to the medical judgment of the pregnant woman's attending physician.

b. For the stage subsequent to approximately the end of the first trimester, the State, in promoting its interest in the health of the mother, may, if it chooses, regulate the abortion procedure in ways that are reasonably related to maternal health.

c. For the stage subsequent to viability, the State, in promoting its interest in the potentiality of human life may, if it chooses, regulate, and even proscribe, abortion except where it is necessary, in appropriate medical judgment, for the preservation of the life or health of the mother (*Roe v. Wade*, 1973).

As a matter of both policy and law, the *Roe* decision has been vigorously criticized (Barzelay & Heymann, 1973; Bopp & Coleson, 1989; Ely, 1979; Regan, 1979). For example, detractors claim that the court improperly made social policy by "finding" an expansive constitutional right to privacy (one broad enough to include the right to terminate a pregnancy) where one did not expressly exist. As a legal matter, many have argued that the decision relied too heavily on medical concepts that would be rendered obsolete as medical technology advanced and that would, in turn, result in a narrowing of the constitutional right advanced in the decision.[8]

Regardless of these and other criticisms, the *Roe* decision was monumental beyond its legal implications. It galvanized political forces opposed to abortion and prompted a movement to create ways to discourage the practice through state policies designed to regulate the factors involved in the abortion decision. For example, as described next, Pennsylvania enacted a law that imposed a series of requirements on women seeking abortion services, and it was this law that nearly 20 years after *Roe* set the stage for another battle at the Supreme Court over abortion and the right to privacy.

The *Planned Parenthood of Southeastern Pennsylvania v. Casey* Decision.

At issue in the 1992 case of *Planned Parenthood of Southeastern Pennsylvania v. Casey* were several amendments to Pennsylvania's Abortion Control Act that made it more difficult for a pregnant woman to obtain an abortion: one provision required that a woman seeking an abortion be provided with certain information at least 24 hours in advance of the abortion; a second stated that a minor seeking an abortion had to secure the informed consent of one of her parents, but included a "judicial bypass" option if the minor did not wish to or could not obtain parental consent; a third amendment required that a married woman seeking an abortion had to submit a signed statement indicating that she had notified her husband of her intent to have an abortion, though certain exceptions were included; and a final provision imposed new reporting requirements on facilities that offered abortion services. The revised law exempted compliance with these requirements in the event of a "medical emergency."

Before any of the new provisions took effect, they were challenged by five Pennsylvania abortion clinics and a group of physicians who performed abortions. The federal trial court struck down all of the provisions as unconstitutional violations under *Roe*. On appeal, the Third Circuit Court of Appeals reversed and upheld all of the provisions, except for the husband notification requirement, as constitutional. The plaintiffs appealed to the Supreme Court, which agreed to hear the case.

The court's 5–4 decision in favor of the plaintiffs in *Casey* expressly acknowledged the widespread confusion over the meaning and reach of *Roe*, and it used its opinion in *Casey* to provide better guidance to legislatures seeking to regulate abortion as a constitutionally protected right. Specifically, the court in *Casey* sought to define more precisely both the constitutional rights of pregnant women and the legitimate authority of states to regulate some aspects of the abortion decision. The deeply divided court wrote the following:

> It must be stated at the outset and with clarity that *Roe*'s essential holding, the holding we reaffirm, has three parts. First is a recognition of the right of the woman to choose to have an abortion before viability and to obtain it without undue interference from the State. Before viability, the State's interests are not strong enough to support a prohibition of

abortion or the imposition of a substantial obstacle to the woman's effective right to elect the procedure. Second is a confirmation of the State's power to restrict abortions after fetal viability, if the law contains exceptions for pregnancies which endanger the woman's life or health. And third is the principle that the State has legitimate interests from the outset of the pregnancy in protecting the health of the woman and the life of the fetus that may become a child. These principles do not contradict one another; and we adhere to each. (*Planned Parenthood of Southeastern Pennsylvania v. Casey*, 1992)

Notice how, in interpreting *Roe*, the court in *Casey* makes some remarkable alterations to the contours of the right to choose to have an abortion. First, trimesters were replaced by fetal viability as the regulatory touchstone. Second, the pregnant woman, not her attending physician, makes the abortion decision. Third, a state's interest in protecting pregnant women and fetuses now attaches "from the outset of the pregnancy," not at the beginning of the second trimester. Fourth, and perhaps most important, the court's invalidation of the trimester framework enabled the establishment of a new "undue burden" standard for assessing the constitutionality of state abortion regulations. Under this new standard, a state may not prohibit abortion prior to fetal viability, but it may promulgate abortion regulations as long as they do not pose a "substantial obstacle" to a woman seeking to terminate a pregnancy. The court did not, however, alter its decision in *Roe* that, post-viability, a state may proscribe abortion except when pregnancies endanger a woman's life or health. Taken together, these alterations both maintain a pregnant woman's basic constitutional right to obtain an abortion pre-viability and enhance state interest in protecting the potentiality for human life.

Once the court established the undue burden standard for assessing the constitutionality of state abortion regulations, it applied the standard to each constitutionally questionable amendment to Pennsylvania's Abortion Control Act. In the end, only the spousal notification provision was struck down as an unconstitutional burden; the court determined that some pregnant women may have sound reasons for not wishing to inform their husbands of their decision to obtain an abortion, including fear of abuse, threats of future violence, and withdrawal of financial support. As a result, the court equated the spousal notification requirement to a substantial obstacle because it was likely to prevent women from obtaining abortions.

The court majority in *Casey* provided a new template for lower courts to use in deciding the constitutionality of state abortion regulations. Likewise, the opinion offered guidance to state legislatures as to what kinds of abortion restrictions were likely to withstand a constitutional attack. Nonetheless, some state legislatures have tested the boundaries of *Casey* by enacting bans on a procedure known as "partial birth" abortion, an issue to which we now turn.

The *Stenberg v. Carhart* Decision. The undue burden standard articulated in *Casey* for assessing the constitutionality of abortion regulations was put to the test in *Stenberg v. Carhart* (2000). At issue in the case was a Nebraska criminal law banning "an abortion procedure in which the person performing the abortion partially delivers vaginally a living unborn child before killing the unborn child and completing the delivery." It further defined "partially delivers vaginally a living unborn child before killing the unborn child" to mean "deliberately and intentionally delivering into the vagina a living unborn child, or a substantial portion thereof, for the purpose of performing a procedure that the person performing such procedure knows will kill the unborn child and does kill the unborn child." The Nebraska law penalized physicians who performed a banned abortion procedure with a prison term of up to 20 years, a fine of up to $25,000, and the automatic revocation of the doctor's license to practice medicine in Nebraska.

Dr. Leroy Carhart, a Nebraska physician who performed abortions, filed a lawsuit seeking a declaration that the Nebraska law violated the constitutional principles set forth in *Roe* and *Casey*. After a lengthy trial, a federal district court agreed with Dr. Carhart and declared the Nebraska law unconstitutional. The Court of Appeals for the Eighth Circuit agreed, concluding that Nebraska's statute violated the Constitution as interpreted by the Supreme Court in *Casey*. The Supreme Court then granted review.

The court was unequivocal in its opinion in *Stenberg* that the case was not a forum for a discussion on the propriety of *Roe* and *Casey*, but rather an application of the rules stated in those cases. In applying the undue burden standard to pre-viability abortions, the court considered trial court testimony from expert witnesses regarding several different abortion procedures that were then current in medical practice to flesh out the procedures' technical distinctions and to determine whether the procedures fell within Nebraska's definition of "partial birth" abortion. The court determined that two distinct abortion procedures were relevant—dilation and evacuation (D&E),

and dilation and extraction (D&X)—and that the Nebraska law's vague definition of "partial birth" abortion effectively banned both procedures.

Again by a 5–4 majority, the Supreme Court struck down the Nebraska law as unconstitutional on two separate grounds. First, the court concluded that the statute created an undue burden on women seeking pre-viability abortions. The court reasoned that banning the most commonly used method for pre-viability second trimester abortions—the D&E procedure—unconstitutionally burdened a woman's ability to choose to have an abortion. Second, the court invalidated the state law because it lacked an exception for the preservation of the health of the pregnant woman. The court rejected Nebraska's claim that the banned procedures were never necessary to maintain the health of the pregnant woman and held that "significant medical authority" indicated that the D&X procedure is in some cases the safest abortion procedure available.

At the time *Stenberg* was decided, nearly 30 states had laws restricting D&E- and D&X-type abortions in some manner. Attempts to enact bans on these abortion procedures, however, have not been made only by state legislatures. Congress has tried numerous times to promulgate a federal ban, and after *Stenberg* was handed down, congressional opponents to abortion vowed to craft a ban that would pass constitutional muster. This effort culminated in the Partial Birth Abortion Ban Act of 2003 (PBABA).

Partial Birth Abortion Ban Act of 2003. PBABA represented Congress's third attempt since 1996 to ban "partial birth" abortions. Previous bills were vetoed by President Bill Clinton in 1996 and 1997, but in late 2003, PBABA easily passed both houses of Congress and was signed into law by President George W. Bush. Immediately, the constitutionality of PBABA was challenged in federal court, and the Supreme Court ultimately decided the law's fate in 2007, as described here.

PBABA establishes criminal penalties for "any physician who . . . knowingly performs a partial birth abortion and thereby kills a human fetus." Attempting to avoid the definitional vagueness that affected the Nebraska law's constitutionality, the drafters of the federal law used more precise language in an effort to ban only D&X procedures, although PBABA does not specifically refer to any medical procedure by name. Instead, the law defines a "partial birth" abortion as

> an abortion in which the person performing the abortion deliberately and intentionally vaginally delivers a living fetus until, in the case of a headfirst presentation, the entire fetal head is outside the body of the mother, or, in the case of a breech presentation, any part of the fetal trunk past the navel is outside the body of the mother, for the purpose of performing an overt act that the person knows will kill the partially delivered living fetus. (PBABA, 2003)

PBABA contains an exception allowing for these otherwise illegal abortions when necessary to protect a pregnant woman's life, but not health. The law's authors claim that the banned procedure is never necessary to protect the health of a pregnant woman and thus that an exception is not required.

Separate lawsuits challenging PBABA were filed in federal courts in California, Nebraska, and New York. All three federal trial courts concluded that the lack of a health exception necessarily rendered the law unconstitutional under Supreme Court precedent. With enforcement of PBABA halted, the federal government appealed all three cases. The appellate courts that examined PBABA all found that substantial medical authority exists supporting the necessity of the banned procedure and declared PBABA unconstitutional because of its lack of a health exception. As noted, the fate of PBABA was then decided by the Supreme Court.

The *Gonzales v. Carhart* Decision. The Supreme Court upheld the constitutionality of the PBABA in *Gonzales v. Carhart*, another 5–4 decision. The court rejected the reasoning of the appellate courts and found that PBABA was not on its face "void for vagueness" (a doctrine that permits courts to reject statutes under which a layperson could not generally understand who is being regulated or what is being prohibited) and did not pose an undue burden on the right to receive an abortion under *Casey*. Although the court reaffirmed again the various basic principles of *Roe* and *Casey*—that women have an unfettered right to an abortion pre-viability, that the government has the power to restrict abortions post-viability, and that the government has an interest from the outset of pregnancy in protecting the health of the woman and the fetus—the court in *Carhart* focused on the latter and held that the government's legitimate interest in promoting fetal life would be hindered if the act was invalidated.

The court first ruled that PBABA was not void for vagueness simply because the law prohibits performing intact D&Es. According to the court, the law puts doctors on notice of the prohibited conduct by adequately describing the intact D&E procedure and requiring that the doctor have knowledge that he is performing the intact D&E for the purpose of destroying the fetus. The court also found that PBABA did not impose an undue burden for being overly broad. To distinguish it from the Nebraska law in *Stenberg*, the court majority stated that PBABA targets extraction of the entire fetus, as opposed to the removal of fetal pieces beyond a specific anatomic point in the pregnant woman.

The court then held that PBABA did not pose a "substantial obstacle" to obtaining an abortion under *Casey*'s undue burden test. According to the court, the ban on partial birth abortions furthers the government's interest in protecting fetal life and the government has the ability to prohibit practices ending fetal life that are similar to condemned practices. Finally, in a major shift that received relatively little attention by the court majority, the court ruled that the fact that PBABA did not contain language protecting the health of the woman did not render the law unconstitutional. Deferring to Congress because there are other safe procedures besides intact D&E that a doctor may use to perform an abortion and because according to the court PBABA promotes fetal life, the court simply declared the law constitutional notwithstanding the missing language.

The Right to Be Free From Wrongful Discrimination

We now transition to the final topic in the discussion of individual legal rights to and within health care—namely, the topic of healthcare discrimination.[h] Like discrimination generally, healthcare discrimination has a lurid and lengthy history in this country. Prior to the *Brown v. Board of Education* decision in 1954 and the civil rights movement of the 1960s, healthcare injustice and exclusion based on race and other factors were commonplace, dating to slavery times and plantation-based racially segregated health care. After the end of the First Reconstruction, states passed so-called Jim Crow laws, cementing in place legally segregated health care. As a result, hospitals, physician practices, medical/nursing/dental schools, and professional medical societies were all separated based on race. In places where Jim Crow laws had not been passed, corporate bylaws and contracts between private parties often had the same discriminatory effect, and these "Jim Crow substitutes" were generally honored and enforced by the courts that interpreted them.

Federal law also played a role in perpetuating racially segregated health care. For example, the Hospital Survey and Construction Act of 1946 (more commonly known as the Hill–Burton Act, after the

key congressional sponsors of the measure) provided federal money to states to build and refurbish hospitals after World War II, but explicitly sanctioned the construction of segregated facilities:

> A hospital will be made available to all persons residing in [its] territorial area…without discrimination on account of race, creed, or color, but an exception shall be made in cases where separate hospital facilities are provided for separate population groups, if the plan makes equitable provision on the basis of need for facilities and services of like quality for each such group. (Hospital Survey and Construction Act, 1946)

This provision was not ruled unconstitutional until the 1963 case of *Simkins v. Moses H. Cone Memorial Hospital*, which has been referred to as the "*Brown v. Board of Education* of health care" (Smith, 1999). *Simkins* also helped fuel the passage of the Civil Rights Act of 1964, this country's most important civil rights legislation of the 20th century. For purposes of health care, Title VI of the 1964 Act was of specific importance. Title VI is discussed in more depth later in this chapter; in sum, this portion of the Civil Rights Act makes it illegal for programs and activities that receive federal funding to discriminate on the basis of race, color, or national origin.

Notwithstanding the healthcare rewards brought about by the civil rights movement—Title VI, the passage of Medicaid and Medicare, the establishment of federally financed community health centers—the focus on healthcare civil rights was waning as early as 1968. Several factors led to this decline, but what is most striking is that compared to the progress made by public and private civil rights efforts over the past 45 years in education, employment, and housing, civil rights enforcement in the healthcare field has been anything but sustained.

Of course, even an enduring and well-funded enforcement effort is no guarantee of wiping out discrimination, regardless of its social context. There are, unfortunately, vestiges of discrimination in many important aspects of American society, including the healthcare system. Moreover, although historically healthcare discrimination on the basis of race and ethnicity has received the most attention, the existence of discrimination in health care on the basis of socioeconomic status, disability, age, and gender also raises troubling questions. The remainder of this section touches briefly on each of these areas, describing laws (where applicable) or legal theories used to combat the particular healthcare discrimination at issue.

BOX 6-4 Discussion Question

If you were asked to distill, down to their most essential parts, the constitutional right to privacy and the right to privacy as it applies to abortion, what elements would you include?

Race/Ethnicity Discrimination

The fact that healthcare discrimination premised on race or ethnicity has dominated the healthcare civil rights landscape should not be surprising, because racist beliefs and customs have infected health care no less so than other areas of life, such as education, employment, and housing. This fact is chronicled to a staggering degree by W. Michael Byrd and Linda A. Clayton, two physician-researchers at the Harvard School of Public Health (2000; 2002). Byrd and Clayton paint a complex and disturbing picture of a healthcare system that itself perpetuates racism in health care in three distinct ways: by not destroying the myth that minority Americans should be expected to experience poorer health relative to Caucasians; by organizing itself as a private, for-profit system that marginalizes the indigent and minorities; and by refusing to acknowledge the historical and ongoing problem of racial exclusion in health care.

One key problem that in part results from the design of the healthcare system is that of racial and ethnic health disparities—differences in healthcare access, treatment, and outcomes between populations of color and Caucasians. In 2003, the Institute of Medicine (IOM; now called the Academy of Medicine) released an influential report that included overwhelming evidence of racial and ethnic health disparities and documented that these disparities could not be explained solely by the relative amount of health care needed by populations of color and nonminority populations (Smedley, Stith, & Nelson, 2003). For example, the report concluded that African Americans are relatively less likely to receive treatment for early-stage lung cancer, publicly insured Latinos and African Americans do not receive coronary artery bypass surgery at rates comparable to publicly insured nonminorities, and Latino and African American children on Medicaid experience relatively higher rates of hospitalization.

Furthermore, the IOM study revealed that even when relevant patient characteristics are controlled for, racial and ethnic differences arise not only in terms of accessing care initially, but also after individuals have entered the healthcare system, a finding that supports the notion that both the system itself and physician practice style contribute to disparities. This notion is, of course, quite controversial, because it suggests that physician decision making and clinical practice can increase the likelihood of racially disparate outcomes.

The key federal law used to combat race and ethnicity discrimination in health care is Title VI of the 1964 Civil Rights Act, which states that "no person in the United States shall, on the ground of race, color, or national origin, be excluded from participation in, be denied the benefits of, or be subjected to discrimination under any program or activity receiving federal financial assistance." Because it attaches only to recipients of federal funding, Title VI does not reach, for example, health professionals who do not directly participate in government-sponsored health programs; nor does it reach physicians whose only participation in federal assistance programs is under Medicare Part B (the basis for this exemption is historical and purely political, and the exemption is not codified in Title VI statutory or regulatory law [Smith, 1999, pp. 115–128]). Nonetheless, Title VI has long had the potential to greatly impact the field of health care, because an enormous amount of federal funding has been poured into the healthcare enterprise over the past 50 years.

The concept of "discrimination" under Title VI applies both to *intentional* acts and to actions or policies that unintentionally have the *effect* of discriminating against racial and ethnic minorities. This is so because federal regulations implementing the Title VI statute (which explicitly prohibits only intentional discrimination) reach actions that, even if neutral on their face, have a disproportionate adverse impact (or effect) on members of minority groups. In the case of healthcare access and delivery, you can imagine several types of conduct that might potentially violate the Title VI disproportionate impact regulations. For example, were a hospital to segregate patients by source of payment—say, by maintaining a ward or floor that treated only patients covered under Medicaid—racial and ethnic minorities may be adversely impacted, given the overall makeup of the Medicaid population. Similarly, the Title VI regulations could be violated if a managed care organization enrolled both privately and publicly insured persons but allowed participating providers to refuse to accept as patients those individuals covered by Medicaid.

The disproportionate impact regulations are crucial to realizing Title VI's full force, because much of the racism in post-1954 America does not take the form of overt, intentional acts. However, as a result of the 2001 Supreme Court decision in *Alexander v. Sandoval*, these regulations were severely undercut.

Under *Alexander*, private individuals were barred from bringing a lawsuit under the disparate impact regulations, leaving the federal government as the sole enforcer when racial or ethnic minorities allege a violation of the regulations.[i]

Physical and Mental Disability Discrimination

Like discrimination based on race or ethnicity, healthcare discrimination premised on disability has a long, sad history in this country and, as with race, the health system itself is partly to blame for its perpetuation. For instance, historically, persons with mental disabilities were viewed from a medical standpoint as having little to offer to society, and they were, as a matter of practice, shipped to mental asylums isolated from communities. Those with physical disabilities were not spared discriminatory practices, either; because individuals with Down syndrome were viewed by medical practitioners as "Mongoloid idiots" and children with cerebral palsy or other serious physical limitations were regularly viewed as unable to contribute to society, they were all simply institutionalized. These historical practices and perspectives resonate even in the modern healthcare system, in which treatment opportunities for the disabled are skewed toward institutional, rather than community, settings, and disease-specific limitations in health insurance are commonplace.

However, passage of the Americans With Disabilities Act (ADA) in 1990 alleviated at least some of the problems associated with disability discrimination in health care. Like Title VI, the ADA is not specifically a "health law"; its intent is to extend to the disabled the maximum opportunity for community integration in many sectors of society, including employment, public services, public accommodations (i.e., privately owned entities open to the public), telecommunications, and more. For this reason, it prohibits discrimination generally against disabled individuals who satisfy the essential requirements of a particular job, or who meet the qualification standards for a program, service, or benefit.

But the ADA's impact on health care for disabled individuals is notable, in large part because the law defines "places of public accommodation" to include private hospitals and other private healthcare providers. So, for example, a dentist in private practice who does not receive any federal funds for his services is nonetheless prohibited from discriminating against a person who is HIV-positive, as the well-known case of *Bragdon v. Abbott* (1990) makes clear. This represents an important expansion of federal disability law because prior to the ADA, only recipients of federal funds were proscribed from discriminating on the basis of disability. Note also how this expanded concept of public accommodations differs from Title VI of the Civil Rights Act, which still requires the receipt of federal money on the part of the offending entity to trigger protections for racial and ethnic minorities.

Although the ADA has dramatically altered the disability law landscape, it is not without limitations. For example, the regulations implementing the ADA's statutory text require entities that implement public programs and services to make only "reasonable modifications"—but not "fundamental alterations"—to those programs and services. Under the ADA, a fundamental alteration is one that would change the essential nature of a public program or service. Whether a requested change to a public program or service by a disabled individual amounts to a "reasonable" or a "fundamental" one is potentially determinative to the outcome of the request. Why? Because if a court determines that the request would alter the essential nature of the program or service at issue, it is powerless under the ADA to order the change. Another way of understanding this reasonable modification/fundamental alteration dichotomy is to recognize that fundamental alterations to public services—alterations that might actually be necessary to achieve at least the spirit of the ADA's loftiest goals and meet the expectations of a modern, enlightened society—could be made only by the political branches of government, not by the courts.

Another important limitation of the ADA (at least as it has been interpreted by most courts) is that it does not prohibit arbitrary insurance coverage limits attached to certain medical conditions. A stark example of this is found in the case of *Doe v. Mutual of Omaha Insurance Company* (1999), in which a federal appellate court ruled that a lifetime benefit limitation in a health insurance policy of $25,000 for AIDS or AIDS-related conditions did not violate the ADA, even though the very same policy set a $1 million lifetime limit for other conditions.

Socioeconomic Status Discrimination

Compared to race or disability discrimination in healthcare access and treatment, healthcare discrimination based on class gains little attention—even though socioeconomic status is independently associated with health status, and the negative effects of poverty on health and healthcare access are incontrovertible. Class-related healthcare discrimination can take many forms. For example, healthcare providers might refuse to accept as patients individuals who are covered under Medicaid, or low-income individuals might fall victim to the practice of redlining, which refers to discrimination based on geographic location when companies offer goods and services to consumers. (Although insufficient data exist to know the extent of redlining in healthcare-related goods and services, industries such as home health care, pharmaceuticals, and managed care have come under particular scrutiny [Perez, 2003].) Another example stems from the fact that healthcare providers (e.g., physician and dental practices, hospitals) sometimes elect to not operate in relatively poor communities, leaving residents of these communities at heightened risk for experiencing a shortage of adequate healthcare resources.

Gender Discrimination

Discrimination against women is also a problem in health care. This bias appears to be of particular concern in the area of coronary heart disease (Bess, 1995), in which delayed or disparate care could have severe consequences. While it may seem that gender discrimination in health care could be remedied under the Equal Protection Clause of the federal Constitution, Equal Protection claims are difficult to win because they require proof of both state action (a sufficient government connection to the discriminatory acts) and proximate causation (a cause-and-effect link between the discrimination and the harm suffered). Also, consider the fact that healthcare practitioners who receive federal funds cannot face suit under Title VI for even obvious gender discrimination, because Title VI's prohibitions relate only to race, color, and national origin discrimination.

Age Discrimination

Finally, the medical care system also seems to be biased against older adults. Just one of several disturbing facts on the treatment front is that older adults sometimes do not receive needed surgical care because health professionals wrongfully assume that the chances of recovery are not good (Smith, 1996). Another concern pertains to insurance coverage, in that many employers are attempting to rescind lifetime health coverage benefits to retired workers, even where the benefits had been promised as part of negotiated labor contracts. At first blush, this may not seem like a critical issue, because many retirees are at or beyond the age required for Medicare eligibility. But some retirees are not yet 65 years old, a retiree's employer-sponsored benefits might provide more or different coverage than Medicare, and employer benefits might cover a retiree's dependents, which Medicare does not do.

▶ Individual Rights in a Public Health Context

The discussion thus far has focused on healthcare legal rights that individuals can claim in the context of access, receipt of services, freedom of choice, and antidiscrimination. In each of these areas, however, the right claimed is not absolute. For example, EMTALA does not make illegal all transfers of indigent patients from private hospitals to public ones; rather, it requires that patients be medically stabilized before a transfer can occur. Even eminent civil rights laws do not provide blanket protections, because they might be triggered only where federal funding is present, or where the assistance requested would not fundamentally alter a government health program.

In this section, we consider restrictions on individual rights and liberties of a different sort: those that derive not from the limitations of specific laws, but rather from governmental police powers used to protect the general public's health and welfare. One simple way to think about individual rights in a public health context is to use a balancing approach—what might the appropriate legal trade-offs be between private rights and public welfare? Public discussion of this trade-off intensified after the terrorist attacks of September 11, 2001, because many government actions taken in their wake—the passage of new laws, the tightening of existing regulations, the detainment of alleged terrorists—starkly raised the question of where to draw the line between individual autonomy and government authority to restrain that autonomy in the name of public welfare and national security. The attacks raised new questions relating to public health law as well, including whether the potential for a bioterrorist attack using smallpox should compel the federal government to vaccinate individuals—even against their will—against the virus in order to protect the public at large in the event of an attack.

Overview of Police Powers

Police powers represent state and local government authority to require individual conformance with established standards of conduct. These standards are designed to promote and protect the public's health, safety, and welfare, and to permit government control of personal, corporate, and other private interests. The government's police powers are broad and take many forms. Healthcare professionals are required to obtain licenses from government agencies. Healthcare facilities face accreditation standards. Food establishments are heavily regulated. Employers are bound by numerous occupational health and safety rules. Businesses are constrained by pollution control measures. Tobacco products can be marketed in only certain ways. The purchase of guns is controlled, buildings have to abide by certain codes, motorcyclists must wear helmets. The list goes on and on.

The government's police powers are oftentimes invasive, a result that stems in part from the fact that the American colonies were battling multiple communicable diseases during the time of the writing of the Constitution, and its drafters were thus well aware of the need for pervasive governmental public health powers. At the same time, the government may not overreach when restricting private autonomy in the name of public health promotion and protection. For example, police powers cannot be used as a form of punishment, they cannot be used arbitrarily and capriciously, and they cannot be used for purposes unrelated to public health and welfare.

A key principle inherent to the use of police powers is that of coercion. This is so because, in a country founded upon the twin ideals of individualism and a limited government, many individuals and businesses do not respond kindly to being told to conform with public health regulations that limit their actions. For example, sometimes a public health concern (e.g., pollution) requires a response (enhanced governmental regulation) that may not be in the best economic interests of an implicated party (a refinery). This is not to say that individuals and businesses do not voluntarily assume responsibilities and measures that are in the public's interest. For instance, one effect of poor exercise habits—obesity—has enormous implications for the public's health and for national healthcare costs. As a result, the government would prefer that all individuals exercise for a minimum amount of time each week, but there is of course no law requiring this; rather, voluntarism is the guiding principle when it comes to personal exercise. Nonetheless, personal coercion and industrial regulation have long been adopted (and accepted) practices of public health officials, and all of the major communicable disease outbreaks have been combated with some combination of compulsory screening, examination, treatment, isolation, and quarantine programs.

The *Jacobson v. Massachusetts* Decision

The fact that government coercion can be justified by important public health goals does not answer the question of where to draw the line between personal/economic freedom on the one hand, and the public welfare on the other. This question was taken up by the Supreme Court in *Jacobson v. Massachusetts* (1905), perhaps the most famous public health law decision in the court's history and the one to which we alluded in the second factual scenario in Box 6-1 at the opening of this chapter.

The facts in *Jacobson* are straightforward enough. At the turn of the 20th century, the state of Massachusetts enacted a law granting local health boards the power to require vaccination when necessary to protect the public's health or safety. In 1902, the Cambridge Board of Health, in the throes of attempting to contain a smallpox outbreak, took the state up on its offer and issued an order requiring all adults in the city to be vaccinated against the disease. Henning Jacobson refused vaccination on the ground that he previously suffered negative reactions to vaccinations. Jacobson was fined $5 for his refusal, a penalty upheld by the state's highest court. Jacobson appealed to the U.S. Supreme Court, setting the stage for a decision that, more than 100 years later, remains both controversial and at least symbolically forceful (Gostin, 2005).

Like the enduring tension between private interests and public welfare underpinning public health law generally, the *Jacobson* decision amounts to "a classic case of reconciling individual interests in bodily integrity with collective interests in health and safety" (Mariner, Annas, & Glantz, 2005). The 7–2 decision went the state's way, with the Supreme Court recognizing that police powers were generally broad enough to encompass forced vaccination. Responding to Jacobson's argument that the Massachusetts law impermissibly infringed on his constitutional right to liberty, the court wrote the following:

> The liberty secured by the Constitution of the United States to every person within its jurisdiction does not import an absolute right in each person to be, at all times and in all circumstances, wholly freed from restraint. There are manifold restraints to which every person is necessarily subject for the common good. On any other basis organized society could not exist with safety to its members. Society based on the rule that each one is a law unto himself would soon be confronted with disorder and anarchy. (*Jacobson v. Massachusetts*, 1905)

Due to this and other language used by the court in the decision, *Jacobson* is often described as sweepingly deferential to public health officials and their use of police powers. And without question, social compact theory (the idea that citizens have duties to one another and to society as a whole) animates the court's decision. However, the *Jacobson* decision also recognizes the individual liberties protected by the Constitution, and in fact requires a deliberative governmental process to safeguard these interests.

According to the *Jacobson* court, public health powers must be exercised in conformity with four standards in order to pass constitutional muster:

- The first standard, that of "public health necessity," requires that government use its police powers only in the face of a demonstrable public health threat.
- The second standard, termed "reasonable means," dictates that the methods used when exercising police powers must be designed in such a way as to prevent or ameliorate the public health threat found to exist under the first standard.
- "Proportionality" is the third *Jacobson* standard; it is violated when a particular public health measure imposes a burden on individuals totally disproportionate to the benefit to be expected from the measure.
- Finally, and axiomatically, the public health regulation itself should not pose a significant health risk to individuals subject to it. This is the standard of "harm avoidance."

These standards have never been explicitly overturned, but it can be argued that they have at the very least been implicitly replaced, given that in the 100-plus years since *Jacobson* was decided, the Supreme Court has developed a much more complex approach to applying constitutional provisions to cases implicating individual autonomy and liberty.

BOX 6-5 Discussion Question

Jacobson v. Massachusetts is a product of the early 20th century, and the public health law principles supporting it are vestiges of an even earlier time. This, coupled with a century of subsequent civil liberties jurisprudence and societal advancement, has led some commentators to question whether *Jacobson* should retain its paradigmatic role in terms of the scope of government police powers. At the same time, other public health law experts call for *Jacobson's* continued vitality, arguing that it is settled doctrine and a still-appropriate answer to the private interest/collective good question. What do you think?

The "Negative Constitution"

The discussion of police powers up to this point might reasonably lead you to believe that the Constitution *obligates* the government to protect the public's health and welfare through affirmative use of its powers. This view, however, has never been adopted by the Supreme Court. Instead, the prevailing view is that the Constitution *empowers* government to act in the name of public health, but does not require it to do so. This interpretation of the Constitution refers to what is known as the "negative constitution"—that is, the idea that the Constitution does not require government to provide any services, public health or otherwise. This approach to constitutional law derives from the fact that the Constitution is phrased mainly in negative terms (e.g., the First Amendment prohibits government abridgment of free speech). Professor Wendy Parmet describes the "negative constitution" this way:

In the century that has witnessed Auschwitz and Chernobyl, it is easy to see the dangers posed by state power. This recognition tempers enthusiasm for public authority and leads us to use law as a limiting device. In our legal tradition, this view of law is integral to constitutional structure, with its emphasis on separation of powers, checks and balances, procedural protections, and individual rights. We rely on the Constitution to limit the power of the government to restrain our freedoms and cause us harm. In this sense, law is a negative force that prevents the state from intruding upon the individual. This negative conception of law, which sees legal rights as a restraint upon the state, has played a dominant role in the formulation of contemporary American public health law. It explains the central pillars of constitutional public health law: the search for limits on governmental authority to restrain individual freedoms in the name of public health, and the concomitant assumption that government has no obligation to promote public health. (Parmet, 1993, pp. 267, 271)

In two important decisions, *DeShaney v. Winnebago County Department of Social Services* (1989) and *Town of Castle Rock, Colorado v. Gonzales* (2005), the Supreme Court has advanced this view of the negative constitution. In the former case, 1-year-old Joshua DeShaney was placed in his father's custody after his parents divorced. Two years later, the father's second wife complained to county officials in Wisconsin that the father had been abusing Joshua physically. Social service workers opened a file on the case and interviewed Joshua's father, but the county did not pursue the matter further after the father denied the charges. One year after that, an emergency department physician treating Joshua alerted social services of his suspicion that Joshua's injuries were the result of abuse. The county again investigated but decided that insufficient evidence of child abuse existed to remove Joshua from his father's custody. This emergency department scenario played out two additional times over the next several months, but Joshua's caseworkers still believed that they had no basis on which to place Joshua in court custody. Some months later, when Joshua was 4 years old, he suffered a beating so severe that he fell into a life-threatening coma. He survived but was left with permanent, severe brain damage, and he was expected to live his life in an institution for the profoundly mentally disabled. Joshua's father was subsequently convicted of child abuse.

Joshua's mother filed a civil rights claim on Joshua's behalf against the county officials who failed to take the boy into their custody. The lawsuit was based on the Due Process Clause of the federal Constitution, which prohibits states from depriving any person of property without due process of law. However, the Supreme Court in *DeShaney* concluded that the "substantive" component of the Due Process Clause— which focuses on challenges to government conduct— could not be read to provide Joshua with a property interest in having state child welfare officials protect him from beatings by his father. For a 6–3 majority, Chief Justice Rehnquist held that state officials had no affirmative constitutional duty to protect Joshua:

> Nothing in the language of the Due Process Clause itself requires the State to protect the life, liberty, and property of its citizens against invasion by private actors. The Clause is phrased as a limitation on the State's power to act, not as a guarantee of certain minimal levels of safety and security. It forbids the State itself to deprive individuals of life, liberty, or property without "due process of law," but its language cannot fairly be extended to impose an affirmative obligation on the State to ensure that those interests do not come to harm through other means. (*Deshaney*, 1989)

The majority further rejected the argument that the state's knowledge of the danger Joshua faced, and its expression of willingness to protect him against that danger, established a "special relationship" that gave rise to an affirmative constitutional duty to protect.

In dissent, three justices in *DeShaney* argued that through the establishment of its child protection program, the state of Wisconsin undertook a vital duty and effectively intervened in Joshua's life, and its failure to live up to its child protection duty amounted to a constitutional violation. According to the dissenters, the majority opinion "construes the Due Process Clause to permit a State to displace private sources of protection and then, at the critical moment, to shrug its shoulders and turn away from the harm that it has promised to try to prevent" (*Deshaney*, 1989).

Sixteen years after *DeShaney*, the Supreme Court in *Castle Rock v. Gonzales* had an opportunity to again consider whether the government has a duty to affirmatively protect its citizens. This time, however, the court was concerned not with substantive due process, but rather with procedural due process, which mandates that when a state establishes a benefit or right for its citizens, it is not entitled to deny individuals the benefit or right in an arbitrary or unfair way.

Unfortunately, the facts in *Gonzales* are as tragic as those in *DeShaney*. In May 1999, Jessica Gonzales received a court order protecting her and her three young daughters from her husband, who was also the girls' father. On June 22, all three girls disappeared in the late afternoon from in front of the Gonzales home, and Jessica suspected that her husband had taken them in violation of the restraining order. This suspicion was confirmed in a phone conversation she had with her husband. In two initial phone conversations with the Castle Rock Police Department, she was told there was nothing the police could do and to wait until 10:00 p.m. to see if her husband brought the girls home.

Shortly after 10:00 p.m., Jessica called the police to report that her children were still missing, but this time she was told to wait until midnight to see what transpired. She called the police again at midnight, reported that her children were still missing, and left her home to go to her husband's apartment. Finding nobody there, she called the police again at 12:10 a.m. and was told to wait for an officer to arrive. Thirty minutes later, after no officer showed up, she went to the police station to submit a report. According to the Supreme Court decision, the officer who wrote up the report "made no reasonable effort to enforce the [restraining order] or locate the three children. Instead, he went to dinner." A couple of hours later, Jessica's husband pulled his truck up to, and began shooting at, the Castle Rock Police Department. After he was killed by police during the gunfight, the three Gonzales daughters were found dead in the back of the truck; they had been murdered by their father hours earlier.

Jessica sued the police department, claiming that her constitutional right to procedural due process was violated by the department's inaction. She argued that the restraining order she received was her "property" under the Constitution's Due Process Clause and that it was effectively "taken" from her without due process. Overturning the federal appellate court that ruled in her favor, the Supreme Court decided by a 7–2 margin that Jessica did not have a property interest in police enforcement of the restraining order against her husband.

The court said it was not clear that *even if* it had found an individual entitlement to enforcement of a restraining order under a Colorado state statute requiring officers to use every reasonable means to enforce restraining orders, that this entitlement would constitute a protected "property" interest that triggers due process protections under the federal Constitution. Justice Antonin Scalia wrote that the Due Process Clause does not protect all government "benefits," including those things that government officials have discretion to grant or deny. Applying this standard, the court ruled that Colorado's protection order law did not create an individual entitlement to police enforcement of restraining orders, explaining that police have discretion to act or not act under many circumstances, including when to enforce a restraining order (e.g., police officers have discretion to consider whether a violation of a protection order is too "technical" or minor to justify enforcement). Furthermore, the court noted that if the Colorado legislature included statutory language making police enforcement of a restraining order "mandatory," even that would not necessarily mean that Mrs. Gonzales had a personal entitlement to its enforcement, given that the statute makes no mention of an individual's power to demand—or even request—enforcement.

In dissent, two justices in *Gonzales* argued that restraining orders amount to a personal, enforceable property interest. They asserted that the majority opinion wrongly ruled that a citizen's interest in government-provided police protection does not resemble a "traditional conception" of property. Looking to the legislative history and text of Colorado's own protection order law and to the purpose of the state's domestic violence legislation, the dissent concluded that a particular class of individuals was indeed entitled beneficiaries of domestic restraining orders.

BOX 6-6 Discussion Questions

The "negative constitution" is a concept over which reasonable people can easily disagree. Notwithstanding the "defensive" manner of some of the Constitution's key provisions, there are several arguments in support of more affirmative action on the part of government health and welfare officials than current Supreme Court jurisprudence requires. For example, the dissent in *DeShaney* argues persuasively that Wisconsin's implementation of a child protection program effectively created a constitutional duty to actually protect children from seemingly obvious danger. As one leading scholar put it,

> If an agency represents itself to the public as a defender of health, and citizens justifiably rely on that protection, is government "responsible" when it knows that a substantial risk exists, fails to inform citizens so they might initiate action, and passively avoids a state response to that risk? (Gostin, 2000)

What do you think of this argument? Can you think of other arguments that call into question the soundness of the negative theory of constitutional law?

▶ Conclusion

This chapter offered a snapshot of the current state of health-related legal rights. But, as alluded to early on in the chapter, there were times in its relatively short history that this country was closer to recognizing broader individual healthcare rights than is currently the case, just as there have been times (as the aftermath of September 11, 2001, proved) when concerns for the public's health and safety have eclipsed the nation's more natural inclinations toward individualism and a deregulated marketplace. That this is so is of no surprise: legal rights are, by nature, subject to shifts in the political and social terrain. For example, the Aid for Families With Dependent Children program (commonly known as AFDC), the federal welfare entitlement program for low-income populations, was dismantled in 1996 after more than 60 years in existence. Originally enacted under a slightly different name as part of the New Deal in 1935, the AFDC was replaced with the Temporary Assistance for Needy Families (TANF) program by a moderate Democrat (President Bill Clinton) and a conservative, Republican-controlled Congress. Compared to the AFDC, TANF dramatically limited the receipt of individual benefits and focused much more heavily on creating work opportunities for needy families. Like legal rights generally, health-related legal rights are similarly subject to changing political currents. For example, at the time of this writing, several state legislatures continue to pass bills that protect health professionals from providing care that conflicts with their personal beliefs, reflecting the current political power of social conservatives.[j]

Of course, changes to legal rights are not always represented by restrictions of those rights. The enactment of Medicaid and Medicare, which created new health-related rights, is an obvious example. Other major examples include EMTALA and expanded state consumer rights for persons in managed care. On a less noticed scale, legal rights for persons with HIV/AIDS have expanded since the 1980s (Halpern, 2004), and federal courts now review the constitutionality of the treatment provided in, and conditions of, psychiatric hospitals (*Wyatt v. Stickney*, 1972). These are just a few of many examples.

Nonetheless, vast challenges remain. After all, many scholars, politicians, and consumers point to the millions of uninsured Americans as just one example of not only a failing healthcare financing and delivery system, but also a failing of the legal system. To reduce this nation's huge uninsured population takes not just political will, but also an enormous undertaking to change the law, as witnessed with the ACA. A "rights revolution" in a health context, like other major legal upheavals, requires something else, too: a substantial amount of general economic and social unrest (Friedman, 1971). As historian Brooks Adams once noted, "Law is merely the expression of the will of the strongest for the time being, and therefore laws have no fixity, but shift from generation to generation" (Nash & Zullo, 1995).

References

Alexander v. Sandoval, 532 U.S. 275 (2001).

Americans With Disabilities Act of 1990, 42 U.S.C. §§ 12101 *et seq.* (1990).

Annas, G. J. (2004). *The rights of patients* (3rd ed.). Carbondale, IL: Southern Illinois University Press.

Barnes, A., & McChrystal, M. (1998). The various human rights in health care. *Human Rights, 25,* 12–14.

Barzelay, D. E., & Heymann, P. B. (1973). The forest and the trees: *Roe v. Wade* and its critics. *Boston University Law Review, 53,* 765–784.

Bess, C. J. (1995). Gender bias in health care: A life or death issue for women with coronary heart disease. *Hastings Women's Law Journal, 6*(1), 41–65.

Blum, J. D., Talib, N., Carstens, P., Nasser, M., Tomkin, D., & McAuley, A. (2003). Rights of patients: Comparative perspectives from five countries. *Medical Law Review, 22*(3), 451–471.

Bopp, J., & Coleson, R. (1989). The right to abortion: Anomalous, absolute, and ripe for reversal. *Brigham Young University Journal of Public Law, 3*(2), 181–355.

Bragdon v. Abbott, 524 U.S. 624 (1998).

Byrd, W. M., & Clayton, L. A. (2000). *An American health dilemma: A medical history of African Americans and the problem of race, beginnings to 1900.* New York, NY: Routledge.

Byrd, W. M., & Clayton, L. A. (2002). *An American health dilemma: Race, medicine, and health care in the United States, 1900–2000.* New York, NY: Routledge.

Canterbury v. Spence, 464 F.2d 772 (D.C. Cir. 1972).

Civil Rights Act of 1964, 42 U.S.C. §§ 2000d (1964).

Claiming Human Rights. (2010). *The Universal Declaration of human rights: Article 25.* Retrieved from http://www.claiminghumanrights.org/udhr_article_25.html

Davis, M. F. (1993). *Brutal need: Lawyers and the welfare rights movement, 1960–1973.* New Haven, CT: Yale University Press.

DeShaney v. Winnebago Cnty., 489 U.S. 189 (1989).

Doe v. Mutual of Omaha Insur. Co., 179 F.3d 557 (7th Cir.1999), cert. denied, 528 U.S. 1106 (2000).

Eisenstadt v. Baird, 405 U.S. 438 (1972).

Ely, J. H. (1979). The wages of crying wolf: A comment on *Roe v. Wade. Yale Law Journal, 82,* 920–949.

Examination and Treatment for Emergency Medical Conditions and Women in Labor, 42 U.S.C. § 1395dd (2011).

Friedman, E. A., & Adashi, E. Y. (2010). The right to health as the unheralded narrative of health care reform. *Journal of the American Medical Association, 304*(23), 2639–2640.

Friedman, L. M. (1971). The idea of right as a social and legal concept. *Journal of Social Issues, 27*(2), 189–198.

Garrow, D. J. (1994). *Liberty and sexuality: The right to privacy and the making of* Roe v. Wade. Berkeley, CA: University of California Press.

Gonzales v. Carhart, 550 U.S. 124 (2007).

Gostin, L. O. (2000). *Public health law: Power, duty, restraint.* Berkeley, CA: University of California Press.

Gostin, L. O. (2005). *Jacobson v. Massachusetts* at 100 years: Police powers and civil liberties in tension. *American Journal of Public Health, 95*(4), 576–581.

Griswold v. Connecticut, 381 U.S. 479 (1965).

Halpern, S. A. (2004). Medical authority and the culture of rights. *Journal of Health Politics, Policy and Law, 29*(4-5), 835–852.

Hospital Survey and Construction Act of 1946, 42 U.S.C. § 291e(f) (1946).

Hurley v. Eddingfield, 59 N.E. 1058 (Ind. 1901).

Jacobson v. Massachusetts, 197 U.S. 11 (1905).

Jost, T. S. (2003). *Disentitlement? The threats facing our public health-care programs and a rights-based response.* New York, NY: Oxford University Press.

Kinney, E. D., & Clark, B. A. (2004). Provisions for health and health care in the constitutions of the countries of the world. *Cornell International Law Journal, 37*(2), 285–355.

Littell, A. (2002). Can a constitutional right to health guarantee universal health care coverage or improved health outcomes? A survey of selected states. *Connecticut Law Review, 35*(1), 289–318.

Loving v. Virginia, 388 U.S. 1 (1967).

Mariner, W. K., Annas, G. J., & Glantz, L. H. (2005). *Jacobson v. Massachusetts*: It's not your great-great-grandfather's public health law. *American Journal of Public Health, 95*(4), 581–590.

Nash, B., & Zullo, A. (Eds.) (1995). *Lawyer's wit and wisdom: Quotations on the legal profession, in brief.* Philadelphia, PA: Running Press.

Navarro, V., & Shi, L. (2003). The political context of social inequalities and health. In R. Hofrichter (Ed.), *Health and social justice: Politics, ideology, and inequity in the distribution of disease.* San Francisco, CA: Jossey-Bass.

Parmet, W. (1993). Health care and the constitution: Public health and the role of the state in the framing era. *Hastings Constitutional Law Quarterly, 20*(2), 267–335.

Partial Birth Abortion Ban Act, 18 U.S.C. §§ 1531 (a)-(b) (2003).

Perez, T. E. (2003). The civil rights dimension of racial and ethnic disparities in health status. In B. D. Smedley, A. Y. Stith, & A. R. Nelson. (Eds.), *Unequal treatment: Confronting racial and ethnic disparities in health care* (pp. 626–663). Washington, DC: The National Academies Press.

Planned Parenthood of Southeasten Pa. v. Casey, 505 U.S. 833 (1992).

President's Commission for the Study of Ethical Problems in Medicine and Biomedical and Behavioral Research. (1983). *Securing access to health care: A report on the ethical implications of differences in the availability of health services.* Washington, DC: The National Academies Press.

Protection of Human Subjects, 45 C.F.R. Part 46 (2009).

Regan, D. H. (1979). Rewriting *Roe v. Wade. Michigan Law Review, 77,* 1569–1646.

Reinhardt, U. (1996). The debate that wasn't: The public and the Clinton health care plan. In H. Aaron (Ed.), *The problem that won't go away: Reforming U.S. health care financing* (pp. 70–109). Washington, DC: Brookings Institution.

Rich, R. F. (2000). Health policy, health insurance and the social contract. *Comparative Labor Law Policy Journal, 21,* 397–421.

Roe v. Wade, 410 U.S. 113 (1973).

Rosenbaum, S. (2011). Realigning the social order: The patient protection and affordable care act and the U.S. health insurance system. *Suffolk Journal of Health and Biomedical Law, 7,* 1–31.

Rosenbaum, S., & Teitelbaum, J. (2003). Civil rights enforcement in the modern healthcare system: Reinvigorating the role of the federal government in the aftermath of *Alexander v. Sandoval. Yale Journal of Health Policy, Law, and Ethics, 3*(2), 215.

Rosenblatt, R. E., Law, S. A., & Rosenbaum, S. (1997). *Law and the American health care system.* Westbury, CT: The Foundation Press.

San Antonio Indep. School Dist. v. Rodriguez, 411 U.S. 1 (1973).

Simkins v. Moses H. Cone Memorial Hospital, 323 F.2d 959 (4th Cir. 1963).

Smedley, B. D., Stith, A. Y. & Nelson, A. R. (Eds.). (2003). *Unequal treatment: Confronting racial and ethnic disparities in health care.* Washington, DC: The National Academies Press.

Smith, D. B. (1999). *Health care divided: Race and healing a nation.* Ann Arbor, MI: The University of Michigan Press.

Smith, G. P. (1996). Our hearts were once young and gay: Health care rationing and the elderly. *University of Florida Journal of Law and Public Policy, 8,* 1.

Smith, P. S. (1997). Addressing the plight of inner-city schools: The federal right to education after *Kadrmas v. Dickinson Public Schools. Whittier Law Review, 18,* 825–835.

Stacy, T. (1993). The courts, the constitution, and a just distribution of health care. *Kansas Journal of Law and Public Policy, 3,* 77–94.

Starr, P. (1982). *The social transformation of American medicine: The rise of a sovereign profession and the making of a vast industry.* New York, NY: Basic Books.

Stein, R. (2006, January 30). Health workers' choice debated: Proposals back right not to treat. *Washington Post.* Retrieved from http://www.washingtonpost.com/wp-dyn/content/article/2006/01/29/AR2006012900869.html

Stenberg v. Carhart, 530 U.S. 914 (2000).

Teitelbaum, J. B. (2005). Health care and civil rights: An introduction. *Ethnicity and Disease, 15*(2, supp. 2), 27–30.

Town of Castle Rock, Colorado v. Gonzales, 545 U.S. 748 (2005).

Vladeck, B. (2003). Universal health insurance in the United States: Reflections on the past, the present, and the future. *American Journal of Public Health, 93*(1), 9–16.

Wailoo, K., & Schlesinger, M. (2004). Transforming American medicine: A twenty-year retrospective on *The Social Transformation of American Medicine. Journal of Health Politics, Policy, and Law, 29*(4–5), 1005–1019.

Wing, K. R. (1993). The right to health care in the United States. *Annals of Health Law, 2,* 161–193.

World Health Organization. (2006). *Constitution of the World Health Organization.* Retrieved from http://www.who.int/governance/eb/who_constitution_en.pdf

Wyatt v. Stickney, 344 F. Supp. 373 (M.D. Ala. 1972).

Yamin, A. E. (2005). The right to health under international law and its relevance to the United States. *American Journal of Public Health, 95*(7), 1156–1161.

▶ Endnotes

a. These competing concepts were given life in Paul Starr's influential 1982 book, *The Social Transformation of American Medicine: The Rise of a Sovereign Profession and the Making of a Vast Industry.* Incidentally, *The Social Transformation of American Medicine* should be read by all students with an interest in the history of medicine; the book's significance across a range of disciplines is hard to overstate. See Wailoo and Schlesinger, 2004.

b. For an interesting article describing the importance of political structures in determining the level of equalities/inequalities in a society, including the level of government-provided healthcare coverage, see Navarro and Shi, 2003.

c. Incidentally, the *Canterbury* decision was authored by Spottswood Robinson, III, who, prior to becoming a highly regarded federal judge, was instrumental in the fight for civil rights, in part as one of the National Association for the Advancement of Colored People (NAACP) lawyers who initially brought suit in one of the cases that eventually morphed into *Brown v. Board of Education.*

d.   A now-famous 1890 *Harvard Law Review* article titled "The Right to Privacy," written by Samuel Warren and Louis Brandeis, is often credited with introducing the constitutional "right to be let alone."

e.   In a health context, this type of privacy is embodied by the Health Insurance Portability and Accountability Act (HIPAA) of 1996, found in large part at 29 U.S.C. §§ 1181–1187, 42 U.S.C. §§ 300gg *et seq.* and 42 U.S.C. §§ 1320a *et seq.*, which creates a federal right to maintain the confidentiality of one's personal health information.

f.   For a compelling look at what the case has meant to society, see Garrow, 1994.

g.   For example, notice how the Supreme Court linked states' power to ban abortions (with certain exceptions) to fetal viability, even though the progression of medical knowledge and technology could push back the point of viability earlier into pregnancy. Also, who appears to hold the power, under "(a)," to decide whether an abortion should occur? The *physician*, a fact often overlooked by those who hail *Roe* as a seminal women's rights case and one that calls into question how the pregnant woman's constitutional right to privacy could be effectuated by her treating physician.

h.   This section was adapted from Teitelbaum, 2005.

i.   For a discussion of the implications of the *Alexander* decision in a healthcare context, see Rosenbaum and Teitelbaum, 2003.

j.   These bills represent a

> surge of legislation that reflects the intensifying tension between asserting individual religious values and defending patients' rights. . . . The flurry of political activity is being welcomed by conservative groups that consider it crucial to prevent health workers from being coerced into participating in care they find morally repugnant—protecting their "right of conscience" or "right of refusal." . . . The swell of propositions is raising alarm among advocates for abortion rights, family planning, AIDS prevention, the right to die, gays and lesbians, and others who see the push as the latest manifestation of the growing political power of social conservatives. (Stein, 2006)

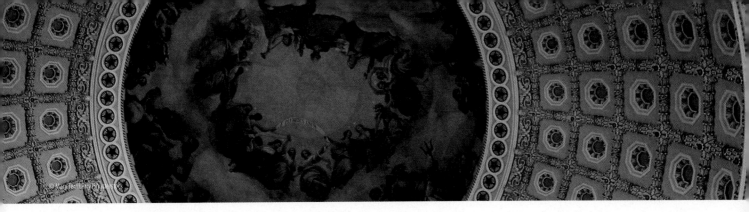

CHAPTER 7

Social Determinants of Health and the Role of Law in Optimizing Health

BOX 7-1 Vignette

Living through brief periods without heat or electricity is a fact of life for most of us, perhaps as a result of a powerful weather system or a blown generator. But have you thought about what it would be like to be without heat or electricity more chronically, due to homelessness, inadequate housing, or an unscrupulous landlord who neglects a property without concern for tenants? Even for the healthiest among us, this social factor would be incredibly challenging; for those with chronic illness, it can mean increased asthma attacks, severe pain associated with sickle cell disease, an inability to refrigerate needed medicine, and much more, including death. The social factors just noted—homelessness, dilapidated homes, slum landlords—and many others have nothing to do with biology, genetics, personal choice, or access to healthcare services, but have a great deal to do with individual and public health.

▶ Introduction

Disparities in health and health care are a systemic and deeply challenging problem in the United States (Smedley, Stith, & Nelson, 2003). While related, the two terms have different meanings. A *health* disparity exists when one population group experiences a higher burden of disability or illness relative to another group; a *healthcare* disparity, by contrast, tends to denote differences in access to healthcare services or health insurance, or in the quality of care actually received (Kaiser Family Foundation, 2012). What makes both types of disparities so invidious—and a major social justice concern—is that they can exist even when patient needs or treatment recommendations do not differ across populations (Hoffman, Trawalter, Axt, & Oliver, 2016). As long as these disparities exist, a society cannot achieve what is known as *health equity*—a situation in which everyone has the opportunity to attain his or her full health potential.

Many different factors can contribute to health and healthcare disparities. Individual behaviors, healthcare provider bias, cultural expectations and differences, the location and financing of healthcare systems, social factors, and more can all be contributors. Furthermore, health and healthcare disparities appear through many different lenses; researchers have documented disparities based on race, ethnicity, socioeconomic status, age, geography, language, gender, disability status, citizenship status, and sexual identity and orientation.

In 2010 the U.S. Department of Health and Human Services developed a series of strategies and goals for eliminating health disparities based on race and ethnicity (National Partnership for Action, n.d.) and, as described most prominently in the Health Reform in the United States chapter, the Affordable Care Act (ACA) includes many provisions aimed at improving the health of vulnerable individuals and populations, including several programs specifically directed at reducing health disparities. In addition, many states, localities, and private organizations have agendas for combating and eliminating various types of health and healthcare disparities.

Too often overlooked in discussions about health and health disparities, however, is a striking fact about American society that both differentiates it from other developed countries and appears to deeply affect individual and population health: aside from expenditures related to the direct provision of individual healthcare services, the United States spends far less on social services (e.g., housing and food programs, support services for older adults, disability and sickness benefits, employment programs, unemployment benefits, homeless shelters, utility assistance programs) than do other developed countries. For every $1 spent on health care, the United States dedicates approximately $0.90 to other social services; in the 33 other Organisation for Economic Co-operation and Development countries (a multinational organization, of which the United States is a member, that strives to fight poverty and achieve economic growth and employment in member countries), the typical spending ratio is $1 on health care to $2 on other social services. As it turns out, the latter ratio is significantly associated with better health outcomes, including less infant mortality, less premature death, longer life expectancy, and fewer low-birth-weight babies (Bradley, Elkins, Herrin, & Elbel, 2011). At the same time, despite spending two to three times more per capita on direct healthcare services than nearly all of our European counterparts, the United States has significantly worse health outcomes in many respects, particularly among the poorest individuals and families (Tobin-Tyler, 2012).

As evidence mounts that interventions targeting social, economic, and environmental factors can account for sizable reductions in morbidity and mortality (Gostin, Jacobson, Record, & Hardcastle, 2011), healthcare payers and policymakers are increasingly aiming to tie these nonmedical interventions to new models of healthcare delivery that create economic incentives for providers to incorporate social interventions into their approach to care by linking payments to overall health outcomes (Bachrach, 2014); for example, "accountable care organizations," or ACOs, are an evolving concept in which various types of healthcare providers collaborate in the provision of care and accept collective accountability for the cost and quality of care delivered to a population of patients. While it will take time to implement and test these new models, early results indicate that these multifaceted approaches to health and health care can result in cost savings, higher patient satisfaction, more provider productivity, and improved employee satisfaction (Bachrach, 2014).

BOX 7-2 Discussion Questions

Do you think trying to achieve wide-scale health equity is a laudable goal? Why or why not? If yes, what do you think are the keys to achieving it? And what about people who are given the opportunity to achieve optimal health but do not take advantage of it; should they face consequences of some sort?

▶ Social Determinants of Health

Defining Social Determinants of Health

According to the federal Centers for Disease Control and Prevention (CDC), determinants of health are "factors that contribute to a person's current state of health" (2013). Included within this broad category are biologic factors (e.g., carrying a genetic mutation that could increase one's chances of developing a particular disease, such as sickle cell anemia), psychosocial factors (e.g., conflicts within one's family that may lead to stress, anger, and/or depression), behavioral factors (e.g., alcohol/drug use, smoking, unprotected sex), and finally, social factors. Social determinants of health (SDH), broadly speaking, are the social conditions into which people are born and that affect their daily lives and overall well-being as they move through the various stages of life. The World Health Organization (WHO) defines SDH as "the conditions in which people are born, grow, live, work and age" (2018), and the CDC notes that SDH are shaped by the distribution of money, power, and resources at both local and national levels.

Resources that enhance the quality of one's life—such as the availability of healthy foods, access to education, and an environment free of toxins—all shape individual and population health. These and many other SDH are transient across the life cycle, with some social determinants becoming more pertinent depending on one's stage of life. For example, proximity to a high-quality school would be more meaningful for a child, while one's actual education level would be more significant to an adult who is either seeking work or to increase his or her income to better support his or her family. Social determinants include factors that may have led to an individual's disadvantaged state to begin with—institutional racism, exposure to crime and violence, a lack of available community-based resources, and many other factors can all be health harming.

As you have likely gleaned already, social factors that influence health cover a wide swath of topics and life events, many of which remain outside the control of individuals and populations affected by them. As a result, it is not always easy to define exactly what role SDH—whether one individual social factor, or many at once—play in shaping health. Researchers have for decades explored such questions as these: Why are some populations more predisposed than others to develop and suffer from certain ailments? Why do differences persist in healthcare quality among racial and ethnic groups? Why do people in low-income families sometimes experience lower-quality care compared to high-income families? Why do studies show incremental improvements in health as one rises in social status? In some capacity, it is likely that social factors are at play in all of these situations, but defining their role is a challenge. Before delving into some of the more specific research findings concerning the health effects of certain social factors, let's take a more detailed look at some different types of SDH.

Types of SDH

The Healthy People 2020 Initiative lists many different examples of SDH (U.S. Department of Health and Human Services, 2018). We summarize several of them here to provide context for the discussion that follows.

- **Access to high-quality educational opportunities:** Individuals with access to consistent, high-quality educational opportunities are more likely to obtain higher-income jobs, and completion of undergraduate and graduate studies affords a sheer greater number of these higher-paying opportunities. Many middle and high schools in low-income areas, however, have high dropout rates or do not adequately prepare students for higher education, and many of these areas do not have adequate access to job training resources for those seeking training in a vocation, which can provide a path to a well-paying career in the absence of a 4-year college degree. Furthermore, many low-paying positions do not offer health insurance as a job benefit, making it all the more difficult for individuals in these positions to access routine and specialty physician services. Overall, educational attainment and corresponding income levels tend to be strong predictors of individual and population health. From an early age, educational attainment and income provide valuable resources that protect individuals against stressors that tend to lead to health complications later in life.
- **Access to medical care services:** Individuals who do not live close to medical care providers (e.g., primary care doctors, clinics, hospitals) are less likely to see a physician regularly and will often seek care only in emergencies, eschewing preventive care. Access is also not just about geography—it entails affordability as well. People who do not receive health insurance coverage as a job-related benefit and cannot purchase it on their own can forgo seeing a doctor for several years before presenting to the emergency department for an acute problem, which can possibly lead to a lengthy hospitalization and/or decreased quality of life.
- **Access to social media and other technologies (e.g., the Internet, cell phones):** The Internet and cell phones are becoming increasingly useful in individual and population health, from

appointment time reminders, to learning more about one's symptoms and diagnoses, to buying insurance through state exchanges established under the ACA, to finding providers who are accepting new patients. In addition, many people connect to support groups or other valuable health-related resources through the Internet, and providers are increasingly making health records available via Internet portals.

- **Availability of community-based resources and opportunities for recreational activities:** Community-based resources can connect residents to local health providers and recreational/physical activities, both of which increase the likelihood that people will lead healthier lives overall. The absence of leisurely activities in one's life can lead to increased stress, which in turn is associated with poorer health outcomes overall.

- **Availability of resources to meet daily needs (e.g., access to local food markets):** The further an individual lives from a grocery store that offers healthy food options, like fruits and vegetables, the more likely it is that the individual will consume fast foods or other relatively unhealthy options. Geographic areas that have no or few healthy food options are referred to as "food deserts." Food deserts tend to be identified based on their shortages of whole food providers and their abundance of "quick marts" and fast-food establishments that stock processed, sugar-heavy, and fat-laden foods that contribute to a poor diet and can lead to higher levels of obesity and other diet-related diseases, such as diabetes and heart disease. Due to the enormous individual and public health effects of food deserts, the U.S. Department of Agriculture has developed a map of the nation's food deserts and many resources aimed at reducing their number (2017).

- **Culture:** By way of example, some cultures rely heavily on time-honored approaches to illness, such as teas and other homemade remedies. While these can be effective, some commonly ingested herbals can in fact be quite dangerous when taken in conjunction with other regularly prescribed medications; for example, St. John's wort—a plant that is used for medicinal purposes in this country and many others—can have drastic effects when taken alongside certain antidepressant medications. So while traditions can have important positive effects in treating illness, cultural norms can also impact health in unseen ways.

- **Language/literacy:** If adequate translation and interpretation services are not in place in healthcare facilities, foreign language–speaking patients may be discouraged from seeking out care. Even when they do, many patients struggle to understand clinicians and medication or other treatment protocols.

- **Public safety:** Individuals who live in dangerous neighborhoods tend to remain indoors, which can close off opportunities for exercise and social interaction. People who must pass through a dangerous neighborhood in order to reach public transportation often have to make a choice between their own safety and attending work or a doctor's appointment. Furthermore, alcohol, drugs, violence, and the adverse health outcomes associated with them tend to be more prevalent in relatively unsafe neighborhoods.

- **Residential segregation:** Physicians may preferentially set up their practices in locations dominated by certain demographics. As a result, some patient populations—often minority and low-income populations—suffer from a lack of healthcare facilities and resources in their neighborhoods, a particularly strident problem in rural areas.

- **Social norms and attitudes (e.g., discrimination, racism, distrust of government):** Discriminatory attitudes remain a cause of health disparities (Tobin-Tyler & Teitelbaum, 2019). Multiple studies have shown that physicians are more likely to recommend medical best practices based on race, gender, and age (Schulman et al., 1999; van Ryn, Burgess, Malat, & Griffin, 2006). These studies demonstrate that bias (unconscious or otherwise) in physicians and other health professionals still plays a significant role in how patients of certain races, ethnicities, social statuses, and education levels are treated. Patient attitudes about the medical professions can also affect health. The most infamous example of discriminatory practice creating negative patient attitudes toward the medical community stems from the Tuskegee syphilis experiment. In this experiment, hundreds of syphilis-infected, African American men in rural Alabama were used as unwitting research subjects by the U.S. Public Health Service, which wanted to study untreated syphilis in humans. The men were given free medical care but were never told they had the disease, nor were any of them treated with penicillin once it became the accepted course of treatment for syphilis. The study lasted a stunning 40 years, from 1932–1972, and has affected the attitudes and healthcare decisions of many African Americans ever since. In 1997 President Bill Clinton issued a formal apology for the Tuskegee Study, but government healthcare programs have been hard-pressed to earn back the trust of millions of patients that was shattered once the study was revealed.[a]

■ **Socioeconomic conditions (e.g., concentrated poverty and the stressful conditions that accompany it):** While the link between poverty and poor health is discussed below, suffice it to say here that the connection between the two is well documented and undeniable, and the health effects of extreme financial hardship in childhood can be lifelong even in the event that people eventually escape poverty. A similar phenomenon, though with far different health effects, can be seen at the other end of the socioeconomic spectrum: greater wealth correlates with lower rates of morbidity and longer life spans.

■ **Transportation options:** Many individuals miss medical appointments because they cannot afford private transportation and live long distances from reliable public transportation. It is common for patients without their own cars to spend hours on buses in an effort to reach medical appointments.

The Link Between Social Determinants and Health Outcomes

While it is well beyond the scope of this chapter to provide a full discussion of the myriad ways in which social factors play important roles in individual and population health, we provide in this section a flavor of the types of links that researchers have drawn in this respect. We note at the outset that these links are not usually linear and directly causative: social determinants do not usually act alone or in "'simple additive fashion,' but rather in concert with one another in complex, interdependent, bidirectional relationships" (McGovern, Miller, & Hughes-Cromwick, 2014, p. 3). Indeed, "most diseases and injuries have multiple potential causes and several factors and conditions may contribute to a single death. Therefore, it is a challenge to estimate the contribution of each factor to mortality" (Mokdad, Marks, Stroup, & Gerberding, 2004, p. 1238). That said, "the overwhelming weight of evidence demonstrates the powerful effects of socioeconomic and related social factors on health, even

when definitive knowledge of specific mechanisms and effective interventions is limited" (Braveman & Gottlieb, 2014, p. 22).

Links can be drawn between social determinants and both physical and mental health. Among many examples on the physical health front, research indicates that while half of all deaths in the United States involve behavioral causes (McGinnis & Foege, 1993), evidence shows that health-related behaviors are strongly shaped by three important social factors: income, education level, and employment (Braveman, Egerter, & Barclay, 2011; Stringhini, et al., 2010). Another study concluded that the number of U.S. deaths in 2000 attributable to low education, racial segregation, and low social support was comparable with the number of deaths attributable to heart attack, cerebrovascular disease, and lung cancer, respectively (Galea, Tracy, Hoggatt, DiMaggio, & Karpati, 2011). The CDC has regularly found that individuals among the lowest levels of income and education suffered the greatest age-adjusted prevalence and incidence rate of diagnosed diabetes (CDC, 2013). Similarly, associations have been demonstrated between lower socioeconomic status and increased prevalence of disease, morbidity, and mortality in persons with arthritis and rheumatic conditions (Callahan et al., 2011).

Access to safe, quality, affordable housing represents one of the most influential SDH. Indeed, for individuals and families trapped in a cycle of housing instability, this determinant can almost completely dictate their ability to achieve and maintain a healthful state (Corporation for Supportive Housing, 2014). Several studies demonstrate that linking healthcare management to supportive housing—an evidence-based practice that combines permanent affordable housing with relevant support services—leads to improved health outcomes. For example, a study out of Denver, Colorado, found that 50% of supportive housing residents experienced improved health status, 43% had better mental health outcomes, and 15% reduced substance use (Perlman & Parvensky, 2006).

Regardless of income or housing cost, living in a predominately minority neighborhood increases the likelihood of having poor access to healthy food choices (Jack, Jack, & Hayes, 2012). For example, one study found that African American urban neighborhoods have only 41% of the chain supermarkets found in comparable white neighborhoods (Powell, Slater, Mirtcheva, Bao, & Chaloupka, 2007), and minority neighborhoods have an overabundance of fast-food restaurants known for relatively inexpensive but unhealthful food options (Fleischhacker, Evenson, Rodriguez, & Ammerman, 2011).

BOX 7-3 Group Activity

Each student should begin by rank-ordering a list of the half-dozen social determinants (from those listed in this chapter or otherwise; broad or specific) that he or she believes most significantly affect individual health. Then get together in groups of three or four people to compare lists, discussing disagreements and making the case for some determinants over others.

As noted, social determinants play a significant role in mental health outcomes, as well. Emotional stressors—such as neighborhood violence, poverty, or familial abuse—during key developmental years in childhood can lead to severe consequences later in life. For example, several studies have been conducted regarding the mental health outcomes of children who have been subject to abuse, including one showing that survivors of childhood sexual abuse have higher levels of both general distress and major psychological disturbances, including personality disorders (Schneiderman, Ironson, & Siegel, 2005). One particularly fascinating but worrisome study demonstrated that the brains of children in low-income families actually had less surface area than did the brains of children from families who were wealthier—specifically, 6% less surface area in children whose families made less than $25,000 a year compared with children whose families made more than $150,000 (Layton, 2015). One theory behind this finding was that children from poor families tend to be malnourished and have less access to high-quality education than their richer peers. Another theory proposed that poorer families tend to lead more chaotic lives, which can inhibit brain development in children.

▶ Law as a Social Determinant of Health

Up to this point, we've described generally various types of SDH and some correlations between those determinants and the health of people who live in communities in which SDH may be relatively more compromised. We turn now to a more nuanced discussion of one very influential SDH: the law. Throughout the nation's history, law has played an integral role in causing, exacerbating, and alleviating health-harming social conditions, from the legally sanctioned, racially segregated—and horribly unequal—medical care systems used during slavery time, to the expansion of building codes in the 1920s, to the War on Poverty legislation of the 1960s, to the ACA's focus on health equity. Because the law's reach in this regard is so expansive, we provide only an overview for purposes of this chapter.

Whether embodied in constitutions, statutes, regulations, executive orders, administrative agency decisions, or court decisions, the law plays a profound role in shaping life circumstances and, in turn, health. The ways in which this occurs can be broken down into five categories.

1. **The law can be used to design and perpetuate social conditions that can have terrible physical, mental, and emotional effects on individuals and populations**. One obvious example in this category is the "separate but equal" constitutional doctrine that allowed racial segregation in housing, health care, education, employment, transportation, and more. Indeed, injustices in healthcare access and quality were commonplace in the United States prior to the civil rights movement. Racially segregated health care dates to slavery times, when plantations had on-site facilities to care for slave laborers. After the slaves were freed but also after the First Reconstruction ended in the late 1870s, Jim Crow laws ushered in a new era of discriminatory healthcare access and delivery through separate hospitals and physician practices; separate medical, nursing, and dental schools; and separate professional medical societies. For example, Alabama once had a law that stated: "No person or corporation shall require any White female nurse to nurse in wards or rooms in hospitals, either public or private, in which Negro men are placed" (Ferris State University, 2012).

2. **The law can be used as a mechanism through which behaviors and prejudices are transformed into distributions of well-being among populations**. By way of example, although black and white people use illicit drugs at approximately the same rate, drug crime incarceration rates are far higher for black people. Thus, who is chosen for surveillance and arrest, and how the arrested are selected for either punishment or treatment, turns out to be an important driver of how a supposedly neutral law differentially impacts people and communities, and in turn their health (Burris, 2011). Healthcare provider discrimination and bias reside in this category, as well. Healthcare discrimination and bias can take many forms: it can be based on race, ethnicity, disability, age, gender, and class (or socioeconomic status). Class-related healthcare discrimination alone can take multiple forms. For example, some healthcare providers might refuse to accept as patients individuals who are covered under Medicaid (because the Medicaid population tends

to be disproportionately poor and of color), or low-income individuals might fall victim to the practice of redlining, which refers to situations in which healthcare entities relocate from poor neighborhoods to wealthier ones (Yearby, 2013).

3. **Laws can be determinative of health through their under-enforcement**. For example, a perfectly good set of housing regulations aimed at keeping housing units safe, clean, and quiet are of little value to individual and group health if there is neither the will, nor the resources, to enforce them. Substandard housing conditions, including the presence of rodents, mold, peeling lead paint, exposed wires, and insufficient heat—all of which are common among low-income housing units—can cause or exacerbate asthma, skin rashes, lead poisoning, fires, and common illnesses, yet none of these housing problems can be "cured" by a clinical encounter. While their consequences can be treated medically, the causes require robust enforcement of existing laws (Tobin-Tyler, Lawton, Conroy, Sandel, & Zuckerman, 2011).

4. **Laws can be determinative of health through their interpretation.** In 2012, the U.S. Supreme Court was asked by half the states in the country to rule on whether the Medicaid expansion in the ACA was unlawfully coercive (*National Federation of Independent Business v. Sebelius*, 2012; note that this decision is discussed in more detail in the Health Reform in the United States chapter). As originally passed into law, the ACA permitted the secretary of the U.S. Department of Health and Human Services to terminate *all* of a state's Medicaid funding if the state failed to implement the Medicaid expansion—even those Medicaid funds that a state would receive that were unconnected to the expansion. While determining that the Medicaid expansion itself was perfectly legitimate, the court ruled that Congress unconstitutionally forced states to potentially have to choose between the Medicaid expansion and a total loss of Medicaid funding. This ruling had the effect of making the ACA's Medicaid expansion optional, rather than mandatory, and states have been deciding individually whether to implement the expansion ever since. At the time of this writing, 33 states and the District of Columbia have adopted the ACA's Medicaid expansion, while 17 states have not; thus, the court's interpretation of a statute has contributed to the fact that otherwise eligible individuals in "non-expansion states" do not have access to Medicaid benefits in the same way that individuals in "expansion states" do.

5. **Finally, the law can be used to structure direct responses to health-harming social needs that result from factors like impoverishment, illness, market failure, and individual behavior that harms others**. For example, the Emergency Medical Treatment and Active Labor Act (EMTALA) requires Medicare-participating hospitals to provide needed stabilization services to individuals who have an emergent condition. Notably, EMTALA's requirements are universal—meaning they have to be fulfilled by hospitals irrespective of the presenting patient's socioeconomic or insurance status—and were written into law because many private hospitals had long turned away emergent patients who were uninsured and could not pay out-of-pocket for their care.

Many financing laws that subsidize healthcare services for vulnerable populations also fit into this category. Medicaid is an obvious example, and the Public Health Service Act includes funding for community health centers, persons with HIV/AIDS, persons with mental illness or substance abuse disorders, and project grants to provide preventive and immunization services, and breast and cervical cancer screening and detection. Title VI of the 1964 Civil Rights Act prohibits discrimination on the basis of race, color, or national origin by any recipient of federal financing, including healthcare providers and facilities. Finally, public health departments funded under state and local legal authority provide primary and preventive healthcare services, such as childhood immunizations, to underserved populations. Programs such as the National Health Service Corps (NHSC) and the Indian Health Service (IHS) were established under federal law to address the lack of providers in rural and other underserved areas. The NHSC was founded in order to incentivize graduates of medical school and other health professions programs to practice primary care in underserved areas, because starting in the 1950s medical graduates began gravitating in large numbers to large cities to practice a medical specialty. The IHS is the principal federal healthcare provider and health advocate for Indian people, providing comprehensive health services to approximately 1.9 million American Indians and Alaska Natives.

Furthermore, through their police powers, states directly regulate individual and corporate behavior in order to protect and promote the public's health. For example, states regulate the food supply and food establishments, enforce occupational safety rules, curb pollution, control the sale of firearms, restrict the marketing of tobacco products, and accredit healthcare professionals and facilities. Indeed, at the local, state, and federal levels, the law has played important roles in all of the 10 most noteworthy public health achievements of the 20th century, as selected by the CDC (1999): control of infectious diseases, motor vehicle safety, fluoridation of drinking water, tobacco use control, vaccinations, decline in deaths due to coronary heart disease and stroke, food safety, improvements in maternal and child health, family planning, and safer workplaces.

Taken together, the preceding discussion illustrates how using law to achieve better health is well suited to what is called a "health in all policies" (HIAP) strategy. This strategy is based on the recognition that several pressing health-related challenges—inequities, chronic disease, skyrocketing costs, the need for insurance reform, and so on—are often complex, multidimensional, and linked to one another. As a result, HIAP relies on a collaborative governmental (and sometimes nongovernmental) approach to health improvement by incorporating health considerations into an array of policy decisions, and by engaging governments and other stakeholders in a multisector approach to shaping the economic, physical, and social environments in which people live, work, and play.

In thinking about how law could be used to foster a HIAP approach, consider the number of rule-making departments and agencies at just the federal level that can (and do) serve healthcare and public health functions even though they are not

---

BOX 7-4 Group Activity

Get together in groups of three or four people. As a group, take 20 minutes to make a list of all the specific ways you can think of that the law has been used to directly respond to health-harming social needs (examples exist in category 5 in this section). When time is up, compare lists across groups, discuss disagreements, and see which group thought of the greatest number of legal interventions.

---

commonly identified as health agencies. The Environmental Protection Agency plays an obviously important role in environmental health. Reducing injuries and hazards in the workplace is the key goal of the Occupational Safety and Health Administration, which is part of the Department of Labor. The Department of Homeland Security protects health when it prepares for and responds to disasters and terrorism. The Department of Agriculture (along with the Food and Drug Administration) plays an important role in the protection of the nation's food supply. The Department of Housing and Urban Development influences the built environment, which in turn influences health. The Department of Energy sets radiation safety standards for nuclear power plants and other sources of energy. Again, these are just federal agencies, and they are all part of the executive branch of government; legislative branch committees at the federal, state, and local levels that are also not typically considered "health" committees could also craft legislation with a HIAP approach in mind. The involvement of multiple branches and agencies in health-related matters plainly shows that the variety of influences impacting individual and population health are outside the control of the health sector alone.

Right to Criminal Legal Representation vs. Civil Legal Assistance

Appreciating the law's power to ameliorate social conditions that negatively affect health requires an understanding of the difference between using law to design broad policies (e.g., Title VI of the Civil Rights Act, firearm regulations, federal housing policy, the ACA) and leveraging the legal system as an individual who is aiming to redress his or her own hardship. In the case of the latter, it helps to understand the difference between rights that attach in the area of criminal legal representation versus those that exist in the realm of civil legal assistance, because it is through civil legal assistance that many types of SDH can been ameliorated.

Criminal Legal Representation

The government is required to provide legal counsel to all federal defendants who are unable to afford their own attorneys; this right is explicit in the Sixth Amendment to the U.S. Constitution. The right to counsel in state criminal prosecutions was established by the U.S. Supreme Court (though only for serious offences) in the famous 1963 case of *Gideon v. Wainwright*. The case arose out of an everyday burglary at a Florida pool hall, for which Clarence Earl Gideon was arrested notwithstanding the flimsy evidence against him. Because Gideon was indigent and could not afford private counsel, he appeared in court alone. He requested counsel but was denied, and as a result acted as his own lawyer at trial. A jury found him guilty and the Florida trial court sentenced Gideon to serve 5 years in state prison.

From prison, Gideon appealed his conviction to the U.S. Supreme Court, arguing that his constitutional rights had been violated when he was denied counsel. The Supreme Court agreed to hear Gideon's constitutional claim and assigned him a well-known lawyer, Abe Fortas, who himself would one day become a U.S. Supreme Court Justice. Building on previous right to counsel cases (for example, in the event of a state prosecution where the death penalty was sought), the court ruled that the assistance of counsel, if desired by an indigent defendant, was a fundamental right under the U.S. Constitution that was required in state prosecutions of serious crimes. Gideon received a new trial and—with the assistance of a lawyer supplied at government expense—was acquitted of all charges just 5 months after the Supreme Court's ruling.

The decision in *Gideon v. Wainwright* spawned many changes in the representation of indigent criminal defendants, including in misdemeanor and juvenile proceedings. The decision effectively created the need for public defenders (lawyers employed at public expense in criminal trials), and it lies at the heart of a series of cases dealing not only with legal representation at trial and on appeal, but also with police interrogation tactics and the right to remain silent.

Civil Legal Assistance

While the right to legal representation exists in criminal matters, no such right exists on the other side of the legal ledger: there is no right to the assistance of a lawyer in civil matters, even when the most basic human needs are at stake. Common civil legal matters involve immigration status, domestic violence, disability law, family law (e.g., child custody cases), housing needs, public benefits (e.g., Medicaid, food stamps, Social Security), employment disputes, and special education needs. In all of these types of disputes—which can be incredibly complex from a legal perspective and which can have life-altering consequences—low-income individuals and families can have no expectation that an attorney will provide them with assistance. (We should note, however, that under some state laws individuals have a right to counsel in limited civil situations, such as with the termination of parental rights or involuntary commitments to mental health facilities.) In civil matters, indigent people (and, increasingly, more members of the middle class and a rising number of small businesses who cannot afford legal fees)[b] can apply for what is known as civil legal aid or civil legal services, which are provided by a network of publicly funded legal aid agencies, private lawyers and law firms practicing on a pro bono basis, law school clinics and professional organizations (the latter group includes organizations such as the American Bar Association, the National Legal Aid and Defender Association, and the American Bar Foundation).

This network is the heart and soul of what is termed the *access to justice* movement, which promotes strategies to address the severe gap in access to both criminal and civil justice for low-income and other vulnerable populations.[c] One of the goals of this movement is to establish a "civil *Gideon*"—in other words, to create a mandate for legal representation of the poor in civil lawsuits. For example, the American Bar Association's House of Delegates passed in 2006 a resolution backing the concept of "civil *Gideon*":

> **RESOLVED,** That the American Bar Association urges state, territorial and federal jurisdictions to provide counsel as a matter of right at public expense to low-income persons in those categories of adversarial proceedings where basic human needs are at stake, such as those involving shelter, sustenance, safety, health or child custody, as determined by each jurisdiction.[d] (American Bar Association, 2006)

Because the combined resources of the civil legal services community are very limited, services are approved on the basis of financial need, meaning that only those individuals with very low incomes receive assistance. Indeed, reports on the legal aid community routinely describe situations in which 80% of civil legal needs for low-income families were not being met, and legal services programs typically turn away over half of the low-income individuals that seek assistance. Congress is most to blame for legal aid's financial predicament; it provides the vast majority of the budget for the Legal Services Corporation (LSC), a not-for-profit corporation established by federal law in 1974 as the single largest funder of civil legal aid for low-income Americans. Considering LSC's annual appropriations from Congress in constant 2015 dollars, its appropriation in 1976 was approximately $386 million; in 2015, its appropriation was $375 million (Legal Services Corporation, 2015).[e] So even as need has soared over time—the U.S. Census Bureau's 2012 statistics on poverty show that over 63 million Americans could qualify for civil legal assistance funded by LSC—the key element of legal aid funding has been treated as an afterthought (Legal Services Corporation, 2018).

The link between civil legal assistance and individual and population health is exemplified by a study of the civil justice experiences of the American public, called the Community Needs and Services Study (Sandefur, 2014). The study uncovers widespread incidence of events and situations that have civil legal aspects and for which people receive no formal or expert legal assistance: fully two-thirds of a random sample of adults in a middle-sized American city reported experiencing at least one of 12 different categories of civil justice situations in the previous 18 months (the average number of situations reported was 3.3, and poor people, African Americans, and Hispanics were more likely to report civil justice situations than were middle- or high-income earners and white people). Unsurprisingly, the most commonly reported situations concerned problems with employment, finances and government benefits, health insurance, and housing. Importantly, respondents indicated that almost half of the civil justice situations they experienced resulted in a significant negative consequence such as feelings of fear, a loss of confidence, damage to physical or mental health, or verbal or physical violence or threats of violence. In fact, adverse impacts on health were the most common negative consequence, reported for 27% of situations. Also important is the fact many of those who responded indicated that they didn't even know that the problems they were experiencing were rightly considered "legal" in nature.

For all of the reasons just discussed—the lack of a right to needed civil legal services, the misunderstandings among those most in need, and the lack of resources in the civil legal aid community—it is paramount that the nation develop and implement innovative, upstream approaches to addressing social conditions that harm health. One such innovation that has taken root is medical-legal partnership.

▶ Combating Health-Harming Social Conditions Through Medical-Legal Partnership[f]

"Do you have any concerns about your housing conditions? Are you concerned about having enough food to eat? Is your child receiving proper supports at school? Do you feel safe at home?" These types of questions are asked of low-income patients with regularity, and their medical care providers know well that the answers speak volumes about patients' health. When the answers come back, however, healthcare providers are too often powerless to do as much as they would like to help remedy these "life circumstances."

Training doctors, nurses, and allied health professionals to reframe these circumstances can help. By now, you probably recognize many of these types of determinants of health for what they are: social conditions whose improvement would benefit from civil legal assistance. Yet despite the connection between poverty, health, and legal needs, and despite the fact that healthcare and civil legal aid professionals commonly provide services to overlapping vulnerable populations, the professions too infrequently attempt to address their populations' needs in a coordinated fashion.

Medical-legal partnership (MLP) aims to bridge this divide. At a practical level, MLPs function as a patient care team that includes both medical and legal professionals; a legal services attorney is literally embedded in a medical care setting (e.g., a hospital, community health center) to address underlying social conditions that negatively affect patient health but whose remediation is outside the expertise of traditional healthcare providers. At a more fundamental level, the goal of the MLP movement is to help create an interconnected care system that focuses on the whole patient (rather than just on biology and behavior), including the ways in which myriad social conditions factor into individual and population health. Thus, the work of MLP lawyers is quite different from that of a general counsel or compliance officer who normally inhabits hospitals and clinics: a general counsel typically provides legal advice to clinicians on matters of medical liability and informed consent and represents them in insurance and disciplinary matters; corporate compliance officers ensure that the facility meets all governmental, environmental, and licensing regulations.

The Evolution of an "Upstream" Innovation

The modern MLP movement has its roots in the late 1960s, when visionary physicians H. Jack Geiger and Count Gibson were funded by the federal government to form the nation's first community health centers in Mississippi and Massachusetts. The government's community health center program grew out of the civil rights movement, when the federal Office of Economic Opportunity (the agency created to administer many of President Lyndon Johnson's War on Poverty programs, and whose programs continue in large part to this day under the auspices of the U.S. Department of Health and Human Services) established "neighborhood health centers" to provide health and social services to medically underserved populations. In designing the earliest centers, Drs. Geiger and Gibson recognized the importance of spending some of their federal funding on lawyers, who assisted African American health center patients battling housing discrimination.

The second prominent instance of the blending of medical and legal services for low-income populations occurred in the early 1980s when, faced with devastating death tolls from HIV/AIDS, some health clinics began providing on-site legal assistance to patients who needed to quickly grapple with end-of-life issues (e.g., medical decision making, asset distribution, family and custody matters). A few pioneering clinics held on to this blended model even after the national AIDS crisis abated, offering comprehensive legal services to all patients in need.

Building on these examples, the first formal MLP was created in the early 1990s in a Boston hospital to intervene on behalf of pediatric patients with chronic conditions who were suffering the consequences of inadequate housing. From that point through 2006, MLPs sprouted up a few at a time, mainly in pediatric healthcare settings, where the model had proven effective in Boston. Since 2006, however, use of the MLP model has expanded considerably. Fueled by the creation of the National Center for Medical-Legal Partnership (NCMLP), the focus by social scientists on the importance of social factors in determining health, and the ACA's focus on disease prevention and professional

collaboration, MLP is now practiced in 46 states by more than 300 hospitals and health centers, in settings as diverse as veteran care facilities, American Indian reservations, and correction facilities (National Center for Medical-Legal Partnership, 2018).

Under the MLP model, public interest lawyers work with healthcare workers to screen for health-related legal problems, often encompassing family matters (divorce, domestic violence), housing problems (eviction, habitability, utility advocacy), special education advocacy, immigration issues, disability issues, employment instability, receipt of public benefits (health insurance, Supplemental Security income), food security concerns, and additional problems that can lead to stress or injury or that can exacerbate existing health problems. **FIGURE 7-1** lays out the key types of patient problems that make up the practice of a typical, comprehensive MLP, using the mnemonic "I-HELP": **I**ncome, **H**ousing and utilities, **E**ducation and employment, **L**egal status, and **P**ersonal and family stability (Marple, 2015).

The MLP approach is built on the understanding not only that many SDH require legal interventions, but that moving "upstream" to assist vulnerable populations with legal needs is preferable to waiting until a legal crisis erupts (for example, remediating a housing problem prior to the receipt of an eviction notice). It is similar to preventive health care: it is often more cost effective—and of course more beneficial to the patient, both physically and emotionally—to help a patient remain healthy, rather than treat the patient post-illness. At MLPs, healthcare and legal professionals are trained side by side about the intersection of health and legal needs and ways to screen for health-harming legal needs. Because MLPs recognize that social determinants contributing to poor health require both health system and public policy change, MLP lawyers utilize on-site legal assistance provided to patients to identify patterns of systemic need, transform institutional practices, and advocate for improved population health policies. **FIGURE 7-2** portrays this upstream MLP approach. Similar to the movement to integrate behavioral healthcare services into primary care, the integration of civil legal aid with healthcare delivery can improve access to services, build team capacity, and promote patient-centered care.

MLPs have become more integrated over time, with healthcare and legal partners sharing patient and institutional data, jointly developing service and training priorities, and establishing cross-sector communication processes. The more collaboration and integration that occurs, the more likely it is that upstream detection of the social conditions that lead to poor health can occur. Deep collaboration and integration also present an opportunity for healthcare

I-HELP ® Issue	Common Social Determinant of Health	Civil Legal Aid Interventions That Help	Impact of Civil Legal Aid Intervention on Health /Health Care
Income	Availability of resource to meet daily basic needs	**Benefits Unit:** Appeal denials of food stamps, health insurance, cash benefits, and disability benefits	1. Increasing someone's income means s/he makes fewer trade-offs between affording food and health care, including medications. 2. Being able to afford enough healthy food helps people manage chronic diseases and helps children grow and develop.
Housing & Utilities	Healthy physical environments	**Housing Unit:** Secure housing subsidies; Improve substandard conditions; Prevent eviction; Protect against utility shut-off	1. A stable, decent, affordable home helps a person avoid costly emergency room visits related to homelessness. 2. Consistent housing, heat and electricity helps people follow their medical treatment plans.
Education & Employment	Access to the opportunity to learn and work	**Education & Employment Units:** Secure specialized education services; Prevent and remedy employment discrimination and enforce workplace rights	1. A quality education is the single greatest predicator of a person's adult health. 2. Consistent employment helps provide money for food and safe housing, which also helps avoid costly emergency healthcare services. 3. Access to health insurance is often linked to employment.
Legal Status	Access to the opportunity to work	**Veterans & Immigration Units:** Resolve veteran discharge status; Clear criminal/credit histories; Assist with asylum applications	1. Clearing a person's criminal history or helping a veteran change their discharge status helps make consistent employment and access to public benefits possible. 2. Consistent employment provides money for food and safe housing, which helps people avoid costly emergency healthcare services.
Personal & Family Stability	Expose to violence	**Family Law Unit:** Secure restraining order for do-mestic violence; Secure adoption, custody and guardianship for children	1. Less violence at home means less need for costly emergency healthcare services. 2. Stable family relationship significantly reduce stress and allow for better decision-making, including decisions related to health care.

FIGURE 7-1 Framing Legal Care as Health Care

Source: Reproduced from: Marple, K. Framing Legal Care as Health Care. National Center for Medical-Legal Partnership. http://medical-legalpartnership.org/new-messaging-guide-helps-frame-legal-care-health-care/. Published January 21, 2015. Accessed August 27, 2015.

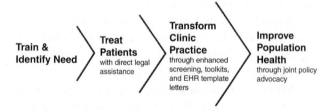

FIGURE 7-2 The Medical-Legal Partnership Approach to the Social Determinants of Health

Source: Reproduced from: The MLP Approach to the Social Determinants of Health. National Center for Medical-Legal Partnership. 2013.

providers and lawyers—two learned professions that, historically, have not been the closest of colleagues— to work together when policymakers design fixes for health-harming social and legal problems.

The Benefits of MLPs

Due to the relatively recent growth of MLPs, the effects of the MLP model have not been regularly tested in formal, large-scale studies. However, several small-scale studies have been conducted (Beeson, McAllister, & Regenstein, 2013; Martinez et al., 2017) and offer preliminary evidence of the benefits of the model in three areas: impact on patient health and well-being, financial impact on partners and patients, and impact on knowledge and training of health providers.

A handful of studies make the case for MLPs by demonstrating the positive impact they can have on patient health and well-being. One such study, focused on home visit/nurse-based interventions for prenatal and postpartum patients, demonstrated better prenatal health behaviors, better pregnancy outcomes, lower rates of child abuse and neglect, and higher rates of maternal employment among participants as a result of MLP services (Williams, Costa, Odunlami, & Mohammed, 2008). A second study found a 91% reduction in emergency department visits and hospital admissions of inner-city asthmatic adults after a medical-legal intervention. In the same study, over 91% of patients also dropped two or more classes in asthma severity (O'Sullivan et al., 2012). Another study focused on cancer patients in an MLP showed a reduction in stress for 75% of the patients, an increase in treatment adherence for 30% of them, and greater ease in keeping appointments for 25% of patients (Fleishman, Retkin, Brandfield, & Braun, 2006). Yet another study showed that by redressing complex social issues through legal advocacy, patients experienced less stress, improved access to preventive health care, and a greater feeling of general well-being (Wang, Conroy, & Zuckerman, 2009).

Several MLP studies have focused on the financial benefits of the model—in other words, on the "return on investment" that accrues to institutions that invest in an MLP. One such study found that an MLP targeting the needs of cancer patients generated nearly $1 million by resolving previously denied health insurance benefit claims (Rodabaugh, Hammond, Myszka, & Sandel, 2013). Similarly, a separate study highlighted four MLP programs, each of which demonstrated successful recovery of previously unreimbursed funds as a result of improperly denied Medicaid or Social Security Disability claims (Knight, 2008). More striking still is evidence of the financial impact that MLPs could have on patients: an MLP in Illinois helped to relieve $4 million in patients' healthcare debt, and claimed $2 million in additional awarded Social Security benefits for patients (Teufel et al., 2012).

Finally, multiple articles have addressed how MLPs can benefit practitioners and patients alike through interdisciplinary training and education. One article, focused on strategies for teaching cultural competence, interdisciplinary practice, and holistic problem solving in legal and medical curricula, describes a legal clinic that increased knowledge about avenues of legal assistance among doctors and of the clinical impact of SDH among lawyers (Tobin-Tyler, 2008). A second paper describes how medical residents working in clinics with social/legal resources were more confident in their knowledge regarding public benefits, and how these same residents were more likely than residents without these resources to ask patients about their social history, use of public benefits, and housing situation (O'Toole, Burkhardt, Solan, Vaughn, &

Klein, 2012). Finally, medical residents who had social work or MLP resources on-site were more confident regarding their personal knowledge of SDH, and as a result were found to screen for them more frequently than other residents (O'Toole et al., 2012).

▶ Conclusion

Recall from the start of this chapter the concept of health equity—essentially, an environment in which all people have an equal opportunity to attain their full health potential. While the nation is far from achieving a state of health equity, it should be everyone's goal to orient society in this direction, even if incrementally. More evidence of whether this is in fact the case will come in a few years, when it will be clearer as to whether most Americans accept the ACA's main goals as ones worth striving for. (Note one final time the law's role as social determinant of health: should the ACA achieve near-complete implementation—and public acceptance along the lines of, say, the Medicare program—the nation, in our view, will be healthier than if the ACA continues to be subjected to political and legal attacks, and to implementation battles in more than a dozen states.)

Whether the nation strives for full health equity aggressively or half-heartedly, there is little doubt that increasing our collective focus on the link between social factors and health would benefit millions of individuals and, in turn, the public more generally. Considering that American children, in particular, experience a high prevalence of social conditions that compromise their care and development—including insufficient family income to meet basic living needs, food insecurity, unstable housing, environmental toxins, and a lack of high-quality child care—this type of reorientation is nothing less than a moral imperative (Miller, Sadegh-Nobari, & Lillie-Blanton, 2011).

One facet of this transformation is reframing civil legal services for vulnerable populations as a critical component of health care. Civil legal aid, after all, is first and foremost about promoting the enforcement of existing laws that protect vulnerable populations (Houseman, 2015). If health is at the core of well-being for all people, then reducing barriers to good health should be an obvious societal goal, and for low-income and other vulnerable populations this means reducing the health-harming effects of social conditions that they struggle with disproportionately. To address this inequality, the civil legal community should closely align its activities and priorities with healthcare and public health partners.

References

American Bar Association. (2006). *Recommendation.* Retrieved from http://www.americanbar.org/content/dam/aba/administrative/legal_aid_indigent_defendants/ls_sclaid_06A112A.authcheckdam.pdf

Bachrach, D. (2014). *Addressing patients' social needs: An emerging business case for provider investment.* Retrieved from http://www.commonwealthfund.org/publications/fund-reports/2014/may/addressing-patients-social-needs

Beeson, T., McAllister, B., & Regenstein, M. (2013). *Literature review: Making the case for medical-legal partnerships.* Retrieved from http://medical-legalpartnership.org/mlp-resources/literature-review/

Bradley, E. H., Elkins, B. R., Herrin, J., & Elbel, B. (2011). Health and social services expenditures: Associations with health outcomes. *BMJ Quality & Safety, 20*(10), 826–831.

Braveman, P., Egerter, S., & Barclay, C. (2011). *What shapes health-related behaviors? The role of social factors.* Princeton, NJ: Robert Wood Johnson Foundation.

Braveman, P., & Gottlieb, L. (2014). The social determinants of health: It's time to consider the causes of the causes. *Public Health Reports, 129*(supp. 2), 19–31.

Bronner, E. (2013, March 15). Right to lawyer can be empty promise for poor. *The New York Times.* Retrieved from https://www.nytimes.com/2013/03/16/us/16gideon.html

Burris, S. (2011). Law in a social determinants strategy: A public health law research perspective. *Public Health Reporter, 126*(supp. 3), 22–27.

Callahan, L. F., Martin, K. R., Shreffler, J., Kumar, D., Schoster, B., Kaufman, J., & Schwartz, T. (2011). Independent and combined influence of homeownership, occupation, education, income and community poverty on physical health in persons with arthritis. *Arthritis Care & Research, 63*(5).

Centers for Disease Control and Prevention. (1999). Ten great public health achievements—United States, 1900–1999. *Morbidity and Mortality Weekly Report, 48*(12), 241–243.

Centers for Disease Control and Prevention. (2013). CDC health disparities and inequalities report. *Morbidity and Mortality Weekly Report, 62*(supp. 3), 1–187.

Corporation for Supportive Housing. (2014). *Housing is the best medicine: Supportive housing and the social determinants of health.* Retrieved from https://www.csh.org/wp-content/uploads/2014/07/SocialDeterminantsofHealth_2014.pdf

Ferris State University. (2012). *What was Jim Crow.* Retrieved from http://www.ferris.edu/jimcrow/what.htm

Fleischhacker, S. E., Evenson, K. R., Rodriguez, D. A., & Ammerman, A. S. (2011). A systematic review of fast food access studies. *Obesity Review, 12*(5), e460–e471.

Fleishman, S. B., Retkin, R., Brandfield, J., & Braun, V. (2006). The attorney as the newest member of the cancer treatment team. *Journal of Clinical Oncology, 24*(13), 2123–2126.

Galea, S., Tracy, M., Hoggatt, K. J., DiMaggio, C., & Karpati, A. (2011). Estimated deaths attributable to social factors in the United States. *American Journal of Public Health, 101*(8), 1456–1465.

Gideon v. Wainwright, 372 U.S. 335 (1963).

Gostin, L. O., Jacobson, P. D., Record, K., & Hardcastle, L. (2011). Restoring health to health reform: Integrating medicine and public health to advance the population's well-being. *University of Pennsylvania Law Review, 159*, 1777–1823.

Hoffman, K. W., Trawalter, S., Axt, J. R., & Oliver, M. N. (2016). Racial bias in pain assessment and treatment recommendations, and false beliefs about biological differences between blacks and whites. *Proceedings of the National Academy of Sciences, 113*(6), 4296–4301.

Houseman, A. (2015). *Civil legal aid in the United States: An update for 2015.* Retrieved from https://repository.library.georgetown.edu/bitstream/handle/10822/761858/Houseman_Civil_Legal_Aid_US_2015.pdf

Jack, L., Jack, N. H., & Hayes, S. C. (2012). Social determinants of health in minority populations: A call for multidisciplinary approaches to eliminate diabetes-related health disparities. *Diabetes Spectrum, 25*(1), 9–13.

Jones, J. H. (1993). *Bad blood: The Tuskegee syphilis experiment.* New York, NY: The Free Press.

Kaiser Family Foundation. (2012). *Disparities in health and health care: Five key questions and answers.* Retrieved from https://kaiserfamilyfoundation.files.wordpress.com/2012/11/8396-disparities-in-health-and-health-care-five-key-questions-and-answers.pdf

Knight, R. (2008). *Health care recovery dollars: A sustainable strategy for medical-legal partnerships?* Retrieved from https://static1.squarespace.com/static/5373b088e4b02899e91e9392/t/53cd59cae4b02facb9407e39/1405966794425/Medical-Legal+Partnership+Health+Care+Recovery+Dollars.pdf

Layton, L. (2015, April 15). New brain science shows poor kids have smaller brains than affluent kids. *The Washington Post.* Retrieved from http://www.washingtonpost.com/local/education/new-brain-science-shows-poor-kids-have-smaller-brains-than-affluent-kids/2015/04/15/3b679858-e2bc-11e4-b510-962fcfabc310_story.html

Legal Services Corporation. (2015). *Congressional appropriations.* Retrieved from http://www.lsc.gov/about-lsc/who-we-are/congressional-oversight/congressional-appropriations

Legal Services Corporation. (2018). *Who we are.* Retrieved from http://www.lsc.gov/about/what-is-lsc

Marple, K. (2015). *Framing legal care as health care.* Retrieved from http://medical-legalpartnership.org/new-messaging-guide-helps-frame-legal-care-health-care/

Martinez, O., Boles, J., Muñoz-Laboy, M., Levine, E. C., Ayamele, C., Eisenberg, R., & Draine, J. (2017). Bridging health disparity gaps through the use of medical-legal partnerships in patient care: A systematic review. *Journal of Law, Medicine and Ethics, 45*(2), 260–273.

McGinnis, J. M., & Foege, W. H. (1993). Actual causes of death in the United States. *Journal of the American Medical Association, 270*(18), 2207–2212.

McGovern, L., Miller, G., & Hughes-Cromwick, P. (2014). *Health policy brief: The relative contribution of multiple determinants to health outcomes.* Retrieved from https://www.rwjf.org/content/dam/farm/reports/issue_briefs/2014/rwjf415185

Miller, W. D., Sadegh-Nobari, T., & Lillie-Blanton, M. (2011). Healthy starts for all: Policy prescriptions. *American Journal of Preventive Medicine, 40*(1 supp. 1), S19–S37.

Mokdad, A. H., Marks, J. S., Stroup, D. F., & Gerberding, J. L. (2004). Actual causes of death in the United States, 2000. *Journal of the American Medical Association, 291*(10), 1238–1245.

National Center for Medical-Legal Partnership. (2018). *Partnerships across the U.S.* Retrieved from http://medical-legalpartnership.org/partnerships/

National Federation of Independent Business v. Sebelius, 567 U.S. 519 (2012).

National Partnership for Action to End Health Disparities. (n.d.). Home page. Retrieved from http://minorityhealth.hhs.gov/npa/

O' Sullivan, M. M., Brandfield, J., Hoskote, S. S., Segal, S. N., Chug, L., Modrykamien, A., & Eden, E. (2012). Environmental improvements brought by the legal interventions in the homes of poorly-controlled inner-city adult asthmatic patients: A proof-of-concept study. *Journal of Asthma, 49*(9), 911–917.

O'Toole, J. K., Burkhardt, M. C., Solan, L. G., Vaughn, L., & Klein, M. D. (2012). Resident confidence addressing social history: Is it influenced by availability of social and legal resources? *Clinical Pediatrics, 51*(7), 625–631.

Perlman, J., & Parvensky, J. (2006). *Denver housing first collaborative cost benefit analysis and program outcomes report.* Retrieved from http://shnny.org/uploads/Supportive_Housing _in_Denver.pdf

Powell, L. M., Slater, S., Mirtcheva, D., Bao, Y., & Chaloupka, F. J. (2007). Food store availability and neighborhood characteristics in the United States. *Preventive Medicine, 44*(3), 189–195.

Rodabaugh, K. J., Hammond, M., Myszka, D., & Sandel, M. (2013). A medical-legal partnership as a component of a palliative care model. *Journal of Palliative Medicine, 13*(1), 15–18.

Sandefur, R. L. (2014). *Accessing justice in the contemporary USA: Findings from the community needs and services study.* Retrieved from http://www.americanbarfoundation.org /uploads/cms/documents/sandefur_accessing_justice_in _the_contemporary_usa._aug._2014.pdf

Schneiderman, N., Ironson, G., & Siegel, S. D. (2005). Stress and health: Psychological, behavioral, and biological determinants. *Annual Review of Clinical Psychology, 1*, 607–628.

Schulman, K. A., Berlin, J. A., Harless, W., Kerner, J. F., Sistrunk, S., Gersh, B. J., . . . Escarce, J. J. (1999). The effect of race and sex on physicians' recommendations for cardiac catheterization. *New England Journal of Medicine, 340*, 618–626.

Smedley, B. D., Stith, A. Y., & Nelson, A. R. (Eds.). *Unequal treatment: Confronting racial and ethnic disparities in health care.* Washington, DC: The National Academies Press.

Stringhini, S., Sabia, S., Shipley, M., Brunner, E., Nabi, H., Kivimaki, M., & Sing-Manoux, A. (2010). Association of socioeconomic position with health behaviors and mortality. *Journal of the American Medical Association, 303*(12), 1159–1166.

Teufel, J. A., Werner, D., Goffinet, D., Thorne, W., Brown, S. L., & Gettinger, L. (2012). Rural medical-legal partnership and advocacy: A three-year follow-up study. *Journal of Health Care for the Poor and Underserved, 23*(2), 705–714.

Tobin-Tyler, E. (2008). Allies not adversaries: Teaching collaboration to the next generation of doctors and lawyers to address social inequality. *Journal of Health Care Law and Policy, 11*, 249–294.

Tobin-Tyler, E. (2012). Aligning public health, health care, law and policy: Medical-legal partnership as a multilevel response to the social determinants of health. *Journal of Health and Biomedical Law, 8*(2), 211–247.

Tobin-Tyler, E., Lawton, E., Conroy, K., Sandel, M., & Zuckerman, B. (Eds.). (2011). *Poverty, health and law: Readings and cases for Medical-Legal Partnership.* Durham, NC: North Carolina Press.

Tobin-Tyler, E., & Teitelbaum, J. (2019). *Essentials of Health Justice: A Primer.* Burlington, MA: Jones & Bartlett Learning.

U.S. Department of Agriculture. (2017). *Food access research atlas.* Retrieved from http://www.ers.usda.gov/data/fooddesert

U.S. Department of Health and Human Services. (2018). *Social determinants of health.* Retrieved from http:// www.healthypeople.gov/2020/topics-objectives/topic /social-determinants-health

U.S. Department of Justice. (n.d.) Office for Access to Justice. Retrieved from https://www.justice.gov/archives/atj

van Ryn, M., Burgess, D., Malat, J., & Griffin, J. (2006). Physicians' perceptions of patients' social and behavioral characteristics and race disparities in treatment recommendations for men with coronary artery disease. *American Journal of Public Health, 96*(2), 351–357.

Wang, C. J., Conroy, K. N., & Zuckerman, B. (2009). Payment reform for safety-net institutions—Improving quality and outcomes. *New England Journal of Medicine, 361*(19), 1821–1823.

Williams, D. R., Costa, M. V., Odunlami, A. O., & Mohammed, S. A. (2008). Moving upstream: How interventions that address the social determinants of health can improve health and reduce disparities. *Journal of Public Health Management and Practice, 14*, s8–s17.

World Health Organization. (2018). *Social determinants of health.* Retrieved from http://www.who.int/social_determinants /sdh_definition/en/

Yearby, R. (2013). Breaking the cycle of "unequal treatment" with health care reform: Acknowledging and addressing the continuation of racial bias. *Connecticut Law Review, 44*(4), 1281–1324.

▶ **Endnotes**

a. For a full account of the Tuskegee Study, see Jones, 1993.

b. According to the World Justice Project, a not-for-profit group promoting the rule of law, the United States ranks 66th out of 98 countries in the access to and affordability of civil legal services (Bronner, 2013).

c. For more information, see, for example, U.S. Department of Justice, n.d.

d. See American Bar Association (2006) for the resolution and an accompanying report on achieving equal justice in the United States.

e. Note that LSC's heyday was back in the late 1970s and early 1980s, when their budget topped $800 million dollars in 2015 terms.

f. In the interest of disclosure, Professor Teitelbaum is co-principal investigator of the National Center for Medical-Legal Partnership at The George Washington University's Milken Institute School of Public Health. For more information about medical-legal partnership and the National Center, visit http://www.medical-legalpartnership.org/

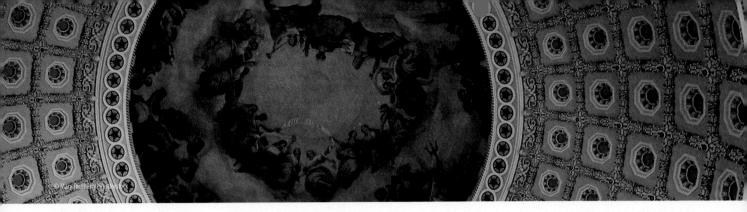

CHAPTER 8

Understanding Health Insurance

LEARNING OBJECTIVES

By the end of this chapter you will be able to:

- Understand the role of risk and uncertainty in insurance
- Define the basic elements of health insurance
- Differentiate various insurance products
- Discuss incentives created for providers and patients in various types of insurance arrangements
- Discuss health policy issues relating to health insurance

▶ Introduction

Unlike many other countries, the United States does not have a national healthcare delivery system; whether individuals have access to healthcare services—and whether they receive health care of appropriate quantity and quality—often depends on whether they are insured. Even if an individual is insured, the kind of coverage he or she has can affect his or her ability to obtain care. Understanding health insurance, however, requires more than understanding its importance to healthcare access.

Policymakers must also know how providers, suppliers, employers, states, and others respond to changes in the health insurance market. For example, if policymakers decide to reduce the number of uninsured by creating a new state health insurance exchange (essentially, an online marketplace) for the sale and purchase of private insurance coverage (as happened under the

ACA), they must know whether providers will participate in the program and what features will make it more or less attractive to providers. Or, if policymakers want to reduce the number of uninsured by mandating that employers offer health insurance (as also happened under the ACA), they must know which requirements will make it more or less likely that more employees will be covered under such a mandate. In either case, policymakers might also want to know whether an initiative will affect the financial viability of public hospitals or health centers.

Several themes emerge when considering these types of health-insurance–related policy questions. First, insurance is rooted in the concepts of uncertainty and risk; reducing uncertainty and risk by, for example, offering a health insurance product, participating as a provider in a health insurance plan, or purchasing health insurance coverage as a consumer creates various incentives for insurers, the insured, providers, and governments to act or refrain from acting in certain ways. As noted in **BOX 8-1**, one goal of the ACA is to reduce the risk of insuring small businesses and individuals by creating a large purchasing pool through state health insurance exchanges (Patient Protection and Affordable Care Act [ACA], 2010). Second, to a large extent, insurance carriers choose the design of their health insurance products, and employers and individuals choose whether to purchase health insurance—and, if so, what type. Indeed, insurance carriers have had wide latitude to determine the individuals or groups that may join a plan, employers have had broad discretion to determine whether to offer

coverage and what type to offer, and individuals have had the choice whether to purchase health insurance coverage, although this choice was often illusory due to the high cost of health care. The ACA attempts to change these choices and incentives. For example, many insurance plans will have to meet new requirements, such as offering a package of "essential health benefits"; most employers will have to provide health insurance coverage or pay a penalty; and most individuals will have to purchase health insurance or pay a penalty. For each choice, the question is: What policy goal (e.g., equity, universal coverage, fiscal restraint, market efficiency) should drive the design and regulation of health insurance?

This chapter begins with a short history of health insurance in the United States and then reviews the health insurance concepts key to understanding the structure and operation of health insurance. It concludes with an overview of managed care, a particular form of health insurance dominant in today's market.

▶ A Brief History of the Rise of Health Insurance in the United States

Although about 88% of people in this country were insured in 2017, health insurance was not always an integral part of our society (Auter, 2018). The initial movement to bring health insurance to the United States was modeled after activities in Europe. In the late 1800s and early 1900s, the European social insurance movement resulted in the creation of "sickness" insurance throughout many countries: Germany in 1883, Austria in 1888, Hungary in 1891, Britain in 1911, and Russia in 1912, to name just a few examples. These programs varied in scope and structure, from a compulsory national system in Germany, to industry-based requirements in France and Italy, to extensive state aid in Sweden and Switzerland. Although the Socialist and Progressive parties advocated for the adoption of similar social insurance systems in the United States in the early 1900s, their efforts were unsuccessful (Starr, 1982).

In the absence of government-sponsored health insurance plans, the private sector insurance industry flourished with the growth of Blue Cross, Blue Shield, and commercial insurance carriers. Blue Cross established its first hospital insurance plan at Baylor University in 1929 by agreeing to provide 1,500 teachers with 21 days of hospital care per year for the price of $6 per person (Starr, 1982, p. 295). The hospital

---

BOX 8-1 Vignette

William owns a small business that sells all kinds of wheels and gears. He has nine employees and has always made it a priority to offer competitive benefits, including health insurance. Unfortunately, last year one of his employees was diagnosed with cancer, which he continues to fight. Due to the sharp increase in use of health services by his employee group, the insurance company doubled his group premiums for the upcoming year. When William contacted other carriers, several of them would not consider insuring his group, and most of the others gave him quotes as expensive as his current carrier. One company gave him a lower quote, but it covered only catastrophic care; his employees would have to pay for the first $5,000 of care out of their own pockets. After reviewing his company's finances, William is left with several unattractive options: stop offering health insurance; offer comprehensive health insurance but pass on the cost increase to his employees, which would make it unaffordable for most of them; offer the bare-bones catastrophic plan only; or significantly lower wages and other benefits to defray the rising health insurance costs. In addition to wanting to offer competitive benefits, William is concerned that adopting any of these options will cause his employees to leave and make it hard to attract others, threatening the sustainability of his company.

The 2010 health reform law, the Patient Protection and Affordable Care Act (ACA), attempts to help small businesses like William's by creating state health insurance exchanges. Starting in 2014, these exchanges were intended to offer a variety of plans to individuals and small businesses that otherwise might not be able to afford health insurance coverage. By creating large groups of purchasers through the exchanges, it is possible to pool risk and keep prices lower than if individuals or small businesses were attempting to purchase insurance coverage on their own.

industry supported the growth of private insurance as a way to secure payment for services during the Depression. Blue Shield, the physician-based insurance plan, began in 1939 as a way to forestall renewed efforts to enact compulsory national health insurance and to avoid growth in consumer-controlled prepaid health plans, both of which would have reduced the type of physician autonomy endemic at that time (Starr, 1982, p. 307).

World War II led to rapid growth in employer-sponsored health insurance. With employees scarce and a general wage freeze in effect, a 1942 War Labor Board ruling that employee fringe benefits of up to 5% of wages did not violate the wage freeze created a strong incentive for employers to provide health benefits to attract new workers and keep their current ones. After the war, labor unions gained the right to bargain collectively, leading to another expansion of employee health plans. In 1954, the Internal Revenue Service declared that employers could pay health insurance premiums for their employees with pre-tax dollars, further increasing the value of the fringe benefit to employers.[a] By 1949, 28 million people had commercial hospital insurance, 22 million had commercial physician insurance, and 4 million had independent hospital plans. At that time, over 31 million had Blue Cross hospital coverage and 12 million had Blue Shield coverage (Starr, 1982, p. 327). Employer-sponsored health insurance, not national health insurance, was well on its way to becoming entrenched as the primary form of health insurance.

The federal government first became a major player in health insurance with the passage of Medicaid and Medicare in 1965. These programs were created, in part, to fill in coverage gaps left by the private insurance market—namely, coverage for the elderly, disabled, and low-income populations who had too little income and too high health risks to be viable candidates for insurance coverage from the insurance carriers' point of view. Like many major policy changes, the passage of these programs was a multilayered compromise. Before the final design of these programs was established, several proposals were considered: the American Medical Association (AMA) supported a combination federal–state program to subsidize private insurance policies for older adults to cover hospital care, physician care, and prescription drugs; Representative John Byrnes (R-WI), ranking Republican on the House Ways and Means Committee, endorsed an AMA-like proposal but with federal, instead of federal–state, administration; the Johnson administration supported hospital insurance for older adults through Social Security; and Senator Jacob Javitz (R-NY) supported federal payments to state programs to provide health care to poor, elderly individuals (Stevens & Stevens, 2003, pp. 46–48). In the end, the Medicare and Medicaid programs were passed in one bill with features from all of these proposals. For example, Medicare was established as a federally funded program with two parts, one for hospital insurance and one for physician insurance, and Medicaid as a state–federal program for the poor.

By the 1970s a number of factors converged to place rising healthcare costs on the national agenda: advances had been made in medical technology, hospitals expanded and became more involved in high-tech care, physician specialties became more common, hospitals and physicians had a large new pool of paying patients due to Medicaid and Medicare, wages for medical staff increased, and an aging population required an increasing amount of services (Starr, 1982, pp. 383–384). In addition, the prevailing fee-for-service (FFS) insurance system rewarded healthcare professionals for providing a high quantity of services. As the name suggests, fee-for-service reimbursement means the providers are paid for each service they provide—the more services (and the more expensive the services) rendered, the more reimbursement the provider receives. From 1960 to 1970, hospital care expenditures tripled from $9.3 billion to $28 billion, and physician service expenditures almost matched that growth rate, increasing from $5.3 billion to $13.6 billion (Sultz & Young, 2001, pp. 257–258). Federal and state governments were also feeling the burden of high healthcare costs. From 1965 to 1970, federal and state governments collectively experienced a 21% annual rate of increase in their healthcare expenditures (Starr, 1982, p. 384).

BOX 8-2 Discussion Questions

Most people in this country obtain health insurance through employer-sponsored plans. Although the historical background you just read explains *how* this system came about, it does not discuss whether it is a good or bad thing. Is our reliance on employer-sponsored health insurance ideal for individuals? Providers? Employers? Society? What are the benefits and drawbacks to having employers as the primary source of health insurance? How different are the benefits and drawbacks when considered from various stakeholder perspectives? Would it be better to have more federal government involvement in providing health insurance? What primary policy goal would you use to decide how to answer these questions?

As is discussed in more detail later in this chapter, managed care moves away from the FFS system by integrating the payment for services and the delivery of services into one place in an attempt to rein in healthcare costs and utilization. The federal Health Maintenance Organization Act of 1973 was intended to spur the growth of managed care by providing incentives to increase the use of health maintenance organizations (HMOs). The act relied on federal loans and grants and a mandate that employers with 25 or more employees offer an HMO option if one was available in their area (Sultz & Young, 2001, pp. 262–263). Even so, managed care did not flourish due to opposition by patients who did not want their provider and service choices restricted, and by providers who did not want to lose control over their practices.

As healthcare cost and quality concerns remained a national priority, the managed care industry eventually found a foothold in the health insurance market. Indeed, enrollment in managed care doubled during the 1990s, with almost 80 million enrollees by 1998. In 2017, only 1% of workers were in conventional, non-managed-care arrangements (Kaiser Family Foundation [KFF], 2017). Although only about 33% of Medicare enrollees choose managed care arrangements (Jacobson, Damico, & Neuman, 2017), some 65% of Medicaid beneficiaries receive some or all of their services through managed care, though for many of them it is mandatory that they receive services through a managed care arrangement (Rudowitz & Garfield, 2018).

▶ How Health Insurance Operates

This section provides an overview of the purpose and structure of health insurance. It begins with a review of basic health insurance terminology, considers the role of uncertainty and risk in insurance, and concludes with a discussion of how insurance companies set their premium rates.

Basic Terminology

As you read earlier, the health insurance industry first developed when the FFS system was standard. Under this system, not only do providers have incentive to conduct more and more expensive services, but patients are unbridled in their use of the healthcare system because FFS does not limit the use of services or accessibility to providers. As we will discuss later in this chapter, managed care developed as a response to the incentives created by the FFS system. However, even though there are numerous differences between FFS and managed care, many of the fundamental principles of how insurance operates are applicable to any type of health insurance contract. The following discussion reviews how health insurance works generally, regardless of the type of insurance arrangement.

The health insurance consumer (also known as the *beneficiary* or *insured*) buys health insurance in advance for an annual fee, usually paid in monthly installments, called a *premium*. In return, the health insurance carrier (or company) pays for all or part of the beneficiary's healthcare costs if she or he becomes ill or injured and has a covered medical need. (A covered need is a medical good or service that the insurer is obligated to pay for because it is covered based on the terms of the insurance contract or policy. As discussed in detail elsewhere, the ACA requires many plans to cover all "essential health benefits.") Insurance contracts cannot identify every conceivable healthcare need of beneficiaries, so they are generally structured to include categories of care (e.g., outpatient, inpatient, vision, maternity) to be provided if deemed medically necessary. Definitions of the term *medically necessary* vary by contract and are important when determining whether a procedure is covered.

Even if the beneficiary never needs healthcare services covered by the insurance policy, he or she still pays for the policy through premiums. The consumer benefits by having financial security in case of illness or injury, and the insurance company benefits by making money selling health insurance.

In addition to premiums, the beneficiary typically pays other costs under most health insurance policies. Many policies have *deductibles*, which is the amount of money the beneficiary must pay on his or her own for healthcare needs each year before the insurance carrier starts to help with the costs. For example, if a policyholder has a $500 deductible, the beneficiary must pay 100% of the first $500 of healthcare costs each year. The insurance carrier is not liable to cover any costs until the individual's healthcare bill reaches $501 in a given year. If the individual does not need more than $500 worth of health care in a specific year, the insurance carrier generally will not help that individual pay his or her healthcare costs.

Furthermore, a beneficiary generally continues to incur some costs in addition to the premiums even after the deductible has been met. Insurance carriers often impose cost sharing on the beneficiary through *co-payment* or *co-insurance* requirements.

BOX 8-3 Discussion Questions

As a general matter, all types of insurance under traditional economic models cover expensive and unforeseen events, not events that have small financial risk or little uncertainty (Council of Economic Advisors, 2004, p. 195). For example, auto insurance does not cover regular maintenance such as an oil change, and home insurance does not protect against normal wear and tear, such as the need to replace an old carpet. Accordingly, many economists argue that health insurance should not cover regular, foreseeable events such as physical exams or low-cost occurrences such as vaccinations. Other economists support a different school of thought. An alternative economic view is that health insurance should insure one's health, not just offer protection against the financial consequences of major adverse health events. Because people without health insurance are less likely to obtain preventive care such as physical exams or vaccinations, these economists believe it is in everyone's best interest, ethically and financially, to promote preventive care. Therefore, it is appropriate for insurance to cover both unpredictable and expensive events as well as predictable and less expensive events. Which theory do you support? What do you think is the best use of insurance? If insurance does not cover low-cost and predictable events, should another resource be available to assist individuals, or should people pay out of their own pockets for these healthcare needs?

families against the financial consequences of these unfortunate and unforeseen events.

Although genetic predisposition or behavioral choices such as smoking or working a high-risk job may increase the chances that an individual will suffer from a health-related problem, in general there is a high level of uncertainty as to whether a particular person will become sick or injured and need medical assistance. Health insurance protects the consumer from medical costs associated with both expensive and unforeseen events. Even if the consumer does not experience a negative event, a benefit exists from the peace of mind and reduced uncertainty of financial exposure that insurance provides.

In terms of health status and wise use of resources, when insurance allows consumers to purchase necessary services they would not otherwise be able to afford, it functions in a positive manner. Conversely, when insurance leads consumers to purchase unnecessary healthcare goods or services of low value because the consumer is not paying full cost, it works in a negative manner. The difficult task is trying to figure out how to set the consumer's share of the burden at just the right point to encourage and make available the proper use of health care, while discouraging improper usage.

BOX 8-4 Discussion Questions

As discussed earlier, risk and uncertainty are important concepts in health insurance. Individuals purchase health insurance policies to protect themselves financially against healthcare costs, and insurance carriers try to set premiums that will cover the cost of the services used by their beneficiaries. Currently (when allowed by law), insurance carriers may consider factors such as medical history, demographics, type of occupation, size of the beneficiary pool, and similar criteria when setting the terms of an insurance policy. Should health insurance carriers also have access to and be able to use genetic testing results when deciding whether to insure an individual, what premiums to charge, or which services to cover? If you think the answer to that question should be "no," why is genetic information different from all of the other kinds of information insurance carriers may take into account when making those decisions? Conversely, what is the strongest argument you can make in favor of allowing insurance carriers to consider an applicant's genetic information? How would allowing genetic testing alter an individual's or a provider's diagnosis and treatment decisions? What is the primary policy goal that affects your view?

A co-payment is a set dollar amount the beneficiary pays when receiving a service from a provider. For example, many HMOs charge their beneficiaries $15 every time a beneficiary sees a primary care provider. Co-insurance refers to a percentage of the healthcare cost the individual must cover. For example, 20% is a common co-insurance amount. This arrangement means the beneficiary pays 20% of all healthcare costs after the deductible has been met, with the insurance carrier paying the other 80%.

Uncertainty

From a traditional economic perspective, insurance exists because of two basic concepts—risk and uncertainty. The world is full of risks—auto theft, house fires, physical disabilities—and uncertainty about whether any such events might affect a particular individual. As a result, people buy various forms of insurance (e.g., automobile insurance, home insurance, life or disability insurance) to protect themselves and their

Risk

Risk is a central concern in insurance. Consumers buy insurance to protect themselves against the risk of unforeseen and costly events. But health insurers are also concerned about risk—the risk that their beneficiaries will experience a covered medical event.

Individuals purchase health insurance to protect themselves against the risk of financial consequences of healthcare needs. Because of differences in risk level, individuals who are generally healthy or otherwise do not anticipate having health expenses may place a lower value on insurance than individuals who are unhealthy or those who are healthy but expect to have medical expenses, such as pregnant women. Therefore, healthy individuals tend to seek out lower-cost insurance plans or refrain from obtaining insurance altogether if it is not, in their view, cost effective. Unhealthy individuals or healthy individuals who often use the healthcare system would obviously prefer a low-cost insurance plan (with comprehensive benefits) but are generally more willing to pay higher premiums because of the value they place on having insurance.

Health insurance carriers are businesses that need to cover their expenditures, including the cost of accessing capital needed to run their company, to stay in the market.[b] They earn money by collecting premiums from their beneficiaries, and they pay out money to cover their beneficiaries' healthcare costs above the deductible amount and to cover the costs of running a business (e.g., overhead, marketing, taxes). One way health insurance companies survive is to make sure the premiums charged to beneficiaries cover these costs. From the insurance carrier's perspective, it would be ideal to be able to charge lower premiums to attract healthy individuals who are less likely to use their benefits, and higher premiums to unhealthy individuals who are more likely to need medical care.

However, insurance companies have difficulty matching healthy people with low-cost plans and unhealthy people with high-cost plans because of the problem of *asymmetric information*. This is the term used by economists when one party to a transaction has more information than the other party. In the case of insurance, the imbalance often favors the consumer because insurance carriers generally do not know as much as the individual does about the individual's healthcare needs and personal habits. Although relatively healthy low-cost individuals want to make their status known because insurance carriers might be willing to sell them an insurance product for a lower price, relatively unhealthy individuals do not want their status known because insurance companies might charge them higher premiums. For this reason,

when an insurance carrier lacks complete information, it is more beneficial to unhealthy beneficiaries than to healthy ones.

Together, uncertainty about risk and the presence of asymmetric information lead to the problem of *adverse selection*. In terms of health insurance, adverse selection is when unhealthy people overselect (that is, select beyond a random distribution) a particular plan. This occurs because people at risk for having high healthcare costs choose a particular plan because of that plan's attractive coverage rules (Penner, 2004, pp. 12–13). The consumer who knows he is a high risk for needing services will be more likely to choose a more comprehensive plan because it covers more services, even though it is probably a more expensive option. This overselection leaves the insurer that offers the comprehensive plan with a disproportionate number of high-risk beneficiaries. As a result of the relatively high-risk pool, beneficiaries will have high service utilization rates, requiring the insurance carrier to raise premiums to pay for the increased cost of covering services for beneficiaries. In turn, some of the healthier individuals might choose to leave the plan because of the higher premiums, resulting in an even riskier beneficiary pool and even higher premiums, and the cycle continues. The healthier consumers may find a lower-cost plan or may choose to go without health insurance (especially since the Tax Cut and Jobs Act of 2017 repealed, as of 2019, the penalty associated with violating the ACA's individual mandate, as described in more detail in a subsequent chapter), while the insurance plan is left with an increasingly higher percentage of relatively unhealthy people. This is the problem of adverse selection.

One instance where adverse selection is a key concern is with an increasingly popular type of health plan, the high-deductible health plan (HDHP). As the name suggests, these plans have very high deductibles (usually defined as at least $1,000 for an individual or $2,000 for a family). In 2017, annual premiums for the average HDHP were $6,024 for individuals and $17,581 for families (KFF, 2017). As with other insurance plans, consumers pay most of their healthcare expenses out-of-pocket until they reach the deductible. HDHPs are often used in conjunction with health reimbursement arrangements (HRAs) or health savings accounts (HSAs), which allow individuals to set aside money for future healthcare needs. Health reimbursement arrangements are funded solely by employers, who usually commit to making a specified amount of money available for healthcare expenses incurred by employees or their dependents, while HSAs are created by individuals, but employers may also contribute to HSAs if the employers offer a qualified HDHP. Individual contributions to HSAs are made with pre-income tax dollars, and withdrawals to pay for qualified healthcare expenses are also not taxed. As shown in **FIGURES 8-1** and **8-2**, HDHPs are increasingly popular with employers and employees.

Those who support HDHPs assert that plans with high deductibles promote personal responsibility because enrollees have a financial incentive to avoid overusing the healthcare system and to choose cost-effective treatment options. As a result, HDHPs are favored by employers and others as a cost-cutting strategy. Others are concerned that HDHPs will have a negative effect on enrollees' health because individuals cannot or will not price shop and are more likely to save money by simply avoiding needed care. As discussed in **BOX 8-5**, researchers continue to evaluate these questions.

An enrollee's experience with a HDHP may depend, in part, on income level. Individuals who are

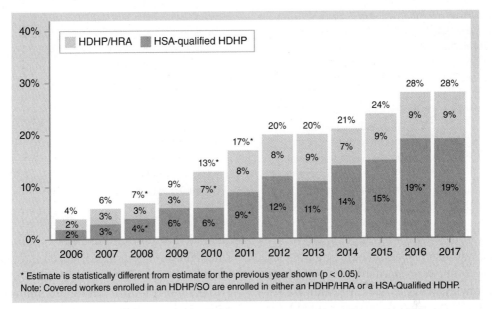

FIGURE 8-1 Percentage of Covered Workers Enrolled in a High-Deductible Health Plan (HDHP) or Health Reimbursement Arrangement, or in a Health Savings Account–Qualified HDHP, 2006–2017

Source: Reproduced from: Kaiser/HRET Survey of Employer-Sponsored Health Benefits, 2017 https://www.kff.org/report-section/ehbs-2017-section-8-high-deductible-health-plans-with-savings-option/

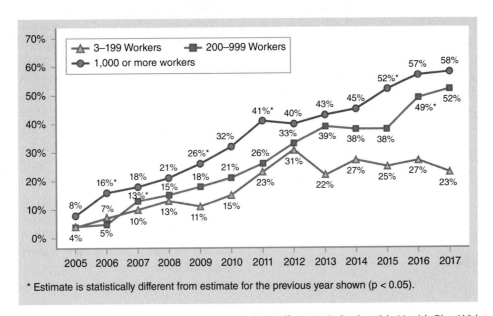

FIGURE 8-2 Among Firms Offering Health Benefits, Percentage That Offer a High-Deductible Health Plan With a Savings Option, 2005–2017

Source: Reproduced from: Kaiser/HRET Survey of Employer-Sponsored Health Benefits, 2017. https://www.kff.org/report-section/ehbs-2017-section-8-high-deductible-health-plans-with-savings-option/

BOX 8-5 Discussion Questions

A literature review of studies relating to consumer behavior with HDHPs found that these plans reduced the use of both appropriate care, such as preventive screenings, and inappropriate care, such as unnecessary emergency department visits (Argwal, Mazurenko, & Menachemi, 2017). To date, research generally has not focused on health outcomes of HDHP users. Some recent studies have shown consumers rarely engaging in price-conscious behavior, instead achieving savings through use of fewer services (Kullgren, Cliff, & Krenz, 2018; Sinaiko, Mehrotra, & Sood, 2016; Sood, Wagner, Huckfeldt, & Haviland, 2013).

Do HDHPs achieve the right balance of providing insurance coverage while incentivizing consumers to use resources prudently? Or are they simply a way to lower employer healthcare costs while making it unaffordable for many consumers to obtain the health care they need? How easy is it for consumers to compare costs for healthcare providers and services? What additional challenges might an HDHP present for individuals who are low-income, live in rural areas, speak a primary language other than English, or have low health literacy?

BOX 8-6 Discussion Questions

In general, people with low incomes or no health insurance (or both) tend to be less healthy than those who are financially better off or insured (or both). As a result, policy proposals that suggest including poor, uninsured individuals in already-existing insurance plans are met with resistance by individuals in those plans and by carriers or employers who operate them. Yet, if an insurance plan is created that subscribes only a less-healthy, poor, or uninsured population, it is likely to be an unattractive business opportunity because beneficiaries are likely to need a high quantity of health care that will be costly to provide. Given what you know about adverse selection and risk, what, in your opinion, is the best way to provide insurance coverage to the poor and uninsured? Should they be included in current plans? Should the government provide financial incentives for private carriers to insure them? Should a separate plan or program be created to serve them? In these various scenarios, what incentives are created for plans, current plan members, government, and so on?

---

wealthier and healthier are likely to have funds to place in a savings account, can afford high out-of-pocket expenses, and are less likely to use the healthcare system (Davis, 2004). As a result, critics contend that the lower service utilization associated with HDHP enrollees is likely due to their better health status, not price sensitivity, undermining one of the main arguments in support of these plans (Davis, 2004). Poorer individuals who may be drawn to the lower premium cost of HDHPs may not be able to afford care when they need it. In fact, a 2018 study found that HDHP enrollees without a savings account were less likely to obtain primary care, preventive services, or specialty care and more likely to be in poor or fair health as compared to enrollees with a savings account (Jetty, Petterson, Rabin, & Liaw, 2018). Finally, if healthier and wealthier individuals flock to HDHPs, poorer individuals in a comprehensive group plan (assuming one is available and affordable), face the possibility of adverse selection due to being part of a relatively high-risk insurance pool (Davis, 2004).

Setting Premiums

Assuming that insurance companies make their decisions in the context of asymmetric information, they cannot determine with certainty the appropriate amount of premium to charge each individual.

Instead, insurance companies rely on making educated guesses about the risk each individual or group of individuals has of needing healthcare services. The two main methods of setting premiums are *experience rating* and *community rating*.

When insurance companies use experience rating to make an educated guess about the risk of someone's needing healthcare services, they are relying on how much a beneficiary or group of beneficiaries spent on medical services previously to determine the amount of the premium for each member or group. Thus, if an individual or group had very high medical costs in a given year, premiums are likely to rise the following year. Conversely, community rating does not take into account health status or claims history when setting premiums. In "pure" community rating, insurers use only geography and family composition to set rates; in "modified" community rating, insurers may be allowed to consider other characteristics, such as age and sex.

Which rating system makes more sense from a policy perspective as a basis for setting premiums may depend on whether you evaluate the insurance market based on efficiency or equity (think back to discussions of competing conceptual frameworks). If the market is judged based on efficiency, then the key issue is whether the optimal amount of risk has shifted from consumers to insurers. If there are individuals willing to pay a higher amount for greater coverage and insurers willing to provide greater coverage for the higher amount, but something in the market prevents this transaction from occurring, then the optimal amount of risk shifting has not occurred. Or, if individuals value a certain level of insurance coverage at a price that is less than the price at which insurers are willing to provide that coverage, but individuals buy coverage anyway at the higher price, the market is not optimally efficient (due to excess coverage).

Conversely, the market may be judged based on equity or fairness. Even the most efficient market may result in some inequities. Some individuals may be uninsured, some may have to pay more than other individuals for the same level of insurance, some may not be able to purchase the level of coverage they desire, and some individuals may not be able to join a particular plan. These inequities are often a concern in the context of the uninsured, especially as uninsurance relates to low-income individuals or those with high health needs due to random events, such as an accident or genetic condition.

Regardless of the underwriting methodology used, premiums are cheaper for people purchasing insurance as part of a large group rather than buying health insurance individually or as part of a small group. Due to the law of averages, larger groups of people are more likely to have an average risk rate. When people join a group for reasons unrelated to health status, such as working for the same company, it is also more likely that the group will have an average risk rate. Groups with average risk rates are attractive to insurers because the cost of insuring a few unhealthy people will probably be offset by savings from insuring many healthy ones. Conversely, in smaller groups it is more likely that the group will have a relatively high risk rate and less likely that the cost of insuring an unhealthy person can be offset by the savings of insuring a few other healthy people. This is the problem faced by William, the small business owner described at the outset of the chapter who has one high-cost employee. Even though he would like to offer health insurance coverage to his employees, William and other small business owners like him often are able to offer only expensive or limited coverage, if they can offer any health insurance benefit at all. To help individuals and small business owners like William, some states require insurers to use a community rating system to set premiums for these groups and in the state health insurance exchanges that were created by the ACA.

Carriers also prefer to insure large groups because most of the administrative costs associated with insurance are the same whether the carrier is covering a few

---

BOX 8-7 Discussion Questions

What populations or types of people pay more under experience rating? Does experience rating create any incentives for individuals to act in a certain way? What populations or types of people pay more under community rating? Does community rating create any incentives for individuals to act in a certain way? Which rating system seems preferable to you? What trade-offs are most important to you? Should the focus be on the good of the individual or the good of the community? Are these mutually exclusive concerns?

---

people or a few thousand (Phelps, 2003, pp. 342–344). In fact, group coverage has traditionally required fewer marketing resources than individual coverage, which targets customers one at a time. However, the proliferation of information on the Internet may change this equation.

Medical Underwriting

The prior discussion about rate setting assumed asymmetric information (i.e., where the insurer has little information about the consumer's health status and the consumer has substantial information about his or her own healthcare needs). Of course, there are ways for insurers to gain information about the medical needs of a consumer looking to join a health plan: physical exams, questionnaires, medical records, occupation, and demographics all provide clues about the health status of the consumer. Although it is much more difficult to accomplish, insurers may also try to predict an individual's future costs through questionnaires that ask, for example, whether an individual engages in risky activities (e.g., riding a motorcycle) or through genetic testing (which is itself an emerging health policy and law issue).

Whether companies are allowed to consider an applicant's medical history or other personal information to help assess risk of healthcare needs in the future—a practice referred to as medical underwriting—is a somewhat complicated legal question that involves both federal and state law. The Health Insurance Portability and Accountability Act of 1996 (HIPAA) includes an important protection for consumers by prohibiting group health plans from excluding or limiting otherwise qualified individuals due to preexisting conditions (a preexisting condition is a medical condition, such as cancer or diabetes, that is present at the time an individual applies to enroll in an insurance plan). The ACA expands this protection by requiring all health insurers to sell policies to all applicants, regardless of preexisting conditions. This requirement was in effect for children shortly after the ACA was signed into law, and took effect for adults in 2014 (as discussed in the Health Reform in the United States chapter, attempts are being made to chip away at this protection).

Prior to HIPAA, many individuals with pre-existing conditions were denied insurance altogether, denied coverage for particular medical care, or charged very high premiums if they sought to purchase a policy. These practices led to a problem referred to as "job lock." Because most Americans receive insurance coverage through their employers, many employees with preexisting conditions could not switch jobs for fear that their new company's insurance policy would be denied to them on account of their preexisting condition. One study estimated that job lock resulted in a 4% reduction in voluntary turnover (Phelps, 2003, p. 341).

Although HIPAA and the ACA do not regulate the amount of premiums that may be charged, all members of a group generally pay the same premium due to the laws' nondiscrimination provisions. In HIPAA, these provisions prohibit plans or insurance carriers from requiring any individual to pay a higher premium or contribution than another "similarly situated" individual (Nondiscrimination in health coverage, 2001, p. 1382) in the plan based on eight health factors: health status, physical or mental medical conditions, claims experience (i.e., the individual has a history of high health claims), receipt of health care, medical history, genetic information, evidence of insurability, and disability (Nondiscrimination in health coverage, 2001, pp. 1378–1384, 1396–1403). However, because those who purchase individual health insurance plans are not covered by HIPAA's protections, the ACA protections were needed as well. The ACA also prohibits plans from charging individuals higher premiums due to their preexisting conditions.

▶ Managed Care

The prior sections reviewed the history, basic structure, and purpose of health insurance generally. In this section, we discuss a specific kind of health insurance structure that has come to dominate the American market: managed care. We will describe why managed care emerged, some of the frequent cost-containment strategies used by managed care organizations, and the most common managed care structures in the market today.

Managed care became the predominant health-care financing and delivery arrangement in the United States because healthcare costs had risen to alarming levels and there were few mechanisms for containing costs under the FFS system. As mentioned earlier, FFS does not create incentives for providers or patients to utilize healthcare services sparingly. Providers have an incentive under FFS to provide more services and more expensive services (but not necessarily higher-quality services) because their income rises with each procedure or office visit and fees are higher for more expensive services. As long as providers are accessible, insured patients can request services and assume their insurance company will pay most or all of the costs to the extent that the services are covered by the health plan and medically necessary.

In addition, the FFS system does not create incentives for providers or patients to use the lowest-cost quality care available. Many people believe specialists provide higher-quality care and turn to them even for minor needs that do not truly require expensive specialty services, and the FFS system does not discourage this behavior. Furthermore, because traditional insurance coverage requires a specific diagnosis for reimbursement, patients are discouraged from seeking preventive services when they are symptom-free under FFS. At the same time, traditional insurance companies do not have the ability to control costs or quality of care under FFS. Their job is limited to determining whether a service is covered and medically necessary and providing the agreed-upon reimbursement. They have little ability to measure or improve the quality of care provided by healthcare professionals and cannot control costs by limiting the amount or type of services received; instead, they can only raise premiums and other rates in the future to cover increasing costs.

To alter the inherent incentives under FFS and to grant insurers some ability to control the quality and utilization of services, managed care integrates the provision of and payment for healthcare services. Through various strategies discussed in the following sections, managed care organizations (MCOs) and managed care plans create incentives to provide fewer services and less expensive care, while still maintaining the appropriate level of healthcare quality. MCOs also attempt to alter patients' decision making through cost-sharing requirements, cost containment tools, utilization restrictions, and free or low-cost coverage for preventive care.

MCOs take various forms, but certain general features apply to all of them to varying degrees. All MCOs provide a comprehensive, defined package of benefits to the purchaser/member for a preset fee (including both monthly premium and cost-sharing requirements). Services are offered to members through a network of providers, all of whom have a contractual relationship with the MCO. The MCOs choose which providers to include in their networks and what services are rendered by network providers. Most notably, they also use financial incentives and other mechanisms to control the delivery, use, quality, and cost of services in ways that are not present in FFS insurance systems (Sultz & Young, 2001, p. 260).

Cost Containment and Utilization Tools

Managed care introduced a variety of tools in its attempt to contain costs and control healthcare service utilization. The cost containment strategies of *performance-based salary bonuses or withholdings*, *discounted fee schedules*, and *capitated payments* shift financial risk or limit payments to providers who, in turn, have an incentive to choose the least costly, but still effective, treatment option. The utilization control strategies of *gatekeeping* and *utilization review* focus on ensuring that only appropriate and necessary care is provided to patients. Another type of strategy, *case management*, is designed to ensure that necessary care is provided in the most coordinated and cost-effective way possible.

Provider Payment Tools

Depending on the structure of the MCO, provider salaries are based on a discounted fee schedule or capitation rate and include incentives to act or not act in certain ways. Providers in what are called staff-model MCOs are employees of the MCO and are paid an annual salary. The salary structure often includes bonuses or salary withholdings that are paid (or withheld) upon meeting (or not meeting) utilization or performance goals, thus shifting some financial risk from the MCO to the provider. A discounted fee schedule is a service-specific fee system, as is used in FFS. However, an MCO-style fee schedule pays lower reimbursement rates than is true in FFS systems; providers agree to accept less than their usual fee in return for the large volume of patients available to them by being a part of the MCO provider network. The MCO retains the financial risk in a discounted fee system, but the costs are lower for the company due to the discounted rate paid to providers. Finally, a capitated payment rate is a fixed monthly sum per member that the MCO uses to determine the provider salary. The capitation rate does not vary regardless of the number or type of services provided to patients. The physician receiving a salary based on a capitated rate is responsible for providing all of the care needed by his or her MCO patients, within the provider's scope of practice. As a result, the financial risk in the case of capitated arrangements is shifted entirely from the MCO to the provider. Depending on the contract between the provider and the MCO, the insurance company may or may not guarantee the provider a minimum number of patients in exchange for accepting a capitated rate. These provider-focused cost containment strategies are summarized in **TABLE 8-1**.

These payment methods lead to very different incentives for providers than is the case under the FFS system. Instead of being paid more for doing more, HMO providers are paid the same amount regardless of the number or type of services they provide. Given the use of bonuses and withholdings,

---

TABLE 8-1 Provider Payment Cost Containment Strategies

Strategy	Provider Payment Method	How Costs Are Controlled	Who Assumes Financial Risk
Salary and bonuses/ withholdings	Provider receives a salary as an employee of an MCO	Incentive for provider to perform fewer and/or less-costly services	MCO and provider
Discounted fee schedule	Provider receives a lower fee than under FFS for each service to members	Pays provider less per service rendered than under FFS	MCO (but also has lower costs)
Capitation	Provider receives a set payment per month for each member regardless of services provided	Incentive for provider to perform fewer and/or less-costly services	Provider

Abbreviations: FFS = fee for service; MCO = managed care organization.

salaried providers may be paid more if they make treatment decisions deemed favorable by an MCO. By using these incentives, MCOs encourage providers to render the fewest and most cost-effective services necessary.

Critics of managed care payment methodologies argue that MCO plan members will not receive all necessary care if providers are incentivized to provide fewer services and less-costly care. Instead of treating patients using both the most cost-efficient and medically necessary services, critics claim MCOs encourage providers to save money by providing fewer services and less specialized care than necessary; MCOs counter that their own incentive is to keep their members healthy so they do not need expensive services in the future. In addition, MCOs point to their ability to impose quality control measures on providers as a way to ensure that patients are properly treated. In response, critics argue that because members switch health plans relatively frequently, MCOs do not have an incentive to keep their members healthy because the MCOs will not realize the long-term savings as members come and go.

Which side has the better argument? There is no definitive answer. On the one hand, studies have found that treatment decisions under MCO arrangements are mostly influenced by clinical factors (not economic ones), that there is little or no measurable difference in the health outcomes of patients in FFS versus managed care plans, and that the quality of care provided under FFS and managed care plans is basically equal (Shi & Singh, 2017, p. 235; Shi & Singh, 2019, p. 382). In fact, patients in areas with a high market share of HMOs are more likely to engage in preventive care, receive diabetes care, and give high provider satisfaction ratings than are patients in areas with low HMO market share (Shi & Singh, 2017, p. 235). Researchers also have not found disparities based on race, ethnicity, and socioeconomic status in MCO versus FFS settings (Shi & Singh, 2017, p. 235; Shi & Singh, 2019, p. 382). While previous studies found that mental health patients did not fare as well in MCOs as in FFS plans, more recent research refutes that conclusion (Shi & Singh, 2019, p. 383).

On the other hand, nonprofit HMOs (a type of MCO) score better on quality measures than do for-profit ones, and HMO enrollees indicate lower patient satisfaction than do non-HMO patients (Shi & Singh, 2017, pp. 235–262; Shi & Singh, 2019, p. 382). Also, due to low reimbursement rates, access is a particular concern for Medicaid MCO enrollees, who appear to have more limited access to certain services, higher emergency department use, and

more unmet prescription drug needs (Shi & Singh, 2019, p. 381).

Utilization Control Tools

MCOs also employ other techniques, not related to provider payment methods, to control use of healthcare services. Once again, the goal in using these tools is to reduce the use of unnecessary and costly services. We review three common utilization control tools: gatekeeping, utilization review, and case management.

Gatekeepers monitor and control the services a patient receives. Members of managed care plans are often required to select a primary care provider from the MCO network upon enrollment. This provider acts as the member's "gatekeeper" and is responsible for providing primary care, referring patients for additional care, and generally coordinating the patient's care. Having a gatekeeper allows the MCO, not the patient or specialty provider, to determine when a patient needs additional or specialty services, diagnostic tests, hospital admissions, and the like. As with the cost containment strategies discussed earlier, there are critics who contend that utilization-based bonuses or salary withholdings give gatekeepers financial incentive not to provide specialty referrals even when it is in the best interest of the patient.

Utilization review (UR) allows an MCO to evaluate the appropriateness of the services provided and to deny payment for unnecessary services. MCO personnel review and approve or deny the services performed or recommended by network providers. UR specialists are often healthcare professionals, and MCOs generally use existing clinical care guidelines to determine whether services are appropriate.

UR may occur prospectively, concurrently, or retrospectively. Prospective UR means that an MCO reviews the appropriateness of treatment before a service is rendered. A request for a recommended service is sent to a UR panel for approval or denial. A denial does not mean a patient cannot move forward with his preferred treatment plan; however, it does mean that the patient will have to pay for the treatment out of his own pocket. Prospective UR is distinguished from concurrent UR, which is when the MCO review of the appropriateness of treatment occurs while treatment is being rendered. For example, a patient may need a procedure that requires hospitalization. Even though the procedure is performed and covered, a UR specialist might still determine the number of days the patient may remain in the hospital or whether certain services, such as home care or physical therapy, will be covered upon discharge from the hospital. Finally, retrospective review means the MCO reviews the appropriateness of treatment (and therefore its coverage) after a service is rendered. In this case, a patient's medical records are reviewed to determine whether the care provided was appropriate and billed accurately; MCOs will not provide reimbursement for services deemed inappropriate or unnecessary. This latter type of review may also be used to uncover provider practice patterns and determine incentive compensation (Shi & Singh, 2019, pp. 373–374). Regardless of when the review occurs, the use of UR is controversial because it may interfere with the patient–provider relationship and allow for second-guessing of provider treatment decisions by a third party who is not part of the diagnosis and treatment discussions.

Case management is a service utilization approach that uses trained personnel to manage and coordinate patient care. Although gatekeeping serves as a basic form of case management for all members, many patients with complex or chronic conditions, such as HIV/AIDS or spinal cord injuries, may benefit from more intensive case management. These patients may have frequent need for care from various specialists and thus benefit from assistance by personnel who are familiar with the many resources available to care for the patient and who are able to provide information and assistance to patients and their families. A case manager works with providers to determine what care is necessary and to help arrange for patients to receive that care in the most appropriate and cost-effective settings (Shi & Singh, 2019, p. 370). Although the general idea of case management is not controversial, some people believe it can be implemented in a manner that acts more as a barrier than an asset to care because additional approval is needed before a patient

receives care and because another layer of bureaucracy is placed between the patient and the provider. **TABLE 8-2** summarizes the three service utilization control strategies just discussed.

As you might imagine, managed care's use of service utilization control mechanisms frequently leads to disputes between patients and their managed care company over whether the company is improperly affecting the provider–patient relationship (and negatively impacting the quality of care provided) by making decisions as to the type or quantity of care a patient should receive. This is both a highly charged health policy issue and a complicated legal issue, and one that is discussed in more detail in a review of individual rights in health care. For purposes of this chapter, it is enough to note that MCOs must have a grievance and appeal process to at least initially handle these sorts of disputes. Although companies' processes differ in their specifics, they generally allow members to appeal a coverage decision, provide evidence to support the appeal, and receive an expedited resolution when medically necessary. The ACA included a number of provisions relating to the appeals process required of insurance plans; these provisions establish a federal standard for state external appeals laws governing products in the individual and group markets and create a new federal appeals process for self-insured plans (the provisions do not affect Medicaid and Medicare, which have their own appeals processes) (National Conference of State Legislatures, 2018). The need for adequate grievance and appeal procedures can be particularly acute for patients with special healthcare needs, such as those with physical or mental disabilities, and patients who otherwise use the healthcare system more frequently than most people.

TABLE 8-2 Service Utilization Control Strategies

Strategy	Description	Potential Concerns
Gatekeeper	Uses a primary care provider to make sure only necessary and appropriate care is provided	Gatekeepers may have financial incentive to approve fewer services or less-costly care
Utilization review	Uses MCO personnel to review and approve or deny services requested by a provider to make sure only necessary and appropriate care is provided	Interferes with patient–provider relationship; someone other than the patient's provider decides whether treatment is appropriate
Case management	Uses MCO personnel to manage and coordinate patient care to make sure care is provided in the most cost-effective manner	May act as a barrier to receiving care if the case manager does not approve a desired service or service provider

Abbreviation: MCO = managed care organization.

Common Managed Care Structures

There are three managed care structures common in the market today: health maintenance organizations (HMOs), preferred provider organizations (PPOs), and point-of-service (POS) plans. All three provide preventive and specialty care, but the rules relating to accessing care differ for each. In general, HMOs have the most restrictive rules pertaining to patients and providers, PPOs have the least restrictive rules, and POS plans fall in the middle.

As shown in **FIGURE 8-3**, PPOs are the most popular type of managed care plan, while very few people are still insured by a conventional FFS plan. In general, the more control an MCO has over its providers and

members, the easier it is to control utilization of services and, therefore, healthcare costs and quality. Conversely, providers and patients prefer to have as much autonomy as possible, so the more restrictive MCO structures may be less desirable in that respect. However, the distinctions among managed care structures have become blurred recently because of the consumer and provider backlash against MCO restrictions.

Health Maintenance Organizations

When managed care first became prominent in the 1970s, HMOs were the most common type of MCO. There are several characteristics shared by all HMOs:

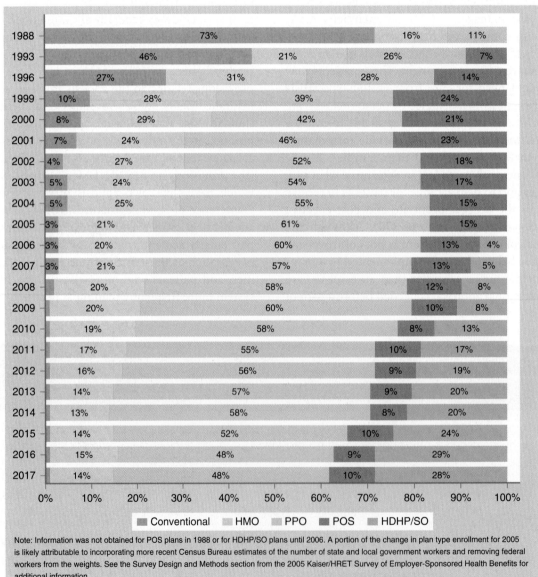

Note: Information was not obtained for POS plans in 1988 or for HDHP/SO plans until 2006. A portion of the change in plan type enrollment for 2005 is likely attributable to incorporating more recent Census Bureau estimates of the number of state and local government workers and removing federal workers from the weights. See the Survey Design and Methods section from the 2005 Kaiser/HRET Survey of Employer-Sponsored Health Benefits for additional information.

FIGURE 8-3 Distribution of Health Plan Enrollment for Covered Workers by Plan Type, 1988–2017

Source: Reproduced from: Kaiser/HRET Employer Health Benefits Survey, 2017. Retrieved from https://www.kff.org/health-costs/report/2017-employer-health-benefits-survey/

- They pay providers a salary to cover the cost of any and all services that beneficiaries need within a provider's scope of practice.
- They negotiate a capitated rate with plan purchasers (e.g., employers) that prices the plan based on a per-member, per-month amount for each type of provider.
- They coordinate and control receipt of services.
- They arrange for care using only their network providers.
- They are responsible for providing care according to established quality standards.

Despite these commonalities, HMOs may be structured through a variety of models, including the staff model/closed-panel model, group model, network model, individual practice association, and direct-contract model (Shi & Singh, 2019, pp. 374–377). Each model has advantages and disadvantages from the perspective of the HMO, its providers, and its members, as shown in **TABLE 8-3**.

Preferred Provider Organizations

As is evident from Table 8-3, every form of HMO is fairly restrictive. In all models, the HMO provides coverage only if members seek care from network providers, and providers may or may not be limited to serving only HMO members. As both patients and providers began rebelling over these restrictions, new

TABLE 8-3 Key Characteristics of Common HMO Models

HMO Model	HMO-Provider Relationship and Payment Type	Provider Employment Arrangement	Must Members Seek Care From Network?	May Providers Care for Nonmembers?	General Comments
Staff model/ closed-panel	HMO employs providers and pays a salary that often includes bonuses or withholdings.	Employed by HMO.	Yes	No	Provides services only in HMO's office and affiliated hospitals. Relatively speaking, HMO has the most control over providers and service utilization, but has fixed costs of building and staff. HMO may contract with outside providers if necessary. Providers and consumers often do not like restrictions imposed by HMO. Providers do not need to solicit patients. Consumers may find it to be the most cost-effective option.
Group	HMO contracts with one multispecialty group for a capitated rate.	Employed by own provider group.	Yes	Depends on terms of contract	HMO has less control over utilization. HMO contracts for hospital care on a prepaid or FFS basis. Providers may prefer this model because they remain independent as opposed to becoming an employee of the HMO and because they may serve nonmembers if their contract permits.

(continues)

TABLE 8-3 Key Characteristics of Common HMO Models *(continued)*

HMO Model	HMO-Provider Relationship and Payment Type	Provider Employment Arrangement	Must Members Seek Care From Network?	May Providers Care for Nonmembers?	General Comments
Network	HMO contracts with several group practices (often primary care practices) for a capitated rate.	Employed by own provider group.	Yes	Depends on terms of contract	The group practices may make referrals but are financially responsible for reimbursing outside providers. HMO has less control over utilization due to greater number of contracts and ability of providers to subcontract. Providers may prefer additional autonomy, but also take on financial risk of providing primary and specialty care. Members may have a relatively greater choice of providers.
IPA	HMO contracts with IPA for a capitated rate.	IPA is intermediary between HMO and solo practitioners and groups. IPA pays providers a capitated rate.	Yes	Depends on terms of contract	HMO has reduced control over providers but may have less malpractice liability because IPA is an intermediary. HMO may contract with specialty physicians as needed and for hospital care on a prepaid or FFS basis. Providers may prefer contracting with IPA instead of HMO to retain more autonomy. Members may have greater choice of providers.
Direct-contract	HMO contracts directly with individual providers for a capitated rate.	Self-employed.	Yes	Depends on terms of contract	HMO has more leverage over providers because it contracts with them as individuals, but its administrative costs are much higher than having one contract or a few contracts with groups. Providers have less leverage regarding practice restrictions when contracting on an individual basis.

Abbreviations: fee for service = FFS; HMO = health maintenance organization; IPA = individual practice association.

BOX 8-8 Discussion Questions

Cost containment strategies embraced by MCOs were a direct result of the FFS experience with ever-increasing utilization and healthcare costs. However, many consumers and providers chafe at the restrictions imposed by MCOs and are concerned that someone other than the provider is making treatment decisions. Are these restrictions appropriate and necessary? Do you favor some of the restrictions over others? Is it appropriate for one entity to be responsible for both paying for and providing care? Should someone other than an MCO—say the federal or state governments—have primary responsibility for making determinations about service utilization?

BOX 8-9 Discussion Questions

In terms of containing healthcare costs and improving healthcare quality, do you think healthcare consumers and professionals need even more restrictions than are currently used in managed care? Are there any reasons to revert back to the FFS system, even knowing its inflationary qualities? If you think that managed care is not the answer to our still-rising healthcare costs and quality concerns, what other tools might help lower costs and improve the quality of care? Should any tools be imposed by government regulation or agreed to voluntarily by insurers and the insured?

forms of MCOs emerged, often formed by providers and hospitals themselves.

Like HMOs, PPOs have a provider network, referred to as preferred providers. Unlike HMOs, however, PPOs provide coverage to patients seeking care from any provider, regardless of whether the provider is part of the member's PPO preferred provider network. However, the amount of the service price that the PPO will cover is greater for an in-network provider than an out-of-network provider. For example, a PPO may agree to cover 80% of the cost for an in-network physician visit, but only 70% of the cost for a similar, but out-of-network, physician visit. PPO patients thus have the option of paying more but choosing among a greater number of providers or paying less but choosing among a more limited number of (in-network) providers. In addition, a PPO member's cost-sharing responsibilities are often higher than is the case for HMO members.

In exchange for being in the network, providers agree to accept a discounted rate for their services, often 25–35% below their usual rates (Shi & Singh, 2019, p. 378). Because PPO members have a financial incentive to seek providers who are in-network, these healthcare professionals find it worthwhile to accept a reduced rate from the PPO in exchange for the higher likelihood that PPO members will select them over non-network providers. Furthermore, unlike the capitation system found in HMOs, PPO providers do not assume financial risk for providing services. Depending on the terms of their contract with the PPO, preferred providers may or may not agree to limit their practice to PPO members. Although it is rare, PPOs may choose to guarantee preferred providers a minimum number of patients.

Even though an MCO has much less control over service utilization in the PPO model than in the HMO

model, PPOs still provide more incentives to use care judiciously than is the case in an FFS system. For example, in-network PPO providers are paid less than their customary rate by the company when they provide care to PPO members and often agree to abide by quality control and UR strategies used by the PPO. In addition, PPO patients have an incentive to use certain providers who will cost them less and have cost-sharing requirements unlike anything found under FFS. The PPO model attempts to locate a middle ground between the very restrictive HMO models and the FFS structure that resulted in very high healthcare utilization and costs.

Point-of-Service Plans

In another effort to contain costs while still providing patients the freedom to choose their provider, POS plans combine features of HMOs and PPOs. Like an HMO, POS plans have a provider network, use a capitated or other payment system that shares financial risk with providers, and require members to use a gatekeeper to help control service utilization. However, designated services may be obtained from out-of-network providers who are paid on an FFS basis, but use of these providers costs the member more money, as with the PPO model. A POS gatekeeper must approve all in-network care and may also have some control over out-of-network care, depending on the terms of the plan. The call by many consumers for increased choice in providers has become forceful enough that some HMOs are now offering POS plans, which they may refer to as open-ended (as opposed to closed-panel) models.

The Future of Managed Care

Managed care is likely to remain an integral part of the health system despite its drawbacks. Patients chafe at utilization restrictions, as is evident by the increase in PPO popularity and the emergence of the hybrid HMO/POS plan. Accurate or not, there is a widespread perception that managed care plans deny necessary care and provide lower-quality care (Shi & Singh, 2017, pp. 218, 235). Providers also complain that managed care interferes with their ability to practice medicine in a manner of their choosing, placing them in ethical dilemmas due to the use of financial incentives and possibly lowering the quality of care they provide due to limits on tests and procedures they order. Yet, the key circumstance that led to the creation of managed care—high healthcare expenditures—has not abated. While the country struggles with ever-growing healthcare costs, even under managed care, the willingness to experiment with various cost and utilization containment strategies is likely to endure.

▶ Conclusion

This introduction to health insurance serves as a building block for additional study, which expands upon many of the key health policy and law themes mentioned here. It should be clear to readers that health policy analysts and decision makers must be particularly attuned to health insurance issues; without knowing both the basic structure of health insurance and how various incentives impact the actions of healthcare consumers, professionals, and insurance carriers, they cannot make informed recommendations and policies addressing the key health issues of the day.

References

Argwal, R., Mazurenko, O., & Menachemi, N. (2017). Health deductible health plans reduce health care costs and utilization, including use of needed preventive services. *Health Affairs, 36*(10), 1762–1768. doi:10.1377/hlthaff.2017.0610

Auter, Z. (2018, January 16). *U.S. uninsured rate steady at 12.2% in fourth quarter of 2017.* Retrieved from https://news.gallup.com/poll/225383/uninsured-rate-steady-fourth-quarter-2017.aspx?g_source=Well-Being&g_medium=newsfeed&g_campaign=tiles

Council of Economic Advisors. (2004). *Economic report of the President.* Washington, DC: U.S. Government Printing Office.

Davis, K. (2004). Consumer-directed health care: Will it improve system performance? *Health Services Research, 39,* 1219–1233.

Health Insurance Portability and Accountability Act of 1996, 42 U.S.C. §§ 18, 26, & 29.

Jacobson, G., Damico, A., & Neuman, T. (2017, June 6). *Medicare Advantage 2017 spotlight: Enrollment market update.* Retrieved from https://www.kff.org/medicare/issue-brief/medicare-advantage-2017-spotlight-enrollment-market-update/

Jetty, A., Petterson, S., Rabin, D. L., & Liaw, W. (2018). Privately insured adults in HDHP with higher deductibles reduce rates of primary care and preventive services. *Translational Behavioral Medicine, 8*(3), 375–385. doi:10.1093/tbm/ibx076

Kaiser Family Foundation. (2017, September 19). *2017 Employer health benefits survey.* Retrieved from https://www.kff.org/health-costs/report/2017-employer-health-benefits-survey/

Kullgren, J. T., Cliff, E. Q., & Krenz, C. (2018). Consumer behaviors among individuals enrolled in high deductible health plans in the United States. *JAMA Internal Medicine, 178*(3), 424–426. doi:10.1001/jamainternmed.2017.6622

National Conference of State Legislatures. (2018). *Right to health insurance appeals process.* Retrieved from http://www.ncsl.org/research/health/right-to-health-insurance-appeals-in-aca.aspx

Nondiscrimination in health coverage in the group market: Interim final rules and proposed rules, 66 Fed. Reg, 1378, 1382 (January, 2001) (codified in 29 C.F.R. pt. 2590.702).

Patient Protection and Affordable Care Act of 2010, Pub. L. No. 111-148 (2010).

Penner, S. (2004). *Introduction to health care economics and financial management: Fundamental concepts with practical application.* Philadelphia, PA: Lippincott, Williams, and Wilkins.

Phelps, C. E. (2003). *Health economics* (3rd ed.). Boston, MA: Addison-Wesley.

Rudowitz, R., & Garfield, R. (2018, April 12). *Ten things to know about Medicaid: Setting the facts straight.* Retrieved from https://www.kff.org/medicaid/issue-brief/10-things-to-know-about-medicaid-setting-the-facts-straight/

Shi, L., & Singh, D. A. (2019). *Delivering health care in America: A systems approach* (7th ed.). Burlington, MA: Jones and Bartlett Learning.

Shi, L., & Singh, D. A. (2017). *Essentials of the U.S. health care system* (4th ed.). Burlington, MA: Jones and Bartlett Learning.

Sinaiko, A. D., Mehrotra, A., & Sood, N. (2016). Cost-sharing obligations, high-deductible health plan growth, and shopping for health care: Enrollees with skin in the game. *JAMA Internal Medicine, 176*(3), 395–397. doi:10.1001/jamainternmed.2015.7554

Sood, N., Wagner, Z., Huckfeldt, P., & Haviland, A. (2013). Price-shopping in consumer-directed health plans. *Forum of Health Economics and Policy, 16*(1), 1–19. doi:10.1515/thep-2012-0028

Starr, P. (1982). *The social transformation of American medicine: The rise of a sovereign profession and the making of a vast industry.* New York, NY: Basic Books, Inc.

Stevens, R., & Stevens, R. (2003). *Welfare medicine in America: A case study of Medicaid.* New Brunswick, NJ: Transaction Publishers.

Sultz, H. A., & Young, K. M. (2001). *Healthcare USA: Understanding its organization and delivery* (3rd ed.). Gaithersburg, MD: Aspen Publishers.

Tax Cut and Jobs Act of 2017, Pub. L. No. 115-97 (2017).

▶ Endnotes

a. Section 106 of the IRS Code of 1954 states that employers who pay a share of premiums for employees' hospital and medical insurance may exclude that amount from the gross income of employees.

b. There are both for-profit and not-for-profit insurance companies. Both types of companies seek to earn enough revenues to cover expenses and the cost of accessing capital. However, for-profit companies return excess revenue to their investors whereas not-for-profit companies put excess revenue back into the company.

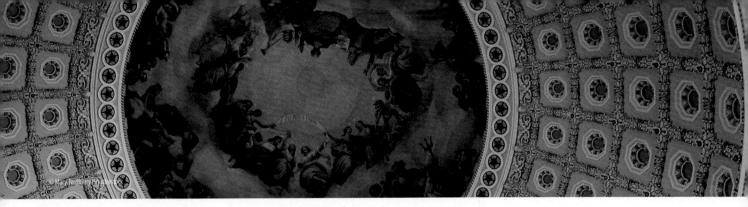

CHAPTER 9

Health Economics in a Health Policy Context

▶ Introduction

There are several disciplines that may be used to assist you in analyzing health policy problems; these include frameworks such as topical domains, historically dominant perspectives, and key stakeholder perspectives, along with political and legal analysis. Furthermore, throughout the text, issues are viewed through a social framework by asking you to consider what policies guide your decision making—in other words, what do you think should happen? This chapter informs you about yet another discipline—economics—that is useful when conducting health policy analysis.

Students just beginning their health policy studies often question why it is necessary to study economics. Most would rather think about and discuss what policies they support and what values should govern decision making, not about competitive markets,

equilibriums, and externalities. What may not be clear initially to students is that economic theory provides one of the fundamental building blocks for making policy choices, both generally and in the context of health care and public health. For instance, economic tools help policymakers predict how consumers and producers will react if they implement certain policies. Knowing this may help policymakers choose the most effective and efficient policy to achieve their goals. The governor's request to Jaia in **BOX 9-1** provides one example of how economic knowledge would prove helpful in health policy decision making. Other examples include the following:

- When federal officials decide which communities should receive grants to support primary care clinics, they need to know if appropriate providers are available to staff clinics. Economic theory can help explain why some providers prefer to locate in urban or suburban Maryland instead of rural

173

West Virginia, why there is a shortage of qualified nurses but an abundance of cardiologists, and how to change this situation and help a rural primary care clinic remain viable.

- In the face of a flu vaccine shortage, the president considers launching an initiative to ensure that every American can be vaccinated against the flu in the case of an epidemic. Economic theory sheds light on why there are so few vaccine producers supplying the United States currently and what could be done to entice manufacturers to participate in the flu vaccine market.

Entire books and courses are devoted to the concept of health economics, and this chapter is not an attempt to distill all the theories and lessons of those texts and courses. Instead, our goal is to introduce you to the basic concepts of health economics, because understanding how economists view health-related problems is one essential component of being a good health policy analyst and decision maker. This chapter

begins with an overview of what health economics is, how economists view health care, and how individuals determine whether obtaining health insurance is a priority in their lives. It then moves to a review of the basic economic principles of supply, demand, and market structure. As part of this discussion, you will learn what factors make supply and demand increase or decrease, how the presence of health insurance affects supply and demand, how different market structures function, and what interventions are available when the market fails to achieve desired policy goals.

▶ Health Economics Defined

Economics is concerned with the allocation of scarce resources, as well as the production, distribution, and consumption of goods and services. Macroeconomics studies these areas on a broad level, such as how they relate to national production or national unemployment levels, while microeconomics studies the distribution and production of resources on a smaller level, including individual decisions to purchase a good or a firm's decision to hire an employee. Microeconomics also considers how smaller economic units, such as firms, combine to form larger units, such as industries or markets (Pindyck & Rubinfeld, 2003, p. 3). Health economics, then, is the study of economics as it relates to the health field.

How Economists View Decision Making

Economists assume that people, given adequate information, are rational decision makers. Rational decision making requires that people have the ability to rank their preferences (whichever preferences are relevant when any sort of decision is being made) and assumes that people will never purposely choose to make themselves worse off. Instead, individuals will make the decision that gives them the most satisfaction, by whatever criteria the individual uses to rate his level of satisfaction. This satisfaction, referred to as *utility* by economists, may be achieved in many ways, including volunteering time or giving money to charities. Utility in a health context takes into account that individuals have different needs for and find different value in obtaining healthcare goods and services, and that whether they purchase health resources—and, if so, which ones they purchase—will depend on the individual's preferences and resources.

Utility Analysis

What does utility mean in terms of health care? Most people do not enjoy going to the doctor or taking medicine. It seems strange to think of individuals as

---

BOX 9-1 Vignette

Jaia is Governor Jara's chief health policy analyst. Governor Jara is interested in improving the health status of residents in the state but is concerned about the impact any new initiative will have on the state's economy. She asks Jaia to compare the economic consequences of three options: tax incentives for individuals to purchase exercise equipment or gym memberships, tax incentives for employers to offer wellness programs, and a mandate requiring that all stores selling food in the state provide fresh food and other healthy options. Fortunately, Jaia has a background in economics and knows that she needs to be concerned with basic principles of supply, demand, and market functions to help her governor make the best choice. This knowledge will lead her to ask questions such as: How big of a tax incentive is necessary to compel individuals or employers to act? Will tax incentives encourage behaviors, such as people joining a gym or employers offering wellness programs, that would not occur otherwise, or will the government simply be subsidizing transactions that would take place anyway? Is the problem that exercise options and healthy foods are not available and affordable, or are individuals simply making the choice not to engage in healthy behavior because they prefer to spend their time and money on other goods and activities? Will a mandate lead to the proliferation of healthy food stores or encourage stores to leave the state? The answers to these questions will help Jaia supply the governor with informed policy recommendations.

being "happy" as a result of, for example, receiving weekly allergy shots or getting chemotherapy treatments. Likewise, it seems odd to think of individuals as undergoing such regimens to "maximize the utility" of the interventions. However, health care can be discussed in terms of utility because most people enjoy being healthy.

Everyone has a different level of health, some due to their status at birth (e.g., infants born prematurely may have problems with their lungs or mental development) and others due to incidents that occur during their lives (e.g., an individual who was in a serious car crash may suffer from back pain). In addition, people have various tolerance levels for being unhealthy. In other words, the willingness to pay for a particular healthcare good or service will vary among individuals based on their circumstances and preferences.

Furthermore, at some point, obtaining additional "units" of a particular good will bring less satisfaction than the previous units did. For example, although icing a sore knee for 20 minutes may reduce swelling, icing the same knee for 40 minutes will not reduce swelling twice as much, or, although buying one pair of glasses may bring high satisfaction, buying two pairs of glasses will not double the consumer's satisfaction, because the second pair of glasses cannot do more than the first. This concept is called *diminishing marginal utility*, and it also affects what goods and services a consumer purchases.

In addition, consumers must consider the *opportunity costs* of their decisions. Opportunity costs refer to the cost associated with the options that are not chosen. For example, if a consumer decides not to purchase any medication to ease his or her back pain, there is zero accounting or monetary cost; that is, it did not cost the consumer any money because he or she did not purchase the medication. However, there may be opportunity costs, monetary or otherwise, because the consumer is not pain-free. The consumer may endure a monetary loss if he or she has to take time off from work due to the injury. Or, the consumer may endure a nonmonetary loss because he or she cannot enjoy walking or exercising due to the back pain. Opportunity costs are the hidden costs associated with every decision, and in order to fully assess the cost and benefits of any decision, these hidden costs must be included in the calculation.

In terms of healthcare goods only, utility can be thought of as a function of individuals' health and the healthcare goods and services they desire. Utility maximization in health care is the ideal set of health-related goods and services that an individual purchases. However, people need to purchase a variety of goods and services, not just those relating to health

care. Overall, consumers maximize their utility by purchasing what they consider to be an ideal bundle of healthcare goods and services, as well as other goods and services, based on their desire for each good and service and subject to the income they have available to make these purchases.

Scarce Resources

In the healthcare arena, consumers have to make choices about the production, distribution, and consumption of healthcare resources. There are many types of healthcare resources. Healthcare goods include items such as eyeglasses, prescription drugs, and hospital beds; healthcare personnel include providers such as physicians, nurses, and midwives, as well as lab technicians, home healthcare workers, and countless others; and healthcare capital inputs (resources used in a production process) include items such as nursing homes, hospitals, and diagnostic equipment (such as an X-ray machine). All of these things (and others) are considered healthcare resources.

If there were unlimited healthcare resources and an unlimited ability to pay for goods and services, the questions confronted by health policy analysts about what healthcare items should be produced and who should have access to them would still exist, but the answers would be less dire because there would be enough health care available for everyone. In reality, however, there is a finite amount of healthcare goods, personnel, and capital inputs. The financial resources are not available to provide all of the health care demanded by the entire population and still provide other goods and services that are demanded. As a result of this scarcity of resources, choices and very apparent trade-offs must be made.

In general, consumer choices are based on individual preference, as discussed earlier, and the concept of efficiency. In economic terms, an efficient distribution of resources occurs when the resource distribution cannot be changed to make someone better off without making someone else worse off. This notion of efficiency in exchange is also referred to as Pareto-efficient, named after the Italian economist Vilfredo Pareto, who developed the concept. There are several types of efficiency, such as *allocative efficiency*, *production efficiency*, and *technical efficiency* (Penner, 2004, pp. 9–10; Santerre & Neun, 2004, p. 5). Allocative efficiency focuses on providing the most value or benefit with goods and services. Production efficiency focuses on reducing the cost of the inputs used to produce goods and services. Technical efficiency focuses on using the least amount of inputs to create goods or services.

The notion of efficiency raises many questions because there are always trade-offs to be made when producing goods and services. For example, should the production be more automated or more labor-intensive? Should the production sites be located in the United States or overseas? Can a service be provided in a less costly setting? Is there any additional or different service or product that will enhance the benefits of the goods or services consumers receive?

Although they may not use this technical economic jargon, public and private policymakers often consider concepts of efficiency when they answer these types of questions. The answers, in turn, help identify which goods and services should be produced overall in society and which of those goods and services should be related to health care. Because there is a finite amount of resources available, the choice to produce more healthcare goods and services would result in the production of fewer non-healthcare goods and services, and vice versa. Similarly, the choice to produce more of one kind of healthcare good or service will lead to the production of fewer healthcare goods and services of other types.

Finally, policymakers must also decide whether equity or fairness concerns should be taken into account, and in response alter their production and distribution decisions in ways that may make some people better off at the expense of others. For example, when a U.S. flu vaccine shortage occurred, some states required that vaccines be given only to individuals in high-risk groups. Individuals who had access to the vaccine, but were not in those high-risk groups, were made worse off by this decision because they were no longer allowed to receive the inoculation. On the other hand, some individuals in the high-risk group who otherwise would not have been able to obtain the vaccine were made better off under the new policy. The point is not that efficiency is more important than equity or vice versa. However, it is important to understand that these are distinct and not always complementary concerns, and whether and how one decides to influence the market will depend, in part, on how much the decision maker values efficiency and equity. In a world of limited resources, balancing consumer preferences, efficiency, and equity concerns can be a very difficult task for policymakers.

How Economists View Health Care

Health economics helps explain how health-related choices are made, what choices should be made, and the ramifications of those choices. Evaluating the consequences of these choices is referred to as *positive* economics. Positive economics identifies, predicts, and evaluates who receives a benefit and who pays for a public policy choice. Positive economics answers the questions, "What is the current situation?" and "What already happened?" *Normative* economics discusses what public policy should be implemented based on the decision maker's values. It answers the question, "What should be?" (Feldstein, 2005, p. 5; Senterre & Neun, 2004, p. 14). For example:

A positive statement: In 2016 approximately 28 million people in the United States did not have health insurance for the entire year.

A normative statement: All people living in the United States should have health insurance.

As shown by the concepts of positive and normative economics, health economists, like other analysts, cannot avoid discussing how health care *should* be perceived. Is health care a good or service like any other good or service such as food, shelter, or clothing that consumers obtain or refrain from obtaining based on availability, price, resources, and preference? Or is health care a special and unique commodity for reasons such as its importance to individuals' quality of life or how the healthcare market is structured? Bear in mind that health policymakers take their own view of health care's place in the market into account when they argue for or against a policy.

The following sections identify two theories of how to view health care. Many economists' views fall somewhere in the middle of these two theories or combine aspects of the two theories to create a hybrid theory. These theories were not presented to be an either/or choice, but to illustrate that even within the field of economics there is a fundamental debate about how to view health care.

▶ Economic Basics: Demand

Consumers, whether an individual, firm, or country, purchase goods and services. *Demand* is the quantity of goods and services that a consumer is willing and able to purchase over a specified time. In the case of health care, for example, demand equals the total demand for healthcare goods and services by all the consumers in a given market.

Demand Changers

In general, as the price of a good or service increases, demand for that good or service will fall. Conversely, as the price of goods or services decreases, demand for those goods or services will rise.

Various factors in addition to price also increase or decrease the demand for a product. Insurance is an important factor relating to demand that is discussed separately later in this chapter. A few of the other factors that may change the demand for a product include the following:

- **Consumer's income:** As a consumer's income increases, demand for a product may increase. For example, a consumer may desire a new pair of eyeglasses but cannot afford it. Once the consumer's income increases, the consumer can purchase the eyeglasses.
- **Quality:** Consumers have preferences based on quality, both actual and perceived. In addition, a change in quality will likely result in a change in demand. A decrease in the quality of a product may result in a decrease in demand because consumers decide the product is no longer worth the price charged. For example, a consumer may discover that the eyeglasses he or she wants fall apart easily, thus may decide not to buy the product.

- **Price of substitutes:** A substitute is a different product that satisfies the same demand. For example, contact lenses may be a substitute for eyeglasses. As the price of contact lenses drops, a consumer may decide he or she prefers contact lenses to eyeglasses.
- **Price of complements:** A complement is a product associated with another product. For example, cleaning solution is a complement to contact lenses. The price and quality of cleaning solution (the complement) may be an important factor when a consumer is debating whether to keep wearing glasses (the original product) or switch to contact lenses (the alternative product). If the price of cleaning solution increases, even though the price of contact lenses stays the same, the consumer may decide to purchase eyeglasses instead of contact lenses. In other words, demand for complements and alternative products shifts in opposite ways, so an increase in the price of a complement will decrease the demand for the alternative product, and vice versa.

BOX 9-2 Discussion Questions

Consider each of the following issues and discuss whether you support Theory X, Theory Y, neither theory, or some combination of them.

Issue	Theory X	Theory Y
Your view about how an individual's health is determined	Whether a person is healthy or sick is determined randomly.	Whether a person is healthy or sick depends on lifestyle choices such as whether a person smokes, drinks, or wears a seatbelt.
Your view of medical practice	Medicine is a science, and experts will ultimately discover the best means for treating every illness.	Medicine is an art and there will never be one best way to treat every illness because illnesses are often patient-specific and because there will always be a demand for lower-cost and less painful treatments.
Your view of medical care	Medical care is a unique commodity.	Medical care is similar to any other good or service.
Your view of the government's role in health care	Government regulations are necessary to protect this unique commodity, to control profiteering at the cost of patient care, to control resources spent on health care, and to improve information sharing.	Government regulations are not necessary, technological advances and more services are desirable, and competition, not regulation, should drive the market.

Source: From Musgrave, GL. Health economics outlook: two theories of health economics. *Bus Econ.* 1995;30:7–13.

The physical profile of a consumer has an impact on demand for healthcare services in some predictable ways. Women generally demand more healthcare services than men do before reaching 65 years of age, primarily due to health needs related to childbearing, whereas men older than 65 years use more care than do women in the same age group. In addition, many diseases are more prevalent in women than in men, resulting in an expected increase in demand for health services by women. Some of these diseases include cardiovascular disease, osteoporosis, and immunologic diseases (Phelps, 2003, pp. 149–150; Senterre & Neun, 2004, p. 111). Regardless of sex, an individual who is born with a medical problem, or who develops one at a relatively young age, can be expected to have a higher than average demand for healthcare services. Aging consumers are more likely to have higher healthcare needs than younger consumers. Of course, any factor that usually leads to increases in demand for healthcare services may be offset by lack of financial resources or lack of access to providers.

In addition to the physical profile of a consumer, interesting research is being conducted in relation to consumers' level of education and their demand for services. Although there is no consensus on the direct impact of general education on demand for health services, some studies show a positive relationship between medical knowledge and demand for healthcare services; that is, the more the consumer knows about medicine, the higher the level of consumption of healthcare services. This association may indicate that consumers without as much medical knowledge underestimate the appropriate amount of health services they need, or it may mean that consumers with more medical education have a greater ability to purchase medical care. Other explanations are possible as well (Agency for Healthcare Research and Quality, n.d.; Cutler & Lleras-Muney, 2006; Senterre & Neun, 2004, p. 127).

Elasticity

Two of the demand changers discussed previously are shifts in price and shifts in income. *Elasticity* is the term used to describe how responsive the change in demand or supply is when there is either a change in price or a change in income. The concept of elasticity is important to understand as a policy analyst because it is essential to know whether changes in consumers' incomes (say, through a tax credit) or changes in the price of a product (perhaps through incentives given to producers) will result in the desired outcome. The desired outcome may be increased consumption,

which might be the case if the service is well-child checkups. Conversely, the desired outcome may be decreased consumption, which might be the case if cigarettes are the product being consumed.

Price Elasticity of Demand

Price elasticity of demand is based on the percentage change in the quantity demanded resulting from a 1% change in price. In other words, does consumer demand for a product, such as a vaccination, increase as the price of a product decreases by 1%, or vice-versa? Elasticity is calculated as follows:

$$\text{Demand elasticity} = \frac{\text{\% change in quantity demanded}}{\text{\% change in price}}$$

(Economists often use the midpoint method which averages the percentage change in quantity and price. This results in the same answer whether there is a price increase or decrease. Price elasticities are always negative because price and demand are inversely related. Even so, elasticities are reported in absolute values, not negative numbers).

Demand for a product is considered elastic if the sum is greater than 1 and inelastic if the sum is less than 1. An elasticity of 0 is perfectly inelastic, meaning the demand does not change in response to a change in price.

For example, suppose a vaccine costs $20 per dose and at that price a family buys four doses, for a total of $80. The next year the price increases 20% to $24 per dose and the family buys only three doses for a total of $72. The mid-point of the two prices is $22 and the mid-point of the two quantities demanded is 3.5. Using the mid-point method, the calculation is as follows

$$\frac{-1/3.5}{2/22} = -3.14 \text{ or } |3.14|$$

Because elasticity equals 3.14, the product is considered elastic (because the result of the elasticity calculation is greater than1). In this example, for every 1% increase in vaccine price, demand decreases by 3.14%. If the price decreases, the quantity demanded would be expected to increase.

Of course, goods may also be inelastic, which means the demand for the good is not as sensitive to a change in price. As a result, when price increases, the quantity demanded will not decrease at the same rate as the price increases. For example, some people will not reduce their consumption of cigarettes even if the price of cigarettes increases. However, at some point the price could become high enough that consumer behavior will change, resulting in a decrease in demand.

Supply elasticity works in much the same way as the price elasticity of demand and uses the same formula, except it refers to the relationship between the quantity of goods supplied and the price of the goods. Supply elasticity is often defined as the percentage change in quantity supplied resulting from a 1% increase in the price of buying the good. The change is usually positive because producers have an incentive to increase output as the price they will receive for the good rises. However, if supply elasticity refers to variables other than the price of the good, such as the cost of raw materials or wages, then the supply elasticity will be negative; that is, as prices of labor or other inputs rise, the quantity supplied will fall (all other things being equal).

Income Elasticity of Demand

Elasticity works in the opposite way in the case of *inferior goods*. An inferior good, as the name suggests, is less desirable than a *normal good*. As a result, as a consumer's income increases, demand for the inferior good will decrease. Instead of buying more of the inferior good, the consumer will prefer to buy the normal good. For example, suppose a generic over-the-counter pain medication is cheaper than a particular prescription pain medication, but the prescription pain medication is more effective. Consumers with low income may choose to purchase the over-the-counter medicine, the inferior good. If their income increases, they will not buy more of the inferior good, but instead will switch to the prescription pain medicine because it is a better good, for their purposes, than the inferior good.

Health Insurance and Demand

In addition to the general economic rules of demand for health services, the presence of health insurance affects demand for healthcare goods and services. Health insurance acts as a buffer between consumers and the cost of healthcare goods and services. In an insured consumer's view, healthcare goods or services cost less because instead of paying full price, the consumer may only have to pay, for example, a co-insurance rate of 20% (after satisfying the deductible). For example, if a surgical procedure normally costs $10,000, the insured consumer may have to pay only $2,000 for the benefit of the surgery because his

or her insurance company pays for the remainder. In this way, the presence of health insurance can have an effect on the consumer—to increase demand—in the same way that an increase in the consumer's income can increase demand.

In general, insured consumers are less sensitive to the cost of healthcare goods and services than uninsured consumers (Penner, 2004, p. 38). Thus, the presence of health insurance creates the problem of *moral hazard*. Moral hazard can occur in a variety of economic situations when consumers buy more goods or services than necessary because they do not have to pay the full cost of acquiring the good or service. In relation to health insurance, moral hazard results when an insured consumer uses more services than he or she would otherwise because part of the cost is covered by insurance.

For example, if a consumer has a $500 health insurance deductible, the consumer pays 100% of the first $500 of health care received. If there is a 20% co-insurance charge after that, the consumer pays only $.20 per dollar for every dollar spent after $500. If the consumer values a particular healthcare service, such as a preventive dental exam, at $50 but the service costs $100, the consumer will not purchase the service before meeting the deductible. However, after the deductible has been met, the dental exam (assuming it is a covered benefit) will cost the consumer $20 (20% of $100), so the consumer will purchase the service because it is under the consumer's $50 value threshold.

As the portion of the healthcare cost that a consumer pays based on co-payments or co-insurance decreases, the consumer becomes less sensitive to changes in the price of the product. Say a consumer decides he or she is unwilling to pay more than $2,500 for surgery. If the consumer owes a 10% co-insurance charge, the consumer will be willing to pay for surgery as long as it is not priced at more than $25,000. At $25,000, the consumer would pay $2,500 and the insurance company would pay $22,500. However, if the same consumer has a 20% co-insurance rate, he or she will not elect surgery once the price rises above $12,500 because the cost to the consumer would be more than the consumer's $2,500 limit; for example, if the surgery costs $15,000, the consumer would owe $3,000 and the insurance company would cover the other $12,000.

The problem of moral hazard is particularly relevant in health care because consumers have an incentive to seek out more medical care: they think it will make them feel better. And, as noted earlier, an insured consumer is more likely to purchase a desirable healthcare good or service because the presence of insurance reduces his or her cost. The same cannot be said of owning a home or auto insurance; although consumers may be a little less careful because of the protection fire or car insurance affords them, it is unlikely that a person will allow an automotive center to replace a working fuel pump on his or her car just because he or she has car insurance.

▶ Economic Basics: Supply

Supply is the amount of goods and services that producers are able and willing to sell at a given price over a given period of time. As with demand, the price of a product is a key factor in determining the level of supply. However, unlike demand, where there is often an inverse relationship between price and demand, an increase in the price a good is sold for usually leads to an increase in quantity supplied. Conversely, as the price consumers will pay for a product decreases, supply will often decrease as well. As with demand, there are many factors that affect the quantity of a good or service being supplied.

Costs

Costs are a key factor in determining the level of supply. Costs refer to what inputs are needed to produce a good or service. For example, the price of cotton may impact the cost of producing medical scrubs or bed linens made out of cotton, or the price of steel may affect the cost of producing an autoclave or X-ray machine made with steel. As the cost of these inputs increases, the cost of producing the final good increases as well. If the price for a good or service does not increase as the cost of inputs increases, the quantity supplied is likely to decrease. Thus, if it costs a manufacturer $100 more to build an X-ray machine because the cost of steel has risen, it is likely that the manufacturer will pass that production cost increase on to the consumer by raising the purchase price of the X-ray machine. Alternately, the manufacturer may choose to absorb the $100 cost increase and not raise the purchase price, which will lead the manufacturer to supply fewer X-ray machines, find a way to produce the good more cheaply using the same method, or find a different way to produce the good.

Costs are counted in many different ways. We focus here on *average costs* and *marginal costs*.

- **Average cost:** The cost of producing one product over a specific period of time. For example, if it costs a manufacturer $2 million to produce 2,000 hospital beds in 1 year, the average cost is $1,000 per bed during that year.

$$\text{Average cost} = \text{Total cost/Quantity}$$
$$= \$2{,}000{,}000/2{,}000 \text{ hospital beds}$$
$$= \$1{,}000 \text{ per hospital bed}$$

- **Marginal cost:** The price of producing one more unit of the output—in our example, one more hospital bed. Whatever additional labor, equipment, and supplies are needed to produce one more hospital bed is the marginal cost of production. As a general matter, the marginal cost increases as output increases.

Supply Changers

Other factors in addition to sale price and cost can increase or decrease the supply of a product. Two common factors are number of sellers and changes in technology:

- **Number of sellers:** As the number of sellers of a good increases, the supply of the good will increase as well because there are more companies producing the good. As long as the market is profitable, new sellers will be enticed to enter the market. This occurs until the market reaches equilibrium, where the quantity demanded equals the quantity supplied.
- **Change in technology:** New technology may mean a new way to produce a desired outcome, which may alter the supply of a good or service. For example, fiberglass has replaced plaster in most casts and the production of each material has shifted accordingly (fiberglass up, plaster down). New technology can also make a product more accessible than before. For example, many surgeries once handled on an inpatient basis may now be performed on an outpatient basis or in a physician's office due to new technology, such as arthroscopy. In addition, evolving technology has led to brand new fields, such as robotic surgery. Technological improvements can increase demand for some services and reduce it for others, leading to a change in the production of these goods and services.

Profit Maximization

Although consumers are driven by the desire to maximize their satisfaction, suppliers are driven by their desire to maximize revenues. For-profit companies seek to make profits to pass on to their shareholders, while not-for-profit companies face a variety of requirements regarding disposing of the revenue they generate in excess of expenses and the cost of acquiring capital to run the company. For ease of explanation, the term *profit* will be used here to discuss supplier incentives, even though the healthcare field includes a large share of not-for-profit companies.

Profit is the price per unit sold less the production cost per unit. In a competitive market, profit is maximized at the level of output where the marginal cost equals the price. If a hospital bed costs $1,000 to produce and is sold for $1,500, the profit per bed is $500. If the marginal cost of producing one more bed is $1,400, the producer will make that additional bed because it can be sold for $1,500, a $100 profit; however, if the marginal cost of producing an additional bed is $1,600, the producer has no incentive to produce that additional bed because it can only be sold at a loss of $100. Due to the profit maximization goal, if the price of a product increases and a competitive market exists for the product, manufacturers will increase production of the product until the output level again reaches the point where the marginal cost equals the price.

When a profitable market exists, new producers will be drawn into the market so they can reap financial benefits. The new producer may price its hospital bed for less than $1,500 to attract consumers, or the new producer may think there is a niche for a higher-priced bed that has additional features. Assume the new producer chooses to market a similar bed as the $1,500 bed but sells it for $1,250. If a consumer can purchase the bed from the competing company for $1,250 with no additional opportunity costs, demand for the $1,500 hospital bed is likely to fall. The manufacturer of the $1,500 bed will have to lower its price or improve the product (or the perception of the product) to increase demand for a higher-priced bed. At the point where there is a balance between the quantity supplied and the quantity demanded and the price is set to the marginal cost of production, there is *equilibrium* in the market.

If such a balance does not occur, there is *disequilibrium* in the market. The disequilibrium could represent a surplus of a good or service due to excess supply or sudden drop in demand, or it could result from a product shortage due to inadequate supply or a sharp increase in demand. Surpluses occur when the market price in a competitive market is higher than the marginal cost of production; as a result, producers lower their prices to increase sales of their product. These price reductions will keep happening until market equilibrium is reached. For example, there could be a sudden drop in demand for a food product due to a news report that eating the product more than three times a week may put people's health at risk. Due to the sudden drop in demand, excess product will be available. Producers will, in turn, lower the price of the product until equilibrium is reached. Shortages occur when the market price is lower than the marginal cost of production. As a result of the shortage, consumers might be willing to pay more for the product, so producers increase their prices until demand stops increasing and market equilibrium is reached. If an opposite news story appeared, hailing the food product as improving health if eaten at least four times a week, there may be a sudden surge in demand. As a result, consumers will likely be willing to pay more for the product and producers will raise the price until equilibrium is reached. Because producers often cannot make significant changes to their production schedule or products in a short amount of time, market equilibrium positions may take some time to achieve.

Health Insurance and Supply

Just as the presence of health insurance affects a consumer's demand for medical goods and services, it also may impact a healthcare provider's willingness to supply goods and services. This is a complicated issue because, on the one hand, a provider is expected to act as the patient's agent and thus should act in the patient's best interests. If providers encourage only appropriate care, insurance is working in a positive way.

On the other hand, providers may have a financial incentive to encourage or discourage the consumption of healthcare goods and services. Providers could recommend against treatment because of financial incentives resulting from the presence or absence of health insurance. For example, financial incentives found in managed care may discourage providers from recommending a particular treatment. Additionally, if a patient is both uninsured and unable to pay for services out-of-pocket, providers have a financial incentive not to provide potentially necessary services due to their inability to receive payment. Similarly, a provider may seek to increase his or her income by encouraging inappropriate or excessive care. This problem—the provider version of moral hazard—is referred to as *supplier-induced demand*. Supplier-induced demand is the level of demand that exists beyond what a well-informed consumer would have chosen. The theory behind supplier-induced demand is that instead of consumer demand leading to an increase in suppliers (healthcare providers), the suppliers create demand in the consumers (patients), often by relying on information only available to the supplier. However, economists debate whether supplier-induced demand actually exists because it is difficult to study empirically and because behavior consistent with supplier-induced demand may also be consistent with appropriate medical treatment (Phelps, 2003, pp. 237–242).

▶ Economic Basics: Markets

To this point, we have reviewed many basic aspects of economic theory—how consumers behave, how suppliers behave, what drives and shifts demand, and what drives and shifts supply. To understand how these theories work in the healthcare industry, it is necessary to explore how health insurance affects markets, what kind of market exists for health care, how market structure relates to the production and distribution of goods and services, and why markets fail and what can be done to alleviate the problems associated with market failure.

Health Insurance and Markets

Before delving into the basics of economic markets, it is necessary to highlight how the presence of health insurance alters the dynamics of a standard economic transaction. In a typical market transaction, such as buying food at the grocery store, there are only two parties involved—the consumer who buys the food and the supplier who sells the food. The cost to the consumer is the cost of the food; the consumer bears full responsibility for paying that cost and pays that cost directly to the supplier, the grocery store.

The typical medical transaction, however, does not follow these rules, both because of the types of events that lead to a medical transaction and because of the presence of health insurance. In health care, there are both routine and expected events (e.g., an annual physical) and unanticipated needs due to an unpredictable illness or injury. The exact diagnosis and treatment are often unknown initially and the patient's response to treatment is not guaranteed, resulting in an inability to predict exactly what resources will be needed. Without knowing what goods and services are required, it is impossible to estimate the cost to be incurred. This makes it very difficult for consumers to weigh their preferences for medical care as compared to other goods and services, and makes it difficult for suppliers to know which goods and services will be demanded and at what price they can sell their goods and services.

Another reason healthcare transactions often do not follow the typical market exchange is because the presence of health insurance means healthcare transactions involve three players, instead of two; these three players are (1) patients (the consumer), (2) healthcare providers (the supplier), and (3) insurers (who are often proxies for employers). Insurers are also known as "third-party payers" because they are the third party involved in addition to the two customary parties. In the public insurance system, the third-party payer is the government, and in the private sector, the third-party payers are private health insurance companies. Having the health insurance carrier as a third party means consumers do not pay the full cost of healthcare resources used and therefore may be less likely to choose the most cost-effective treatment option, to reduce the information gap between themselves and providers, or be as vigilant against supplier-induced demand as they might in other circumstances.

Market Structure

Understanding markets begins with the notion of a *perfectly competitive* market, because in economic theory a perfectly competitive market serves society by efficiently allocating the finite resources available. Due to specific market conditions that make up a perfectly competitive market, a competitive equilibrium is reached once quantities supplied equal the quantities demanded.

There are numerous types of market structures, ranging from perfectly competitive markets with many buyers and sellers to *monopolistic* markets with a single seller controlling the market. Other common market structures include oligopolies, which have a few dominant firms and substantial but not complete barriers to entry, and monopsonies, which have a limited number of consumers who control the price paid to suppliers. Based on the market structure, consumers and producers have varying degrees of power in terms of setting prices, choosing among products, and deciding whether to participate in the market. **TABLE 9-1** reviews the characteristics of three market structures that are most useful to understanding healthcare markets: perfectly competitive markets, monopolistic markets, and monopolistically competitive markets.

You know from the discussion of supply and demand that the healthcare market cannot be perfectly competitive based on the description in Table 9-1. (In fact, no markets are truly perfectly competitive.) Some consumers, such as the federal government, may have extensive market power as well as the ability to set prices. Producers of patent-protected healthcare products are provided with supply power for a limited period of time, which gives them an ability to control

TABLE 9-1 Characteristics of Key Market Structures

	Perfectly Competitive	**Monopoly**	**Monopolistically Competitive**
Number of firms	Many	One (in a pure monopoly)	Many
Market share	No dominant firms	One firm has all market share and price and output.	There may be many firms with market share and or a few dominant firms. Firms can set price because of product differentiation.
Barriers to entry for new firms into market	No	Yes—absolute barriers; no new firms may enter market.	Some barriers, due to differentiation of product, licensure, etc.
Product differentiation	No. Products are for each other.	No. Only one product; no substitutes are available.	Yes. Many products; they are not substitutes for each other (brand loyalty).
Access to information and resources	Consumers and producers have perfect information.	One firm controls all information (asymmetric information).	All firms have equal access to resources and technology unless there are a few dominant firms with more access to resources.
Cost of transaction	Consumers bear cost of consumption, and producers bear cost of production.	Higher price to consumer because firm has ability to reduce quantity, retain excess profits.	Blend of costs in perfectly competitive market and monopoly market.

prices. Consumers do not have perfect information regarding healthcare needs and healthcare costs, and providers and insurers do not have perfect information regarding patient illnesses. Given the presence of health insurance, consumers do not bear all the cost of using healthcare services. With these characteristics, the healthcare market is monopolistically competitive. In many areas of the healthcare market, there are a few dominant firms with a lot of market power and many smaller firms who participate in the market, but the smaller firms do not have the power to shape market conditions.

Market Failure

A *market failure* means resources are not produced or allocated efficiently. As you recall, we defined efficiency generally as the state of least cost production where the resource distribution cannot be changed to make someone better off without making someone else worse off, and we also described a few specific types of efficiency. When something about the structure of the market prohibits it from being efficient, it is referred to as market failure; the question then becomes what interventions in the market, if any, should occur in an attempt to alleviate the market failure.

Before we turn to why markets fail, we must address one additional issue: Does an inequitable distribution of resources constitute a market failure? Under the traditional economic school of thought, the answer is no; a market failure refers to inefficiency, and concerns about equity are not part of the efficiency calculation. However, some economists consider equity a valid factor when evaluating the functioning of a market. Regardless, whether an inequitable distribution of resources fits under the economic designation of "market failure" is not as important as whether policymakers choose to intervene in a market based on equity concerns.

Some of the most salient reasons that market failures occur in health care include concentration of market power, imperfect information (producers or consumer not having complete and accurate information), the consumption of *public goods*, and the presence of *externalities*. We have already discussed concentration of market power and imperfect information; the next sections focus on public goods and externalities.

Public Goods

Public goods have two main features. First, public goods are *nonrival*, meaning that more than one person can enjoy the good simultaneously. An example of a rival private good would be a single pen, as two people may not use the same pen at the same time. Second, a public good is *nonexclusive*, because it is too costly to try to exclude nonpaying individuals from enjoying public goods (Senterre & Neun, 2004, p. 230).

Classic examples of public goods are national defense measures and lighthouses. Everyone simultaneously benefits from national defense, and it is not economically feasible to exclude nonpaying individuals (e.g., tax evaders) from enjoying the benefits. In the same way, multiple ships may benefit at the same time from a warning provided by a lighthouse, and it would be very difficult to exclude a particular ship from enjoying the benefit. In the health field, examples of local public goods include clean water in a free public swimming area or a public health awareness campaign on city streets. Everyone enjoys the clean water (at least until it is overcrowded), and it would be costly to exclude nonpayers. Similarly, multiple people can benefit from a public health campaign simultaneously, and exclusion of nonpayers would be impossible or quite costly.

Public goods can be transformed into other types of goods. For example, a public good could be made exclusive by charging a fee; these are called *toll goods* (Weimer & Vining, 1999, p. 81). The public swimming water could be fenced off and a fee charged for admission, or the public health campaign could be placed in the subway, which would exclude those who could not afford the fare. Once public goods are transformed into toll goods, concerns arise about whether the price is set at the most efficient level. Toll goods may still lead to market failure if the cost of using the good excludes users who would gain more from enjoying the good than they would cost society by consuming the good (Weimer & Vining, 1999, pp. 81–82).

In addition, goods provided by local, state, and federal governments may be, but are not necessarily, public goods in the economic sense. For example, if a state funds a free healthcare clinic, it is not funding a public good. Even though nonpayers are, by definition, included, the benefits generally inure to the individual and, in most cases, more than one individual cannot enjoy the same healthcare good or service. It is possible, however, that other people will benefit from a healthcare service they do not receive; for example, if your neighbor receives a service that helps him quit smoking, you will receive the benefit of no longer being exposed to your neighbor's secondhand smoke.

Public goods also create the *free rider* problem, making it unprofitable for private firms to produce and sell goods due to the high cost of excluding nonpayers (Santerre & Neun, 2004, p. 230). The free rider is one who enjoys the benefit of the good without paying for the cost of producing the good. Because it is impossible to exclude users or force consumers to reveal their true demand for the public good, they do not have incentive to pay for the units of the good they use (Weimer & Vining, 1999, p. 86). For example, an individual cannot be prevented from gaining knowledge from a public health awareness campaign, so if a private company were responsible for providing the education campaign, it could not force a consumer to pay for it. Eventually, even though many people would like to take advantage of clean air or health education, the lack of people paying for it would result in an underproduction of these services unless some action were taken to alter the market dynamics.

Externalities

Externalities are much more common than public goods in the healthcare market. An *externality* is "any valued impact (positive or negative) resulting from any action (whether related to production or consumption) that affects someone who did not fully consent to it through participation in a voluntary exchange" (Weimer & Vining, 1999, p. 94). In a typical economic transaction, the costs and benefits associated with a transaction impact only those involved in the transaction. For example, remember our consumer buying food at the grocery store? The only two people affected by that transaction are the consumer, who pays money and receives food, and the grocer, who provides food and receives money. Situations with externalities, however, are different. Externalities exist when the action of one party impacts another party *who is not part of the transaction*; in other words, the parties to the transaction will find there is an "unpriced by-product" of producing or consuming a good or service (Santerre & Neun, 2004, p. 231).

Externalities may be positive or negative. An example of a positive externality is when one person gets vaccinated against the chicken pox and other people benefit because chicken pox is less likely to be transmitted in that community. If enough people get vaccinated, "herd immunity" will exist in the community.[a]

In this case, the positive unpriced by-product is the additional protection received by others who were not vaccinated. An example of a negative externality is represented by illegal hazardous waste disposal. Say a hospital dumps biologic waste such as blood, syringes, gauze with infected material on it, and the like into a public water source. The unpriced by-product is paid by the general public, who face an increased risk of illness from using the contaminated water source. The costs to the general public may not have been included in the hospital's cost–benefit analysis when it decided to dump the biologic waste.

With both positive and negative externalities, the cost and benefits of production or consumption are borne by individuals who do not participate in the transaction. Due to the unpriced by-products, there are external costs and benefits that are not considered when deciding whether to make the transaction, leading to an under- or overproduction of the resource from society's perspective.

Government Intervention

When market failures occur, the government may intervene to promote efficiency or to promote equity (of course, it may also choose not to intervene at all). Some examples of government interventions include financing or directly providing public goods, creating incentives through tax breaks and subsidies, imposing mandates through regulation, prohibiting activities, and redistributing income. We discuss these options in the following sections.

Government Finances or Directly Provides Public Goods.
When market failure occurs, the government may choose to finance or provide a good or service directly instead of attempting to influence the actions of private producers. For example, if the government wanted to increase access to health care, it could create new government-run health centers or provide financing to privately run health centers.

These are two different paths—direct provision or financing—with different sets of issues. The main difference when the government provides or finances care instead of a private sector is the lack of profit motive on the part of the government (Santerre & Neun, 2004, p. 252). Instead of focusing on the financial bottom line, public providers may focus on other goals, such as equity or assuring the presence of a particular good or service for everyone or for specific populations.

When the government creates or expands a public program, there is concern that *crowd-out* may occur. Whenever a program is established or expanded, the program has a particular goal and targets a particular audience. For example, the government may try to reduce the number of people without insurance by expanding an existing public program such as the Children's Health Insurance Program. Crowd-out occurs when instead of reaching only the target audience (in this case, the uninsured), the public program also creates an incentive for other individuals (in this case, privately insured people) to participate in the public program. Because the program has a finite amount of resources, some of the target audience (the uninsured) may be crowded out from participating in the program by the presence of the other, nontargeted individuals (the privately insured). This unintended development prevents programs from maximizing cost-effectiveness because instead of obtaining the largest change (in this case, the reduction in the number of uninsured) for the public dollar, some of the change is simply a result of a cost shift from a private payer (the privately insured) to a public payer (the expanded program). Crowd-out may also change incentives for other providers of services. In this example, the presence of the new or expanded government program may reduce the incentive for private employers to provide the same good or service (in this case, health insurance).

Government Increases Taxes, Tax Deductions, or Subsidies.
Taxes and subsidies can be used to alter the price, production, or consumption of goods in an effort to fix a market failure. For example, increasing a tax on a good raises the price of that good and discourages consumption; this strategy is often employed to discourage consumption of harmful products, such as cigarettes. Similarly, the government could choose to tax cigarette producers as a way to encourage them to produce less of the harmful product or leave the market altogether.

Conversely, the government could subsidize a good, directly or through a tax deduction, when it wants to encourage the consumption and production of the good. For example, if the government wanted more low-income individuals to purchase healthy foods, it could choose to subsidize their purchase of fruits and vegetables by allowing individuals who use public benefits, such as food stamps, to purchase more fruits and vegetables than would normally be allowed by the face value of the food stamps (for example, $1 in food stamps would allow for the purchase of $2 of fruits or vegetables). Similarly, if the government wanted to encourage vaccine manufacturers to produce more vaccine doses, it could accomplish this goal through direct subsidies to or tax deductions for the manufacturers.

Note that the government has an economic incentive to tax goods that are price inelastic. This incentive exists because the amount purchased declines by a smaller percentage than the price increase. For example, if cigarettes are price inelastic, a 10% cigarette tax increase will result in less than a 10% decrease in cigarette consumption, meaning the cigarette tax will be a good revenue producer for the government because consumers will continue to purchase cigarettes despite the tax. However, taxing price-inelastic goods is less effective as a public health tool for the same reason. If the government desires a 10% reduction in cigarette consumption, the tax must be much higher than 10% if cigarettes are price inelastic. Of course, the government may choose to impose a higher cigarette tax, but it is likely that, for political reasons, a higher tax increase will be harder to obtain than a smaller one.

Government Issues Regulatory Mandates. Regulations may be used to fix a market failure by controlling the price, quantity, or quality of goods and services, or the entry of new firms into the market (Santerre & Neun, 2004, p. 241). For example, healthcare consumers often have imperfect information when making their healthcare decisions. As a result, the government may choose to create a requirement that a type of provider, such as nursing homes, supply information to the public about the quality of care in their facilities to aid in consumers' decision making. The government may also promulgate regulations that restrict entry of new firms into a market and regulate prices because it is cheaper for one or a few firms to produce a high level of output. Of course, government regulations could also be used to achieve a policy goal like reducing carbon emissions by mandating that public transportation systems use alternative fuels that result in lower emissions.

The government could also set a cap on the price of a good and prohibit producers from selling that good above the set price. This will keep the good at a price the government deems socially acceptable. However, if the price is set below the market price, some unfavorable market consequences may occur because it is no longer profitable for the producer to supply the product. Possible consequences include the following:

- Suppliers exiting the market or reducing the quantity of the good supplied, resulting in a shortage
- Suppliers reducing the quality of the good by making cheaper products or providing less care
- Suppliers shifting cost from one product to another
- Suppliers engaging in unethical behavior because some consumers will be willing to pay more than the government price ceiling

Furthermore, regulations aimed at increasing the quality of a good or service will likely impose additional costs on producers of the good. As the cost of inputs rise, the price charged to consumers is likely to rise as well. As a result, some consumers will be priced out of the market for that good or service.

Government Prohibits Goods or Services. Prohibiting the production of goods and services often is ineffective and leads to a "black market" for such products. Because the prohibited goods or services are not available legally, consumers may be tempted to purchase goods or services that are not protected by price or quality controls. This situation may occur with the use of drugs or supplements not approved by the Food and Drug Administration, including unapproved drugs from other countries entering the United States via the Internet or other sources. In addition, because other countries are producing the good or service, the United States may be at a competitive disadvantage. For example, if stem cell research is permitted abroad but not in this country, some scientists may leave the United States to work abroad and domestic companies may not remain competitive in certain fields.

Redistribution of Income

In the case of market failure, the government may also act to redistribute income. Remember, efficient allocation of resources is not the same as equitable allocation of resources. A government may decide that every member of society should obtain a certain minimum level of income or resources or health status. Redistributing income may occur by taxing

BOX 9-3 Discussion Questions

Some people argue that the government should not intervene in the case of a market failure because the government itself is inefficient and will simply create new problems to replace the ones it is trying to fix. In addition, critics contend that the government is usually less efficient than private sectors. Do you think the government is less efficient than the private sector? Does it depend on the issue involved? If you think it is inefficient in a particular area, does that lead you to recommend against government intervention, or is there a reason that you would still support government intervention? If you think the government should intervene, which intervention options do you prefer and why?

the wealthier members of society and using the revenue to provide resources to poorer members of society. If the government sought to create more market equity through voluntary donations, it is likely that a free rider problem would exist because some citizens would volunteer to contribute resources while others would not, but the latter would still receive a benefit from the redistribution. For example, wealthier citizens who should be in the "donor group" but do not contribute may benefit from the donations given by other wealthy citizens that lead to increased productivity and welfare of those in the recipient group. Both the notion of income redistribution and the decisions as to who should be providing versus receiving resources is open to debate. In addition, it is important to remember that income redistribution may reduce efficiency or have other undesirable market effects.

References

Agency for Healthcare Research and Quality. (n.d.). *Population health: Behavioral and social science insights.* Retrieved from https://www.ahrq.gov/professionals/education/curriculum -tools/population-health/zimmerman.html

Cutler, D., & Lleras-Muney, A. (2006). *Education and health: Evaluating theories and evidence* (National Bureau of Economic Research Working Paper 12352). Retrieved from http://www .nber.org/papers/w12352.pdf

Feldstein, P. (2005). *Health care economics* (6th ed.). Clifton Park, NY: Thomas Delmar Learning.

Gordis, L. (2000). *Epidemiology* (2nd ed., p. 19). Philadelphia, PA: WB Saunders.

Penner, S. J. (2004). *Introduction to health care economics and financial management: Fundamental concepts with practical applications.* Philadelphia, PA: Lippincott, Williams, & Wilkins.

Phelps, C. E. (2003). *Health economics* (3rd ed.). Boston, MA: Addison-Wesley.

Pindyck, R. S., & Rubinfeld, D. L. (2003). *Microeconomics* (5th ed.). Upper Saddle River, NJ: Prentice Hall.

Senterre, R. E., & Neun, S. P. (2004). *Health economics: Theories, insights, and industry studies* (3rd ed.). Mason, OH: Thomas South-Western.

Weimer, D., & Vining, A. (1999). *Policy analysis: Concepts and practice* (3rd ed.). Upper Saddle River, NJ: Prentice-Hall.

▶ Conclusion

This introduction to economic concepts illustrates why health policy analysts and decision makers must understand how economists analyze healthcare problems. We have taken a broad look at the issues of supply, demand, and market structure with a focus on concerns that are relevant in the health policy field. In particular, it is essential to understand how health insurance affects both consumer and producer decisions. Although we only scratched the surface of healthcare economics in this chapter, you should now realize that without an understanding of the economic ramifications of a policy decision, a health policy analyst cannot know, for example, whether to recommend addressing a problem through a government-run program, subsidy, or the like, or if it would be better to let the free market set the production level and price of a resource.

▶ Endnotes

a. *Herd immunity* is "the resistance of a group to an attack by a disease to which a large proportion of the members of the group are immune" (Gordis, 2000). Once a certain portion of the group is immune, there is only a small chance that an infected person will find a susceptible person to whom the disease may be transmitted.

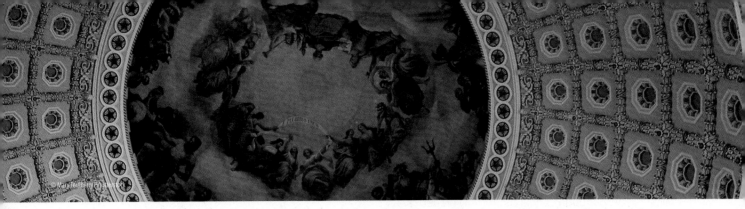

CHAPTER 10

Health Reform in the United States

LEARNING OBJECTIVES

By the end of this chapter you will be able to:

- Describe previous national health reform attempts
- Understand why national health reform has been difficult to achieve in the United States
- Analyze why national health reform succeeded in 2010 when so many previous attempts had failed
- Understand the key components of the Patient Protection and Affordable Care Act
- Understand the core rulings of multiple U.S. Supreme Court decisions related to the Affordable Care Act
- Evaluate the political climate regarding repealing and replacing the Affordable Care Act, and understand the main features of legislation drafted toward that end
- Describe key issues going forward related to implementation of the Affordable Care Act

▶ Introduction

The Patient Protection and Affordable Care Act of 2010 (generally referred to as the Affordable Care Act, or ACA) is the most monumental piece of U.S. federal health policymaking in nearly 50 years. It reorders not only many aspects of the health insurance and healthcare delivery systems but also longstanding relationships that underpin those systems. Yet beyond the sheer scope and content of the ACA and the policy trade-offs that led to its passage lies another story: its implementation and subsequent effect on the lives of tens of millions of Americans. Implementation of the ACA is an ongoing, dynamic process for the federal government, states, employers, insurers, providers, patients, and others. In addition,

there have been and, no doubt, will continue to be state and federal court decisions across the country that alter the trajectory of the law and its implementation.

The vignette in **BOX 10-1** describes just a few of the competing viewpoints about the ACA and its role in creating a new and potentially more equitable health insurance system. As ACA implementation moves forward, bear in mind the many different ways that this round of health reform can be perceived and how it affects people differently.

Furthermore, the future of the ACA was made even more uncertain by the monumental election cycle in 2016. Unexpectedly, Donald Trump was elected president in November of that year, and the Republicans maintained control of both the U.S. House of Representatives and the Senate. Having control of

A group of friends were talking about the ACA, illustrating the wide-ranging viewpoints about the law. Katherine, whose friend Sophia is struggling to make a living as an artist, is pleased that Sophia has health insurance for the first time since graduating from college. Although Sophia cannot stay on her parents' insurance because she just turned 27 years old, she can now afford a good health insurance plan that she found on her state's health exchange. While Katherine has not noticed much of a change in her own health insurance coverage, which she obtains through her government employer, her cousin Mia is upset about health reform. She does not want the government forcing her to purchase health insurance (although she always chose to be insured in the past), and she recently found out that her old plan was cancelled because it did not meet the law's requirements. Mia found several new plan options to choose from, but none had her former plan's exact combination of benefits, providers, and price. In addition, Katherine's uncle, Ethan, is 55 years old and self-employed. He purchases his health insurance on his state's exchange and because he has preexisting conditions, he is grateful to be able to find a plan. Even so, Ethan's premiums will increase by 15% this year and his deductible is $5,000, making health care difficult to afford even with insurance. Katherine's husband, Calvin, thinks we should all be willing to pay a little more or change some aspects of our plans to help the millions of people who can now afford insurance for the first time as a result of the ACA. After witnessing her uncle's experience, however, Katherine is doubtful that the government will be able to keep its promises.

Congress and the White House gives Republicans a chance to fulfill a promise they have campaigned on for years—to repeal and replace the ACA. Even if they are not successful in passing a repeal and replacement bill, President Trump can use his executive powers to rewrite existing regulations and implement new policies. Indeed, he has already started to do so, as will be discussed in this chapter.

The interplay between legal and political decisions makes it difficult to discern how implementation of the law will be carried out, assuming it is not repealed entirely. By way of example, the U.S. Supreme Court's landmark 2012 decision upholding the constitutionality of the ACA and 2015 decision upholding subsidies provided through the ACA to the federal insurance exchange are described in the pages that follow, and there are currently dozens of lawsuits challenging the ACA's coverage mandate related to contraceptive and other family planning services. The practical consequences and legal rulings that actually manifest as a result of ACA implementation—not just the changes to American health care contemplated by Congress when they put pen to paper with the ACA—will, for years to come, need to be studied and understood by students across a range of disciplines, not just for academic purposes, but for healthcare and public health job market purposes as well.

Although there has been general agreement about the problems facing the U.S. healthcare system—high costs, high uninsured rates, health disparities, quality concerns—politicians and voters have disagreed about the best solutions. As a result, numerous attempts to pass national health reform legislation did not succeed. What was different in 2010? Why was the Obama administration successful when several previous attempts had failed? This chapter begins with a discussion of why it has been so difficult to achieve broad health reform in this country and then examines the numerous failed attempts at national health reform over the last century. It then analyzes how health reform was enacted in 2010, provides an overview of the law that eventually emerged, and covers the U.S. Supreme Court decision upholding its constitutionality. Finally, the discussion turns to the current political climate and what it means for health reform going forward, including a discussion of key political and implementation issues. Throughout this chapter we examine several key themes: choosing between state flexibility and national uniformity; determining the appropriate role for government, the private sector, and the healthcare financing and delivery entities; defining a primary decision-making goal (e.g., fiscal restraint, equity/social justice, improved health outcomes, uniformity); and settling on the appropriate scope of coverage to offer beneficiaries.

▶ Difficulty Achieving Health Reform in the United States

The array of problems facing the healthcare system has led to numerous health reform proposals and implemented policies. The concept of health reform can have several different meanings. Given the patchwork health insurance system, health reform often refers to changes that seek to reduce the number of uninsured. Due to the high and increasing cost of healthcare services, health reform might also include changes that seek to contain costs and control utilization. The notion of health reform could also address other shortcomings, such as trying to reduce medical errors, strengthening patient rights, building the public health infrastructure, and confronting the rising cost of medical malpractice insurance. Unsurprisingly, the ACA touches on many of these issues.

We begin with a discussion about why health reform is difficult to achieve in the United States and then introduce some of the reforms that have been attempted, with varying degrees of success, on a national level. Numerous authors have addressed the main factors that deter significant social reform in this country, including health reform (Blake & Adolino, 2001; Gordon, 2003; Jost, 2004). Factors that are prominently discussed include the country's culture, the nature of U.S. political institutions, the power of interest groups, and path dependency (i.e., the notion that people are generally opposed to change).

Culture

This country's culture and lack of consensus about health reform have impeded attempts to create universal coverage health plans. The twin concepts of entrepreneurialism and individualism have had a real impact on health policy decisions: Americans generally oppose government solutions to social welfare problems (Jost, 2004, p. 238). In addition, there is no agreement about the overall scope of the healthcare problems we face (Kaiser Family Foundation [KFF], 2008). Prior to the passage of the ACA, most Americans believed the extant health system needed major changes, yet 22% believed only minor changes were required and another 17% thought the system should basically stay the same (KFF, 2009b).

Americans have a complicated and partisan view of the proper role of the federal government in the healthcare arena. On one hand, 60% of respondents to a 2017 survey felt that the federal government has a responsibility to ensure healthcare coverage for all Americans (Kiley, 2017). This is much higher than the 47% who shared that view in 2010, at the height of the health reform debate (Newport, 2010). Of those who supported federal intervention in the 2017 survey, 33% reported they would like to see a single-payer system developed (Kiley, 2017).

At the same time, there was a stark difference of opinion based on the respondents' political views. While 85% of Democrats and Democrat-leaning independents believed the federal government was responsible for ensuring healthcare coverage, only 32% of Republicans and Republican-leaning independents agreed (Kiley, 2017). Even so, over half (57%) of Republican/Republican-leaners supported the continuation of Medicaid and Medicare, the country's largest public health insurance programs. Furthermore, only

5% of respondents thought the federal government should not have any role in ensuring healthcare coverage (Kiley, 2017).

It is accepted political dogma that it is difficult to take away benefits once they are established, and this has proven to be true with healthcare coverage (Steinhauer, 2017). The popularity of the ACA has increased since the Republicans gained power in the 2016 elections and the threat of repealing the ACA became a realistic possibility. A June 2017 Kaiser Tracking poll showed the ACA's favorability ratings above 50% for the first time since the poll began in 2010 (KFF, 2017b), and a separate poll taken a couple months later showed 64% of respondents preferred to either keep the ACA as it is or make fixes to it that would shore up problems and weaknesses (Kahn & Erman, 2017). Furthermore, the public is clearly opposed to the proposed Republican replacement plans. A majority of respondents opposed both the House (56% opposed) (Magness, 2017) and Senate (55% opposed) (Wynn, 2017) bills. Even though many Republicans also opposed the replacement options (only 21% have a very favorable view) (KFF, 2017b), most Republicans (about 75%) would still like to see the ACA repealed and replaced at some point (Kahn & Erman, 2017).

U.S. Political System

The country's system of government also has made it difficult to achieve universal coverage. Traditionally, social welfare programs—including the provision of health care—have been the responsibility of the states. Initially, there was almost no federal involvement in the provision of health care, and when the federal government became more heavily involved in 1965, Medicaid continued to keep the locus of decision making at the state level. Of course, there are select populations, such as older adults (Medicare) and veterans (Veterans Health Administration), who have a federalized health insurance system. However, support for federal involvement in health care depends on what language is used to describe the change. For example, "single-payer" or "socialized" health care was backed by less than half of the public in a 2017 poll, while "universal health coverage" and "Medicare-for-all" was supported by over 60% (KFF, 2017c).

Although states are generally home to social welfare changes, it is difficult to provide universal health care on a state-by-state basis. If state health reform efforts lead the way, the country could have a patchwork of programs and policies that vary from state to state, with the potential to make health coverage even more complex and inefficient than it is currently.

In addition, states must consider whether they are making policy decisions that will give employers an incentive to choose to locate in another state with fewer or less onerous legal requirements. If employers leave the state, it could result in loss of jobs and have downstream effects on the state's economy.

The federal government also has resource advantages over states, making it easier for the federal level to be the engine for health reform. Individual states have a much smaller tax and revenue base than the federal government to draw from to implement health reform plans. In addition, once the federal government decides to tax a good or service, a state's ability to tax that same good or service is constrained by the individual's willingness and ability to pay a higher price. Unlike the federal government, most states have some type of balanced budget requirement (Garrett, 2011). While state legislatures may use accounting gimmicks and other maneuvers to avoid balanced budget requirements, states more often must make difficult choices about resource allocation that federal policymakers often avoid (and thus generate enormous deficits). These restrictions, however, also may help with reform efforts by forcing states to a crisis point where a decision must be made to avoid an untenable situation. The federal government rarely reaches such a crisis point, which means tough decisions are often left for the next Congress, executive branch administration, or generation.

State reform efforts are also constrained by the Employee Retirement Income Security Act of 1974 (ERISA). ERISA is a federal law that regulates "welfare benefit programs," including health plans, operated by private employers. ERISA limits ability of states to reform because it broadly preempts state laws that "relate to" employer-sponsored plans and because it applies to nearly all individuals who receive health benefits through a private employer. One effect of the law, for example, is that states have little regulatory control over the benefits covered in employer-sponsored health plans, because ERISA accords employers near-total discretion over the design of their benefit packages (Weissert & Weissert, 2002, p. 237).

Despite these hurdles, it is also important to recognize that a health reform strategy focusing on states has benefits as well. At its best, reform at the state level can be accomplished more rapidly and with more innovation than at the federal level. State legislatures may have an easier time convincing a narrower band of constituents important to the state than Congress has in accommodating the varied needs of stakeholders nationwide. Along the same lines, states are able to target reforms to meet the particular needs of their population, instead of covering more diverse needs across the entire country. Additionally, through the use of "direct democracy" (e.g., referenda, ballot initiatives), it is easier for citizens to have an impact on decisions by state-level policymakers than by federal legislators. Finally, because the healthcare delivery system is run primarily on the state level, states have the expertise and ability to implement many parts of healthcare reform.

Other aspects of the U.S. political system also make it difficult to institute sweeping reform. For example, although presidents have significant influence on setting policy agenda and proposing budgets, they have limited power to make changes without the assistance of Congress. The federal government is often politically divided, with different parties holding power in the executive and legislative branches. This division often results in partisanship and policy inaction due to different policy priorities and views.

Furthermore, although members of Congress may ride the coattails of a popular president from their own party, they are not reliant on the president to keep their jobs. The issues and views their constituents care about most may not align with the president's priorities. In those cases, members of Congress have a strong incentive to adhere to the wishes of those who vote for them, instead of simply following the president's lead. Barring an overwhelming wave of discontent, as occurred in the 2010 midterm elections when Democrats suffered historic losses in Congress, it is usually difficult to unseat incumbents. Even when there is a historic level of turnover, reelection rates remain very high. For example, 97% of House incumbents successfully defended their seats in 2016; even in the Senate, where turnover is relatively more common, 93% of incumbents won reelection in 2016 (Kondick & Skelley, 2016). As a result, legislators in Congress may have confidence in focusing on their district's or state's needs before those of the entire nation.

Federal legislative rules also support inaction or incremental reform over sweeping changes. In the Senate, 60 (of 100) votes are needed to break a filibuster in most cases. Thus, even the political party in the majority can have difficulty effecting change. One exception to the filibuster rule is the "reconciliation" process, which allows bills to pass with only 51 votes. Reconciliation is used as part of the budgetary process, and bills passed via reconciliation may not be filibustered (so can pass with 51 votes), can pertain only to federal revenue and spending issues, must comply with spending and revenue targets set forth in the budget resolution, and must adhere to other budgetary rules (Tax Policy Center, n.d.). The reconciliation process is being increasingly used when one party maintains a slim majority and that party cannot find 60 votes to pass a bill. For example, the Democrats used a reconciliation bill to pass the ACA in 2010 after they lost their filibuster-proof majority, and likewise, the Republicans attempted to use a reconciliation bill to pass their ACA repeal-and-replace bills. Also, because both the House and the Senate have to pass bills containing the same policies and language to have any chance at becoming law, a large political majority in one chamber or the other does not guarantee the ability to enact a policy. As a result, in many cases members of Congress have to work together, at least to some degree, to devise a consensus policy that satisfies enough members to pass a bill. This need to build consensus makes radical change unlikely.

Interest Groups

Interest groups often influence the decisions of politicians. The role of interest groups is to represent their members' interests in policy decisions. These groups can be corporate for-profit entities or nonprofit consumer-oriented organizations. They lobby politicians and the general public about the virtues or vices of specific proposals, work to improve proposals on the policy agenda, and attempt to defeat proposals they believe are not in the best interest of their group. By contributing to political campaigns or by helping to draw supportive voters out on Election Day, interest groups gain the ear, and often the influence, of politicians who vote on issues that are important to the group.

In terms of health reform, interest groups representing various providers, businesses, employer groups, insurance companies, and managed care organizations often have been opposed to comprehensive health reform (Jost, 2004, pp. 438–439). There are numerous points along the path—from developing a policy idea to voting for or against a bill—when interest groups can attempt to affect politicians' views. The more radical the policy proposal, the more interest groups are likely to become engaged in the political decision-making process, making it difficult to pass a bill that includes comprehensive reform.

In general, it is easier to oppose a proposal than to develop one and pass a bill. Opponents of proposals are not required to provide a better alternative to whatever is on the table. Instead, they can simply point to aspects of the policy idea that are unpopular and call for the proposal to be rejected. This was the tactic used by the Health Insurance Association of America in their well-known "Harry and Louise" television ads that opposed the Clinton administration's comprehensive health reform bill in 1993, the Health Security Act. In the ad, Harry and Louise, two "average" Americans, are seen discussing the healthcare system over breakfast. Although they both agree the system needs to be improved, they highlight certain aspects of the Clinton plan that were particularly controversial, such as an overall cap on funds for healthcare needs and restrictions on provider choice. The tag line for the ad was, "There's got to be a better way" (West, Heith, & Goodwin, 1996). Similarly, before the 2016 elections, many Republicans promised to "repeal and replace" the health reform bill without specifying their favored replacement option. To be effective in opposing health reform, opponents did not have to propose an alternative that was scrutinized and compared with the existing proposal. Simply saying "the country can do better" was enough to help create significant opposition to the plan.

Path Dependency

Finally, the concept of path dependency has been a hindrance to major health reform. "The notion of path dependency emphasizes the power of inertia within political institutions" (Jost, 2004, p. 439). That is, once a certain way of doing things becomes the norm, it is hard to change course. Yet this theory does not mean that health reform is impossible. Inertia may be overcome at "critical moments or junctures" that open a window for change (Jost, 2004, p. 439). For example, the passage of Medicaid and Medicare in 1965 was a radical change from the past pattern of limited federal government involvement in health care. The catalysts for this change were the growing social pressure for improving the healthcare system and the landslide victory of Democrat Lyndon Johnson as president and of liberal and moderate Democrats in Congress.

The 1992 election of Democrat Bill Clinton, who ran on a platform emphasizing broad health reform, coupled with the Democratic majority in Congress (until 1994), also presented a window of opportunity. Although Clinton's plan was not ultimately successful, it appeared that the American public and politicians were open to changing the course of the healthcare "path" that had been taken to date. In 2010 another "critical moment" appeared, and President Obama took advantage of the circumstances to push through the health reform bill. Although path dependency suggests that inertia and fear of change have made broad reform difficult, it is not impossible to achieve.

Path dependency is also evident on the individual level; that is, once individuals are accustomed to having things a certain way, it is difficult for them to accept change. In 2010, prior to the passage of the ACA, about 84% of Americans had health insurance, most through employer-sponsored coverage (U.S. Census Bureau [Census], 2010). It was assumed that comprehensive health reform would likely change the condition of the insured population to some degree by changing either their source of coverage, the benefits included in coverage, the cost of coverage, or some other factor. During the debate over the ACA, about one-third of people surveyed reported that the bill would probably make them worse off, and another third thought it would not make any difference to them (KFF, 2008). Professor Judith Feder refers to this problem as the "crowd-out" politics of health reform: "The fundamental barrier to universal coverage is that our success in insuring most of the nation's population has 'crowded out' our political capacity to insure the rest" (Feder, 2004, p. 461). In other words, many of the insured do not want a change in the healthcare system that will leave them worse off to make the uninsured better off.

According to Professor Feder, the way to solve the political crowd-out dilemma is by changing the very nature of American culture. The focus on individualism must be replaced with a concern for the community and recognition that all Americans are part of a single community. "The challenge to improving or achieving universal coverage is to decide whether we are a society in which it is every man, woman or child for him/herself or one in which we are all in it together" (Feder, 2004, p. 464). Clearly, the country remains divided about the extent to which "we are all in it together." Shortly before the ACA passed, over half of people surveyed (54%) said they would not be willing to pay more so others could have access to health insurance (KFF, 2009a). The continued debate over the future of the ACA has highlighted fundamental disagreements about how our health system should be structured and the proper role of individuals and governments in ensuring the country's good health.

▶ Unsuccessful Attempts to Pass National Health Insurance Reform

Since the early 1900s, when medical knowledge became advanced enough to make health care and health insurance desirable commodities, there have been periodic attempts to implement universal coverage through national health reform. The Socialist Party was the first U.S. political party to support health insurance in 1904, but the main engine behind early efforts for national reform was the American Association for Labor Legislation (AALL), a "social progressive" group that hoped to reform capitalism, not overthrow it (Starr, 1982, p. 243). In 1912, Progressive Party candidate Theodore Roosevelt supported a social insurance platform modeled on the European social insurance tradition that included health insurance, workers' compensation, old-age pensions, and unemployment insurance. After his loss to Woodrow Wilson, the national health insurance movement was without a strong national leader for three decades.

The AALL continued to support a form of health insurance after Roosevelt's defeat and drafted a model bill in 1915. This bill followed the European model, limiting participation to working class employees and their dependents. Benefits included medical aid, sick pay, maternity benefits, and a death benefit. These costs were to be financed by employers, employees, and the state. The AALL believed that health insurance for the working population would reduce poverty and increase society's productivity and well-being through healthier workers and citizens.

Opposition to AALL's bill came from several sources (Starr, 1982, pp. 247–249). Although some members of the American Medical Association (AMA) approved of the bill conceptually, physician support rapidly evaporated when details emerged about aspects of the plan that would negatively impact their income and autonomy. The American Federation of Labor (a labor union) opposed compulsory health insurance because it wanted workers to rely on their own economic strength, not the state, to obtain better wages and benefits. In addition, the federation was concerned that it would lose power if the government, not the union, secured benefits for workers. Employers were generally opposed to the bill, contending that supporting public health was a better way to ensure productivity. In addition, they feared that providing health insurance to employees might promote malingering instead of reducing lost workdays. After experiencing the high cost associated with workers' compensation, employers also were not eager to take on an additional expensive benefit. Of course, the part of the insurance industry that had already established a profitable niche in the death benefit business was strongly opposed to a bill that included a death benefit provision. Employers, healthcare providers, and insurers have, in general, remained staunch opponents of national health reform over the years, whereas unions have supported national reform efforts. However, this dynamic has changed recently with more provider groups, employers, and even some insurers calling for a national solution to the problems of rising healthcare costs and the uninsured.

The country's entry into World War I in 1917 also changed the health reform debate. Many physicians who supported the AALL bill entered the military, shifting their focus away from the domestic health policy debate. Anti-German sentiment was high, so opponents of the bill gained traction by denouncing compulsory health insurance as anti-American. One pamphlet read as follows: "What is Compulsory Social Health Insurance? It is a dangerous device, invented in Germany, announced by the German Emperor from the throne the same year he started plotting and preparing to conquer the world" (Starr, 1982, p. 253).

The next time national health insurance might have taken hold was from the mid-1930s through the early 1940s as the country was coping with the difficulties of the Great Depression. During this time there was a significant increase in government programs, including the creation of Social Security in 1935, which provided old-age assistance, unemployment compensation, and public assistance. Yet the fourth prong of the social insurance package, health insurance, remained elusive. President Franklin Roosevelt heeded his staff's advice to leave health insurance out of Social Security because of the strong opposition it would create (Starr, 1982, p. 267). Opposition from the AMA was particularly strong. The AMA believed that "socialized medicine" would increase bureaucracy, limit physician freedom, and interfere with the doctor–patient relationship.

Even so, members of Roosevelt's administration continued to push for national health insurance. The Interdepartmental Committee to Coordinate Health and Welfare Activities was created in 1935 and took on the task of studying the nation's healthcare needs. This job fell to its Technical Committee on Medical Care. Instead of supporting a federal program, the committee proposed subsidies to the states for operating health programs. Components of the proposal included expanding maternal and child health and public health programs under Social Security, expanding hospital construction, increasing aid for medical care for the indigent, studying a general medical care program, and creating a compensation program for those who lost wages due to disability.

Although President Roosevelt established a National Health Conference to discuss the recommendation, he never fully supported the medical care committee's proposal. With the success of conservatives in the 1938 election and the administration's concerns about fighting the powerful physician and state medical society lobbies, national health reform did not have a place on Roosevelt's priority list. Senator Robert Wagner (D-NY) introduced a bill that followed the committee's recommendations in 1939, and although it passed in the Senate, it did not garner support from the president or from the House.

World War II provided another opportunity for the opposition to label national health insurance as socialized medicine. But once the war neared an end, President Roosevelt finally called for an "economic bill of rights" that included medical care. President Truman picked up where Roosevelt left off, strongly advocating for national health insurance. President Truman's proposal included expanding hospitals, increasing public health and maternal and child health services, providing federal aid for medical research and education, and, for the first time, a single health insurance program for all (Starr, 1982, p. 281). Heeding lessons from earlier reform failures, Truman emphasized that his plan was not socialized medicine and that the delivery system for medical and hospital care would not change.

Again, there was strong opposition to the proposal. The AMA vehemently rejected the proposal, and most other healthcare groups opposed it as well. Although the public initially approved of it, there was no consensus about how national health insurance should be structured, and more people preferred modest voluntary plans over a national, compulsory, comprehensive health insurance program (Starr, 1982, p. 282). Additional opposition came from the American Bar Association, the Chamber of Commerce, and even some federal agencies concerned about losing control over their existing programs. In the end, only the hospital construction portion of the proposal was enacted.

When Truman won reelection on a national health insurance platform in 1948, it appeared the tide had turned. However, the AMA continued its strong opposition and its attempts to link national health insurance to socialism. Congress considered various compromises but never reached a consensus. The public remained uncertain about what kind of plan to favor. Employers maintained their opposition to compulsory insurance. In addition, one large group of potential supporters—veterans—was disinterested in the debate because they had already secured extensive medical coverage through the Veterans Administration. As the Korean War moved forward, Truman's focus shifted away from national health insurance and toward the war effort and other priorities.

National health insurance did not return to the national policy agenda until the 1970s. The landscape then was quite different from Truman's era. Medicaid and Medicare had been created, healthcare costs had begun to rise exponentially, and the economy was deteriorating. In 1969, President Nixon declared that a "massive crisis" existed in health care and that unless it was fixed immediately, the country's medical system would collapse (Starr, 1982, p. 381). The general public seemed to agree, with 75% of respondents in one survey concurring that the healthcare system was in crisis (Starr, 1982, p. 381). Democrats still controlled Congress by a significant margin, and Senator Edward Kennedy (D-MA) and Representative Martha Griffiths (D-MI), the first woman to serve on the powerful House Committee on Ways and Means, proposed a comprehensive, federally operated health insurance system.

At the same time, a movement supporting health care and patient rights was gaining momentum. This movement included rights to informed consent, to refuse treatment, to due process for involuntary commitment, and to equal access to health care (Starr, 1982, p. 389). The public was both anxious to obtain care and willing to challenge the authority of healthcare providers.

The Nixon administration's first attempt at health reform focused on changing the healthcare system's financing from one dominated by a fee-for-service system, which created incentives to provide more and more expensive services, to one that promoted restraint, efficiency, and the health of the patient. The result was a "health maintenance strategy" intended to stimulate the private industry to create health maintenance organizations (HMOs) through federal planning grants and loan guarantees, with the goal of enrolling 90% of the population in an HMO by the end of the 1970s (Starr, 1982, pp. 395–396). Ironically, group health plans, often labeled socialized medicine, had become the centerpiece of a Republican reform strategy.

Nixon's proposal included an employer mandate to provide a minimum package of benefits under a National Health Insurance Standards Act, a federally administered Family Health Insurance Program for low-income families that had a less generous benefit package than the one required by the National Health Insurance Standards Act, reductions in Medicare spending to help defray the costs, a call for an increase in the supply of physicians, and a change in how medical schools were subsidized. Opponents were plentiful, and this plan did not come to fruition. Some believed the plan was a gift to private insurance companies. Advocates for the poor were outraged at the second tier of benefits for low-income families. The AMA was concerned about HMOs interfering with physician practices and supported an alternative that provided tax credits for buying private insurance.

After the 1972 election, Nixon proposed a second plan that covered everyone and offered more comprehensive coverage. Private insurance companies would cover the employed and a government-run program would cover the rest of the population, with both groups receiving the same benefit package. Senator Kennedy and Representative Wilbur Mills (D-AR) supported a similar plan, and it appeared a compromise was close at hand. However, labor unions and liberal organizations preferred the original Kennedy plan and resisted compromising with the hope of gaining power in the 1974 post-Watergate elections. Fearing the same political shift, insurance companies actually supported a catastrophic insurance plan proposed by Senator Russell Long (D-LA), believing it was better than any plan that would come out of a more liberal Congress after the elections. Once again, there was no majority support for any of the bills, and a national health insurance plan was not enacted.

Although President Jimmy Carter gave lip service to national health reform, he never fully supported a proposal. It was not until the election of Bill Clinton in 1992 that the next real attempt at national health insurance was made. The Clinton administration plan, dubbed the Health Security Act, was designed to create national health insurance without spending new federal funds or shifting coverage from private to public insurance. It relied on the concept of "managed competition," which combined elements of managed care and market competition.

Under the Health Security Act, a National Health Board would have established national and regional spending limits and regulated premium increases. "Health alliances" would have included a variety of plans that were competing for the business of employees and unemployed citizens in each geographic area. All plans were to have a guaranteed scope of benefits and uniform cost-sharing. Employers would have been required to provide coverage for their workers at a defined high level of benefits, and those with 5,000 employees or fewer would have had to purchase plans through the health alliance. Subsidies were provided for low-income individuals and small businesses. Funding was to be provided from cost-containment measures that were reinvested. Forced by the Congressional Budget Office to provide an alternative funding strategy should the cost containment not create enough funds, the plan also included the option of capping insurance premium growth and reducing provider payments.

Like the national health insurance plans before it, the Health Security Act had opponents from many directions. The health alliances were attacked as big government, employers resisted mandates and interference with their fringe benefits, some advocates feared that cost containment would lead to care rationing, the insured were concerned about losing some of their existing benefits or cost-sharing arrangements, older adults feared losing Medicare, and academic health centers were concerned about losing funds based on new graduate medical education provisions (Starr, 1982, p. 463). In addition, the usually strong support from unions was missing because of an earlier disagreement with the president on trade matters. It is also generally accepted that the Clinton administration made several political mistakes that made a difficult political chore nearly impossible. The Health Security Act never made it to a vote.

▶ The Stars Align (Barely): How the ACA Became Law

In many ways, 2010 was a very unlikely year to pass a national health reform plan. The country had been growing increasingly ideological, with the popular and electoral votes almost evenly split in both the 2000 and 2004 presidential elections. George W. Bush beat Al Gore despite losing the popular vote in 2000, and Bush beat John Kerry in 2004 with only 51% of the popular vote. Even though Barack Obama won the electoral vote in a landslide over John McCain (365 to 173), only 53% of the population voted for Obama in 2008 (National Archives and Records Administration, n.d.).

In addition to the ideological divide, a financial crisis erupted toward the end of the 2008 presidential election. In October 2008, President Bush signed into law the Emergency Economic Stabilization Act, which included the $700 billion Troubled Asset Relief Program (TARP) that allowed the federal government to take over distressed assets, primarily bad mortgage loans, from private financial institutions (Emergency Economic Stabilization Act of 2008). It was argued that TARP was necessary to save the financial industry from collapsing, which could have led to another Great Depression. Even with TARP, the United States (and many other countries) entered into a recessionary period. Many individuals lived in homes they could no longer afford, banks limited lending opportunities, and employers laid off millions of workers due to the drop in consumer spending. In an effort to improve

the economy, Obama signed into law the American Recovery and Reinvestment Act of 2009, also known as the stimulus bill. This almost $800 billion effort was intended to save existing jobs, create new jobs, and spur long-term growth of the U.S. economy. Although TARP was not popular with politicians or the general public, it was seen as necessary by members of both political parties and signed into law by a Republican president. Unlike TARP, however, the stimulus bill was not a bipartisan effort. Republicans in the House unanimously opposed the stimulus bill, and only three Republicans voted for the bill in the Senate.

Not surprisingly, health care was not the only issue on voters' minds during the election campaign. Shortly before the election, 43% of registered voters ranked the economy as their number one priority. Economic concerns trumped health care, which ranked second, by an almost two-to-one margin (Jones, 2010). Although voters from both political parties ranked the economy as their top priority, differences emerged along party lines regarding the next most important issue. Democratic voters ranked health care second, whereas both Republican and Independent voters were more concerned about the size and power of the federal government. These results were not surprising; Democrats have ranked health care as a higher priority than Republican and Independent voters in every presidential election from 1988 to 2012 (Blendon et al., 2008, p. 2053; Jones, 2010).

It was against this backdrop of a faltering economy, partisan differences, and the recent passage of two massive government spending bills that President Obama pursued a national health reform plan. Given the history of failed reform efforts, it would have been an accomplishment to pass health reform in the best of times, and clearly this was not the best of times. How did Obama and the 111th Congress succeed? It was a combination of having commitment, exhibiting leadership, applying lessons from past failures, and being pragmatic that led to the passage of health reform.

Commitment and Leadership

It is highly unlikely that the 2010 health reform effort would have succeeded without a passionate and committed president willing to make health reform a priority. Health care has long been a priority for Democrats, and President Obama was no exception. Perhaps Obama's dedication to passing health reform stemmed in part from his personal experience: Obama's mother died of ovarian cancer, and he had seen her worry about paying her medical bills as much as beating the disease (Kornreich, 2007). Thus, for

Obama, signing comprehensive health reform legislation into law would represent the opportunity to make sure others would not endure the same experience.

Some of Obama's political advisors suggested waiting to tackle health reform until after taking action to address the poor economy and rising unemployment. Even voters who supported Obama were split over what his priorities should be during his first days in office (Appleby, 2008). Just days before the election, Obama suggested that the economy and energy independence were higher priorities than health reform. To Obama, that meant he should tackle several majors issues at once, not put health reform on the back burner.

Health reform efforts did not begin smoothly. President Obama initially wanted former U.S. senator Tom Daschle to run both the Department of Health and Human Services (HHS) and the White House Office on Health Reform. It was thought that his experience in the Senate and relationships with legislators were the right combination to take the lead on health reform. When his nomination was derailed due to personal tax problems, it was not a good omen. As deliberations in Congress lagged, Democrats were not able to present a bill to President Obama before recessing for the summer. During the summer of 2009, members of Congress went home to their constituents and held town hall meetings to discuss health reform. Some of the meetings erupted in vocal opposition to health reform, and the media focused on these town hall meetings throughout the summer. Obama and the Democrats were criticized for losing the momentum for reform by letting the debate linger.

At the same time, there were several instances when the health reform effort appeared politically doomed, and President Obama's leadership made a clear difference. Obama attempted to reclaim the upper hand on health reform with a speech to a joint session of Congress in September 2009. He memorably proclaimed, "I am not the first president to take up health reform, but I intend to be the last" (White House, 2009b). Although public support for health reform had been on the decline for several months, September 2009 polls showed that 62% still thought it was important to address health reform at that time, and 53% thought the country as a whole would be better off if health reform passed (KFF, 2009c). Less support existed for the Democrats' specific reform proposal, however, with 46% in support of the proposed change and 48% opposed to it (Cohen & Balz, 2009).

In January 2010, an event occurred that some assumed was the death knell of health reform. In the 2008 elections, Democrats had made significant gains in Congress, earning a 59–41 majority in the Senate and a 257–178 majority in the House. Furthermore, Senator Arlen Specter of Pennsylvania switched parties, giving Democrats the crucial 60th vote needed for a filibuster-proof majority. Although the numbers were now in their favor, President Obama, Senate Majority Leader Harry Reid (D-NV), and House Speaker Nancy Pelosi (D-CA) would have to balance the competing interests of conservative Democrats who were concerned with having too much government intervention, progressive Democrats who sought a public insurance option to compete with private companies, Blue Dog Democrats who were most concerned with fiscal discipline, and pro-life and pro-choice factions who would battle over whether and how abortion services would be included in any health reform bill.

Then, in August 2009, Senator Ted Kennedy (D-MA) died. In office for 47 years, Kennedy was not only a lifelong supporter of health reform but also an expert negotiator who could work with Republicans and possibly achieve a bipartisan consensus. The January 2010 special election to fill his seat was won by Republican Scott Brown, who campaigned against the Democrats' health reform plan. In a postelection poll, 42% of voters said they voted for Brown to stop health reform from moving ahead (Condon, 2010).

Despite this setback and concerns by some that health reform efforts should be abandoned, Obama, along with Reid and Pelosi, remained strong in his conviction to pursue reform. President Obama's senior advisors said it would be a "terrible mistake" to walk away from the process based on Brown's victory, and Pelosi reminded her caucus how detrimental it was when Democrats abandoned the health reform effort during the Clinton administration (Brown & O'Connor, 2010). In his State of the Union address just a week after Senator Brown claimed the special election, President Obama tied his health reform efforts to fixing the economy and reiterated his commitment to the issue:

> And it is precisely to relieve the burden on middle class families that we still need health reform. Now let's be clear, I did not choose to tackle this issue to get some legislative victory under my belt. And by now it should be fairly obvious that I didn't take on health reform because it was good politics.... Here is what I ask of Congress though: Do not walk away from reform. Not now. Not when we are so close. Let us find a way to come together and finish the job for the American people. (White House, 2010)

Obama was not alone in providing leadership on health reform. Reid's and Pelosi's determination to see health reform succeed, and their skill in mobilizing and controlling their caucuses, were essential to the passage of the ACA. It is likely that health reform would not have passed without the skillful efforts of all three leaders working together. Even so, it is clear that the health reform effort would not even have begun without a president who put health reform at the top of the agenda and stuck with it despite the pitfalls and political opposition.

Lessons From Failed Health Reform Efforts

The Obama administration tried to avoid events that doomed earlier health reform efforts. Although the failed effort by the Clinton administration probably provided the most relevant lessons, Obama confronted some of the same obstacles that reformers had faced decades earlier. At times, President Obama was accused of learning some of the lessons too well, swinging the pendulum too far to the other side. Although that debate may continue, clearly the way in which the Obama administration applied those lessons brought him success where others had failed before him.

President Clinton was criticized for not moving quickly enough to try to enact health reform after he was elected in 1992. He did not present a plan to Congress until a year into his presidency, having been sidetracked by other issues such as the economy, including a budget showdown with Republicans, and whether gays should be allowed to serve in the military. Even after he finally sent his healthcare proposal to Congress, Clinton was preoccupied with other issues that sapped his political capital, such as passing the North American Free Trade Agreement and the fallout from the deaths of 18 American soldiers in Somalia.

President Obama, over the objection of some aides, chose to address health reform as quickly as possible, despite also having to tackle the poor economy and possible collapse of the financial sector. Obama was elected into office with a 70% approval rating, and he moved to capitalize on his popularity (Saad, 2008). It was almost inevitable that his approval rating would decline as he tried to turn the promise of a campaign into the reality of running the country. As Lyndon Johnson said after winning the 1964 election in a landslide, "Every day while I'm in office, I'm gonna lose votes" (Blumenthal & Morone, 2009, p. 172). In addition, it is almost universally expected that the president's party will lose seats in the midterm elections due to both lower voter turnout that gives more clout to partisan voters and a loss of popularity as the president moves from candidate to elected official (Wihbey, 2014). Obama was correct to assume his Democratic majorities in Congress would not last long. After the 2010 midterm elections, the Democrats lost control of the House and several seats in the Senate.

President Obama also dealt with interest groups in a different way from his predecessors. Previous failed efforts at health reform have shown that those vested interests can be important players in the debate. In general, though not in all instances, provider groups, insurers, and employers have opposed health reform, whereas unions have supported health reform efforts. All of these stakeholders have been known to devote significant resources and apply pressure on their representatives to support their point of view. During its reform effort, the Clinton administration warred with many stakeholder groups, with insurance companies and small businesses taking a leading role (West & Heith, 1996).

Obama took a different approach than Clinton by making deals with various stakeholders at the outset of the health reform debate. The lure of millions of newly insured customers helped convince the Pharmaceutical Research and Manufacturers of America and the American Hospital Association to contribute to health reform financing through reduced Medicare and Medicaid payments. In addition, the health insurance industry supported universal insurance coverage under health reform. After being credited with helping derail the Clinton health plan, the Health Insurance Association of America favored the general idea of health reform, though it differed with Obama and the Democrats on some of the specifics. To be fair, Clinton may not have been able to broker deals with these stakeholders in the 1990s no matter how hard he tried. A combination of a changing healthcare environment, the likelihood that some type of health reform was likely to pass, and the uncertain future of employer-sponsored insurance made it more palatable for interest groups to try to influence instead of oppose the 2010 legislation (Oberlander, 2010).

Clinton was also criticized for failing to master the legislative process. The Clinton administration chose to design the health reform plan itself and developed a complicated and secretive process, headlined by the Health Care Task Force run by Hillary Clinton, to do so. Although naming Hillary Clinton as the leader of the task force signaled the administration's commitment to the issue, she became a lightning rod for criticism, and questions about the appropriateness of the First Lady taking on such a significant policy role detracted from the substance of the health reform debate.

Instead of negotiating with Congress, the administration debated the specifics of health reform among its own advisors and then asked Congress to pass the bill they had developed. Shutting out members of Congress instead of negotiating with them and taking over Congress's role in developing legislation was not, it turned out, a formula for success.

President Obama learned from Clinton's mistakes as well as from other presidents' legislative achievements. Instead of presenting a detailed plan or written legislation to Congress, success has often been found in outlining ideas and principles and letting Congress work through the details. When President Johnson was trying to get a Medicare bill passed, he told key members of Congress that he would not delve into the details of the bill but generally pushed for a larger package. When President George W. Bush was pursuing a new Medicare prescription drug benefit, he outlined his desire for an approach that worked with the private sector and encouraged competition, but let Congress find the exact formula that would pass (Morone, 2010, p. 1097).

Similarly, Obama set out his principles but left the work of drafting a bill and fleshing out the details to Congress. On June 2, 2009, President Obama sent a letter to Senators Kennedy and Baucus, two leaders in the health reform effort, outlining his "core belief" that Americans deserved better and more affordable health insurance choices and that a health reform bill must not add to the federal deficit (White House, 2009a). Although he let the negotiators know what his priorities were, Obama stayed above the fray during the legislative process. Whereas he preferred a public option to compete with private insurers, he did not insist on it. Although Obama campaigned against an individual mandate as a presidential candidate, he was open to including it in the bill. The president refused to be drawn into the debate over taxing generous health plans or creating a Medicare cost-containment commission. Instead, he focused his efforts on persuading Congress not to give up on the effort, bringing together various factions of the Democratic caucus, and reaching out to the public to garner support for health reform.

The legislative process for completing the bill was long, rocky, and ultimately partisan. The House of Representatives moved more quickly and with less fractious debate than the Senate. Instead of having multiple House committees work on competing bills, as occurred during the Clinton administration, House Democratic leaders created a "Tri-Committee" bill jointly sponsored by Charles Rangel (D-NY), Henry Waxman (D-CA), and George Miller (D-CA), the

chairmen of the House Ways and Means, Energy and Commerce, and Education and Labor (later renamed the Education and Workforce committee) committees, respectively. On November 7, 2009, the House passed its health reform bill with only two votes to spare, 220–215 (Affordable Health Care for America Act, 2009). Only one Republican voted for it, and 39 conservative Democrats voted against it. The bill from the then-more-liberal House contained several provisions that were likely to be rejected by the Senate: a public health insurance option to compete with private plans, a national health insurance exchange instead of state-based exchanges, more generous subsidies for low-income individuals, a broader expansion of Medicaid, and higher taxes on wealthier Americans.

Finance Committee Chairman Max Baucus (D-MT) led the effort in the Senate. The legislative process he established was lengthy, and some observers believed he compromised on too many issues in an attempt to forge a bipartisan bill. For a time Senator Charles Grassley (R-IA) actively participated in the health reform deliberations, and a few other Republican senators appeared willing to consider a bipartisan measure. Ultimately, however, a bipartisan agreement could not be reached. In a 2009 Christmas Eve vote, the Baucus bill passed 60–39, with all Democrats and two Independents voting for the measure and all Republicans voting against it (ACA, 2010).

Shortly after the New Year, members of the House and Senate began meeting to resolve differences between the bills passed in the House and the Senate. Before those differences were resolved, however, Scott Brown was elected to fill Kennedy's seat in the Senate and the Democrats no longer had a filibuster-proof majority. Before the special election that led to Brown's victory, it was assumed that after the Senate passed a health reform measure, House and Senate negotiators would work out their differences in a conference committee, with each chamber then voting to pass the compromise bill. With Brown's election and his opposition to health reform, however, this plan became unworkable. Democratic congressional leaders were left with few options, all of them unpalatable: the House could pass the Senate version of the bill; Democrats could try to use the reconciliation process—which does not allow for the use of filibusters and requires only a simple majority vote—to pass a new comprehensive bill; the House and Senate could compromise on a much smaller, more incremental health reform bill that focused on areas where a bipartisan agreement could be reached; or Democrats could abandon their efforts to pass a health reform bill. The day after Brown's election, House Speaker Pelosi appeared to eliminate the easiest (legislatively speaking) of these paths by declaring that the House would not pass the Senate version of the bill: "I don't think it's possible to pass the Senate bill in the House. I don't see the votes for it at this time" (Murray & Kane, 2010).

In the end, a compromise was reached. House and Senate leaders agreed to use the budget reconciliation process to amend the Senate bill. The House then passed the Senate version of the bill along with a companion reconciliation bill that amended certain aspects of the Senate bill. The reconciliation bill included more generous subsidies for individuals to purchase insurance than existed in the stand-alone Senate bill, the closure of the Medicare Part D doughnut hole, a tax on more generous insurance plans, changes to the penalties on individuals who would not buy insurance and for employers that would not offer insurance, and an increase in Medicare and investment taxes for higher earners. The Senate then passed the reconciliation bill. Once again, the final vote to approve the bills was along party lines. The House approved the Senate bill by a vote of 219–212, with all Republicans and 34 Democrats voting against it (Khan, 2010). President Obama signed the bill into law on March 23, 2010 (ACA, 2010).

Some observers argue that Obama may have overlearned the lesson about working with Congress and that in doing so he did not provide enough guidance to legislators and allowed the debate over health reform to linger for too long (Morone, 2010, p. 1097). On the one hand, it is difficult to criticize Obama's approach because he was ultimately successful. On the other hand, could the problems stemming from the 2009 town halls and Scott Brown's election have been avoided, and would public opinion of the health reform effort be higher, if the process had been better managed? Only time will tell whether Obama was successful over the long term (e.g., Is the law effective? Will the public support it over time? Will it be repealed?) and whether the political cost of the lengthy battle hurt the Democrats more than passing the bill helped them.

Political Pragmatism

President Obama is both credited and criticized for being as pragmatic as necessary to help ensure that a health reform law came to fruition. He was comfortable making deals with industry stakeholders even though those agreements limited the savings and other changes that could have been achieved in the health reform bill. Obama ultimately signed a bill that did not include a public option, even though he preferred that

one be included, and his liberal base thought health reform without such an option was not true reform. An argument over abortion nearly derailed the bill in its final days, and Obama supported a compromise on abortion language to keep enough Democrats in the fold. Even his goal of creating universal insurance coverage was not recognized. Yet Obama's willingness to be pragmatic instead of staunchly principled, taking some victories instead of an all-or-nothing approach, allowed him to succeed in passing a health reform bill where others had failed (Oberlander, 2010, p. 1116). Some people argued it was worse to pass a flawed bill than not pass a bill at all, but Obama believed the promise of reducing the uninsured rate and gaining numerous health insurance market reforms were worth the compromises he made.

▶ Overview of the ACA

As noted earlier, while President Obama left the details of health reform legislation to Congress, he set forth what he believed to be the most important principles that should guide the legislation's development. Soon after becoming president in 2009, Obama delineated those principles, saying that any health reform measure should do the following:

1. Protect families' financial health (slowing the growth of out-of-pocket expenses and protecting people from bankruptcy due to catastrophic illness)
2. Make health insurance coverage more affordable (reducing administrative costs, wiping out unnecessary tests and services, limiting insurers' ability to charge higher premiums for certain populations)
3. Aim for insurance coverage universality
4. Provide portability of insurance coverage
5. Guarantee choice of health plans and providers (including keeping current ones)
6. Invest in disease prevention and wellness initiatives
7. Improve patient safety and healthcare quality
8. Maintain long-term fiscal sustainability (reducing cost growth, improving productivity, adding new revenue sources)

The extent to which these principles were brought to life in what eventually became the ACA lives along a spectrum. For example, health insurance was absolutely made more affordable for millions of people; disease prevention and wellness initiatives seem to be gaining momentum, though slowly; and universal insurance coverage was absolutely not achieved. Whatever the case with any particular principle, it is instructive to look to four key reforms that became law under the ACA as having paved the way for President Obama's overall vision to come to fruition. These four reforms essentially reordered long-standing relationships among health system stakeholders, including individuals, providers, insurers, employers, and governments. As a result of this reordering, all of these stakeholders were legally obligated to alter normative behaviors.

The first major change, known as the individual mandate, is a requirement that individuals maintain "minimum essential health coverage" (i.e., health insurance) or face financial penalties that are spelled out in the ACA. This requirement was a critically important beam in the ACA architecture because it created a new, large pool of individuals who pay premiums to insurance companies, and it created leverage for policymakers who were eager for the private insurers to accept many of the ACA's other insurance reforms that may otherwise have been unpalatable. For certain individuals whose socioeconomic status makes it impossible for them to purchase (or gain through an employer) the type of minimum coverage mandated by the ACA, and who do not qualify for Medicaid (even under the ACA expansion), federal subsidies are made available under the law. As discussed in more detail below, in 2017 Congress repealed the penalties associated with the individual mandate as part of the Tax Cut and Jobs Act.

The second fundamental change results from reforms that prohibit or curtail existing health insurer and health plan practices (these are the types of reforms, noted in the preceding paragraph, that all insurers—not just those who sell products through the new exchanges, described in the following paragraph—were forced to accept to reciprocate for the new group of premium payers they would insure as a result of the individual mandate). For example, the ACA prohibits insurers from considering an applicant's preexisting conditions when determining whether to insure the applicant, guarantees the renewability of an individual's existing insurance plan, requires insurers to cover certain preventive and immunization services, and guarantees coverage for dependent children who are 26 years old or younger.

The third key change is the creation of health insurance "exchanges" or "marketplaces" in each state. These are essentially online shopping sites, the purpose of which is to make it easier for individuals and small employers to compare and purchase health insurance. Because the ACA requires everyone to carry health insurance, and because the insurance marketplace has not historically been easy to navigate, policymakers forced the creation of regulated state-based exchanges to help with the purchase of individual and small-group insurance plans.

The final major reform is an expansion of the existing Medicaid program (which is discussed in detail in the Government Health Insurance Programs: Medicaid, CHIP, and Medicare chapter). This reform has the potential to dramatically increase the number of individuals who can gain access to insurance coverage—and thus access to better and more appropriate health care. Because states cannot be forced to implement this expansion (more on this to follow in the discussion of the U.S. Supreme Court's decision around the constitutionality of the ACA), and many states have thus far declined to implement the expansion, this potential has yet to become a reality. Although the ACA does not completely alter the way health insurance is provided by, say, establishing a single-payer system or even a large government-run insurance plan to compete with private insurers, the law makes significant philosophical and practical changes in how health insurance is regulated, structured, and administered. Indeed, as a result of the reforms and reordering just described, the ACA has resulted in 19 million people gaining insurance between 2010 and 2017, dropping the uninsured rate from 16% in 2010 to 11.1% in early 2017 (Blumberg, Holahan, Karpman, & Elmendorf, 2018). In addition, as a result of the essential health benefits requirement, there is a large segment of the population that is no longer underinsured because of insurance plans that do not offer comprehensive benefits.

Even so, many people contend that the ACA falls short in its reform of the healthcare delivery system. And in many cases they are correct. The ACA is most notable for the transformations it makes to health insurance—both access to it and its content—rather than for structural reforms made to the delivery system. Many provisions that focus on improving the healthcare delivery system, increasing the quality of care received by patients, reducing healthcare costs, and incentivizing providers to reconsider traditional methods of delivering care, often exist in the form of temporary pilot programs that may never be enacted permanently even if they prove to be valuable. Other analysts contend that these provisions were written as strongly as they could be at the time, given the political environment and data available to policymakers. According to this view, the ACA provides the secretary of HHS with unprecedented authority to make the pilot programs permanent, and it would have been irresponsible to implement more permanent, wholesale changes without more evidence. In any case, as sweeping as the ACA is, it is far from being the last step that needs to be taken to improve how health care is provided in the United States.

President Trump's proclamations about the ACA have vacillated from supporting efforts to repeal and then replace the law, to repeal and replace it simultaneously, to let the ACA "implode" to force the Democrats to negotiate, to keep the existing law but make improvements to it (Graham, 2017). His administration's actions, however, have consistently undermined the ACA, making it more likely that the uninsured rate will increase, premiums will rise, and consumer protections will diminish. Examples of these actions are highlighted in **BOX 10-2**. In general, the administration's strategy appears to focus on (1) providing states with flexibility to interpret ACA requirements and (2) weakening the marketplaces by deterring insurers from participating in the exchanges and increasing prices for consumers purchasing products through the exchanges (Tworney, Berger, & Brady, 2018). We turn now to a more detailed discussion of the ACA's key components, including a review of how

the administration's efforts have altered the law even though Congress has been unsuccessful in its efforts to repeal and replace the ACA.

Individual Mandate

An individual mandate is a requirement that individuals purchase health insurance. This is not a new idea. President Clinton proposed an individual mandate in 1993 as part of his Health Security Act, and other competing proposals at the time, including those supported by Republicans, also included an individual mandate. Massachusetts, the only state in the country to require that everyone older than 18 years have health insurance, included an individual mandate as one way to achieve that goal. A number of other countries, including the Netherlands, Switzerland, Germany, Japan, and Australia, have some form of an insurance mandate in their healthcare systems (Eibner & Nowak, 2018). During the 2008 election, Obama originally supported a mandate for children to be covered but suggested waiting to see if a mandate was necessary for adults after implementing other major health reform changes.

BOX 10-2 Select Trump Administration Executive Actions Relating to the ACA

- Issued Executive Order ordering federal agencies to begin dismantling the ACA "to the maximum extent permitted by law" and to grant exemptions or delay implementation of ACA provisions that impose a tax, fee, or other costs (January 2017)
- Issued an insurance regulation that made it more difficult for individuals to sign up for insurance during a special enrollment period, shortened the length of the enrollment period, lowered premium tax credits, made it easier for insurers to collect back premiums, and provided states more flexibility to define Essential Health Benefits (April 2017)
- Ended contracts to navigators that provided one-on-one enrollment assistance to consumers, slashed funding for enrollment outreach efforts, and limited weekend access to online enrollment functions (July–August 2017)
- Created an expanded option for employers who choose not to provide contraceptive coverage due to religious or moral reasons (October 2017)
- Ceased cost-sharing reduction payments to insurers (October 2017)
- Signed the Tax Cut and Jobs Act, which eliminated individual mandate penalties (December 2017)
- Proposed Association Health Plan (AHP) rules that would allow these plans to offer insurance products that are exempt from many ACA provisions, such as the Essential Health Benefits provision and another one that limits the charging of higher premiums based on one's age, gender, or occupation (January 2018)
- Issued guidance allowing work requirements to be applied to Medicaid recipients. Approved Kentucky's Medicaid waiver that includes work requirements, higher premiums, and coverage lockouts (January 2018) (Note that this waiver was subsequently vacated by a federal court and the question of whether states can mandate work requirements for Medicaid recipients is the subject of ongoing litigation.)
- Proposed rules to extend short-term limited duration health plans (that do not need to meet many of the ACA's requirements) from 3 months to 1 year (February 2018)
- Filed a brief in *Texas v. United States* declining to defend the constitutionality of the ACA (June 2018)
- Delayed risk-adjustment transfers that provide payments from insurers with low-risk pools to insurers with high-risk pools (July 2018)
- Slashed the budget (again) for enrollment outreach and navigation efforts (July 2018)

Source: Center on Budget and Policy Priorities, 2018.

While the individual mandate is not a new idea and has been championed by both Republicans and Democrats at different times in history, it has proven to be a politically perilous route to reducing the number of uninsured. Opposition to the individual mandate has softened over time, but public opinion remains split and partisan. A 2017 poll taken during the debate about the Republican ACA repeal and replacement efforts found that 50% of respondents supported retaining the individual mandate, while 48% preferred to eliminate this provision (Agiesta, 2017). This represents a shift in favor of the mandate over a 2013 poll that found 58% of respondents opposed (Burke, 2013). Over half of Republicans (55%) opposed the individual mandate in 2017 as compared to 84% in 2013. Democrats remained supportive of the individual mandated, with 60% preferring to keep the mandate in place in 2017, similar to the 57% who felt that way in 2013 (Agiesta, 2017).

It appears that some individuals do not prefer to be told they have to purchase health insurance by the government, even if it is a choice they made on their own prior to the passage of the ACA. But issues such as affordability or difficulty using the federal exchange website were more likely to be cited as reasons for not having health insurance than political opposition to the mandate. A poll conducted shortly after the first enrollment period closed found that most people who remained uninsured cited affordability (39%) or job-related reasons (22%), while only 9% felt they did not want or need health insurance (Hamel, Firth, & Brodie, 2014). Understandably, affordability remains a top issue for the public. In a recent poll, all respondents (regardless of political leanings) ranked limiting the amount individuals pay for health care as their top priority (DiJulio, Kirzinger, Wu, & Brodie, 2017). Almost half (49%) were very worried or somewhat worried about not being able to afford healthcare services in the future (DiJulio et al., 2017).

Individual mandates can be set up in a variety of ways, but usually individuals who do not comply will be required to pay some sort of penalty. The penalty is intended to provide both an incentive to comply with the law and to raise funds to cover the cost of health care for those individuals who choose not to carry health insurance. Individual mandates are considered to be a cornerstone of health reform efforts because they ensure that everyone covered by the mandate will be in an insurance pool to help cover costs and share risk.

Starting in 2014, the ACA's individual mandate required that almost everyone purchase health insurance or pay a penalty. This penalty is phased in over time, beginning at the greater of $95 or 1% of taxable income per person in 2014 and growing to the greater of $695 or 2.5% of taxable income per person in 2016 and 2017. In subsequent years, the penalty amount increases through cost of living adjustments. The maximum penalty is the cost of the national average bronze plan sold through the marketplace.

The mandate is considered essential because without it people who are in poor health or otherwise expect to use more healthcare services will be more likely to purchase health insurance, whereas healthier people will be more likely to opt out of insurance coverage. This situation would lead to an insurance pool that is relatively sick and thus more expensive, a problem referred to as *adverse selection*. Adverse selection leads to a so-called "death spiral" as the insurance pool gets continually sicker and more expensive, encouraging more healthy people to opt out of coverage.

While there remains for now uncertainty about the exact impact of the recent decision to remove the penalties associated with the individual mandate, it is generally agreed that the uninsured rate and premiums will increase due to adverse selection. For example, the Congressional Budget Office estimates that eliminating the penalty associated with the mandate will reduce the number of people with insurance by 3 to 6 million and will increase individual market premiums by 10% between 2019 and 2021 (Eibner & Nowak, 2018). The Rand Compare microsimulation model found that by 2020 there would be 2.8 to 13 million fewer insured individuals and a premium change of a 1% decrease to a 13% increase, depending on the plan type and modeling assumptions (Eibner & Nowak, 2018).

Some policy experts consider the ACA's mandate to be too weak to be effective in any event, thus reducing, in their view, the impact of eliminating the penalties. In 2016, 6.5 million people paid an average fine of $70 for lack of coverage (Scott, 2018). Under the ACA, the penalties may not have been significant enough, nor the premium subsidies generous enough, to compel people to buy insurance. In addition, the United States does not enforce the mandate as vigorously as other countries do (Scott, 2018).

Due to fears of adverse selection, analysts have been closely watching how many young adults (ages 18–34 years), who are more likely to be healthy, sign up for health insurance. While ideally 40% of enrollees would be in this age range in order to prevent adverse selection, only about 28% of the 8 million enrollees signed up at the end of the first enrollment period in April 2014 were young adults (Galewitz, n.d.). About 45% of taxpayers who either paid a penalty for not having insurance or claimed an exemption from the mandate that year were younger than 35 years (Mills, 2016). While young adults have experienced a dramatic reduction in their uninsured rate, they still accounted for 37.9% of the uninsured in 2017 (Blumberg et al., 2018).

The individual mandate is also an essential feature of health reform because healthy individuals who choose not to purchase health insurance but then later need health care will likely receive some care even though they are uninsured. This is especially true if the individuals have the resources to pay for healthcare services. These individuals are referred to as *free riders* because they avoid paying premiums for health insurance during their healthy years but then enjoy the benefits of healthcare services when they become sick. In 2015, over 7 million people who earned more than $75,000 were uninsured (Census, 2015). Because it is likely that many of these individuals could have afforded to purchase health insurance, some analysts consider this evidence of the free-rider problem.

Politically, the individual mandate was essential to passing the ACA because it was the carrot that enticed health insurers to support health reform. The ACA includes a prohibition against excluding individuals who have preexisting conditions as a way to make health insurance available for those with health needs. Health insurers would have balked at being forced to enroll sicker individuals without a mandate intended to draw in healthier consumers as well. In addition, the mandate guaranteed new premium dollars from the new enrollees.

There are a number of exceptions to the individual mandate requirement. Individuals are exempt from purchasing insurance if their income is below the tax-filing threshold (in 2017 this was $10,400 for single people younger than 65 years and $20,800 for couples younger than 65 years), the lowest-cost plan option exceeds 8% of their income, they qualify for a religious exemption, they are incarcerated, they are undocumented immigrants, they were without coverage for less than 3 months, they are Native Americans, or they qualify as having a hardship. Based on a June 2013 HHS rule, hardship exemptions must be granted for individuals who experience an event that resulted in an unexpected increase in expenses such that purchasing health insurance would make it impossible to pay for necessities, such as food and shelter. The rule cites circumstances that would be considered under this exemption: homelessness, eviction, domestic violence, death of a close family member, bankruptcy, substantial recent medical debt, and disasters that substantially changed the individual's property (Exchange Establishment Standards, 2013). Hardship exemptions are also allowed for individuals who would have qualified for Medicaid had their state chosen to expand the program under the ACA, and other exemptions exist based on projected low income (Jost, 2013). In 2018, the Trump administration created four new exemption categories (Center for Consumer Information, 2018; HHS Notice of Benefit and Payment Parameters [HHS Benefit and Payment Rule], 2018). Individuals may apply for a hardship exemption if they (1) live in counties without marketplace plans, (2) live in counties with a single insurer, (3) object to abortion coverage, or (4) meet additional hardship circumstances, such as needing specialty care out-of-network (Keith, 2018b). Some have criticized the exemptions for being so broad as to swallow the individual mandate.

To some, the individual mandate remains controversial. In addition to believing that it represents unwarranted government intrusion into private decision making, opponents of the individual mandate argued after the ACA was passed that Congress did not have the legal authority to impose such a requirement. This argument is grounded in jurisprudence relating to the federal Constitution's Commerce Clause, which gives Congress the power to "regulate commerce with foreign nations, and among the several states, and with the Indian tribes" (U.S. Const. art. I, §8). Since the 1940s, the Supreme Court has interpreted the Commerce Clause to permit Congress to regulate economic activity that carries across state lines or local concerns that substantially affect interstate commerce, and several Commerce Clause cases have allowed the regulation of individual conduct (for example, the Supreme Court has upheld laws that prohibit an individual from refusing to interact with a minority and laws that regulate an individual's ability to grow wheat or marijuana for home consumption [*Heart of Atlanta Motel v. United States*, 1964]), and the regulation of health insurance has also been deemed within the scope of the Commerce Clause (*Gonzales v. Raich*, 2005; *Wickard v. Filburn*, 1942).

Notwithstanding these cases, those who argued against the individual mandate contended that the Commerce Clause does not permit Congress to require an individual to purchase a service or good such as health insurance. In other words, the argument goes, an individual's decision not to purchase health insurance cannot be considered "economic activity" that Congress may regulate. Instead, it is argued, Congress is trying to regulate economic *in*activity—the decision not to purchase health insurance—and that this is not permitted under the Commerce Clause (Shapiro, 2010).

On the other hand, those who contend the Commerce Clause permits Congress to establish an individual mandate to purchase health insurance argue that everyone uses healthcare services at some point in their lives. Decisions regarding health insurance are an economic activity because no one can opt out of the healthcare market; that is, the decision individuals make is not whether to participate but how to participate in it. People will participate by purchasing health insurance now to cover the cost of future services or by paying out-of-pocket later at the time services are needed.

In the end, the Supreme Court upheld the individual mandate as a valid exercise of congressional *taxing* power; the court did, however, agree with those who maintained that the mandate was not permitted under the Commerce Clause. This outcome is described more fully later, when we provide an overview of the Supreme Court's June 2012 ruling on the constitutionality of the ACA.

State Health Insurance Exchanges/Marketplaces

The ACA established a new series of entities called health insurance exchanges (also referred to as marketplaces in federal documents) that are intended to create a more organized and competitive market for purchasing health insurance. These exchanges are state-based and geared toward those who purchase health insurance as individuals (through American Health Benefit Exchanges) or through small businesses (through the Small Business Health Options Program, or SHOP).

The SHOP exchange struggled from the start with implementation delays and much lower than anticipated enrollment (Aron-Dine, 2017). The Trump administration announced a rule that will effectively end the federally facilitated SHOP exchange as of January 2018 (HHS Notice of Benefit and Payment, 2018; Jost, 2017; Luhby, 2017b). The small employer tax credit will remain in place, but businesses will purchase

SHOP-qualified plans directly from insurers instead of on the exchange. According to the new rule, Centers for Medicare and Medicaid Services (CMS) will be working to find more efficient and effective ways to increase insurance coverage for small business employees.

Starting in 2014, the exchanges for individuals began offering a variety of health insurance plans that meet ACA criteria regarding plan benefits, payments, and consumer information. The Congressional Budget Office (CBO) projects that by 2028, 8 million individuals will purchase their own health insurance through an exchange (CBO, 2018). This is significantly lower than earlier CBO estimates. Much of the difference is because fewer individuals are now projected to purchase unsubsidized plans on the exchange instead of directly from insurers in the nongroup market (Centers for Medicare and Medicaid Services, 2017). Because fewer employers than anticipated dropped their employee coverage, CBO overestimated the number of individuals who would shift from employer coverage to marketplace plans (CBO, 2017c; Jost, 2016). In addition, CBO expects 5 million fewer individuals to purchase nongroup coverage, including marketplace coverage, as a result of the individual mandate penalty repeal (CBO, 2017d).

The exchanges are a critical component of health reform because it would be untenable to require individuals to purchase health insurance without also making comprehensive and affordable health insurance options available. Individuals often face expensive and less comprehensive health insurance choices because their insurance pools are not extensive enough that the premiums paid by healthy individuals offset the costs associated with sicker individuals. The exchanges are intended to create a new market by bringing together large numbers of individuals to create wider insurance pools. Individuals are eligible to purchase health insurance through an exchange if they live in the state where the exchange operates, are U.S. citizens or legal immigrants, and are not incarcerated. Additional requirements must be met, however, to obtain subsidies that reduce the cost of health insurance. Subsidies are available to individuals who meet the previously mentioned requirements and who also do not have access to affordable (as defined by the ACA) employer-sponsored insurance, meet specified income requirements, file taxes jointly (if married), and are not eligible for Medicaid, Medicare, or the Children's Health Insurance Program (CHIP) (KFF, n.d.).

Under the ACA, states have three main options when it came to exchanges: they can build their own, enter into a partnership with the federal government, or ignore the process altogether and thus default into what is referred to as a federally facilitated market-place (FFM; this federally facilitated exchange was mandated by the ACA for states that were not willing or able to establish a state exchange or a partnership exchange). In a state-run exchange, the state either handles all functions or may use the federal information technology (IT) platform; in a partnership exchange, states may administer plan management functions, in-person consumer assistance functions, or both, with HHS performing remaining responsibilities; and in the FFM, HHS performs all functions. Whatever the structure, the exchanges for individuals were required to be up and running by January 1, 2014. At the time of this writing, the breakdown is as follows: 17 states and the District of Colombia built their own exchange (with 5 of the states using the federal IT platform); 6 set up partnership exchanges; and 28 states defaulted to the FFM (KFF, 2018). States also may form a regional exchange with other states or allow multiple exchanges within one state as long as each exchange covers a distinct geographic area. In addition, the federal Office of Personnel Management is required to offer at least two multistate plans within each exchange to provide individuals and businesses with additional choices.

The ACA requires the exchanges to ensure that plans meet other requirements of participating in the exchange. These requirements relate to marketing practices, provider networks, outreach and enroll-ment, insurance market regulations, and the provision of information in plain language. In addition, the entity running the exchange must provide a call center for customers, maintain a website, develop uniform applications, provide information regarding eligibility for public programs, assist individuals in calculating their tax credits, and certify individuals who are exempt from the individual mandate requirement.

As noted earlier, the Trump administration actions undermining the ACA have focused on strategies that weaken the ACA marketplaces. One way to accomplish this goal is to allow cheaper alternatives for individuals to purchase health insurance in the nongroup market outside of the exchanges. In general, a cheaper alternative is likely to have less comprehensive benefits and/or higher cost-sharing for the individual. The administration's rule expanding both Association Health Plans (AHPs) and short-term limited-duration plans are part of this strategy. AHPs allow business associations and other organizations to join together to provide fringe benefits, including health insurance (CBO, 2018). Short-term plans were designed to fill in a temporary insurance coverage gap and are not renewable (Pollitz, Long, Semanskee, & Kamal, 2018).

Both types of plans are likely to "limit benefits, be priced on the basis of an individuals health status, and impose lifetime and annual spending limits, and insurers could reject applicants on the basis of their health and any preexisting condition" (CBO, 2018, p. 10). One review of short-term plans found that 71% did not cover outpatient prescription drugs, 62% did not cover substance abuse services, 43% did not cover mental health services, and no plans covered maternity care (Pollitz et al., 2018). By allowing insurers to offer nongroup plans that do not have to comply with these ACA provisions, it is possible to create cheaper and skimpier insurance products. As a result, adverse selection is likely to occur in the exchange plans as healthier individuals who do not believe they need a comprehensive plan—or do not want to pay a higher premium to participate in one—will leave the exchange plan and move to a cheaper nongroup option. CBO estimates that 6 million people will enroll in AHPs or short-term plans by 2023 (CBO, 2018).

Another way to weaken ACA marketplaces is to make it more difficult to enroll in marketplace plans. Several Trump administration policies create barriers to enrollment. These policies include shortening the enrollment period, limiting advertising and other outreach during the enrollment period, reducing the budget for "navigators" who assist consumers in understanding and enrolling in marketplace plans, and limiting weekend online enrollment functions through the official HealthCare.gov website (Center for American Progress, 2018).

Essential Health Benefit Requirement

All qualified health plans that participate in an exchange (as well as individual and small-group plans outside of the exchanges) must offer a standard benefit package called essential health benefits (EHBs) (**BOX 10-5**) (Giovannelli, Lucia, & Corlette, 2014). This requirement represents the first time private health insurance plans have been subject to a federal standard regarding what benefits must be offered. The ACA requires the secretary of HHS to ensure the scope of benefits is equal to the benefit level found in a "typical employer plan." Plans may not design their benefit or reimbursement packages in ways that discriminate based on age, disability, or expected length of life (Rosenbaum, Teitelbaum, & Hayes, 2011).

While the ACA outlines 10 categories of services that must be provided in the EHB package, the federal regulatory process left states with significant discretion about how they implemented this requirement. States have a choice of 10 federally approved health plans to serve as a benchmark to determine the breadth of

BOX 10-4 Provider Networks

An emerging policy and care delivery issue has been the question of whether provider networks available in plans offered in the exchanges are adequate. Prior to the ACA, insurers could control costs through a variety of mechanisms, including limiting benefits, excluding consumers with preexisting conditions, and using medical underwriting to charge higher premiums to higher-risk individuals and groups. Plans would compete with each other based on price, benefits, cost-sharing, and other features. The ACA includes a variety of rules that eliminate these options, such as prohibition of exclusions based on preexisting conditions, guaranteed issue requirements, community rating requirements, essential health benefit requirements, and actuarial tiering of plans. As a result of ACA restrictions, many plans are trying to control costs by limiting provider networks and/or provider reimbursement. Of course, some providers may choose not to participate in exchange plans if the reimbursement is not sufficient.

Many consumers who purchase plans in an exchange choose plans based on the premium price and indicate they would prefer cheaper plans with narrow networks as opposed to expensive plans with broader networks. On the other hand, consumers who purchase plans through employer-sponsored insurance often prefer broader networks, even if the coverage is more expensive. Complaints about narrow networks range from consumers being disappointed that their usual doctor or local hospital is not in network, to questions about access to care, network transparency, and quality of care. Several lawsuits have been filed against plans regarding network transparency and provider terminations. In 2014 the Office of the Insurance Commissioner issued federal rules regarding network adequacy in individual and small-group plans, and CMS continues to issue guidance regarding network adequacy for qualified health plans. State responses to network adequacy concerns have spanned the gamut, from Massachusetts requiring plans to develop tiered and narrow networks to promote cost savings, to several failed attempts by state legislatures to pass "any willing provider" laws that require insurers to include any provider willing to accept the insurers' terms.

Source: Data from: McDermott Will & Emery. Challenges facing "narrow" provider networks on the ACA health insurance exchanges. http://www.mwe.com /files/Uploads/Documents/News /Challengs-Facing-Narrow-Provider-Networks.pdf. Published April 20, 2015. Accessed July 7, 2015.

BOX 10-5 Essential Health Benefits

All plans in the state exchanges must offer the following benefits:

- Ambulatory patient services
- Emergency services
- Hospitalization
- Maternity and newborn care
- Mental health services and substance use disorder services, including behavioral health treatment
- Prescription drugs
- Rehabilitative and habilitative services and devices (rehabilitative therapies improve, maintain, or prevent deterioration of functions that have been acquired [e.g., after an adult has surgery], whereas habilitative therapies are provided to achieve functions and skills never acquired [e.g., as with a developmentally disabled child])
- Laboratory services
- Prevention and wellness services and chronic disease management services
- Pediatric services, including vision and dental services

the services covered under the EHB categories. These approved benchmark plans include the largest three small-group plans available in the state, the largest three state-employee health plans in the state, the largest three Federal Employee Health Benefit Program plan options for federal employees, or the state's largest commercial HMO (Giovannelli et al., 2014). In 2017, 26 states did not choose a benchmark plan and were defaulted to the largest small-group plan offered in that state (Keith, 2017). Whether by choice or default, most states are using small-group plans,

which are often less generous than large-group plans, as their benefit benchmark (Giovannelli, Volk, Lucia, William, & Connor, 2015). The Trump administration added another benchmarking option through its definition of a "typical employer plan," effective in 2020. In addition to the 10 benchmark plans discussed, states may also use any of the five largest (by enrollment) group health insurance products in the state that meet certain requirements (Keith, 2018b). The administration further expanded state choice in 2020 by allowing states to select annually whether to (1) use another state's entire 2017 benchmark plan, (2) replace one or more of its EHB categories with another state's EHB categories, or (3) choose a new EHB benchmark plan (Keith, 2018b).

Benchmark plans are subject to minimum and maximum standards. At a minimum, the benchmark plans must meet the "typical employer plan" standard. At a maximum, also known as the generosity test, the benchmark plan cannot be more generous than the most generous comparison plan (Keith, 2018b). The comparison plans are the state's 2017 benchmark and the state's three or four largest (by enrollment) small-group health plans (Keith, 2018b). The federal government will defer to the state's interpretation of plan benefits and limits (Keith, 2018b).

The Trump administration has also changed the rules regarding substituting benefits. Under the Obama administration, insurers were allowed to substitute benefits *within* an EHB category, but not *across* EHB categories, as long as the substitution was actuarially equivalent to the benefit it was replacing. Under the Trump administration, states may substitute actuarially equivalent benefits both *within* and *across* EHB categories (Keith, 2018b). An example of a *within* EHB substitution could be replacing a blood screen (lab test) for ovarian cancer with coverage of a blood screen for high cholesterol, a different, but actuarially equivalent, laboratory test (Giovannelli et al., 2014). An *across* EHB substitution would be replacing one type of service (e.g., an inpatient hospital service) with a completely different type of service (e.g., an outpatient physician service). Substitution is not permitted for prescription drugs.

Critics of the *across* substitution rule are concerned that plans will substitute out select benefits so that they do not appeal to certain high-risk individuals. In addition, once a service is not considered an EHB, it is no longer subject to ACA protections, such as lifetime or annual dollar limits, nor is it used to calculate premium subsidies and cost-sharing reductions (Keith, 2018b). Nine states and the District of Columbia prohibited *within* category substitution in 2014 (Giovannelli et al., 2014). As with many of the Trump administration changes, states will have the final say over whether and how they choose to take advantage of this flexibility.

Further variation across the states may occur with habilitative service coverage and state benefit mandates. Habilitative services assist individuals with gaining or maintaining functional skills (e.g., speaking, walking). Prior to ACA passage, coverage for and the definition of habilitative services varied significantly. As part of ACA implementation, federal regulators permitted states to use the habilitative services

definition in their benchmark plan (if there was such coverage), create their own coverage definition, or let the insurers define the coverage benefit (Giovannelli et al., 2014). As a result, the definition of habilitative services may differ across states and within states. Finally, some states passed laws that required insurers in their states to cover a particular benefit, such as obesity management services. Any benefit mandates that were in place before 2012 were incorporated into that state's EHB package, meaning the variation that was in place prior to health reform is likely to continue. It is less likely that states will add new benefit mandates at this time because if a state plans to include any services beyond the essential health benefits package that were not mandated prior to 2012, the state must defray the cost of the additional service through a payment to the enrollee or the plan. In addition, the new generosity test means that it may be more difficult for states to choose a benchmark that includes an expensive mandate (Keith, 2018b).

In the lead-up to passage of the ACA, there was significant debate about whether to allow or require plans to offer abortion and contraceptive services. In fact, the abortion debate was so divisive it almost doomed the entire health reform bill at the 11th hour. A compromise was reached with the intent of keeping the status quo regarding federal funding for abortion services (i.e., limit federal funding for abortion services to cases where the life of the pregnant woman is in danger or the pregnancy is a result of rape or incest). Under the compromise, states may enact a law that prohibits plans that participate in their state exchanges from providing abortion services.

The ACA also provides coverage, without any cost-sharing, for all contraception methods approved by the Food and Drug Administration. While contraception is considered a preventive service under the EHB standard, it is not specifically listed in the statute (nor are other preventive services; instead the statute references guidelines such as the U.S. Preventive Services Task Force A and B recommendations). Contraceptive coverage is part of a separate provision that includes women's preventive services identified by the Health Resources and Services Administration. Because this guideline is created by an administrative agency, each successive administration has the power to change the list of approved women's preventive services without needing congressional approval. The Obama administration exempted certain entities from being required to provide contraception coverage due to religious objections (Coverage Preventive Services, 2013). The required breadth of this exemption is the subject of numerous lawsuits and remains unsettled at this time. The Trump administration is considering a new administrative rule that would significantly broaden the group of employers and insurers who would qualify for the exemption based on religious or moral grounds (Pear, 2017).

Given the Trump administration's policies intended to restrict access to abortion services (e.g., supporting the defunding of Planned Parenthood) and contraceptive devices (e.g., by broadening the religious objection exemption), it is worth noting what actions states have taken on these issues. As of June 2018, 11 states have enacted laws that restrict abortion coverage in all private plans in the state, 25 states restrict abortion coverage in private plans offered through their exchange, and 21 states restrict abortion coverage in public employee plans (Guttmacher Institute, n.d.; Guttmacher Institute, 2018a). If a state does not enact such a law and a plan chooses to offer abortion services in other circumstances, the plan must create separate financial accounts to ensure that federal premium and cost-sharing subsidies are not used toward those abortion services. In addition, at least one of the multistate plans is required not to provide abortion services beyond those that are currently allowed with federal funding. As with most compromises, neither side was entirely pleased with the outcome. Those who want more restrictive abortion policies found the separate accounting process to be a meaningless exercise, whereas those who want more permissive abortion policies were disturbed by the ability of states to prohibit plans from offering abortion services. As of June 2018, 29 states require insurance plans to cover the full range of contraceptive drugs, 9 states prohibit cost-sharing for contraceptives, and 5 states prohibit other restrictions and delays by insurers. At the same time, 21 states exempt select employers and insurers from providing contraceptive coverage based on religious objections (Guttmacher Institute, 2018b).

The ACA also created a "catastrophic coverage" option that must include EHBs (KFF, n.d.). A catastrophic plan may be offered only to individuals younger than 30 years who would be exempt from the individual mandate requirement due to hardship or affordability exemptions. These plans require coverage of EHBs, certain preventive services without cost-sharing, and at least three primary care visits each year before meeting the deductible (KFF, n.d.). Individuals may not use premium tax credits to subsidize catastrophic plans, which typically have low premiums but very high deductibles.

Premium and Cost-Sharing Subsidies

One key difference among the exchange plans is the cost to the enrollee. Four levels of plans may be offered,

and they are distinguished by their actuarial value. Actuarial value is the average share of covered benefits generally paid by the insurer based on the cost-sharing provisions in the plan. The higher the actuarial value, the more the plan pays for a given set of services. For example, in a plan with 70% actuarial value, the plan pays 70% of the cost of services on average across all enrollees, while enrollees pay 30%. Actuarial value is set by average cost, but any single enrollee in that plan may pay more or less than 30% of the cost of services. In general, plans with a higher actuarial value will also have higher premiums to cover the cost of providing services to enrollees. A plan with lower premiums could have higher cost-sharing (co-pays or deductibles) to offset the lower premium. The four ACA-approved plan levels by actuarial value are bronze (60% actuarial value), silver (70% actuarial value), gold (80% actuarial value), and platinum (90% actuarial value). Plans must offer at least one silver-level and one gold-level option in each exchange in which they participate.

The ACA includes premium tax credits and cost-sharing subsidies (CSRs) to help make it affordable for people to purchase health insurance in a state exchange. Given the mandate to purchase insurance, it was necessary to include some assistance to make it possible for low-income individuals to comply with the new requirement. The tax credits and subsidies were available starting in 2014, the same year the individual mandate and the state health insurance exchanges went into effect. In 2017, 8.7 million people (84% of marketplace enrollees) received a premium tax credit, and 5.9 million people (57% of marketplace enrollees) received a CSR (KFF, 2017a).

Premium tax credits are available to individuals who are eligible to purchase health insurance in state exchanges; have incomes between 100% and 400% of the federal poverty level; are not eligible for Medicaid, CHIP, or Medicare; and do not have access to affordable employer-sponsored health insurance. (An employer plan is not considered affordable if it does not cover at least 60% of covered benefits or if the employee's share of premium contributions exceeds 9.5% of the employee's income.) In 2018, 400% of the poverty level was $48,560 for an individual and $100,400 for a family of four (Office of Assistant Secretary for Planning and Evaluation, 2018). The tax credits are advanceable and refundable, meaning they are available when health insurance is purchased and regardless of whether the individual owes any taxes. CSRs (i.e., federal funds provided to assist individuals with the purchase of insurance) are available to people who earn between 100% and 250% of the poverty level. Under the ACA, individuals with income less than 133% of the poverty level will be eligible for Medicaid beginning in 2014 in those states that elected to implement the ACA's Medicaid eligibility expansion.

The amount of the premium tax credit is tiered based on income and set so individuals will not have to pay more than a certain percentage of their income on premiums (**TABLE 10-1**). The tax credit amount is based on the cost of the second-lowest-cost silver plan in the exchange and location where the individual is eligible to purchase insurance. Individuals who want to purchase a more expensive plan have to pay the difference in cost between the second-lowest-cost silver plan and the plan they prefer to purchase. Under the ACA, HHS will adjust the premium people are expected to pay to reflect that premium costs typically grow faster than income levels.

For example, assume Bob's income is 250% of poverty (about $31,000 for an individual), and the cost of the second-lowest-cost silver plan in Bob's area is $5,700. Under the premium tax credit schedule, Bob will pay no more than 8.05% of his income, or $2,495. Bob's tax credit is $3,205, which is $5,700 minus $2,495 (KFF, n.d.).

CSRs are available to help low-income people reduce the amount of out-of-pocket spending on health insurance (**TABLE 10-2**). The subsidies are tiered by income level and set so that plans pay a higher percentage of service costs. In other words, they are set to increase the actuarial value of the plan for low-income individuals.

Under the ACA, insurers receive payments from the federal government to cover the expense of providing CSRs to their low-income enrollees. Nearly 6 million enrollees qualified for CSRs in 2017, which was expected to cost the federal government $7 billion (Liptak, Luhby, & Mattingly, 2017). These payments to insurers have been the subject of litigation brought by House Republicans, originally during the Obama administration (the case was first known as *House v. Burwell*, then it was retitled *House v. Price* to account for a new HHS Secretary, and currently the case has been retitled *House v. Azar* for the same reason). Initially, the federal trial court agreed with the plaintiffs' claim that the subsidies should not be funded because Congress did not appropriate money for that purpose. The Obama administration appealed, after which the case was put on hold during multiple delays. In October 2017, the Trump administration announced that it would no longer make CSR payments to insurers, and as a result the various parties to the lawsuit—House Republicans, the Trump administration, and several states (which had been granted a request along the way to intervene in the case)—started to negotiate a settlement. Having reached a conditional settlement in December 2017, the parties asked the original trial judge to issue an "indicative ruling" that she would vacate her original order on CSR payments if the case

TABLE 10-1 Premium Tax Credit Schedule

Income Level by Federal Poverty Level (FPL)	Premium as a Percentage of Income
100–133% FPL	2% of income
133–150% FPL	3–4% of income
150–200% FPL	4–6.3% of income
200–250% FPL	6.3–8.05% of income
250–300% FPL	8.05–9.5% of income
300–400% FPL	9.5% of income

TABLE 10-2 Cost-Sharing Subsidy Schedule

Income Level by Federal Poverty Level (FPL)	Actuarial Value
100–150% FPL	94%
150–200% FPL	87%
200–250% FPL	73%

were sent back to her from the appellate court (to which the Obama administration had appealed some years earlier) without a ruling on the merits. At the request of the parties, the appellate court did just that; it dismissed the appeal and sent the case back to the trial court. In turn, the trial judge vacated her initial decision. That said, the CSR saga is not over: several state attorneys general filed a lawsuit against HHS over its decision to end the CSR payments, and some insurers have done the same.

The ACA requires insurers to offer low-income enrollees reduced deductibles and co-payments. Without CSR payments to cover the costs of those reductions, insurers will increase premiums to make up for lost revenue and/or leave the insurance market altogether (Liptak et al., 2017). While the amount varies by state, it is estimated that cessation of CSR payments led to an average premium increase of 19% in 2018 (Kamal, Semanskee, Long, Claxton, & Leavitt, 2017). Many insurers are targeting their premium increase just to the silver plan, a strategy known as "silver loading" (Keith, 2018c). By doing so, they are maximizing premium tax credits they receive, which are tied to silver plan costs. In addition, since consumers may use their tax credits for any plan, many could enroll in a bronze or gold plan at a lower cost than in prior years. While the Trump administration could prohibit silver loading, they have not done so to date (Keith, 2018c). Ironically, it is estimated that the cost to the federal government for not making the CSR payments is $2 billion *more* than it would be if it simply made the payments, because of the higher premium tax credits owed (Fise, 2017).

In addition to the premium tax credits and CSRs, the ACA limits the overall amount of out-of-pocket costs paid by individuals with incomes up to 400% of poverty (**TABLE 10-3**). The limits are based on the maximum out-of-pocket costs for health savings accounts ($6,650 for single coverage, $13,300 for family coverage in 2018) and will be indexed annually.

The insurance subsidies have been at the center of litigation and political maneuvering and are discussed

BOX 10-7 Discussion Questions

CBO estimates that premium subsidies and CSRs will cost the federal government $760 billion over the years 2019–2028 (CBO, 2018). Is this a good use of resources? Are these subsidies well designed? Are they sufficient to make health insurance affordable? Do they cover people with incomes that are too high? Should they cover more people?

later. These subsidies—and, in turn, the viability of the ACA overall—were at risk due to a lawsuit that challenged the legality of subsidies provided to the millions of people in the states that use a federally operated insurance exchange instead of setting up a state-based exchange (Taylor, Saenz, & Levine, 2015). Congress wrote in the ACA that federal subsidies were available to individuals who purchased health insurance through exchanges that were "established by the State." As part of the law's implementation process, the Internal Revenue Service (IRS) issued a regulation indicating that federal subsidies were available to individuals who purchased health insurance in either state-run or federally operated exchanges (Health Insurance Premium, 2012). The individuals who brought the lawsuit argued that the IRS regulation was unlawful because it contradicted the language of the ACA. In essence, the court case boiled down to the meaning of the four words "established by the State": when read contextually against the rest of the ACA, were federally operated exchanges included in exchanges "established by the State," or were federal subsidies reserved only for individuals in states that established their own state-run exchange?

In a 6–3 decision in *King v. Burwell*, the U.S. Supreme Court upheld the ACA's statutory and regulatory scheme, allowing federal subsidies to flow to individuals who purchase insurance in both state-run and federally operated exchanges. Instead of reading the four words in question in a vacuum, Chief Justice Roberts, writing for the majority, viewed the phrase "established by the State" in the context of the overall purpose of the law. Doing otherwise, according to the court, would bring about "the type of calamitous result [insurance market failure] that Congress plainly meant to avoid" in crafting the ACA in the first place. Noting that the court's duty is to construe statutes as a whole, not "isolated provisions," Chief Justice Roberts wrote the following:

Congress passed the Affordable Care Act to improve health insurance markets, not to destroy them. If at all possible, we must interpret the [ACA] in a way that is consistent with the former, and avoids the latter. [The IRS

TABLE 10-3 Out-of-Pocket Spending Limits	
Income Level by Federal Poverty Level (FPL)	**Out-of-Pocket Limit**
100–200% FPL	2/3 of maximum
200–300% FPL	1/2 of maximum
300–400% FPL	1/3 of maximum

regulation] can fairly be read consistent with what we see as Congress's plan, and that is the reading we adopt. (*King v. Burwell*, 2015)

In upholding the subsidies, the court differed in its reasoning from some lower federal courts that nonetheless also upheld the subsidies across all exchanges. These lower courts found the ACA's subsidy language ambiguous and therefore deferred to the agency (the IRS) that was tasked with interpreting the statute. In a critical move, the Supreme Court instead ruled that because the availability of tax credits was an issue with "deep economic and political significance" to the country, the meaning of the subsidy language should be interpreted by the court itself, rather than left to agency discretion. This decision means that the only way the subsidy language can be altered in the future is through congressional action, rather than by a future president whose administration might reinterpret the language more narrowly. Thus, it is far more likely that the subsidies will remain available in all exchanges—regardless of whether a state or the federal government operates them—going forward.

In addition to saving insurance subsidies for millions of Americans, the decision in *King v. Burwell* could have additional ramifications. Taken in conjunction with *NFIB v. Sebelius* (the 2012 Supreme Court decision upholding the constitutionality of the ACA), lower courts may read *King's* direction to interpret the ACA as a congressional effort to improve insurance markets as a signal to forestall future litigation against the law. Furthermore, in states that have had difficulty setting up or operating their own exchange, the decision may encourage them to rely on the federal exchange apparatus; because there is no longer the threat that insurance subsidies could be easily untethered from federally facilitated exchanges, the use of such an exchange could become relatively more attractive.

Employer Mandate

As written in the ACA, employers with 50 or more employees and at least 1 employee who qualifies for a tax credit were required to offer affordable health insurance or pay a penalty beginning in 2014. The Obama administration twice delayed implementation of the mandate to smooth the transition, but the mandate itself did not change. Under the mandate, covered employers have three options: (1) provide affordable health insurance and not pay a penalty, (2) provide health insurance not considered affordable and pay a penalty, or (3) do not provide health insurance and pay a penalty. The penalties are based on whether an employer offers health insurance and whether any

full-time employees take a premium tax credit. The amount of the penalty increases over time based on the national increase in premium costs. The employer mandate was put in place to encourage employers to continue offering or start offering health insurance. Without such a mandate, employers may have found it profitable not to offer health insurance and let their employees purchase health insurance through state exchanges, shifting more of the costs of health reform to the public sector and taxpayers.

For employers that do not offer health insurance and have at least one full-time employee who takes the premium tax credit, the penalty is $2,000 per employee after the first 30 employees. In other words, if such an employer has 50 employees, the employer would pay a $40,000 penalty ($2,000 × 20 employees).

Employers that offer health insurance do not pay a penalty if the insurance is considered affordable. Insurance is affordable if the plan has an actuarial value of at least 60% or if the premiums do not cost more than 9.5% of an employee's income. Employees who would have to pay more than 9.5% of their income on premiums have the option to purchase insurance through an exchange and receive a premium tax credit.

Employers who provide unaffordable insurance have to pay a penalty for each employee who takes a tax credit, not counting the first 30 employees (the 30-employee exception was included in the law due to Congress's concern about the impact of the employer mandate on small businesses). The penalty is $3,000 per employee who takes a tax credit but may not exceed $2,000 times the number of employees over 30. For example, if the employer has 50 employees and offers unaffordable coverage, the employer would pay a maximum penalty of $40,000 ($2,000 × 20). If only 10 employees take a tax credit, the penalty would be $30,000 ($3,000 × 10). If all 50 employees take a tax credit, the penalty would be $40,000, which is the maximum penalty allowed, not $150,000 ($3,000 × 50).

Given their smaller pool of employees, small businesses have often found it quite expensive to offer health insurance to their employees. In addition to exempting businesses with fewer than 50 employees from the employer mandate (and creating a health insurance exchange for small businesses), Congress also included a small business tax credit to encourage these employers to provide coverage. Employers are eligible for the tax credit if they have fewer than 25 full-time-equivalent employees, average annual wages under $50,000, and pay for at least half of the cost of health insurance coverage for their employees. The tax credit covers a portion of the cost of the employer's contribution toward employees' premiums. The credit is capped based on the average premium costs in the employer's geographic area and phases out as firm size and annual wages increase.

Because the employer mandate (and other provisions) will lead to increased costs for certain employers, some of these employers may be influenced to offset new costs by employing more part-time workers (at the expense of full-time employment) and/or capping the number of workers they hire at 49 to avoid the mandate (Blumberg, Holahan, & Buettgens, 2014). While several analyses indicate that the ACA's effects to the labor market may in fact be modest (Abraham & Royalty, 2017; Blumberg et al., 2014), the authors of one study (Blumberg et al., 2014) nonetheless go so far as to advocate for eliminating the employer mandate altogether. They argue that doing so would actually not reduce overall insurance coverage significantly, would eliminate any market distortions that could result from changes in employer hiring practices, and would have the added benefit of lessening employer opposition to the ACA (Blumberg et al., 2014).

Changes to the Private Insurance Market

In addition to creating a new marketplace for private insurance through state exchanges, the ACA includes a variety of changes to private health insurance rules and requirements. These requirements cover everything from rate setting, to benefits, to who must be covered. Although the overall health reform law is controversial, many of these private market reforms have overwhelming support. Together, these changes filled in gaps left by the private market that many people believed were unfair to consumers.

The following coverage changes took effect in 2010:

- **Preexisting conditions:** Individual and group plans may not exclude children due to their health status or based on preexisting conditions.
- **Dependent coverage:** Individual and group plans must provide dependent coverage up to age 26 years.
- **Preventive services:** New health plans may not impose cost-sharing for certain preventive services, including the following:
  - Preventive services with an A or B rating from the U.S. Preventive Services Task Force
  - Immunizations recommended by the Centers for Disease Control and Prevention's Advisory Committee on Immunization Practice
  - Preventive care and screening for women based on guidelines to be issued by the Health Resources and Services Administration
- **Coverage limits:** Individual and group plans may not impose lifetime dollar limits on coverage (and

the ability to impose annual limits on the dollar value of coverage is prohibited as of 2014).

- **Rescission:** Individual and group plans may not rescind coverage except in the case of fraud.
- **Appeals:** New health insurance plans must have an effective appeals process that includes an external review option.

Congress also focused on the issue of how insurers determine premium rates and what they spend those resources on within their plans. The ACA charged HHS with establishing an annual process to review "unreasonable" increases in premiums (ACA, 2010, §1003). The 2019 benefit and payment rules change the definition of "unreasonable" from a 10% to a 15% increase and exempt student health services from the review requirements (Keith, 2018d). As of 2016, 43 states and the District of Columbia had some type of rate review law in place for all of their insurance markets, and the federal process is intended to work with, not preempt, those state laws (National Conference of State Legislators, 2016). These states must post all proposed increases at the same time and all final rate increases at the same time and must provide CMS with 5 days' notice of rate increases (Keith, 2018d).

In addition, the ACA requires that plans spend at least 85% (large-group plans) or 80% (small-group or individual plans) of their premium dollars on medical care and quality improvement services, not administrative or other expenses (e.g., profits). Regulations clarifying this medical loss ratio (MLR), as it is called, took effect on January 1, 2011 (Health Insurance Issuers, 2010). Insurers must provide enrollees with a rebate if they do not spend the requisite percentage on clinical and quality improvement services. Initially, insurers paid significant rebates to consumers ($1 billion in 2011), but by 2016 only 1.5% of enrollees received rebates as insurers improved their MLR to 92% in the individual market and 86% in the small-group market (Keith, 2018d). Under the 2019 benefit and payment rules, insurers may automatically claim 0.8% of earned premiums for quality improvement without supplying verifying documentation. This will raise the MLR rate for most insurers (Keith, 2018d). The rule also eases standards for seeking an MLR adjustment in the individual market. CMS projects that 22 states will seek such an adjustment, resulting in consumer rebate reductions of $52 to $64 million annually (Keith, 2018d).

A number of significant insurance changes took place in 2014 alongside implementation of the individual mandate and health insurance exchanges:

- **Guaranteed issue and renewability:** Individual and group plans may not exclude or charge more to individuals based on preexisting conditions or health status in the individual market, small-group market, and exchanges.

- **Rate variation limits:** Premium rates may vary based only on age, geographic area, family composition, and tobacco use in the individual market, small-group market, and exchanges.
- **Coverage limits:** Individual and group plans may not place annual dollar limits on coverage.
- **Essential health benefits:** Insurers providing coverage to small businesses or individuals and in the exchanges have to provide essential health benefits through one of four plan categories (bronze, silver, gold, or platinum) and adhere to annual cost-sharing limits.
- **Wellness plans:** Employers may offer rewards that reduce the cost of coverage to employees for participating in a wellness plan.

These private market changes do not affect all plans equally. Plans in small-group or nongroup markets must follow these rules whether or not they are offered in an exchange. However, the ACA included two significant exceptions to these reforms. First, insurance plans that were in existence when the ACA was signed into law are referred to as "grandfathered plans" and are subject to some, but not all, of the new rules. The grandfathered plans must follow new requirements relating to preexisting conditions, lifetime and annual limits, waiting period limits, and dependent coverage rules. These plans are exempt, however, from having to provide essential health benefits, preventive services without co-pays, and limited cost-sharing, although many of the large employer plans already have some of these features (Healthcare. gov, n.d.). A plan may retain its grandfathered status as long as it does not make significant changes to plan benefits or cost-sharing rules. If it loses its grandfathered status, the plan will have to meet all applicable requirements. In 2017, 23% of all employers offered at least one grandfathered plan, and 17% of covered workers were enrolled in a grandfathered plan (KFF and Health Research and Educational Trust [HRET], 2017, Section 13).

The second major exception is for self-funded plans. In these plans, an employer does not buy insurance from a company but instead takes on the insurance risk itself. Self-funded plans are exempt from state law and subject to federal rules under ERISA. Self-funded plans must adhere to ACA rules regarding dependent coverage, cost-sharing for preventive services, annual and lifetime limits, and waiting period limits, but do not need to comply with essential health benefit requirements (Commercial Insurance, 2012)

Financing Health Reform

Congress financed health reform primarily through Medicare and Medicaid savings, excise taxes and fees on the healthcare industry, changes to the income tax code, a tax on some health insurance plans, and expected individual and employer payments for violating insurance mandates. Several of these financing changes were made as part of the deals the Obama administration struck with various stakeholders.

The ACA's main financing features are as follows:

- **Medicare provider reimbursement:** Reduces "market basket" or cost updates for inpatient and outpatient hospital reimbursement and reduces payments for preventable hospital readmissions and hospital-acquired infections. This feature includes productivity adjustments (an adjustment in the Medicare physician fee schedule pertaining to physician productivity) for certain providers that will result in lower reimbursement rates.
- **Medicare Advantage payments:** Reduces reimbursement rates and imposes cost-sharing limits for Medicare's managed care plans.
- **Medicare Part A (hospital insurance):** Increases Medicare Part A tax rate for high-income earners.
- **Medicare premiums:** Reduces Medicare Part D (prescription drug) premium subsidy for high-income beneficiaries.
- **Medicare employer subsidy:** Eliminates tax deduction for employers who receive a Medicare Part D (prescription drug coverage) subsidy.
- **Disproportionate share hospital (DSH) payments:** Reduces Medicare payments to DSH hospitals. Payments may increase over time based on the percentage of uninsured served and uncompensated care provided. This feature reduces Medicaid DSH payments and requires HHS to develop a new funding formula. The effective date of the reduction was delayed until 2018, but the amount of reduction increased from $18 billion to $43 billion through 2025 (Kardish, 2015).
- **Medicaid prescription drugs:** Increases rebates that drug manufacturers give to state Medicaid programs
- **Income tax code provisions:** Increases the threshold from 7.5% to 10% of adjusted gross income to claim deduction for unreimbursed medical expenses, prohibits purchasing over-the-counter drugs with tax-free savings accounts, increases the tax burden on distributions not used for qualified medical expenses, and limits the amount individuals may put in accounts toward medical expenses.

■ **Health industry fees:** Imposes a 10% tax on indoor tanning services, 2.3% tax on all taxable medical devices, annual fees on the pharmaceutical manufacturing sector, and fees on the health insurance sector.

■ **Health insurance plans:** Imposes a tax on employer-sponsored health insurance plans with aggregate expenses that exceed $10,800 for individual coverage or $29,050 for family coverage.

Although it is the responsibility of the CBO to estimate the cost of legislation as it is written, time-bound cost estimates (e.g., a 10-year estimate) have their limitations. First, the CBO must assume that all the provisions in the bill will be implemented as written. One of the most unpopular cost-saving tools—a tax on more generous health insurance plans—is not slated to take effect until 2018. Second, because the 10-year estimate, by design, does not consider costs beyond the first decade, some expected costs are not included in the estimate. Third, different methodologies may be used to calculate costs. Fourth, cost estimates cannot account for provisions that are left out of a bill. For these reasons, cost estimates should not be taken as the final word on the cost of any bill, because changes in political will can undermine the best projections.

Public Health, Workforce, Prevention, and Quality

The ACA also includes a variety of programs and pilot projects that focus on improving quality of care and increasing access to preventive care. These provisions show both a commitment to these issues and the limitations of that commitment. For example, the Prevention and Public Health Fund was created to improve the nation's public health and is scheduled to provide $14 billion to support these activities from 2018 to 2027 (HHS, 2016). Congress, however, has the ability to redirect resources, and the prevention fund lost over $6 billion in 2012 when money intended for the fund was used to offset a scheduled reduction in Medicare physician payments, and it lost another $68 million in 2016 due to budget sequestration (HHS, 2017; Trust for America's Health, 2017). In addition, while task forces and pilot programs can be useful tools to try out new ideas and gather data to inform future changes, their temporary nature can also mean that progress ends once the experiment is over, especially in tight budget times. Whether these steps lead to lasting reform and needed change in the delivery of health care and in public health practice remains to be seen.

The ACA includes a tax on insurers for more generous health plans. Because it is likely insurers will pass on the cost of the tax to consumers, the idea behind the tax is to provide incentives for people to choose lower-cost plans. In theory, the less money employers spend on healthcare costs (and other fringe benefits), the more they will spend on wages. The income tax paid for by workers on their higher wages will provide revenue that can be used to pay for health reform. In addition, people may be less likely to obtain unnecessary care if fewer services are covered by their plan or if cost-sharing is higher.

Is it likely that employers will trade lower benefits for higher wages? Are there times or industries where this trade-off is more or less likely to occur?

In 2017 the average cost of premiums for an employer plan was $6,690 for single coverage and $18,764 for family coverage (KFF & HRET, 2017, Section 1). Beginning in 2020, plans that exceed $10,800 for individual coverage and $29,050 for family coverage are taxed. Congress rejected lower thresholds for the tax ($8,500/$23,000) that would have raised an estimated $149 billion. Did Congress pick the right thresholds for the tax? Should they be higher or lower?

Why did Congress delay implementation of the tax until 2020? What are the pros and cons to having the tax start well after the main provisions of health reform are in place?

The ACA includes a wide range of quality improvement activities that fall into three main categories: evaluating new models of delivering health care, shifting reimbursement from volume to quality, and improving the overall system (Abrams et al., 2015). New models of healthcare delivery include accountable care organizations, which combine a variety of providers who collectively assume responsibility for the cost and quality of patient care, and patient-centered medical homes, which provide comprehensive and coordinated primary care. Reimbursement reforms include strategies such as penalizing hospitals with high rates of hospital-acquired infections or providing bonuses or penalties based on performance on quality measurements. Finally, overall system improvement efforts are highlighted by the National Strategy for Quality Improvement and the Patient-Centered Outcomes Research Institute (PCORI). The priorities of the National Strategy for Quality Improvement include improving delivery of healthcare services, patient outcomes, and population health. PCORI, a comparative effectiveness institute, was created to consider the clinical effectiveness of medical treatments. The idea behind comparative effectiveness is to determine which procedures, devices, and pharmaceuticals provide the best value for a given outcome. The institute is designed to supply information to help providers, patients, and others make decisions; Congress has stipulated, however, that findings from the institute may not be construed as mandates or recommendations for payment, coverage, or treatment decisions.

The ACA also provides funds to promote public health, wellness, and a stable and high-quality healthcare workforce. In addition to the Public Health and Prevention Fund, the law calls for the creation of a new regular corps and ready reserve corps to assist when public health emergencies occur. Also, a variety of programs and incentives are in place to promote employer wellness programs. Finally, the workforce shortage is addressed through graduate medical education reforms that promote primary care training; increases in scholarships and loans to support primary care providers and workforce diversity; and education, training, and loan repayment programs to address the primary care nursing shortage.

▶ The U.S. Supreme Court's Decision in the Case of *National Federation of Independent Business v. Sebelius*

In November 2011, in the first of what would be several ACA-related decisions, the U.S. Supreme Court agreed to decide four issues related to the legality of the ACA, two of which remain relevant for purposes of this text: (1) whether Congress had the power under the federal Constitution to enact the individual insurance coverage requirement and (2) whether it was unconstitutionally coercive for Congress, through the ACA, to threaten to take away existing federal Medicaid funding from states that did not want to implement the Medicaid expansion.

In June of the following year, the court handed down a remarkable 5–4 decision in the case of *National Federation of Independent Business, et al., v. Sebelius, Secretary of Health and Human Services, et al.* The opinion was surprising for two reasons: it defied expectation—few people thought that the entirety of the ACA would be found constitutional by a majority of the court—and Chief Justice Roberts, a conservative, ended up in the majority with the court's relatively liberal members (Justices Ginsburg, Breyer, Sotomayor, and Kagan).

BOX 10-9 Discussion Questions

There is a debate about the proper age at which to start regular mammogram screenings to detect breast cancer in women who do not have specific risk factors for the disease. As of 2009, the U.S. Preventive Services Task Force recommends waiting until age 50 years to begin mammogram screening for breast cancer and further recommends that screening should occur every 2 years. It also stated, however, that the final decision about the initial timing and frequency of breast cancer screening should be made by the patient and her physician. In making its recommendations, the Task Force found that physicians would need to screen 1,000 women to save 1 woman's life and concluded that earlier and/or more frequent screening was not worth the harm associated with false positives (anxiety, unnecessary biopsies, overtreatment). Other organizations disagree with the U.S. Preventive Services Task Force and conclude that the lifesaving effects of more routine mammogram screening outweigh the potential harm. Thus, the American Cancer Society recommends having routine annual mammograms from age 45 to 54 years (or 40 if the patient so chooses) and then every 2 years thereafter. The American College of Obstetricians and Gynecologists recommends starting annual mammograms at age 40 years.

The idea of comparative effectiveness research is to provide information about the value of different tools. Once that information is available, however, who should make the decisions about whether to provide coverage and reimbursement for a particular good or service? Can one objectively assess the potential harms and benefits associated with mammograms or other services or medications? Should decisions be made solely by the patient and treating provider? Does it matter if decisions affect taxpayers (for example, if a patient is covered by a government program such as Medicare or the Veterans Administration)?

Sources: United States Preventive Services Taskforce. (2016, January). Breast cancer: Screening. Retrieved from https://www.uspreventiveservicestaskforce.org/Page /Document/UpdateSummaryFinal/breast-cancer-screening1?ds=1&s=breast%20cancer; American College of Obstetricians and Gynecologists. (2016, January 11). ACOG statement on breast cancer screening guidelines. Retrieved from https://www.acog.org/About -ACOG/News-Room/Statements/2016/ACOG-Statement-on-Breast-Cancer-Screening -Guidelines; American Cancer Society (n.d.). American Cancer Society guidelines for the early detection of cancer. Retrieved July 19, 2018 from https://www.cancer.org/healthy /find-cancer-early/cancer-screening-guidelines/american-cancer-society-guidelines-for -the-early-detection-of-cancer.html

The court first tackled the question of whether Congress exceeded its authority in effectively forcing most everyone to carry health insurance. It concluded, not totally unexpectedly given the outcome of the court's more recent Commerce Clause decisions (*United States v. Lopez*, 1995), that the "individual mandate" amounted to an unconstitutional reach on the part of federal legislators:

> The individual mandate . . . does not regulate existing commercial activity. It instead compels individuals to become active in commerce by purchasing a product, on the ground that their failure to do so affects interstate commerce. Construing the commerce clause to permit congress to regulate individuals precisely because they are doing nothing would open a new and potentially vast domain to congressional authority. (*NFIB*, 2012, p. 2587)

Surprisingly, however, the court's analysis of the constitutionality of the individual mandate did not end there. The court majority pivoted to Congress's power to tax, and ruled that under this separate power, the individual mandate passed constitutional muster. The court wrote:

> The exaction the Affordable Care Act imposes on those without health insurance [i.e., the financial penalty assessed on those who do not obtain minimum health insurance coverage] looks like a tax in many respects. . . . In distinguishing penalties from taxes, this Court has explained that "if the concept of penalty means anything, it means punishment for an unlawful actor omission." While the individual mandate clearly aims to induce the purchase of health insurance, it need not be read to declare that failing to do so is unlawful. Neither the Act nor any other law attaches negative legal consequences to not buying health insurance, beyond requiring a payment to the IRS. (*NFIB*, 2012, p. 2595)

Read together, the Supreme Court's analysis of the individual mandate under the Commerce Clause and the Taxing and Spending Clause leads to the following conclusion: although Congress could not outright *command* Americans to buy health insurance, it could *tax* those who choose not to.

Next, the court turned its attention to whether the ACA's Medicaid expansion was structured in a way that effectively, and unlawfully, coerced states into adopting it. Fully half of the states in the country—the 26 that sued to halt implementation of the ACA—believed the answer to be "yes." As originally passed into law, the ACA allowed the secretary of HHS to terminate *all* of a state's Medicaid funding in the event that the state failed to implement the Medicaid expansion—even

those Medicaid funds that a state would receive that were unconnected to the expansion. This, the states argued, amounted to a coercively unacceptable choice: either adopt the ACA Medicaid expansion or potentially receive no federal Medicaid financing at all. As a result, they asked the court to rule that the Medicaid expansion itself was unconstitutional.

The court responded to this argument in two ways. On the one hand, it determined that the Medicaid expansion itself was perfectly constitutional; on the other hand, the court ruled that it was indeed unconstitutional for HHS to penalize states that did not adopt the expansion by terminating all Medicaid funding:

> The Constitution simply does not give Congress the authority to require the States to regulate. That is true whether Congress directly commands a State to regulate or indirectly coerces a State to adopt a federal regulatory system as its own. . . . When, for example, such conditions take the form of threats to terminate other significant independent grants, the conditions are properly viewed as a means of pressuring the States to accept policy changes. . . . Nothing in our opinion precludes Congress from offering funds under the Affordable Care Act to expand the availability of healthcare, and requiring that States accepting such funds comply with the conditions on their use. What Congress is not free to do is to penalize States that choose not to participate in that new program by taking away their existing Medicaid funding. (*NFIB*, 2012, pp. 2602–2607)

This twin ruling had the effect of making the ACA Medicaid expansion optional rather than mandatory, and states have been deciding individually whether to implement it. As of the time of this writing, 33 states and the District of Columbia have adopted the ACA's Medicaid expansion, while 17 states have not adopted the expansion (though note that the latter number is noticeably lower than the number of states [26] that originally argued in *NFIB v. Sebelius* that the Medicaid expansion was unconstitutionally coercive) (Advisory Board, 2018).

▶ States and Health Reform

Before the ACA and in the wake of numerous failed attempts at national health reform, states had been active players in health reform. Filling the gap left by the lack of federal action, states took steps to experiment with individual mandates, employer mandates, small business pools, and programs to reduce the number of uninsured. Although the ACA is a federal law, it is full of state obligations and opportunities for state innovation. Even though governors in many states have expressed opposition to health reform, numerous states will expend significant efforts toward continued implementation of the ACA over the next several years. States will have their hands full developing and running health insurance exchanges, regulating the private health insurance market, and implementing Medicaid changes.

The Supreme Court's decision to transform the ACA's Medicaid expansion from a mandatory program change to a state option has significant ramifications. As noted above, 33 states and the District of Columbia have chosen to expand Medicaid. As a result, by February 2017 there were 16 million more enrollees than prior to the ACA, with most new enrollment occurring in expansion states (Medicaid CHIP Payment and Access Commission, n.d.). Not surprisingly, expansion states have witnessed significant increases in Medicaid enrollment, both among newly eligible enrollees and individuals who were previously eligible but nonetheless unenrolled. This latter group is a result of the "welcome mat" or "woodwork" effect, when increases, incentives, and outreach result in more previously eligible individuals joining the program (Antonisse, Garfield, Rudowitz, & Artiga, 2018). The number of new Medicaid beneficiaries will ultimately depend on how many states eventually choose to expand their Medicaid program.

The court's decision drastically changed the blueprint of health reform. The ACA was designed assuming Medicaid expansion in every state, meaning there would be uniform coverage across the country for individuals earning below 138% of the federal poverty level. Under this plan, Medicaid would provide insurance for the lowest-income individuals, while state exchanges (with the assistance of federal subsidies) and employer-sponsored insurance would provide coverage for those who had higher earnings. It is now estimated that in states that do not expand their Medicaid program, 2.2 million people with incomes below the poverty line will remain uninsured because their incomes are too high to qualify for the state's traditional Medicaid program, yet too low to be able to afford private insurance in the exchanges because they do not qualify for subsidies (because it was assumed Medicaid would be expanded nationally, premium subsidies are available only for individuals earning at least 100% of poverty). The vast majority of them (89%) live in the South, reflecting that region's population demographics (e.g., more poor uninsured adults,

higher uninsured rate) and resistance to Medicaid expansion (Garfield, Damico, & Orgera, 2018).

As noted earlier, the Trump administration's policy choices have put states at the center of health reform. The administration is providing states with a variety of tools that increase a state's ability to mold its health insurance market and Medicaid program. For example, political leaders in states that embrace more liberal positions may counter the administration's policies by using state insurance regulations to block short-term plans, implement a state-based individual mandate, and maintain a generous definition of EHBs. Discussions in some left-leaning states involve creating a public option to compete with private insurers and allowing uninsured individuals to buy into Medicaid (Brownstein, 2018). In states with more conservative leaders, it is likely that health insurance products that are not required to meet ACA requirements will flourish and that Medicaid waivers that include features such as work requirements and provisions that allow beneficiaries to be locked out for administrative reasons will be implemented (Brownstein, 2018; Quinn, 2018). As a result, the health insurance landscape is moving closer to pre-ACA days, when the cost and content of one's insurance plan depended on where one lived.

▶ Key Issues Going Forward

At the time of this writing, the Republican effort to repeal and replace the ACA has stalled. Many in the party want to keep working toward that goal, while others, including the Senate leadership, appear ready to focus on other matters. President Trump appears to support efforts to continue to reform health reform but does not any longer seem to be making it a priority. Of course, the political landscape could change dramatically after the 2018 midterm elections. If Democrats gain control of either the House or the Senate, or even gain a significant number of seats, it is unlikely Congress would pass a major reform bill. If Republicans maintain a sizeable majority in the House and pick up a few seats in the Senate, a new Congress may approve the bills that were defeated in 2017. Assuming Congress does not repeal and replace the ACA, it is unclear whether the Trump administration's executive actions will result in the ACA's "death by 1,000 cuts," or whether Congress's inability to repeal the law will eventually cement the ACA as an accepted part of the fabric that holds together our healthcare and public health systems. Until the ACA's future becomes clearer, we discuss here a few major political and implementation issues that will likely dominate the health reform discussion in the near term.

Congressional Activity

The Republicans gained control of both chambers of Congress and of the White House in the 2016 election and spent the better part of the spring and summer in 2017 wrestling with ACA repeal and replacement bills. After 7 years of campaigning on (and winning with) a platform that included repealing and replacing the ACA, Republican legislators felt a strong obligation to keep their promise. While the party was unified in its opposition to the ACA, it was less successful agreeing on a replacement plan. With a slim majority in the Senate (52 Republicans, 48 Democrats) and no Democrats supporting this effort, Republicans found it impossible to meet the demands of moderate Republicans who wanted to protect the ACA's insurance gains and conservative Republicans who wanted to eliminate as many ACA requirements, regulations, and taxes as possible. Republicans faced a similar dilemma in the House, but were able to succeed in passing a reform bill because they had a little more room for disagreement. They could tolerate 21 Republican defectors and still pass a bill without support from the Democrats. Even though Republicans were not successful in 2017 in passing a bill the House and Senate could agree on, it is worthwhile to consider the substance and politics of that debate to understand what Republicans hope to achieve when altering the ACA and how the 2018 midterm elections could affect the future of health reform.

After much political drama, including one failed vote, the House passed its ACA replacement bill, the American Health Care Act of 2017 (AHCA), on May 4, 2017 by a narrow 217–213 margin. Every Democrat and 20 Republicans voted against the bill. In the Senate, Republicans drafted the Better Care Reconciliation Act of 2017 (BCRA) as a substitution amendment to replace the AHCA. The BCRA followed the same general contours of the AHCA. After barely mustering sufficient support to proceed with debate on the bill, the Senate voted against the BCRA on July 25, 2017. All Democrats and nine Republicans opposed the bill (Fox, Lee, Mattingly, & Barrett, 2017). The next day, all Democrats and seven Republicans also voted against a bill that would have simply repealed the ACA (effective in 2 years) and did not include any type of replacement (Lee & Mattingly, 2017). This repeal-only bill actually passed Congress while President Obama was in office, but because members of Congress who voted for repeal knew that Obama would veto the bill,

it was considered a protest vote more than an agreement on a policy position.

During the 2017 Senate debate, Sen. John McCain (R-AZ), who at the time had been recently diagnosed with aggressive brain cancer (and who died in late August 2018 while still a member of the Senate), provided a moment of high drama. His "no" vote was the third Republican vote (along with those of Sens. Lisa Murkowski [R-AL] and Susan Collins [R-ME]) that ultimately doomed what was referred to as the "skinny repeal" option (Fox, 2017). The skinny repeal option eliminated just the individual and employer mandates as well as a tax on medical devices. It was a bill that few actually wanted to become law, and it was projected to increase premiums and drastically reduce the number of insured individuals. Even the senators who voted for the bill did so only after assurances that the House would not pass it. Why, then, move forward with a bill few supported? The goal was to reach a "conference committee" wherein the House and Senate could work to reach a repeal-and-replace compromise, which would then be sent back to each chamber for approval. At that point, the political pressure to support a compromise bill would have been immense. The vote for the skinny repeal bill was a vote to keep the health reform debate alive, but risked a result that few desired. In voting against this strategy, the three Republican senators who voted "no" urged their colleagues to move forward in a bipartisan manner and to follow regular order in the Senate (e.g., holding hearings, passing bills through committee).

Even though the primary legislative bills—the AHCA and BCRA—did not have sufficient support across Congress to become law, and some of their provisions may not have been allowed under reconciliation rules, it is worth considering the main features of the bills to understand the type of health reform changes many Republicans support (**TABLE 10-4**). Overall, these bills reduced taxes, eliminated government mandates, lowered federal government spending, lowered premiums for some people while increasing them for others, phased out the Medicaid expansion under the ACA, and ended Medicaid as an entitlement program. According to the CBO, the effect of the bills would be to significantly increase the number of uninsured, significantly reduce the deficit, lower costs for young and healthy consumers, and increase costs for older and poorer consumers (CBO, 2017a; CBO, 2017b).

Major industry players and a clear majority of the public opposed the proposed bills to repeal and replace the ACA. Industry groups such as hospitals, physicians, safety net providers, and insurers were concerned about the health and financial effects of

TABLE 10-4 Comparison of U.S. House and Senate Bills Designed to Replace the Affordable Care Act

	American Health Care Act (House)	**Better Care Reconciliation Act (Senate)**
Premium tax credits	Replaces with tax credits based on age only, not income or geographic area	Keeps tax credits, lowers eligibility to 350% FPL, includes those under 100% FPL, tied to less expensive benchmark, changes individual contribution levels so older consumers pay more
Individual mandate	Eliminates penalties, replaces with 1-year 30% premium surcharge if lapse in coverage	Eliminates penalties, replaces with 6-month waiting period if lapse in coverage
Employer mandate	Eliminates penalties	Eliminates penalties
Medicaid expansion	Phases out at end of 2019	Phases out by end of 2024
ACA taxes	Eliminates most key taxes	Eliminates many key taxes, keeps Medicare surtax and investment tax on high-income earners
Essential health benefits	Allows state waivers to redefine	Allows state waivers to redefine
Medicaid program	Changes to block grant or per-capita allotment in 2020, allows work requirements	Changes to block grant or per-capita allotment in 2020, allows work requirements
CSR funds	Funds through 2019, repeals in 2020	Funds through 2019, repeals in 2020
Women's health services	Defunds Planned Parenthood for 1 year; redefines qualified plan to exclude plans that provide abortion services except for rape, incest, or life of mother in danger	Defunds Planned Parenthood for 1 year; redefines qualified plan to exclude plans that provide abortion services except for rape, incest, or life of mother in danger
Private market rules	Keeps guaranteed issue, dependent coverage until 26; keeps preexisting condition protection	Keeps guaranteed issue, dependent coverage until 26; keeps preexisting condition protection; permits sale of noncompliant plans as long as selling one ACA-compliant plan
State stabilization pool	Provides $123 billion over 9 years	Provides $182 billion over 9 years
Public health prevention fund	Eliminates	Eliminates
Age rating band	Changes to 5-to-1 but allows for state variation	Changes to 5-to-1 but allows for state variation
CBO estimate—uninsured	23 million more uninsured by 2026	22 million more uninsured by 2026
CBO estimate—federal savings	$119 billion	$321 billion

ACA = Affordable Care Act; CBO = Congressional Budget Office; FPL = federal poverty level.

the bills, while key conservative groups (e.g., Heritage Foundation, Club for Growth) did not think the bills made sufficient changes (Watkins, 2017). While 64% of respondents in one poll indicated either a preference to keep the ACA as it is or to modify it, a clear partisan divide existed (Kirzinger, DiJulio, Wu, & Brodie, 2017). Nine out of 10 Democrats supported keeping or modifying the ACA, while only 3 out of 10 Republicans agreed. Most Republicans (about 75%) indicated they wanted the ACA repealed and replaced at some point (Kahn & Erhman, 2017). For these reasons, it is not surprising that many Republican legislators feared the ramifications of disappointing their conservative base and donors by not repealing the ACA more than they feared whatever hazards awaited if they supported a bill that was unpopular with their constituencies.

One thing Congress has not tried yet is a bipartisan approach. A clear majority of the public (71%) strongly prefers for Republicans and Democrats to work together on health reform, and a number of legislators from both sides of the aisle have indicated a desire to do so (Kirzinger et al., 2017). While a partisan divide remains here as well, 41% of all Republicans and 46% of Trump supporters would like to see the parties work together (Kirzinger et al., 2017). After the failed Senate efforts, Sen. Lamar Alexander (R-TN), Chair of the Senate committee on Health, Education, Labor and Pensions, agreed to open bipartisan hearings on fixing the individual marketplace (Park, 2017). In addition, a group of bipartisan legislators from the House announced a plan to improve the ACA. Their strategy includes paying low-income CSRs to insurers, providing federal funds to the states to create reinsurance funds and other programs to lower premiums, applying the employer mandate to employers with 500 (instead of 50) or more employees, redefining full-time employees as those who work 40 hours per week, obtaining clarification from HHS about a section 1332 waiver process, and repealing the medical device tax (Lee, 2017). They also recommend offsetting the federal funds spent on these ideas, but do not indicate how current funding should be cut.

The political difficulty of repealing and replacing the ACA is not surprising. It is always difficult to take away benefits once people have started to use them. Supporting a bill that would result in over 20 million people losing insurance is clearly more politically perilous than not supporting legislation (i.e., the ACA) that would deliver health insurance to 20 million people for the first time. This is particularly true for federal legislators who hail from states that (1) implemented the ACA's Medicaid expansion and (2) have Republican governors. Why? Much of the savings

from the House and Senate bills came from reduced Medicaid spending, both through the elimination of the expansion and by changing the entire program from an entitlement program to a block grant or per-capita allotment. In turn, states would either have had to absorb the federal spending reductions in their own budgets or absorb the healthcare costs of having more uninsured residents. Indeed, the proposed changes to Medicaid, which went well beyond repealing and replacing the ACA, resulted in many of the biggest criticisms from moderate Republicans. Also, Medicaid has become even more important to the nation now that it is grappling with an opioid epidemic, because Medicaid and CHIP cover approximately one-third of individuals with an opioid addiction. This is nearly double the share covered by Medicaid in 2005, and the increase is mostly due to the ACA Medicaid expansion (KFF, 2017d).

The Senate Republican leadership also made a difficult political situation even harder by alienating several of their own members when the leadership decided that the ACA repeal bills would be drafted in relative secret, ignored regular process (by not holding hearings, debates, mark-ups), used reconciliation to avoid a filibuster, and expected their members to vote on bills they had little time to review. Sen. John Cornyn (R-TX), the second-ranking Republican in the Senate, went so far as to say that knowing prior to the start of debate which bill the Republicans would be voting on was "a luxury we don't have" (Sullivan, 2017). This was a hard pill to swallow for many Republicans who vilified the Democrats for their partisan approach to passing the ACA and who mocked then-House Speaker Nancy Pelosi (D-CA) for saying, "we have to pass the healthcare bill so that you can find out what's in it" (Capehart, 2010). While ultimately Republican leaders were not successful in getting the legislation passed, they decided that the negative ramifications of these hardball tactics were easier to survive than the negative publicity of a drawn-out process where opposition groups could mobilize their resources.

Insurance Plan Premium Rates

One of the key issues to monitor going forward is the affordability of health insurance plans under the ACA. Most people were pleasantly surprised by premium rates for 2014 and 2015, although there was a lot of variation across the country. Insurers had incentive to keep premiums low because they wanted to encourage people to enroll in their health plans. In addition, there was limited information about who would be in the insurance pools that could have assisted insurers with premium rate setting, and many plans contracted with a narrower set of providers as a way to keep premiums low. After moving past the initial enrollment period, will insurance companies hike premiums in future years?

Going into 2018, insurers were faced with significant uncertainty due to the political landscape. With Congress reviewing a variety of repeal-and-replace plans and the Trump administration threatening to let ACA reforms fail, insurers did not know what to expect in the upcoming year, and uncertainty is not something that makes for a stable health insurance market. As a result, insurers asked for delays in submitting premium rates, and some even submitted two rates depending on the outcome of certain political decisions (Mangan, 2017). Many insurers submitted requests for double-digit increases. For example, insurers in Maryland asked for rate increases ranging from 18% to 60%, and in Connecticut the range was 15% to 34%. Nevada requested an average rate hike of 38%, and Colorado's request was similar, with an average increase of 41% (Livingston, 2017; Luhby, 2017a). On average, 2018 premiums were expected to increase by 17% for bronze plans, 32% for silver plans, and 18% for gold plans (Semanskee, Claxton, & Leavitt, 2017).

There is continuing uncertainty going into 2019. Insurers have to contend with the unknown effect of factors that might lead to higher costs. Primary concerns that could lead to premium increases include the individual mandate penalty repeal, the defunding of CSR payments, policy changes (e.g., expanded short-term limited duration plans) that may result in sicker marketplace pools as healthier enrollees leave plans, varying estimates of medical inflation, and changes to the ACA's risk adjustment program (Corlette, 2018). Other factors may reduce premium costs, including suspension of a tax on health insurers, reduction of the corporate tax rate for insurers, the ability to offer less generous benefits, and state policies limiting short-term plans (Corlette, 2018). Based on limited early plan filings, it is estimated that silver plan premiums will increase 15% in 2019, with wide variation across the country. For example, the average silver plan is expected to decrease by 5% in Minnesota, increase by 16% in New York, and increase by 53% in Maryland (Brantley & Brooker, 2018).

The fate of the risk adjustment program is an issue insurers are watching closely. This program was created to remove incentives for insurers to try to enroll healthy consumers over unhealthy ones. The program transfers funds from non-grandfathered plans in the small and individual market with healthier enrollees to those plans with less healthy enrollees. While states may choose to run their own risk adjustment program, none have chosen to do so at this time (Keith, 2018a).

Due to conflicting court decisions regarding the risk adjustment formula, CMS suspended risk adjustment payment transfers from 2014 to 2018 (Keith, 2018a). About 3 weeks later, the Trump administration reversed course due to fears over the financial consequences for insurers. This type of uncertainty makes it difficult for insurers to establish viable operations in the health insurance market.

Reinsurance is another tool that could help insurers reduce premiums. Insurers or companies may purchase reinsurance to protect themselves against losses from high-cost enrollees—losses that would lead to premium increases for everyone in the pool (Swartz, 2017). Essentially, insurers take out a policy to protect against costs in a certain segment of an individual's coverage (e.g., costs between $100,000 and $200,000). As with most insurance, the health insurer will pay an annual premium for this reinsurance, a deductible before reinsurance takes effect, and a co-payment once the deductible is met (Swartz, 2017). Even so, it is cheaper for the insurer to pay the costs of reinsurance instead of the full cost of care for a high-risk enrollee. By keeping costs down, insurers reduce not only premiums for enrollees, but also premium tax credits paid by the federal government. For that reason, the federal government has an incentive to promote reinsurance programs. The Trump administration appears to favor reinsurance programs and sent a letter to the governors encouraging them to establish one through an ACA section 1332 State Innovation waiver (Clark, n.d.).

In the last few years, 19 states either introduced legislation to create their own reinsurance program (9 enacted) or applied for a §1332 waiver (Clark, n.d.). Section 1332 waivers allow states to finance part of the reinsurance program with a "federal pass-through" from the savings attributed to lower premiums (Clark, n.d.). As of July 2018, only Alaska, Minnesota, and Oregon have an approved waiver, with the federal government covering 97% (AK), 61% (MN), and 48% (OR) of the costs, respectively (Clark, n.d.). The programs are effective, with premium increases in Alaska dropping from 42% to 7% and premiums in Minnesota going from a 67% increase to a 15% decrease (Clark, n.d.). While these results are promising, many states cannot afford to establish a program because they have to front the entire cost and wait for the federal government to reimburse its share. The programs are indeed expensive; Minnesota's program cost $271 million and Oregon's cost $90 million (Clark, n.d.). Even if states are able to establish a program and obtain federal funding, there is always the concern whether state and federal funding will be available in future years.

In the end, the political uncertainty relating to the ACA, the various executive actions that have the potential to undermine the marketplaces, and the uncertainty surrounding ongoing litigation have created a difficult business environment for health insurance plans. There remains debate about whether the exchanges are collapsing or stabilizing in the wake of these concerns. While several analyses show a stabilizing market, continued subsidy support and increased enrollment of healthier individuals are key factors to the long-term success of the exchanges (National Academy for State Health Policy, 2018; Semanskee, Cox, & Leavitt, 2018; Zeitlin, 2017).

ACA Litigation

Legal challenges to and about the ACA have been a fixture since the law's passage in 2010; there have been countless ACA cases brought in both state and federal courts. A small handful of them even reached the U.S. Supreme Court, a rarity for a law that is relatively young. First there was the Supreme Court's decision in *NFIB v. Sebelius*, which was described earlier in this chapter (*NFIB v. Sebelius*, 2012). Then the court decided a case that answered whether, under a federal statute called the Religious Freedom Restoration Act (RFRA), closely held private corporations have a legal right to refuse to comply with provisions of the ACA that require them to provide certain contraceptive coverage to employees (*Burwell v. Hobby Lobby Sores, Inc.*, 2014). (A closely held corporation is one that has a limited number of shareholders; in the *Hobby Lobby* case, the plaintiffs were two private, for-profit companies owned by members of a single family—Hobby Lobby Stores [owned by Evangelical Christians] and Conestoga Wood Specialties [owned by Mennonites]). In a 5–4 decision, the court majority determined that the ACA's contraception mandate imposed a significant enough burden on the plaintiff companies' exercise of their beliefs so as to violate RFRA. Just a year later, the Supreme Court ruled that subsidies available under the ACA to help individuals and small businesses buy insurance were available whether the insurance was purchased through a state-run or federally facilitated insurance exchange (*King v. Burwell*, 2015).

Then just a year after that, the court heard a case that is an offshoot of its earlier decision in *Burwell v. Hobby Lobby* (*Zubik v. Burwell*, 2016). After the *Hobby Lobby* decision, the Obama administration offered an accommodation to religious entities that objected to the requirement to provide contraceptive coverage without cost-sharing: the religious organization could simply inform HHS of its objection and identify its insurer, at which point HHS would take responsibility for ensuring that contraceptive services are provided

by the insurer without the involvement of the religious organization. The accommodation, however, was not acceptable to a number of religious entities, which filed their own RFRA lawsuits. Over time, nine federal appellate courts ruled that the accommodation did not substantially burden the entities' exercise of religion; however, one appellate court ruled the opposite way, creating a division that the Supreme Court wanted to clear up. Eventually, the Supreme Court—likely split 4–4 on the merits by this time (i.e., after Justice Scalia died and the Senate failed to hold hearings on his replacement) and hoping to spark a compromise among the litigants—remanded the cases to the lower courts without a definitive answer.

At the time of this writing, this issue is still being litigated. In October 2017, the Trump administration issued interim final rules offering any for-profit or nonprofit employer or insurer that objected to contraceptives for religious reasons an absolute exemption (i.e., without the need to notify the government or insurers) from providing contraceptive coverage to its employees. However, the legality of these rules has been called into question. One federal judge held (1) that the administration unlawfully bypassed a law (the Administrative Procedure Act, or APA) requiring federal agencies to adopt rules only after notice and an opportunity for public comment and (2) that the rules were likely substantively improper as well, because they lacked sufficient clarity and a proper legal basis. A different federal judge has also found that the rules violated the APA. Appeals by the Trump administration are likely.

At the time of this writing, two other ACA-related lawsuits bear mentioning (space limitations prevent us from discussing *all* of the ongoing ACA litigation). The first is a lawsuit brought by 20 Republican-led states that effectively contends that given the repeal of the individual mandate financial penalty (discussed previously), the entire ACA must fall (*Texas v. United States*, 2018). How do Texas and their counterparts reach this conclusion? They argue that absent the monetary fine for not having health insurance, the requirement to buy insurance has no legal basis, and because the insurance mandate is central to the ACA architecture, the entire law should be thrown out.

As if the lawsuit itself was not enough of a threat to the ACA, a different type of threat emerged in June 2018 when the Trump administration alerted the federal trial court hearing the case that it would not defend the ACA in court. While politically speaking this might not seem like a big deal to most readers, this decision in fact represents a dramatic break from the executive branch's tradition of defending existing statutes. While the Justice Department's filing with the trial court acknowledges that the decision not to defend an existing law deviates from history, it contends that its decision is not unprecedented. In turn, Democratic state attorneys general from 16 states and the District of Columbia have been allowed to intervene in the case to defend the ACA. Needless to say, this case will probably be on the legal radar for the foreseeable future, given the likely appeals that will follow decisions in both the federal trial and appellate courts.

The second case worth noting is perhaps more theoretical than *Texas v. United States*, but it is interesting because it stands in stark contrast to that lawsuit. In early August 2018, four cities filed a lawsuit arguing that President Trump's attempts to undermine the ACA violate his duties under the federal Constitution (*City of Columbus v. Trump*, 2018). According to the plaintiffs, a president's obligation under Article II of the Constitution to "take Care that the laws be faithfully executed" is violated by President Trump's "sabotage" of the ACA. Plaintiffs further contend that HHS is complicit in this sabotage, and that this violates both the Administrative Procedure Act and President Trump's duty under the Constitution to ensure that laws passed by Congress are faithfully executed.

To be sure, the Constitution's "take care" clause, as it is known, is rarely invoked, much less successfully. Cases of this sort are rare because the president is granted discretion with respect to how he and his administration enforce a law, and thus drawing lines that separate "faithful" from unreasonable discretion can be extremely difficult. Nonetheless, in these incredibly politicized times, this case is also worth following.

Given these and other lawsuits (both pending and still to come), it is unlikely that the Supreme Court

has cleared the ACA from its docket. However, irrespective of whether the Supreme Court hands down ACA-related cases in the future, what bears keeping in mind is that judicial decisions may continue to shape the contours of the ACA for years to come.

▶ Conclusion

After decades of trying and against the predictions of numerous experts, the United States passed a health reform law that provides insurance coverage on a more universal scale than ever before, includes protections for individuals who have been historically excluded from the insurance market, and shows a concern for improving healthcare quality and access to preventive care. From a philosophical perspective, the ACA moves America toward a society where (almost) everyone is expected to have adequate access to affordable health insurance. Under this perspective, health insurance is considered both an obligation and a right: individuals are required to obtain insurance and the government is obligated to make it affordable and accessible.

At the same time, there remains in some quarters strong philosophical and political opposition to the ACA, which continues to be challenged both legislatively and in the courts. The Republican control of both Congress and the White House, and the Trump administration's policies undermining the ACA, have created a very uncertain future for health reform. Because of this opposition and because the ACA is still not close to engendering the type of support reserved for, say, Medicare, the full story of the ACA is far from being completed.

References

Abraham, J., & Royalty, A. B. (2017, January 19). *How has the Affordable Care Act affected work and wages?* Retrieved from https://ldi.upenn.edu/brief/how-has-affordable-care-act-affected-work-and-wages

Abrams, M. K., Nuzum, R., Zezza, M. A., Ryan, J., Kiszla, J., & Guterman, S. (2015, May 7). *The Affordable Care Act's payment and delivery reforms: A progress report at five years.* Retrieved from https://www.commonwealthfund.org/publications/issue-briefs/2015/may/affordable-care-acts-payment-and-delivery-system-reforms

Advisory Board. (2018, June 8). *Where the states stand on Medicaid expansion.* Retrieved from https://www.advisory.com/daily-briefing/resources/primers/medicaidmap

Affordable Health Care for America Act of 2009, H.R. 3962, 111th Cong. (2009).

Agiesta, J. (2017, March 7). *CNN/ORC poll: Public splits on revoking individual mandate.* Retrieved from https://www.cnn.com/2017/03/07/politics/health-care-replacement-poll/index.html

American Health Care Act of 2017, H.R. 1628, 115th Cong. (2017).

American Recovery and Reinvestment Act of 2009, Pub. L. No. 111-5, 123 Stat. 115 (2009).

Antonisse, L., Garfield, R., Rudowitz, R., & Artiga, S. (2018, March 28). *The effects of Medicaid expansion under the ACA: Updated findings from a literature review.* Retrieved from https://www.kff.org/medicaid/issue-brief/the-effects-of-medicaid-expansion-under-the-aca-updated-findings-from-a-literature-review-march-2018/

Appleby, J. (2008, December 20). Health reform up in the air as economy sinks. *USA Today.* Retrieved from https://usatoday30.usatoday.com/news/health/2008-12-18-health_N.htm

Aron-Dine, A. (2017, May 30). *CBO correctly predicted historic gains under ACA.* Retrieved from https://www.cbpp.org/blog/cbo-correctly-predicted-historic-coverage-gains-under-aca

Better Care Reconciliation Act of 2017, H.R. 1628, 115th Cong. (2017).

Blake, C. H., & Adolino, J. R. (2001). The enactment of national health insurance: A Boolean analysis of twenty advanced industrial countries. *Journal of Health Politics Policy and Law, 26*(4), 670–708. doi:10.1215/03616878-26-4-679

Blendon, R. J., Altman, D. E., Benson, J. M., Brodie, M., Buhr, T., Deane, C., & Buscho, S. (2008). Voters and health reform in the 2008 presidential election. *New England Journal of Medicine, 359*(19), 2050–2062. doi:10.1056/NEJMsr0807717

Blumberg, J., Holahan, J., & Buettgens, M. (2014, May 9). *Why not just eliminate the employer mandate?* Retrieved from https://www.urban.org/research/publication/why-not-just-eliminate-employer-mandate

Blumberg, J., Holahan, J., Karpman, M., & Elmendorf, C. (2018). *Characteristics of the remaining uninsured: An update.* Retrieved from https://www.urban.org/sites/default/files/publication/98764/2001914-characteristics-of-the-remaining-uninsured-an-update_0.pdf

Blumenthal, D., & Morone, J. A. (2009). *The heart of power: Health and politics in the Oval Office.* Berkeley, CA: University of California Press.

Brantley, K., & Brooker, C. (2018, June 21). *Double-digit premium increases expected in the exchange market in 2019.* Retrieved from http://avalere.com/expertise/managed-care/insights/double-digit-premium-increases-expected-in-the-exchange-market-in-2019

Brown, C. B., & O'Connor, P. (2010, January 21). The fallout: Democrats rethinking health care bill. *Politico.* Retrieved from https://www.politico.com/story/2010/01/fallout-dems-rethinking-health-bill-031693

Brownstein, R. (2018, March 8). The health care gap between red and blue America. *The Atlantic.* Retrieved from https://www.theatlantic.com/politics/archive/2018/03/obamacare-trump/555131/

Burke, C. (2013, December 17). *Rasmussen poll: Most Americans oppose ACA's individual mandate.* Retrieved from https://www.newsmax.com/Newsfront/Obamacare-majority-oppose-Rasmussen/2013/12/17/id/542447/

Burwell v. Hobby Lobby Stores, Inc., 134 S. Ct. 2751 (2014).

Capehart, J. (2010, June 12). Pelosi defends her infamous health care remark. *The Washington Post.* Retrieved from https://www.washingtonpost.com/blogs/post-partisan/post/pelosi-defends-her-infamous-health-care-remark/2012/06/20/gJQAqch6qV_blog.html?utm_term=.566e5b909d99

Center for Consumer Information and Insurance Oversight, Centers for Medicare and Medicaid Services. (2018, April 9). *Guidance on hardship exemptions from the individual shared responsibility provision for persons experiencing limited issuer options or other circumstances.* Retrieved from https://www.cms.gov/CCIIO/Resources/Regulations-and-Guidance/Downloads/2018-Hardship-Exemption-Guidance.pdf

Center on Budget and Policy Priorities. (2018). *Sabotage watch: Tracking efforts to undermine the ACA.* Retrieved from https://www.cbpp.org/sabotage-watch-tracking-efforts-to-undermine-the-aca

Centers for Medicare and Medicaid Services. (2017, May 15). *The future of SHOP: CMS intends to allow small businesses in SHOPs using Healthcare.gov more flexibility when enrolling in healthcare coverage.* Retrieved from https://www.cms.gov/CCIIO/Resources/Regulations-and-Guidance/Downloads/The-Future-of-the-SHOP-CMS-Intends-to-Allow-Small-Businesses-in-SHOPs-Using-HealthCaregov-More-Flexibility-when-Enrolling-in-Healthcare-Coverage.pdf

City of Columbus v. Trump, No. 18-cv-2364 (2018). Retrieved from https://democracyforward.org/wp-content/uploads/2018/08/ACA-Complaint.pdf

Clark, K. (n.d.). *States return to reinsurance to stabilize ACA marketplaces.* Retrieved from https://www.lexisnexis.com/communities/state-net/b/capitol-journal/archive/2018/05/11/states-return-to-reinsurance-to-stabilize-aca-marketplaces.aspx

Cohen, J., & Balz, D. (2009, September 14). Opposition to Obama's health reform plan is high, but easing. *Washington Post.* Retrieved from http://www.washingtonpost.com/wp-dyn/content/article/2009/09/13/AR2009091302962.html

Commercial Insurance. (2012, July). *Self-insured plans under health care reform.* Retrieved from http://www.ciswv.com/CIS/media/CISMedia/Documents/Self-Insured-Plans-Under-Health-Care-Reform-070312_1.pdf

Condon, S. (2010, January 20). *Scott Brown win shakes up health care fight.* Retrieved from https://www.cbsnews.com/news/scott-brown-win-shakes-up-health-care-fight/

Congressional Budget Office. (2017a). *American Health Care Act: Cost estimate.* Retrieved from https://www.cbo.gov/system/files?file=115th-congress-2017-2018/costestimate/americanhealthcareact.pdf

Congressional Budget Office. (2017b). *Better Care Reconciliation Act of 2017: Cost estimate.* Retrieved from https://www.cbo.gov/publication/52941

Congressional Budget Office. (2017c). *Federal subsidies under the Affordable Care Act for health insurance coverage related to the expansion of Medicaid and nongroup health insurance: Tables from CBOs January 2017 baseline.* Retrieved from http://acasignups.net/sites/default/files/CBO-2017-01-healthinsurance.pdf

Congressional Budget Office. (2017d). *Repealing the individual health insurance mandate: An updated estimate.* Retrieved from https://www.cbo.gov/system/files?file=115th-congress-2017-2018/reports/53300-individualmandate.pdf

Congressional Budget Office. (2018). *Federal subsidies for health insurance coverage for people under age 65: Tables from CBOs spring 2018 projections.* Retrieved from https://www.cbo.gov/system/files?file=2018-06/51298-2018-05-healthinsurance.pdf

Corlette, S. (2018, May 21). *The effect of federal policy: What early premium rate filings can tell us about the future of the Affordable Care Act.* Retrieved from http://chirblog.org/what-early-rate-filings-tell-us-about-future-of-aca/

Coverage of Certain Preventive Services Under the Affordable Care Act, 78 Fed. Reg. 127, 29870-29899 (July 2, 2013).

Department of Health and Human Services. (2016, December 16). *Prevention and public health fund.* Retrieved from https://www.hhs.gov/open/prevention/index.html

DiJulio, B., Kirzinger, A., Wu, B., & Brodie, M. (2017, March 2). *Data note: Americans' challenge with health care costs.* Retrieved from https://www.kff.org/health-costs/poll-finding/data-note-americans-challenges-with-health-care-costs/

Eibner, C., & Nowak, S. (2018, July 11). *The effect of eliminating the individual mandate penalty and the role of behavioral factors.* Retrieved from https://www.common wealthfund.org/publications/fund-reports/2018/jul/eliminating-individual-mandate-penalty-behavioral-factors

Emergency Economic Stabilization Act of 2008, Pub L. No. 110-343, 122 Stat. 3765 (2008).

Employee Retirement Security Income Act of 1974, Pub. L. No. 93-406, 88 Stat. 829 (1974).

Exchange establishment standards and other related standards under the Affordable Care Act, 177 Fed. Reg. 11718, 2012

Feder, J. (2004). Crowd-out and the politics of health reform. *Journal of Law, Medicine, and Ethics, 32*(3), 461-464. doi:10.1111/j.1748-720X.2004.tb00158.x

Fise, P. (2017, June 8). *Cost sharing reduction subsidies: What happens if they aren't paid?* Retrieved from https://bipartisanpolicy.org/blog/cost-sharing-reduction-subsidies-what-happens-if-they-arent-paid/

Fox, L. (2017, July 28). *John McCain's maverick moment.* Retrieved from https://www.cnn.com/2017/07/28/politics/john-mccain-maverick-health-care/index.html

Fox, L., Lee, M. J., Mattingly, P., & Barrett, T. (2017, July 26). *Senate rejects proposals to repeal and replace Obamacare.* Retrieved from http://cnnphilippines.com/world/2017/07/26/senate-rejects-proposal-to-repeal-and-replace-obamacare.html

Galewitz, P. (n.d.). *HHS targets young adults for Obamacare enrollment.* Retrieved from https://www.webmd.com/health-insurance/news/20160621/hhs-targets-young-adults-in-2017-obamacare-enrollment-plan

Garfield, R., Damico, A., & Orgera, K. (2018, June 12). *The coverage gap: Uninsured poor adults in states that do not expand Medicaid.* Retrieved from https://www.kff.org/medicaid/issue-brief/the-coverage-gap-uninsured-poor-adults-in-states-that-do-not-expand-medicaid/

Garrett, T. A. (2011, October 19). *State balanced-budget and debt rules.* Retrieved from https://files.stlouisfed.org/files/htdocs/publications/es/11/ES1133.pdf

Giovannelli, J., Lucia, K. W., & Corlette, S. (2014, October 31). *Implementing the Affordable Care Act: Revisiting the ACA's essential health benefits requirements.* Retrieved from https://www.commonwealthfund.org/publications/issue-briefs/2014/oct/implementing-affordable-care-act-revisiting-acas-essential

Giovannelli, J., Volk, J., Lucia, K. W., Williams, A., & Connor K. (2015, October 27). *States revisit insurer benefit requirements, but have little data on consumers' experiences.* Retrieved from https://www.commonwealthfund.org/blog/2015/states-revisit-insurer-benefit-requirements-have-little-data-consumers-experiences

Gonzales v. Raich, 545 U.S. 1 (2005).

Gordon, C. (2003). *Dead on arrival: The politics of health care in twentieth-century America.* Princeton, NJ: Princeton University Press.

Graham, D. A. (2017, July 28). "As I have always said": Trump's ever-changing positions on health care. *The Atlantic.* Retrieved from https://www.theatlantic.com/politics/archive/2017/07/as-i-have-always-said-trumps-ever-changing-position-on-health-care/535293/

Guttmacher Institute. (n.d.). *Abortion: Insurance coverage.* Retrieved from https://www.guttmacher.org/united-states/abortion/insurance-coverage

Guttmacher Institute. (2018a, June 1). *An overview of abortion laws.* Retrieved from https://www.guttmacher.org/state-policy/explore/overview-abortion-laws

Guttmacher Institute. (2018b, June 11). *Insurance coverage of contraceptives.* Retrieved from https://www.guttmacher.org/state-policy/explore/insurance-coverage-contraceptives

Hamel, L., Firth, J., & Brodie, M. (2014, April 29). *Kaiser health tracking poll—April 2014.* Retrieved from https://www.kff.org/health-reform/poll-finding/kaiser-health-tracking-poll-april-2014/

Health Insurance Issuers Implementing Medical Loss Ratio Requirements Under the Patient Protection and Affordable Care Act, 75 Fed. Reg. 74864 (2010).

Health Insurance Premium Tax Credit, 77 Fed. Reg., 30377 (2012, May 23).

Healthcare.gov. (n.d.). *Grandfathered health insurance plans.* Retrieved from https://www.healthcare.gov/health-care-law-protections/grandfathered-plans/

Heart of Atlanta Motel, Inc. v. United States, 379 U.S. 241 (1964).

HHS Notice of Benefit and Payment Parameters for 2019. 83 Fed. Reg. 74, 16930-17071 (2018, April 17).

Jones, J. M. (2010, October 26). *Economy top issue for voters: Size of gov't may be more pivotal.* Retrieved from https://news.gallup.com/poll/144029/economy-top-issue-voters-size-gov-may-pivotal.aspx

Jost, T. S. (2004). Why can't we do what they do? National health reform abroad. *Journal of Law, Medicine, and Ethics, 32*(3), 433–441. doi:10.1111/j.1748-720X.2004.tb00154

Jost, T. S. (2013). *Implementing health reform: Exemptions from the individual mandate.* Retrieved from https://www.healthaffairs.org/do/10.1377/hblog20130627.032474/full/

Jost, T. S. (2016, January 26). *CBO lowers marketplace enrollment predictions, increases Medicaid growth projections (updated).* Retrieved from https://www-healthaffairs-org.proxygw.wrlc.org/do/10.1377/hblog20160126.052850/full/

Jost, T. S. (2017, May 15). *CMS announces plans to effectively end the SHOP exchange.* Retrieved from https://www.healthaffairs.org/do/10.1377/hblog20170515.060112/full/

Kahn, H. (2010, January 22). Health care bill aftermath: Rep. Patrick Kennedy hails dad's dream; Sen. John McCain sees heavy price. *ABC News.* Retrieved from https://abcnews.go.com/GMA/HealthCare/health-care-congress-passes-landmark-reform-obama-sign/story?id=10167139

Kahn, C., & Erman, M. (2017, July 29). Exclusive: Majority of Americans want Congress to move on from health reform. *Reuters.* Retrieved from https://www.reuters.com/article/us-usa-healthcare-poll-idUSKBN1AE0RY

Kaiser Family Foundation. (n.d.) *Health reform FAQs.* Retrieved from https://www.kff.org/health-reform/faq/health-reform-frequently-asked-questions/#question-who-is-eligible-for-marketplace-premium-tax-credits

Kaiser Family Foundation. (2008). *Findings of Kaiser health tracking poll: Election 2008—October 2008.* Retrieved from https://www.kff.org/health-reform/poll-finding/findings-of-kaiser-health-tracking-poll-election/

Kaiser Family Foundation. (2009a). *Chartpack: Kaiser health tracking poll: November 2009.* Retrieved from https://www.kff.org/health-costs/poll-finding/chartpack-kaiser-health-tracking-poll-november-2009/

Kaiser Family Foundation. (2009b). *Kaiser health tracking poll: August 2009.* Retrieved from https://www.kff.org/health-costs/poll-finding/kaiser-health-tracking-poll-august-2009/

Kaiser Family Foundation. (2009c). *Key findings: Kaiser health tracking poll—September 2009.* Retrieved from https://www.kff.org/health-costs/poll-finding/key-findings-kaiser-health-tracking-poll-september/

Kaiser Family Foundation. (2017a, August 18). *Counties at risk for having no insurer on marketplace (Exchange) in 2018.* Retrieved from https://www.kff.org/interactive/counties-at-risk-of-having-no-insurer-on-the-marketplace-exchange-in-2018/

Kaiser Family Foundation. (2017b). *Kaiser health tracking poll—June 2017: ACA, replacement plan, and Medicaid.* Retrieved from https://www.kff.org/health-reform/poll-finding/kaiser-health-tracking-poll-june-2017-aca-replacement-plan-and-medicaid/

Kaiser Family Foundation. (2017c). *Kaiser health tracking poll - Novmber 2017: The politics of health insurance coverage, ACA open enrollment*. Retrieved from https://www.kff.org/health-reform/poll-finding/kaiser-health-tracking-poll-november-2017-the-politics-of-health-insurance-coverage-aca-open-enrollment/

Kaiser Family Foundation. (2017d). *The opioid epidemic and Medicaid's role in treatment: A look at changes over time*. Retrieved from https://www.kff.org/slideshow/the-opioid-epidemic-and-medicaids-role-in-treatment-a-look-at-changes-over-time/

Kaiser Family Foundation. (2018). *State health insurance marketplace types, 2018*. Retrieved from https://www.kff.org/health-reform/state-indicator/state-health-insurance-marketplace-types/?currentTimeframe=0&sortModel=%7B%22colId%22:%22Location%22,%22sort%22:%22asc%22%7D

Kaiser Family Foundation and Health Research Educational Trust. (2017, September 19). *2017 Employer health benefit survey*. Retrieved from https://www.kff.org/health-costs/report/2017-employer-health-benefits-survey/

Kamal, R., Semanskee, A., Long, M., Claxton, G., & Leavitt, L. (2017, October 27). *How the loss of cost sharing subsidy payments is affecting 2018 premiums*. Retrieved from https://www.kff.org/health-reform/issue-brief/how-the-loss-of-cost-sharing-subsidy-payments-is-affecting-2018-premiums/

Kardish, C. (2015, April 17). *Medicare deal delays but deepens hospital cuts*. Retrieved from http://www.governing.com/topics/health-human-services/gov-medicare-deal-delays-hospital-cuts.html

Keith, K. (2017, October 31). *Proposed 2019 Affordable Care Act payment rules: A big role for states*. Retrieved from http://chirblog.org/proposed-2019-affordable-care-act-payment-rule-big-role-states/

Keith, K. (2018a, July 17). *ACA round up: New risk adjustment guidance, New Jersey 1332 application, GAO report on Association Health Plans*. Retrieved from https://www.healthaffairs.org/do/10.1377/hblog20180717.450336/full/

Keith, K. (2018b, April 10). *New guidance on exemptions from the individual mandate*. Retrieved from https://www.healthaffairs.org/do/10.1377/hblog20180410.721972/full/

Keith, K. (2018c, July 19). *States' lawsuit over cost-sharing reductions is dismissed*. Retrieved from https://www.healthaffairs.org/do/10.1377/hblog20180719.822849/full/

Keith, K. (2018d, April 11). *Unpacking the 2019 final payment notice (part 2)*. Retrieved from https://www.healthaffairs.org/do/10.1377/hblog20180411.618457/full/

Kiley, J. (2017, June 23). *Public support for "single payer" health coverage grows, driven by Democrats*. Retrieved from http://www.pnhp.org/news/2017/june/new-gallup-and-pew-surveys-show-concern-and-hope-for-health-care

King v. Burwell, 135 S. Ct. 2480 (2015).

Kirzinger, A., DiJulio, B., Wu, B., & Brodie, M. (2017, July 14). *Kaiser health tracking poll—July 2017: What next for Republican ACA repeal and replacement plan efforts?* Retrieved from https://www.kff.org/health-reform/poll-finding/kaiser-health-tracking-poll-july-2017-whats-next-for-republican-aca-repeal-and-replacement-plan-efforts/

Kondick, K., & Skelley, G. (2016, December 15). *Incumbent re-election rates higher than average in 2016*. Retrieved from http://www.rasmussenreports.com/public_content/political_commentary/commentary_by_kyle_kondik/incumbent_reelection_rates_higher_than_average_in_2016

Kornreich, L. (2007, September 21). *Obama talks about mother's cancer battle in ad*. Retrieved from http://politicalticker.blogs.cnn.com/2007/09/21/obama-talks-about-mothers-cancer-battle-in-ad/

Lee, M. (2017, July 31). *Bipartisan coalition looks to solve problem of individual market*. Retrieved from http://www.modernhealthcare.com/article/20170731/NEWS/170739986

Lee, M. J., & Mattingly, P. (2017, July 26). *Health care debate: Senate rejects full Obamacare repeal without replacement*. Retrieved from http://www.wowt.com/content/news/Health-care-debate-Senate-rejects-full-Obamacare-repeal-without-replacement-436817863.html

Liptak, K., Luhby, T., & Mattingly, P. (2017, October 13). *Trump will end health care cost sharing subsidies*. Retrieved from https://www.cnn.com/2017/10/12/politics/obamacare-subsidies/index.html

Livingston, S. (2017, May 10). *Health insurers proposed 2018 rate hikes are early warning signs*. Retrieved from http://www.modernhealthcare.com/article/20170510/NEWS/170519999/

Luhby, T. (2017a, July 29). *Repeal is dead (for now). But will Obamacare survive?* Retrieved from https://money.cnn.com/2017/07/29/news/economy/obamacare-repeal/index.html

Luhby, T. (2017b, March 12). *What CBO got right—and wrong—on Obamacare*. Retrieved from https://money.cnn.com/2017/03/09/news/economy/cbo-obamacare/index.html

Magness, J. (2017, March 30). *America's opposition to repealing Obamacare grows, particularly among Republicans*. Retrieved from https://www.mcclatchydc.com/news/politics-government/article141562849.html

Mangan, D. (2017, April 28). *California will allow insurers to file two sets of rates: One for "Trumpcare" the other for "Obamacare."* Retrieved from https://www.cnbc.com/2017/04/28/california-will-allow-health-insurers-to-file-two-sets-of-rates-one-for-trumpcare-other-for-obamacare.html

Medicaid, CHIP Payment and Access Commission. (n.d.). *Medicaid enrollment changes following the ACA*. Retrieved from https://www.macpac.gov/subtopic/medicaid-enrollment-changes-following-the-aca/

Mills, D. (2016, June 29). *Young adults targeted in this fall's Obamacare enrollment drive*. Retrieved from https://www.healthline.com/health-news/young-adults-targeted-in-obamacare-drive

Morone, J. A. (2010). Presidents and health reform: From Franklin D. Roosevelt to Barack Obama. *Health Affairs, 29*(6), 1096–1100. doi:10.1377/hlthaff.2010.0420

Murray, S., & Kane, P. (2010, January 22). Pelosi: House won't pass Senate bill to save health-care reform. *Washington Post*. Retrieved from http://www.washingtonpost.com/wp-dyn/content/article/2010/01/21/AR2010012101604.html

National Academy for State Health Policy. (2018, February 7). *Individual marketplace enrollment remains stable in the face of national uncertainty*. Retrieved from https://nashp.org/individual-marketplace-enrollment-remains-stable-in-the-face-of-national-uncertainty/

National Archives and Record Administration. (n.d.). *Historical election results: Electoral college box scores 2000–2016*. Retrieved from https://www.archives.gov/federal-register/electoral-college/scores2.html

National Conference of State Legislators. (2016, June 17). *States with effective rate review programs*. Retrieved from http://www.ncsl.org/research/health/health-insurance-rate-approval-disapproval.aspx

National Federation of Independent Business v. Sebelius, 132 S. Ct. 2566 (2012).

Newport, F. (2010, November 18). U.S. still split on whether gov't should ensure healthcare. *Gallup*. Retrieved from https://news.gallup.com/poll/144839/Split-Whether-Gov-Ensure-Healthcare.aspx

Oberlander, J. (2010). Long time coming: Why health reform finally passed. *Health Affairs, 29*(6), 1112–1116. doi:10.1377/hlthaff.2010.0447

Office of Assistant Secretary for Planning and Evaluation. (2018). *HHS poverty guidelines for 2018*. Retrieved from https://aspe.hhs.gov/poverty-guidelines

Park, M. (2017, August 2). *Senator announces bipartisan hearing on Obamacare*. Retrieved from https://www.cnn.com/2017/08/02/politics/senate-health-care-hearing-bipartisan/index.html

Patient Protection and Affordable Care Act of 2010, 42 U.S.C. § 18001 (2010).

Pear, R. (2017, June 1). Trump rule could deny birth control coverage to hundreds of thousands of women. *The New York Times*. Retrieved from https://www.nytimes.com/2017/06/01/us/politics/birth-control-women-trump-health-care.html

Pollitz, K., Long, M., Semanskee, A., & Kamal, R. (2018, April 23). *Understanding short-term limited duration health insurance*. Retrieved from https://www.kff.org/health-reform/issue-brief/understanding-short-term-limited-duration-health-insurance/

Quinn, M. (2018, April 12). *Trump's new Obamacare rules give states more power. Will they take it?* Retrieved from http://www.governing.com/topics/health-human-services/gov-trump-obamacare-states.html

Rosenbaum, S., Teitelbaum, J., & Hayes, K. (2011). Crossing the Rubicon: The impact of the Affordable Care Act on the content of insurance coverage for persons with disabilities. *Notre Dame Journal of Law, Ethics, and Public Policy, 25*(2), 527–562. Retrieved from https://scholarship.law.nd.edu/ndjlepp/vol25/iss2/16

Saad, L. (2008, November 10). Obama and Bush: A contrast in popularity. *Gallup*. Retrieved from https://news.gallup.com/poll/111838/obama-bush-contrast-popularity.aspx

Scott, D. (2018, April 13). *A requiem for the individual mandate*. Retrieved from https://www.vox.com/policy-and-politics/2018/4/13/17226566/obamacare-penalty-2018-individual-mandate-still-in-effect

Semanskee, A., Claxton, G., & Leavitt, L. (2017, November 29). *How premiums are changing in 2018*. Retrieved from https://www.kff.org/health-reform/issue-brief/how-premiums-are-changing-in-2018/

Semanskee, A., Cox, C., & Leavitt, L. (2018, June 26). *Individual insurance market performance in 2018*. Retrieved from https://www.kff.org/private-insurance/issue-brief/individual-insurance-market-performance-in-early-2018/

Shapiro, I. (2010). State suits against health reform are well grounded in law—and pose serious challenges. *Health Affairs, 29*(6), 1229–1233. doi:10.1377/hlthaff.2010.0449

Starr, P. (1982). *The social transformation of American medicine: The rise of a sovereign profession and the making of a vast industry*. New York, NY: Basic Books.

Steinhauer, J. (2017, July 17). Old truths trip up G.O.P. on health law: A benefit is hard to retract. *The New York Times*. Retrieved from https://www.nytimes.com/2017/07/17/us/politics/republican-party-health-care-law-obamacare.html

Sullivan, P. (2017, July 20). *Cornyn: Knowing health plan ahead of vote is "luxury we don't have."* Retrieved from http://thehill.com/policy/healthcare/342980-cornyn-knowing-health-plan-ahead-of-vote-is-luxury-we-dont-have

Swartz, K. (2017, August 14). *"Reinsurance" program critical to shoring up the ACA*. Retrieved from https://www.hsph.harvard.edu/news/features/reinsurance-aca/

Tax Cut and Jobs Act of 2017, Pub. L. No. 115-97, 131 Stat. 2054 (2017).

Tax Policy Center. (n.d.). *Briefing book: What is reconciliation?* Retrieved from https://www.taxpolicycenter.org/briefing-book/what-reconciliation

Taylor, A., Saenz, A., & Levine, M. (2015, June 25). *Supreme Court upholds Obamacare subsidies, President says ACA is "here to stay."* Retrieved from https://abcnews.go.com/Politics/supreme-court-upholds-obama-health-care-subsidies/story?id=31931412

Texas v. United States, No. 4:18-cv-00167 (2018). Retrieved from https://www.law360.com/cases/5a9498d53206a62437000003

Trust for America's Health. (2017, August 8). *Prevention and Public Health Fund detailed information*. Retrieved from http://healthyamericans.org/report/134/

Tworney, M., Berger, S., & Brady, M. (2018, April 10). *Tracking Trump's sabotage of the ACA*. Retrieved from https://www.americanprogressaction.org/issues/healthcare/reports/2018/04/10/167820/tracking-trumps-sabotage-aca/

United States v. Lopez, 514 U.S. 549 (1995).

U.S. Census Bureau. (2010). *Income, poverty, and health insurance coverage in the United States: 2009*. (Current Population Reports, P60-238). Washington, DC: U.S. Government Printing Office.

U.S. Census Bureau. (2015). *Health insurance coverage in the United States: 2015*. (Current Population Reports, P60-257). Washington, DC: U.S. Government Printing Office.

U.S. Const. art I, §8.

Watkins, E. (2017, March 9). *Groups lining up in opposition to GOP health plan*. Retrieved from https://www.cnn.com/2017/03/08/politics/interest-groups-politicians-american-health-care-act/index.html

Weissert, C. S., & Weissert, W. G. (2002). *Governing health: The politics of health policy* (2nd ed.). Baltimore, MD: Johns Hopkins University Press.

West, D. M., Heith, D., & Goodwin, C. (1996). Harry and Louise go to Washington: Political advertising and health care reform. *Journal of Health Politics, Policy, and Law, 21*, 35–68. doi:10.1215/03616878-21-1-35

White House. (2009a, June 3). *Letter from President Obama to Chairmen Edward M. Kennedy and Max Baucus*. Washington, DC: Office of the Press Secretary.

White House. (2009b, September 9). *Remarks by the President to a joint session of Congress on health care*. Washington, DC: Office of the Press Secretary.

White House. (2010, January 27). *The 2010 State of the Union address*. Washington, DC: Office of the Press Secretary.

Wickard v. Filburn, 317 U.S. 111 (1942).

Wihbey, J. (2014, October 1). *Midterm Congressional elections explained: Why the president's party typically loses*. Retrieved from https://journalistsresource.org/studies/politics/elections/voting-patterns-midterm-congressional-elections-why-presidents-party-typically-loses

Wynn, B. (2017, March 27). *Five lessons from the AHCA's demise*. Retrieved from https://www.healthaffairs.org/do/10.1377/hblog20170327.059388/full/

Zeitlin, J. (2017, February 16). *Are the ACA exchanges really in a death spiral? We asked the experts*. Retrieved from https://www.advisory.com/daily-briefing/2017/02/16/death-exchange-market

Zubik v. Burwell, 136 S. Ct. 1557 (2016).

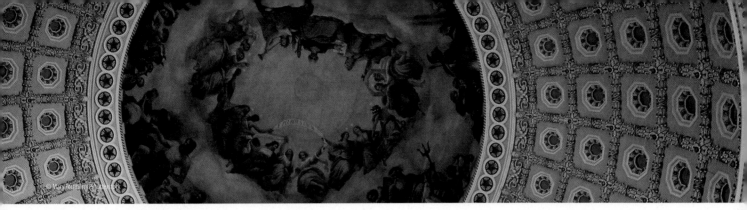

CHAPTER 11

Government Health Insurance Programs: Medicaid, CHIP, and Medicare

LEARNING OBJECTIVES

By the end of this chapter you will be able to:

- Describe the basic structure, administration, financing, and eligibility rules for:
  - Medicaid
  - The Children's Health Insurance Program (CHIP)
  - Medicare
- Understand how the Patient Protection and Affordable Care Act alters Medicaid, CHIP, and Medicare
- Discuss key health policy questions and themes relating to each of these public programs

BOX 11-1 Vignette

Governor Jadyn is in a quandary. She believes everyone should have access to health care and would like to support state policies that make care accessible and affordable. While she supported President Obama's goal of reducing the number of uninsured, she is concerned that some of the provisions in the Patient Protection and Affordable Care Act are too burdensome on the states, particularly in a fragile economy. The governor wonders how her state can afford the mandated Medicaid expansion when the recent trend has been to cut services across the board. How will state agencies cope with their new responsibilities when positions are being defunded and employees are being furloughed? Should she spend her state's time and resources to establish a health insurance exchange when the federal government will step in if she does not act? At the same time, does she want to leave decisions about how the exchange will be operated in her state to bureaucrats in Washington, DC?

▶ Introduction

In prior chapters we discussed in detail the significant role of employer-sponsored health insurance in financing health care, the flexibility that private insurers have in designing health insurance coverage and selecting who they will cover, why private insurers do not have incentive to cover high-risk populations, and how the Patient Protection and Affordable Care Act (ACA) has changed the health insurance and healthcare delivery landscape. Here, we focus on Medicaid, the Children's Health Insurance Program (CHIP), and Medicare, which were established in part because the private health insurance market was not developing affordable, comprehensive health insurance products for society's low-income, older, and disabled populations. Federal and state governments chose to fill some of those gaps through these public programs. The insurance coverage gaps were substantial, as shown by the over 130 million beneficiaries served by these three programs today (Department of Health and Human Services [HHS], 2017; Medicaid.gov, n.d.c). Due to the needs of vulnerable populations and the requirements necessary to make health insurance coverage for them viable, these programs are quite different from standard private health insurance plans.

There are numerous other important health insurance and direct service programs funded by federal, state, and local governments. Just a few examples include the Ryan White Care Act, which provides HIV/AIDS services to infected individuals and their families; the Women, Infants, and Children Supplemental Nutrition Program, which provides nutritional supplements and education to poor women and their children; and the Indian Health Service, which provides federal health services to American Indians and Alaska Natives. Although these and many other health programs are vital to the health of our population, this chapter focuses only on the three major government health insurance programs in this country, because in addition to providing health insurance to millions, these programs are also influential in terms of setting healthcare policy. For example, when Medicare, a program serving almost 60 million people, makes a decision to cover a certain treatment, private insurance companies often follow suit, establishing a new standard for generally accepted practice in the insurance industry (HHS, 2017). Conversely, states may decide to try healthcare innovations with their Medicaid programs that, if successful, may become commonplace across the country. Thus, understanding these three major programs is essential in terms of both how this country finances and delivers health care and how it makes health policy decisions.

The ACA made wide-ranging changes to Medicaid, CHIP, and Medicare. In general, the ACA included a significant Medicaid eligibility expansion, altered which children are eligible for Medicaid and CHIP, added new benefits to Medicare, and included a host of changes intended to produce savings in the Medicare program. Overall, the ACA expansion has created a two-tier Medicaid program, with newly eligible individuals falling under one set of eligibility, financing, and benefit rules, and the rest of Medicaid beneficiaries adhering to different standards.

As you learn about specific rules for each program, keep in mind the numerous tensions that are present throughout the healthcare system as policymakers decide how to design and implement public insurance programs. This chapter touches on several recurring themes relating to these tensions, which were evident during the debate that led to passage of the ACA: choosing between state flexibility and national uniformity; determining the appropriate role for government, the private sector, and individuals in healthcare financing and delivery; defining a primary decision-making goal (e.g., fiscal restraint, equity/social justice, improved health outcomes, uniformity); and settling on the appropriate scope of coverage to offer beneficiaries.

Before delving into the details of each program, it is necessary to explain the difference between entitlement and block grant programs. Medicaid and Medicare are *entitlement* programs, whereas CHIP is a *block grant* program. Some of the themes listed earlier, such as the appropriate role of government and primary decision-making goals, are implicated in the decision of whether to establish a program as an entitlement or a block grant.

In an *entitlement* program, everyone who is eligible for and enrolled in the program is legally entitled to receive benefits from the program. In other words, the federal or state governments cannot refuse to provide program beneficiaries all medically necessary and covered services due to lack of funds or for other reasons. Because everyone who is enrolled has a legal right to receive services, there cannot be a cap on spending. The absence of a spending cap has the advantage of allowing funds to be available to meet rising healthcare costs and unexpected needs, such as increased enrollment and use of services during recessions or natural or man-made disasters.

Opponents of entitlement programs focus on the open-ended budget obligation that entitlements create. With healthcare costs straining federal and state budgets, critics would prefer to establish a cap on the funds spent on entitlement programs such as Medicaid. It is impossible to determine how many people will enroll in the program or how many and what kind of healthcare

Do you think it makes more sense to structure government healthcare programs as entitlements or block grants? What are the economic and healthcare risks and benefits of each approach? Does your answer depend on who is paying for the program? Who the program serves? What kinds of benefits the program provides? Do you think various stakeholders would answer these questions differently? How might the answers change if you ask a member of the federal government, a governor, a state legislator, an advocate, or a tax-paying citizen who is not eligible for benefits under the program?

services they will use in any given year, so governments cannot establish exact budgets for their Medicaid program. In addition to these fiscal objections, many opponents reject the notion that government should play a large role in providing health insurance, preferring to leave that function to the private market.

Entitlement programs are often contrasted with *block grant* programs such as CHIP. A block grant is a defined sum of money that is allocated for a particular program (often, but not always, from the federal government to the states) over a certain amount of time. If program costs exceed available funds, additional money will not be made available and program changes have to be made. Such changes could include terminating the program, capping enrollment in the program, reducing program benefits, or finding additional resources. Unlike entitlement programs, individuals who qualify for block grant programs may be denied services or receive reduced services due to lack of funds.

The arguments for and against block grant programs are similar to those found with entitlement programs. Proponents of block grant programs laud the limited and certain fiscal obligation and reduced role of government in providing health insurance. Opponents of block grant programs object to the lack of legal entitlement to services and the finite amount of funds available to provide health insurance.

▶ Medicaid

Medicaid is the country's federal–state public health insurance program for the indigent. In this section, we discuss fundamental aspects of the Medicaid program, including its structure, eligibility, benefits, and financing, as well as changes to Medicaid made by the ACA. Unlike private health insurance plans, which are based on actuarial risk, the Medicaid program is designed to ensure that funds are available to provide healthcare services to a poorer and generally less-healthy group of beneficiaries; to do so, Medicaid has several features not found in private health insurance plans.

Program Administration

Medicaid is jointly designed and operated by the federal and state governments. The Centers for Medicare and Medicaid Services (CMS) is the federal agency in charge of administering the Medicaid program. Each state, the District of Columbia, and certain U.S. territories,[a] as defined in the Social Security Act (SSA) of 1935, have the option to participate in the Medicaid program, and all have chosen to do so. The federal government sets certain requirements and policies for the Medicaid program though statutes (SSA, Title 19), regulations (Grants to States, 1988), a *State Medicaid Manual* (Medicaid.gov, n.d.e), and policy guidance such as letters to state Medicaid directors (Medicaid.gov, n.d.e). Each state has its own Medicaid agency that is responsible for implementing the program in the state. States file a Medicaid State Plan with the federal government outlining the state's own eligibility rules, benefits, and other program requirements; this plan is effectively a contract between states and the federal government and between states and program beneficiaries.

The federal and state governments jointly set rules concerning who is covered and which services are provided by Medicaid. The federal government outlines which populations must be covered (*mandatory populations*) and which ones may be covered (*optional populations*), as well as which benefits must be covered (*mandatory benefits*) and which ones may be covered (*optional benefits*). Between these floors and ceilings, states have significant flexibility to determine how Medicaid will operate in their particular state. In general, states must cover mandatory populations and benefits, and they may choose to cover any combination of optional populations or benefits, including the choice not to offer any optional coverage at all. In addition, states may seek a waiver from federal rules, allowing states to experiment with coverage and benefit design while still drawing federal funds to operate their program. Given all of these possible permutations, it is often said that "if you have seen one Medicaid program, you have seen one Medicaid program"; in other words, within the broad federal parameters, every state (and territory) has a unique Medicaid structure—no two programs are exactly alike. As a result, similarly situated individuals in different states may have very different experiences in terms of the generosity of benefits they are entitled to or even if they are eligible for the program at all.

Eligibility

Traditionally, Medicaid has covered low-income pregnant women, children, adults in families with dependent children, individuals with disabilities, and older adults. About 43% of all Medicaid beneficiaries are children, and another 40% are individuals with disabilities and older adults (Rudowitz & Garfield, 2018). Approximately 11 million people are called *dual enrollee* or *dual-eligible* older adults, meaning they qualify for both Medicaid and Medicare (Accius, Flowers, & Finn, 2017). Although most dual enrollees are eligible for full Medicaid benefits, a small portion of them receives only premium and/or cost-sharing assistance to help them pay for Medicare, not full Medicaid benefits.

Among all people with health insurance, members of ethnic or minority groups are more likely than Caucasians to have coverage through Medicaid. As shown in **FIGURE 11-1**, about 43% of Medicaid beneficiaries are white, non-Hispanic beneficiaries, 30% are Hispanic, and 18% are Black. **FIGURE 11-2** shows that Medicaid provides assistance to a variety of vulnerable populations.

BOX 11-3 Discussion Questions

What are the benefits and drawbacks of having a health program that varies by state versus having one that is uniform across the country? Do you find that the positives of state flexibility outweigh the negatives, or vice versa? Does your analysis change depending on what populations are served? Does your analysis change depending on whose point of view you consider? Is it fair that similarly situated individuals may be treated differently in different states? Does this occur in other aspects of society?

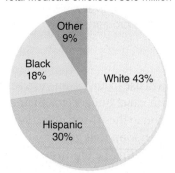

Total Medicaid enrollees: 58.9 million

Kaiser Family Foundation, Distribution of the non-elderly with Medicaid by Race/Ethnicity, 2016.

FIGURE 11-1 Medicaid Beneficiaries by Race/Ethnicity, 2016

Source: Kaiser Family Foundation, Distribution of the non-elderly with Medicaid by race/ethnicity, 2016. Retrieved from https://www.kff.org/medicaid/state-indicator/distribution-by-raceethnicity-4/?currentTimeframe=0&selectedDistributions=white--black--hispanic--other&selectedRows=%7B%22wrapups%22:%7B%22united-states%22:%7B%7D%7D%7D&sortModel=%7B%22colId%22:%22Location%22,%22sort%22:%22asc%22%7D

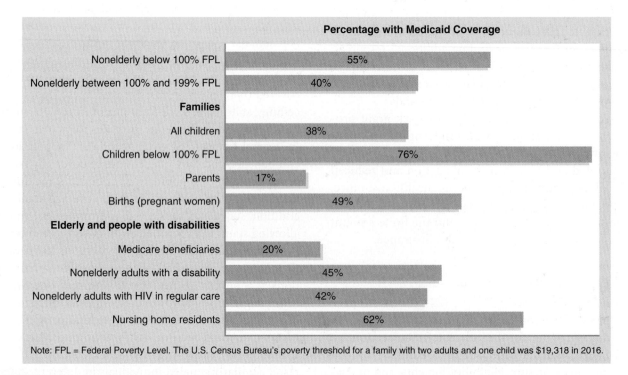

FIGURE 11-2 Medicaid Plays a Key Role for Selected Populations, 2017

Source: KFF Analysis of 2017 Current Population Survey, Annual Social and Economic Supplement; Birth data - Implementing Coverage and Payment Initiatives: results from a 50-State Medicaid Budget Survey for State Fiscal Years 2016 and 2017, KFF, October 2016.; Medicare data - Medicare Payment Advisory Commission, *Data Book: Beneficiaries Dually Eligible for Medicare and Medicaid* (January 2018); 2013 data. Disability - KFF Analysis of 2016 ACS; Nonelderly with HIV - 2014 CDC MMP; Nursing Home Residents - 2015 OSCAR/CASPER data. Retrieved from https://kaiserfamilyfoundation.files.wordpress.com/2015/05/medicaid_s-role-for-selected-populations.png

Federal poverty guidelines are determined annually and calculated based on the number of individuals in a family. The guidelines are commonly referred to as the *federal poverty level*, but the U.S. Department of Health and Human Services (HHS) discourages the use of this term because the Census Bureau also calculates, using different methods, a figure referred to as the *federal poverty thresholds*. However, because the term federal poverty level is still commonly used when discussing eligibility for federal and state programs, we use it here. The poverty guidelines are somewhat higher for Alaska and Hawaii due to administrative procedures adopted by the Office of Economic Opportunity.

While Medicaid covers both children and adults, coverage for children and pregnant women typically has been more generous than coverage for nonpregnant adults. Prior to ACA implementation, Medicaid covered 75% of children who lived below the poverty line, but only 35% of adults below that income level (Paradise, Lyons, & Rowland, 2015, p. 3). Of adults who were covered by Medicaid, states were more generous when it came to pregnant women. While half the states provided coverage to pregnant women up to 200% of the federal poverty level (FPL; **BOX 11-4**), the median income eligibility limit for working parents was 61%, and many states did not cover childless adults at all (Paradise, 2015, p. 8; Paradise et al., 2015, p. 3). Traditionally left out of the program have been low-income adults without disabilities, women who are not pregnant, and the near-poor who earn too much money to qualify for Medicaid. However, the ACA included a significant eligibility expansion. As of August 2017, there were 16 million more Medicaid enrollees than prior to passage of the ACA (Medicaid and CHIP Payment and Access Commission [MACPAC], n.d.a). States that adopted the ACA Medicaid expansion option experienced an average enrollment increase of 37% as compared to non-expansion states, with an average increase of 12.6%. In 2016, the newly eligible enrollees comprised 20.4% of enrollees across all states (MACPAC, n.d.a). As discussed later in more detail, the expansion is designed to include the low-income groups that have been traditionally excluded from Medicaid.

Traditional Medicaid Eligibility Requirements

Eligibility requirements (as well as financing rules and benefits) differ for the groups that have been traditionally covered by Medicaid and those that are covered under the ACA expansion option. To help clarify these differences, when referring to the rules that existed prior to the ACA, we use the term *traditional Medicaid*, and when referring to rules that attach to the ACA, we use the term *expansion Medicaid*. It is important to remember that states may follow both traditional and expansion Medicaid rules; the ACA expansion did not replace traditional Medicaid, but rather added to it.

Under traditional Medicaid rules, everyone must meet *all five* of the following requirements to be eligible:

1. **Categorical:** An individual must fit within a category (e.g., pregnant women) covered by the program.
2. **Income:** An individual/family must earn no more than the relevant income limits, which are expressed as an FPL percentage (e.g., 133% of the FPL).
3. **Resources:** An individual/family must not have nonwage assets (e.g., car, household goods) that exceed eligibility limits.
4. **Residency:** An individual must be a U.S. resident and a resident of the state in which they are seeking benefits.
5. **Immigration status:** Immigrants must meet certain requirements, including having been in the country for at least 5 years (for most immigrants).

As shown in **TABLE 11-1**, under traditional rules it is necessary to consider both categorical eligibility and income limits for all populations to understand who is covered by Medicaid and which populations are mandatory and which are optional. The groups in Table 11-1 represent some of the larger and more frequently mentioned categories of Medicaid beneficiaries, but it is not an exhaustive list. There are approximately 50 categories of mandatory and optional populations in the Medicaid program, with each state picking and choosing which optional populations to include and at what income level.

Medically Needy

Medicaid's *medically needy* category is an option that has been picked up by 32 states and the District of Columbia as of 2016 (MACPAC, n.d.b). As its name implies, this category is intended to cover individuals who have extremely high medical expenses. These individuals fit within a covered category but earn too much money to be otherwise eligible for Medicaid. Given who is in this population, it is not surprising that the medically needy experience

TABLE 11-1 Select Medicaid Mandatory and Optional Eligibility Groups and Income Requirements Prior to ACA

Eligibility Category	Mandatory Coverage	Optional Coverage
Infants <1 year	≤133% FPL	≤185% FPL
Children 1–5 years	≤133% FPL	>133% FPL
Children 6–19 years	≤100% FPL	>100% FPL
Pregnant women	≤133% FPL	≤185% FPL
Parents	Below state's 1996 AFDC limit	May use income level above state's 1996 AFDC limit
Parents in welfare-to-work families	≤185% FPL	
Older adults and disabled SSI beneficiaries	SSI limits	Above SSI limits, below 100% FPL
Certain working disabled	May not exceed specified amount	Variable, SSI level to 250% FPL
Older adults—Medicare assistance only[a]	Variable, up to 175% FPL	Variable up to 175% FPL
Nursing home residents		Above SSI limits, below 300% SSI
Medically needy		"Spend down" medical expenses to state-set income level

[a]Medicare assistance only = payment for Medicare cost-sharing requirements.

Abbreviations: AFDC = Aid to Families With Dependent Children; FPL = federal poverty level; SSI = Supplemental Security Income (a federal program that provides cash assistance to older adults and individuals who are blind or disabled who meet certain income and resource requirements).

high medical expenses: in 2009, this population accounted for only 5% of Medicaid beneficiaries but 11% of Medicaid expenditures (Kaiser Family Foundation [KFF], 2012b).

Medically needy programs have both income and asset requirements. In terms of income requirements, states subtract the costs of individuals' medical expenses from their income level. States have the choice of deducting the medical expenses as they are incurred each month, every 6 months, or any time in between. As soon as otherwise qualified individuals "spend down" enough money on medical expenses, they are eligible for Medicaid through the medically needy option based on their reduced income level for the remainder of the period.

The following is a simplified example of how the "spend down" process works. Let's say a state calculates incurred medical expenses every 3 months to determine eligibility for the medically needy option, and in this state an individual (who we'll call Peter)

must earn no more than $8,500 a year to qualify as medically needy. Peter earns $11,000 per year and has $6,000 each year in medical expenses, incurred at a rate of $500 per month. After 3 months, Peter has spent $1,500 on medical expenses. Instead of considering the income level to be the annual amount earned ($11,000), the state subtracts Peter's medical expenses as they occur. So, after 3 months the state considers Peter to earn $9,500 annually ($11,000–$1,500). Because this amount is still over the $8,500 limit, Peter is not eligible under the medically needy option. In another 3 months, Peter will have spent $3,000 in medical expenses over the past 6 months. At that time, the state considers Peter to earn $8,000 annually ($11,000 – $3,000), making him eligible because he earns less than the $8,500 limit. For the rest of this period (i.e., 3 months), Peter is eligible for Medicaid. After another 3 months, the state recalculates his earnings and medical expenses. Each year, this entire calculation starts over. In the end, Peter

Does the medically needy category make sense to you? Do you think it is a good idea to discount medical expenses of high-need individuals so they can access the healthcare services they need through Medicaid? If so, is the process described above cumbersome and likely to result in people being on and off Medicaid (and therefore likely on and off treatment) because their eligibility is based on their spending patterns? Why should individuals with high medical needs have an avenue to Medicaid eligibility that is not available to other low-income people who have other high expenses, such as child care or transportation costs? Would it make more sense to simply raise the eligibility level for Medicaid so more low-income people are eligible for the program? Politically, which option would likely have more support? Does your view about the medically needy category vary depending on your primary decision-making goal (e.g., fiscal restraint, equity, improved health outcomes)?

will not be eligible for Medicaid for the first 6 months of the year but will be eligible for Medicaid for the second 6 months of the year.

Immigrants

There are also special Medicaid eligibility rules relating to immigrants. The Personal Responsibility and Work Opportunity Reconciliation Act of 1996 (PRWORA) severely restricted immigrant eligibility for Medicaid (and most of the same rules in PRWORA were later applied to CHIP eligibility in 1997). Prior to PRWORA, legal immigrants followed the same Medicaid eligibility rules as everyone else, but undocumented immigrants were not eligible at all. PRWORA instituted a 5-year bar, meaning that most immigrants who come to the United States after August 22, 1996, are not eligible for Medicaid (or CHIP) for the first 5 years after their arrival. After 5 years, legal immigrants are eligible on the same basis as U.S. citizens, while undocumented immigrants remain ineligible for full Medicaid (or CHIP) benefits. However, both legal and undocumented immigrants who are otherwise eligible for Medicaid may receive emergency Medicaid benefits without any temporal restrictions. Immigrant eligibility eased slightly when CHIP was reauthorized through the Children's Health Insurance Program Reauthorization Act of 2009. States now have the option to cover legal immigrant children and/or pregnant women through Medicaid and CHIP in the first 5 years that they are in the United States.

Proponents of the immigrant restrictions believe they discourage people who cannot support themselves from coming to the United States and prevent immigrants from taking advantage of publicly funded programs they did not support through taxes before their arrival. In addition, some proponents believe that healthcare resources should go first to U.S. citizens, not noncitizens.

Opponents of the restrictions assert that most immigrants pay taxes once they arrive in this country and therefore deserve to receive the full benefits of those taxes (Fremstad & Cox, 2004, p. 15). They also find the restriction ill-suited as a deterrent because immigrants often come to the United States for economic opportunities, not social benefits (Passel, 2005). Furthermore, restricting immigrants' access to health care may be a public health hazard for all members of the community because contagious diseases do not discriminate by immigration status. Finally, opponents contend that having higher numbers of uninsured individuals in the United States will further strain the ability of providers to care for all vulnerable populations in a community and lead to rising healthcare costs because uninsured immigrants are much less likely to obtain preventive care or early treatment for illnesses or injuries (Fremstad & Cox, 2004, p. 15). As of 2017, 31 states cover legal immigrant children under Medicaid and/or CHIP, and 5 states and the District of Columbia use state-only funds to cover children who qualify based on income, but not immigration status (Brooks, Wagnerman, Artiga, Cornachione, & Ubri, 2017). Sixteen states use CHIP funding to cover pregnant women under the unborn child option, which allows for coverage regardless of immigration status. Also, 23 states cover legal immigrant pregnant women under Medicaid without the 5-year bar. Two states and the District of Columbia use state-only funds to cover pregnant women who qualify based on income, but not immigration status (Brooks et al., 2017). Even with these reforms and the ACA, 16% of the 30 million individuals who remained uninsured in 2017 were illegal immigrants (Blumberg, Holahan, Karpman, & Elmendorf, 2018).

Medicaid Eligibility Expansion Under the ACA

As mentioned earlier, the ACA significantly expanded Medicaid eligibility. As of 2014, all non-Medicare-eligible individuals younger than 65 years, with incomes up to 133% FPL,[b] are eligible for Medicaid in states that choose to expand its program. This eligibility expansion option marks a drastic departure from how Medicaid has generally been structured.

Unlike Medicaid's traditional eligibility structure, individuals eligible through the expansion only have to satisfy an income threshold and do not have to meet a resource test or fit within a preapproved category. In addition, in traditional Medicaid, states have significant flexibility to determine how individual income and other personal resources are calculated. Under the ACA expansion, however, all states are required to accept newly eligible individuals using the federal income level calculation and without accounting for other assets.

As discussed in detail in the Health Reform in the United States chapter, the ACA Medicaid expansion was intended to be mandatory in all states, but the Supreme Court's decision in *National Federation of Independent Business v. Sebelius* held that the federal government could not force states to expand Medicaid in this way. As of June 2018, 33 states and the District of Columbia have chosen to expand their Medicaid program under the ACA, resulting in 16 million new enrollees (Advisory Board, 2018; MACPAC, n.d.a.).

Lawmakers built the ACA coverage options assuming that all states would be required to expand Medicaid. After the Supreme Court ruled that Medicaid expansion was optional, coverage gaps emerged in those states that have not chosen to expand their Medicaid program. In non-expansion states there are approximately 2 million poor adults who remain ineligible for Medicaid and who are also too poor to obtain subsidies to purchase health insurance through their state exchanges (Garfield, Damico, & Orgera, 2018). Eligibility for these subsidies begins at 100% FPL, resulting in the illogical situation in which a poorer individual (e.g., one who earns 75% FPL) cannot obtain a subsidy while an individual who earns more (e.g., 115% FPL) is able to purchase subsidized insurance in the state exchange.

In addition to the Medicaid expansion rule just described, the ACA also requires that children ages 6 to 19 years must be covered up to 133% FPL, instead of up to only 100% FPL as under pre-ACA rules. Undocumented immigrants, as well as legal immigrants who have resided in the United States for fewer than 5 years, will not be eligible for Medicaid under the expansion, although states have the option to cover legal immigrant pregnant women and children who have been in the country fewer than 5 years (matching the new rules put in place under CHIP).

Benefits

Medicaid benefits are structured in the same way as Medicaid eligibility: some are mandatory and some are optional, and the newly eligible individuals under

---

BOX 11-6 Discussion Questions

Looking at Medicaid's traditional eligibility rules, you notice numerous value/policy judgments: pregnant women and children are favored over childless adults, the medically needy are favored over other low-income individuals with high costs, non-immigrants are favored over immigrants. Under the ACA expansion, these distinctions mostly disappear and eligibility depends purely on income level in the case of the biggest expansion group. Which approach do you prefer? If the ACA approach were expanded beyond 133% of FPL, the costs of the Medicaid program would soar. Given limited resources, do you think it would be better to cover more people at a higher poverty level across the board or continue to favor some groups over others through the categorical requirement? Should we decide that, for some populations, the government should step in and provide coverage regardless of the cost? In other words, is there a point where equity trumps financial constraints?

BOX 11-7 Discussion Questions

What are the implications of a two-tiered Medicaid system? Is there justification for offering some beneficiaries a less generous benefit package than others? Is it fair to impose additional requirements (categorical, asset test) on only some beneficiaries? Why do you think policymakers created these distinctions? Do you think they will remain in place over time?

---

the ACA expansion have their own set of rules. Again, this means that no two Medicaid programs are alike, as each state picks its own menu of optional benefits to provide.

Traditional Medicaid Benefits

Historically, Medicaid programs have offered a rich array of benefits, including preventive services, behavioral health services, long-term care services, supportive services that allow people with disabilities to work, institutional services, family planning services, and more. In fact, the coverage provided by traditional Medicaid generally has been more generous than the typical private insurance plan, particularly in the case of children. While federal Medicaid regulations exclude very few services, there are prohibitions. Since 1977, Congress has prohibited the use of federal funds to pay for the costs of an abortion or mifepristone (commonly known as RU-486), a drug that induces

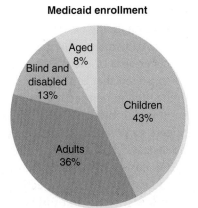

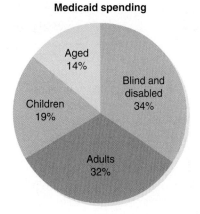

FIGURE 11-3 Enrollment and Spending in Medicaid

Source: Spending and enrollment estimates for FY2015 from the Congressional Budget Office's March 2016 Medicaid baseline. Center on Budget and Policy Priorities. Retrieved from cbpp.org.

children and adults are fairly inexpensive to cover, whereas older adults and individuals with disabilities use more, as well as more expensive, services. In 2015, almost half of spending went to care for older adult and disabled beneficiaries even though they constituted less than one-fifth of all enrollees (Center on Budget and Policy Priorities, 2016). One of the biggest reasons these groups account for a high proportion of Medicaid expenditures is their use of long-term care services, such as nursing homes and home- and community-based services, which takes up over 20% all Medicaid spending (KFF, 2016a). In addition, they are heavy users of prescription drugs and are relatively more likely to be hospitalized. **FIGURE 11-4** shows Medicaid's significant role in funding home health and nursing home care in this country, along with a variety of other services.

In addition to expanding eligibility, the ACA included a few changes to Medicaid benefits. States will have new options relating to community-based care, home health care, and family planning. Further, all states will have to cover tobacco cessation programs for pregnant women. The ACA also includes a variety of demonstration programs that target key health issues such as obesity, high cholesterol, high blood pressure, diabetes, and tobacco use.

Medicaid Financing

The Medicaid program is jointly financed by the federal and state governments, with about 63% of the total program costs paid for by the federal government and the rest by the states (KFF, 2016f). Even with the federal government picking up over half the tab, states have found their share of Medicaid costs to be increasingly burdensome, accounting for over 25% of state funds nationally in 2016 (Rudowitz & Garfield, 2018).

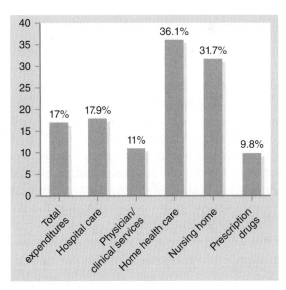

FIGURE 11-4 Medicaid Percentage of National Spending by Type of Service, 2016

Source: Data from Medicaid and CHIP Payment and Access Commission. (2017, December). MACSTATS: Medicaid and CHIP data book. Retrieved from https://www.macpac.gov/wp-content/uploads/2015/12/MACStats-Medicaid-CHIP-Data-Book-December-2017.pdf

Program financing occurs through a matching payment system that divides the amount paid by the federal and state governments. The matching rate for most medical services, called the Federal Medical Assistance Percentage (FMAP), is determined by a formula that is tied to each state's per-capita income. Poorer states—those with lower per-capita incomes—receive more federal money for every state dollar spent on Medicaid, while the wealthier states receive less. In addition, the ACA allows for a 1% increase in FMAP for states that cover certain preventive services and immunizations without any cost-sharing requirements. The FMAP rate may not be lower than 50% for any state, meaning the costliest scenario for a state government is that it splits program costs evenly with the federal government. In 2016, FMAP rates ranged from 50% to 76.3% (KFF, 2016g). Given the variation in matching rates and state programs' size, federal funds are not distributed evenly among the states. In fact, in 2016, four states (California, New York, Pennsylvania, and Texas) accounted for over one-third of all federal Medicaid spending (KFF, 2016g).

Medicaid is also partially financed through beneficiary co-payments, co-insurance, and premiums. In traditional Medicaid, cost sharing is extremely limited. States may not charge any cost sharing for emergency services, family planning services, pregnancy-related services, or preventive services for children. In addition, states can charge only nominal cost sharing for individuals under 100% FPL, such as $4 for a physician visit or $8 for non-emergency use of an emergency department (Medicaid.gov, n.d.d). The DRA included drastic changes to Medicaid's cost-sharing rules that now apply to ABPs through section 1937. These changes allow for higher cost sharing for individuals who earn over 100% FPL, although out-of-pocket costs may not exceed 5% of a family's income. For example, beneficiaries between 101% and 150% FPL can pay up to a 10% co-pay for a physician visit, and beneficiaries over 151% FPL can pay up to a 20% co-pay for the same service (Medicaid.gov, n.d.d.). Also, prior to the DRA, cost-sharing requirements were "unenforceable," meaning health professionals could not refuse to provide services if a beneficiary did not pay a required cost-share amount. Now states can deny services if enrollees do not pay the higher out-of-pocket costs. As with the DRA benefit changes, many groups and services are excluded from the new cost-sharing options.

As noted earlier, the federal government is picking up the bulk of the cost of the ACA Medicaid expansions.

From 2014 to 2016, the federal government paid 100% of the cost of financing newly eligible enrollees. While the federal government's share will lessen over time, it will still cover 90% of the cost in 2020 and beyond. It was also expected that the Medicaid expansion would reduce the uncompensated care burden of states—because fewer individuals will be uninsured—and this appears to be the case. Between 2013 and 2015, uncompensated care costs fell from 3.9% to 2.3% of hospital costs, for a savings of over $6 billion. Hospitals in expansion states treating the highest proportion of low-income and uninsured patients experienced the largest savings (Dranove, Garthwaite, & Ody, 2017). Even so, many states are concerned about the financial burden of the Medicaid expansion, and greater-than-expected increases in enrollment already have several states reconsidering their commitment to the ACA Medicaid expansion. The ACA included a maintenance-of-effort (MOE) rule forbidding states from reducing their own eligibility rules. States must keep the eligibility rules they had in place in March 2010 (when the law was enacted) until 2019 in the case of children, and until 2014 in the case of adults. This requirement was included to prevent states from rolling back coverage expansions and from simply replacing state dollars with federal dollars without actually expanding coverage. There is, however, a significant exception to the MOE rule: states with a documented budget deficit may reduce eligibility for nonpregnant, nondisabled adults earning over 133% FPL.

Medicaid Provider Reimbursement

Medicaid's complex design also extends to its provider reimbursement methodology. States have broad discretion in setting provider rates. Not only do reimbursement rates vary by state, but they also vary by whether services are provided in a fee-for-service

(FFS) or managed care setting and by which type of provider (e.g., physicians, hospitals) renders a service.[c]

FFS Reimbursement

When reimbursing FFS care under Medicaid, states are required to set their payment rates to physicians at levels that are "sufficient" to ensure Medicaid patients have "equal access" to providers compared to the general population (SSA § 1396a(a)(30)(A)). Despite this language, Medicaid reimbursement is much lower than both Medicare and private practice rates, and a 2015 U.S. Supreme Court decision found that providers cannot sue a state to raise Medicaid reimbursement rates (*Armstrong v. Exceptional Child Center*, 2015).

Low reimbursement is one reason that many providers are wary of treating Medicaid patients; in addition, physicians decline to participate in Medicaid due to extensive program requirements, delays in payment, and the burden of treating a complex patient population (Rosenbaum, 2014). The Centers for Disease Control and Prevention reported that in 2013 68.9% of physicians would accept new Medicaid patients, as compared to 84.7% and 83.7% who would accept new privately insured and Medicare patients, respectively (Hing, Decker, & Jamoom, 2015). There was wide variation across the country, with only 38.7% of New Jersey providers indicating they would accept new Medicaid patients as compared to 96.5% in Nebraska (Hing et al., 2015). Not surprisingly, providers have been more willing to accept Medicaid patients in states with higher reimbursement levels (Decker, 2012).

Physicians who treat Medicaid patients are demographically different from those who serve privately insured patients. Medicaid patients are more likely to be seen by physicians who are younger, work in large practices, are graduates of foreign medical schools, are graduates from lower-ranked medical schools, and are not board-certified (Decker, 2018). Overall, relatively few physicians see the bulk of Medicaid patients across the country: from 2013 to 2015, approximately 20% of physicians saw 60% of Medicaid patients (Neprash, Zink, Gray, & Hempstead, 2018).

Prior to the ACA, Medicaid reimbursement was 59% of Medicare rates (Decker, 2018). The ACA included a temporary bump in primary care payment rates for services provided in both FFS and managed care settings. For 2013 and 2014, primary care payment rates equaled 100% of Medicare payment rates, with the federal government covering the cost of the increased reimbursement. On average, this change resulted in a 73% increase in Medicaid payments, but there was wide variation across the country (Decker, 2018). While this measure was intended to support primary care providers and boost access to primary care services, its temporary nature means it is unlikely to have a lasting effect. While a few limited studies suggested there may have been a positive effect on access from the temporary fee bump, a recent study based on nationally representative data from the National Center for Health Statistics found no significant increase in physician participation in Medicaid after the fee bump (Decker, 2018).

Hospital FFS plans are reimbursed at a rate that is "consistent with efficiency, economy, and quality of care" (SSA, § 1902(a)(30)(a)). However, there is no specified minimum reimbursement level that states are required to meet, resulting in rates that are lower than what hospitals receive from Medicare and private insurance. While it is difficult to estimate Medicaid payments to hospitals due to data issues and differences in state payment methodologies, it appears Medicaid pays hospitals about 90% to 93% of costs on average, with significant variation across the country (Cunningham, Rudowitz, Young, Garfield, & Foutz, 2016). Hospitals that serve a high number of Medicaid and uninsured individuals may receive additional Medicaid payments, called disproportionate share hospital (DSH) payments. Under the ACA, however, these payments will be reduced significantly. The effective date of the reduction was delayed until 2018, but the amount of reduction increased from $18 billion to $43 billion through 2025 (Kardish, 2015).

Managed Care Reimbursement

As with the rest of the healthcare system, managed care has become an increasingly important part of the Medicaid program. In 2016, over two-thirds of all Medicaid beneficiaries—mostly children and parents—obtained their care through comprehensive managed care organizations (MCOs), including over half of enrollees in 37 states (**FIGURE 11-5**) (Medicaid. gov, 2018). In addition, almost 7% of enrollees used a "medical home" or primary care case management model that year (Medicaid.gov, 2018). These models pay a provider to coordinate care for beneficiaries, whether it is only primary care services or a range of services, such as physical, behavioral, long-term care, social supports, and so on. ACA expansion states also relied on MCOs to serve 12.5 million new beneficiaries in 2016 (Medicaid.gov, 2018). States may require managed care enrollment for all beneficiaries except children with special healthcare needs, Native Americans, and Medicare recipients (SSA, § 1936u-2).

MCOs that enroll Medicaid beneficiaries receive a monthly capitated rate per member and assume financial risk for providing services. In 2015, managed

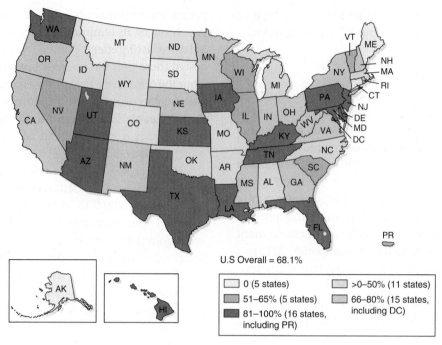

U.S Overall = 68.1%

- ☐ 0 (5 states)
- ☐ 51–65% (5 states)
- ☐ 81–100% (16 states, including PR)
- ☐ >0–50% (11 states)
- ☐ 66–80% (15 states, including DC)

Note: Comprehensive managed care includes risk-based managed care organizations (MCOs) and Programs of All-inclusive Care for the Elderly (PACE).

FIGURE 11-5 State Comprehensive Managed Care Penetration as of July 1, 2016

Source: Medicaid.gov. (2018). Medicaid managed care enrollment and program characteristics, 2016. Retrieved from https://www.medicaid.gov/medicaid/managed-care/downloads/enrollment/2016-medicaid-managed-care-enrollment-report.pdf

care payments to comprehensive MCOs accounted for 46% of Medicaid spending (CMS.gov, 2016). States and MCOs agree upon a set of services the MCOs will provide for the capitated rate. If there are any Medicaid-covered services that are not included in a state's managed care contract with MCOs, states reimburse them an amount in addition to the capitated rate or reimburse non-MCO providers on an FFS basis to provide those services. In other words, beneficiaries are still entitled to all Medicaid services, even when they are enrolled in a managed care plan.

States are required to pay MCOs on an "actuarially sound basis," a term that is not defined in the Medicaid statute (SSA, § 1396b(m)(2)(iii)). As with other types of provider rates, capitation rates vary widely among states. However, it is difficult to compare capitation rates across states because of the variation in Medicaid programs generally and in the types of services and populations covered by the managed care contracts.

With the rapid growth of Medicaid managed care services, CMS issued new rules in 2016 to improve the managed care component of the program. These rules covered a wide variety of issues, such as strengthening beneficiary protections, aligning Medicaid and CHIP requirements as necessary, improving payment provisions and program integrity, promoting quality of care, and creating network adequacy standards (Paradise & Musumeci, 2016).

BOX 11-13 Discussion Questions

Is higher Medicaid cost sharing a good idea? What are the strongest arguments you can make for and against higher cost sharing? Should Medicaid beneficiaries have the same cost-sharing responsibilities as privately insured individuals, or should the government bear more of the cost because Medicaid beneficiaries are low-income individuals? What is the primary decision-making goal that led to the exclusion of so many populations and services from the new cost-sharing options?

BOX 11-14 Discussion Questions

Who should determine Medicaid provider reimbursement rates, and how should they compare to other insurance programs or plans? Should the federal government play a stronger role in setting provider rates? Is this an area where it is better to have state variation or national uniformity? Should the federal or state governments be required to ensure that Medicaid reimbursement rates match private insurance reimbursement rates? What might occur if poorer states were required to provide higher reimbursement rates? What is the risk if reimbursement rates are very low?

Medicaid Waivers

Much of the previous discussion about Medicaid highlighted both the numerous requirements placed on states and the enormous amount of flexibility states have in operating their program. Medicaid *waivers* provide still another level of flexibility for states. There are several different types of waivers under Medicaid; here, we focus only on the broadest one—the "section 1115" waiver. Under section 1115 of the SSA, states may apply to the secretary of HHS to waive certain requirements of health and welfare programs under the SSA, including both Medicaid and CHIP. The secretary may grant section 1115 waivers, also called demonstration projects, as long as the proposal "assists in promoting the objectives" of the federal program.[d] This broad standard has not been defined and leaves the secretary with enormous discretion to approve or reject waiver applications.

The Medicaid statute describes one main purpose of the program as furnishing medical assistance to those who cannot afford necessary care (SSA, § 1901). CMS developed criteria in 2015 to ensure waiver approvals meet this standard. Under this guidance, waiver projects should (1) increase and strengthen coverage for low-income individuals; (2) increase access to, strengthen, and stabilize Medicaid provider networks; (3) improve health outcomes for Medicaid beneficiaries and other low-income individuals; or (4) improve efficiency and quality of care for Medicaid beneficiaries and other low-income individuals through healthcare delivery reforms (Solomon & Schubel, 2017).

The issue of defining the objectives of the Medicaid program has taken center stage under the Trump administration. To achieve its goal of reshaping the Medicaid program, the administration replaced the 2015 guidance with its own program objectives. The administration acknowledges that the "core" mission of Medicaid is to "serve the health and wellness needs of our nation's vulnerable and low income" populations (Medicaid.gov, n.d.a). As a means of achieving this goal, the administration invited states to submit waivers that "support upward mobility" and "greater independence," promote "responsible decision making," and prepare beneficiaries for private coverage (Medicaid.gov, n.d.a). By identifying these goals as meeting objectives of the program, the administration is trying to lay a foundation to support waivers that limit eligibility and place additional requirements on beneficiaries. For example, the administration has approved or is considering approving waivers that allow states to impose work requirements, require drug screening, institute eligibility time limits, allow coverage lockouts for failing to meet administrative requirements, eliminate retroactive eligibility, and charge higher premiums with disenrollment allowed for nonpayment (KFF, 2018b).

As of July 2018, 37 states have been granted section 1115 waiver approvals, and 21 states have waivers that are pending (KFF, 2018b). The Trump administration has approved four waivers (Arizona, Indiana, Kentucky, and New Hampshire) that include work requirements and other elements, but a federal court recently vacated Kentucky's waiver. In *Stewart v. Azar*, the court held, in part, that the Secretary of HHS did not consider how Kentucky's waiver would promote affordable coverage, a key objective of the Medicaid program (Musumeci, 2018). The outcome of this and other court decisions will dictate how much leeway the administration has in changing the contours of the Medicaid program.

BOX 11-15 Discussion Questions

Should states be allowed to impose work requirements as a condition for receiving Medicaid benefits? Do work requirements promote independence and upward mobility, and, if so, are those two goals legitimate objectives of the Medicaid program? Are work requirements unnecessary barriers to care?

Those who oppose work requirements argue that they do not further the objective of the program, which is to provide coverage to those who cannot afford it. As a practical matter, most beneficiaries are already working, and most of those who are not working are in poor health or disabled, are acting as caregivers, or are students. Many of the nonworkers would be exempt even under the recently approved waivers. In addition, work requirements create extensive administrative obligations for beneficiaries and administrators alike. Of the 1 to 4 million beneficiaries estimated to lose coverage if work requirements are imposed broadly, most would be disenrolled due to lack of reporting.

Those who support requirements contend that everyone who can work should be working, both to reduce the burden on the Medicaid program and to support personal upward mobility. According to this view, the ultimate goal should be to wean people off of Medicaid and promote work requirements. Some states with Republican legislatures, such as Virginia, would not support expanding Medicaid under the ACA without work requirements.

Do you support work requirements? Even if you oppose work requirements, is it better to expand coverage with work requirements than to not expand coverage at all?

One of the most important aspects of a waiver is the "budget neutrality" requirement. A state must show that the waiver project will not cost the federal government more money over a 5-year period than if the waiver had not been granted. The MOE rule under the ACA also applies to waivers. Although the amount of money spent remains the same, by seeking a waiver, a state is agreeing to use itself as a "policy laboratory" in exchange for being able to operate its Medicaid program with fewer requirements. Ideally, other states and the federal government will learn from these demonstration projects and incorporate their positive aspects, while avoiding negative ones.

In 2001, the Bush administration created a specific type of section 1115 waiver called the Health Insurance Flexibility and Accountability (HIFA) demonstration. These waivers differ from traditional section 1115 waivers in that they encourage integration of Medicaid and CHIP with private insurance through premium assistance programs and other means. HIFA waivers also allow states to achieve budget neutrality by reducing the amount, duration, and scope of optional benefits and increasing cost-sharing requirements for optional eligibility groups (changes that may now be possible under section 1937 without the need for a formal waiver). Although states may reduce optional benefits and populations under HIFA, mandatory populations must remain covered and mandatory benefits may not be reduced. Given these rules, HIFA waivers often involve a trade-off between covering more people with fewer services or fewer people with more services.

The Future of Medicaid

Due to the high cost of the Medicaid program, the large federal deficit, other pressures on federal and state budgets, and ideological differences among policymakers, Medicaid reform has been a hot topic in recent years. Although the ACA included a significant Medicaid expansion, the Supreme Court's decision to make expansion optional has ensured that the battle over Medicaid and other entitlement programs will continue. Curtailing the Medicaid expansion and transforming Medicaid from an entitlement program to a block grant program were central features of the recent Republican ACA repeal and replacement efforts.

Even if Medicaid remains effectively intact, with the newly eligible Medicaid population operating under different rules than traditional Medicaid enrollees, the administrative complexity of running a two-tiered system will undoubtedly lead to calls for further reforms to simplify the program. It appears that many policymakers are moving away from viewing Medicaid

---

BOX 11-16 Discussion Questions

What type of Medicaid reform, if any, do you support? Should Medicaid beneficiaries be treated like privately insured individuals, meaning increased cost-sharing requirements, fewer legal protections, and fewer guaranteed benefits than in the current Medicaid program? Is it fair to provide a more generous package of benefits to publicly insured individuals than most privately insured people receive? Can the country afford a more generous Medicaid program? Can it afford not to provide adequate health insurance and access to care for the poor and near poor? Is it best to let states experiment with new ideas? If you could design a new Medicaid program, what would be your primary decision-making goal?

---

as a social insurance program that provides a certain set of healthcare benefits and specific legal protections to vulnerable populations. Instead, they are envisioning Medicaid as a program that more closely mirrors private insurance plans in terms of their use of risk, cost sharing, and comparatively limited benefits and in their lack of extra protections that ensure fairness and access to care. As noted previously, some states are implementing these types of changes through waivers granted by HHS.

While the high number of Medicaid enrollees in expansion states speaks to the need for an affordable insurance option for many low-income individuals, the cost of the expansion is already making states question their ability to support a larger Medicaid program. Nonetheless, Medicaid remains quite popular with the public, with 74% of respondents in one poll indicating a favorable view of the program; there is also relatively little support for curtailing funding (Rudowitz & Garfield, 2018). These competing political views about what form Medicaid should take makes the future of the program uncertain at best.

▶ Children's Health Insurance Program

Congress created the Children's Health Insurance Program (CHIP) in 1997 as a $40 billion, 10-year block grant program, codified as Title XXI of the SSA. When the program expired in 2007, Congress tried to extend it by passing two versions of the Children's Health Insurance Program Reauthorization Act (CHIPRA). Despite the bipartisan support for these bills, then-president George W. Bush vetoed both versions and instead signed a temporary extension of the program. In 2009, Congress again passed CHIPRA, and newly elected President Obama signed it into law as one of his first acts in office. CHIPRA included $33 billion in federal funds for children's coverage and extended the program and its funding through 2013 (KFF, 2012a). The ACA further extended the program until 2019, but only included funding through fiscal year 2015. In April 2015, Obama signed the Medicare Access and CHIP Reauthorization Act of 2015, which provided 2 more years of funding (through 2017) for CHIP. After a short lapse in funding, Congress extended funding until 2023 through the HEALTHY KIDS Act of 2018 and until 2027 through the Bipartisan Budget Act of 2018.

CHIP is designed to provide health insurance to uninsured low-income children whose family income is above the eligibility level for Medicaid in their state. Overall, CHIP has been successful at insuring low-income children, enrolling more than 8.9 million children in 2016 (MACPAC, 2018). Nonetheless, 5.4% of children younger than 19 years remained uninsured as of 2016, and many of them live in low-income families (U.S. Census, 2017, p. 2).

CHIP Structure and Financing

CHIP is an optional program for the states, but all 50 have chosen to participate. States have three options regarding how their CHIP is structured:

1. States may incorporate CHIP into their existing Medicaid program by using CHIP children as an expansion population.
2. States may create an entirely separate CHIP program.
3. States may create a hybrid program in which lower-income children are part of Medicaid and higher-income children are in a separate CHIP program.

In 2017, 2 states had a separate program, 8 states and the District of Columbia had a Medicaid expansion program, and 40 states had a hybrid program (MACPAC, 2018).

As with Medicaid, federal CHIP funds are disbursed on a matching basis, although the federal match is higher for CHIP than for Medicaid. It is known as the E-FMAP, for enhanced-FMAP. Historically, the CHIP match rate ranged from 65% to 81.5% (MACPAC, 2018). The ACA included a significant increase in the CHIP match for states from 2015 to 2019 that raised the minimum match from 65% to 88% (but not to exceed 100%). In 2018, the E-FMAP matching rate ranged from 88% to 100%. The federal

government covered 92.5% of the $15.6 billion in CHIP spending in 2016 (MACPAC, 2018). The HEALTHY KIDS Act added a phase-down year for the ACA E-FMAP, extending it through 2020. After that, the E-FMAP reverts to the pre-ACA rate.

The matching formula is set by law and was changed when CHIPRA was enacted. Originally, allotments were for 3 years and were based on state-specific estimates of the number of low-income uninsured children, the number of low-income children generally, and healthcare costs relative to other states. Under CHIPRA, allotments are for 2 years and state allotments will increase annually to account for growth in healthcare spending, increases in the number of children in the state, and state program expansions. Every 2 years, state allotments will be rebased to reflect actual use of CHIP funds (Ryan, 2009). If states exhaust their funding and they exceed target enrollment levels, they are eligible for contingency funding (MACPAC, 2011; MACPAC, 2018).

The changes to the CHIP allotment formula were intended to allow for more predictable budgeting and to account for state program expansions. In addition, they address a recurring problem under the old formula. Previously, if states did not use their full allotment, the unused money reverted to the federal treasury and could be used by the federal government for any purpose. This system led to frequent fights to keep the money in the CHIP and over how the unused funds would be redistributed. Many states became dependent on receiving redistributed funds to keep their CHIP afloat. The new formula and process should help avoid this problem through better budgeting predictability and shorter allotment time frames. In addition, under CHIPRA, all unused funds are designated to go to Medicaid performance bonuses for increased enrollment and outreach, instead of reverting to the federal treasury (MACPAC, 2011; Ryan, 2009).

TABLE 11-4 highlights a number of differences between Medicaid and CHIP. One very important difference is that whereas Medicaid is an entitlement program, CHIP is a block grant. As mentioned earlier, as a block grant, the federal matching funds are capped (through the allotments). Thus, a state is not entitled to limitless federal money under CHIP, and children, even if eligible, are not legally entitled to services once the allotted money has been spent. If a state runs out of funds and operates its CHIP separate from Medicaid, it will have to cut back its CHIP program by eliminating benefits, lowering provider reimbursement rates, unenrolling beneficiaries, or wait-listing children who want to enroll in the program. A state with a Medicaid expansion CHIP or a hybrid structure would not receive new CHIP money but would

TABLE 11-4 Comparing Key Features of Medicaid and CHIP

Feature	Medicaid	CHIP
Structure	Entitlement	Block grant
Financing	Federal–state match	Federal–state match at higher rate than Medicaid
Use of funds for premium assistance	No (without a waiver)	Yes
Benefits	Federally defined, with option to use benchmark or benchmark-equivalent benefits package; broad EPSDT services for children	Benefits undefined; use benchmark package; limited "basic" services required
Cost sharing	Limited or prohibited for some populations and services, higher amounts allowed for some populations and services	Cost sharing permitted within limits, but prohibited for well-baby and well-child exams
Antidiscrimination provision	Yes	No

Abbreviations: CHIP = Children's Health Insurance Program; EPSDT = early and periodic screening, diagnosis, and treatment.

BOX 11-17 Discussion Questions

Why do you think that Medicaid was created as an entitlement program but CHIP was established as a block grant? Both programs are federal–state insurance programs for low-income individuals, so does the distinction make sense? Does it matter that one program is for children and the other is broader? Should one program be changed so they are both either entitlements or block grants? Which structure do you prefer?

---

continue to receive federal funds for Medicaid-eligible children as allowed under the Medicaid rules and at the Medicaid matching rate.

CHIP Eligibility

Children are eligible for CHIP if they meet their state's income requirement, are younger than 19 years, do not have other health insurance coverage, and are not eligible for Medicaid (MACPAC, 2018). CHIP originally allowed states to cover children up to 200% FPL, but CHIPRA expanded coverage to 300% FPL with the enhanced matching rate (KFF, 2012a).[e] If states go above 300% FPL, they receive the state's regular Medicaid match rate instead of the enhanced CHIP rate.

Because CHIP coverage is built on a state's Medicaid eligibility rules, when CHIP eligibility begins depends on when Medicaid eligibility ends. For example, if a state covers a child up to 150% FPL, CHIP eligibility in that state would start at over 150% FPL. If another state Medicaid program covers children at 200% FPL, CHIP eligibility would start at over 200% FPL. CHIP eligibility ranges from 170% in North Dakota to 400% in New York. Twenty-three states cover children in families with income between 200% and 249% FPL, and 25 states cover children in families with incomes at or above 250% FPL (MACPAC, 2018). In 2013, most CHIP children (88.8%) were in families with incomes at or below 200% FPL (MACPAC, 2018).

Under the ACA, states must cover all children ages 6 to 19 years up to 133% FPL in their Medicaid program, and children in families with incomes up to 133% who are currently in CHIP programs must be moved to the state's Medicaid program.[b] Variations may still exist above that level. As a result, children in families with the same income levels could be in CHIP in one state and in Medicaid in another state. States also have an MOE requirement under CHIP. They are required to maintain their 2010 eligibility levels through 2019. The MOE requirement remains in place from 2020 through 2027 for children in families with income at or below 300% FPL (MACPAC, 2018).

Originally, pregnant women were not eligible for coverage under CHIP without a waiver. CHIPRA explicitly allows for coverage of pregnant women, and 5 states have used that option as of January 2017 (MACPAC, 2018). In addition, 16 states have adopted an option to cover unborn children as a way to indirectly allow pregnant women to access the program (MACPAC, 2018). As noted earlier in this chapter, CHIPRA also expanded eligibility by allowing states to cover lawfully residing immigrant pregnant women and children, even if they have not been in the United States for 5 years. Prior to CHIPRA, states could cover these populations only with state dollars. As of 2018, 33 states cover immigrant children and 25 states cover immigrant pregnant women without a 5-year waiting period (KFF, 2018a).

CHIPRA included a number of provisions to streamline enrollment and improve outreach. While states must verify the citizenship status of CHIP enrollees, just as they must for Medicaid enrollees, states must do so through an electronic data match in most cases. They may request paper documentation only when electronic data are not available or are not "reasonably compatible" with information provided by the individual (Georgetown University, 2017). This option eases the administrative burden of the citizenship verification and other documentation requirements and makes it much less likely that eligible individuals will be dropped from the program. CHIPRA also allows states to use "express lane eligibility," which permits states to take information provided when individuals apply for other public programs and use that information to assess eligibility for CHIP. In addition, the ACA limited eligibility determinations to once every 12 months and created a continuous eligibility option that allows states to provide 12 months of coverage regardless of changes in income (Georgetown University, 2017). Finally, CHIP includes performance bonuses and other financial incentives to states that adopt various enrollment simplification and outreach policies (Ryan, 2009).

CHIP Benefits and Beneficiary Safeguards

States must provide "basic" benefits, including inpatient and outpatient hospital care, physician services (surgical and medical), laboratory and X-ray services, well-baby and well-child care, and age-appropriate immunizations. Under CHIPRA, states must now provide dental coverage and may provide dental-only supplemental coverage for otherwise eligible children who have health insurance without dental coverage. States may also choose to provide additional benefits such as prescription drug coverage, mental health services, vision services, hearing services, and other services needed by children. CHIPRA requires that states that choose to provide mental health or substance abuse services offer the same level of coverage as they do for medical and surgical benefits (KFF, 2012a). States that use the Medicaid expansion structure must provide full Medicaid benefits, including EPSDT, and follow Medicaid cost-sharing rules (MACPAC, 2018).

Various standards may be used for the CHIP benefit package (Georgetown University, 2017). The law outlines the following benchmarks that states may use when designing their programs:

- The health insurance plan that is offered by the HMO that has the largest commercial, non-Medicaid enrollment in the state
- The standard Blue Cross Blue Shield preferred provider plan for federal employees
- A health plan that is available to state employees
- A package that is actuarially equivalent to one of the above plans
- A coverage package that is approved by the HHS secretary

(Do these benchmark plans sound familiar? Clearly, the DRA revisions to Medicaid were modeled on the existing CHIP program.) Under a stand-alone CHIP program, the benefit package may be the same

---

BOX 11-18 Discussion Questions

When designing CHIP, policymakers chose to follow the private insurance model instead of the Medicaid model. Although states have the choice to create a generous Medicaid expansion program for their CHIP beneficiaries, they also have the choice to implement a more limited insurance program with fewer protections. Similar choices were made when the DRA options were created for Medicaid. These decisions raise essential questions about the role of government in public insurance programs. Does the government (federal or state) have a responsibility to provide additional benefits and protection to its low-income residents? Or, is the government satisfying any responsibility it has by providing insurance coverage that is equivalent to major private insurance plans? What if the standard for private insurance plans becomes lower—does that change your analysis? Is it fair for low-income individuals to receive more comprehensive health insurance coverage than other individuals? Is there a point where fiscal constraints trump equity or the likelihood of improved health outcomes when designing a public insurance program?

as the state's Medicaid package or equal to one of these benchmarks. States with separate CHIP programs commonly create benefit packages that are less generous than the ones available in their Medicaid programs (Ryan, 2009).

In addition to the benefit package options, there are other areas where CHIP provides states with more program flexibility and beneficiaries with less protection than is the case under Medicaid. CHIP does not have the same standards regarding reasonableness, benefit definitions, medical necessity, or nondiscrimination coverage on the basis of illness (though, as noted earlier, states may opt out of or alter some of these protections in Medicaid under section 1937 plans). States, however, may not exclude children based on preexisting conditions. Also, like the section 1937 cost-sharing option, states with separate CHIP programs may impose cost-sharing requirements up to 5% of a family's annual income for families with incomes at or above 150% FPL (MACPAC, 2018).

CHIP and Private Insurance Coverage

In devising CHIP, Congress was concerned that Medicaid-eligible children would enroll in CHIP instead of Medicaid without reducing the overall number of uninsured children in a state. To avoid this outcome, CHIP requires that all children be assessed for Medicaid eligibility and, if eligible, enrolled in Medicaid instead of CHIP (MACPAC, 2018). With Medicaid expansion under the ACA, it is likely that some children in stand-alone CHIP programs will now be eligible for Medicaid. In addition, Congress wanted to make sure the government did not start funding health insurance coverage that was previously being paid for in the private sector. In other words, it did not want to give individuals or employers an incentive to move privately insured children to the new public program. To avoid private insurance crowd-out, Congress allowed states to institute enrollment waiting periods and impose cost-sharing requirements as a disincentive to switch to CHIP. As of 2017, 15 states have established waiting periods before enrollment (Georgetown University, 2017).

CHIP Waivers

States may apply to the secretary of HHS to waive CHIP requirements in exchange for experimenting with new ways to increase program eligibility or benefits. Initially, the most common use of CHIP waivers was to expand eligibility for uncovered populations, such as childless adults and parents and pregnant women who are not eligible under a state's Medicaid program. Using CHIP funds to provide coverage for adult populations was controversial because the program was designed to provide health insurance to children. While CHIPRA expands eligibility options for pregnant women, it also prohibits states from obtaining new waivers to cover adults with CHIP funds (Ryan, 2009).

In addition, seven states have used CHIP waivers and other pathways to create premium assistance programs (CHIPRA and the ACA also provide premium assistance options) (Department of Labor, 2018). Premium assistance means that public subsidies (in this case, CHIP funds) are available to help beneficiaries cover the cost of private health insurance premiums for employer-sponsored coverage or other health insurance plans that are available to them. States favor premium assistance programs as a way to reduce the state's cost of providing a child with health insurance. Premium assistance programs may also reduce crowd-out by providing an incentive for people to keep their children in private coverage instead of enrolling them in CHIP. States must abide by numerous rules when creating a premium assistance program, and the combination of these rules and the high cost of private insurance has led to low enrollment in CHIP premium assistance programs in the states that have initiated them. The use of premium assistance programs may increase in the future, as CHIPRA and the ACA include provisions to help reduce these barriers (KFF, 2013).

The Future of CHIP

The future of CHIP is clouded by the politics ensnaring the ACA. CHIP has been a very successful program, with consistent bipartisan support. CHIP could be strengthened by eliminating waiting periods for lower-income beneficiaries, reducing cost sharing, continuing to fund outreach efforts, and developing policies to ensure seamless transitions as children move among various insurance products (MACPAC, 2017). Many policy experts argued that CHIP remained necessary even with robust implementation of health reform that was supposed to include widespread expansion of Medicaid and strong marketplaces.

There are several reasons that CHIP remains vital in an ACA era: CHIP was designed for children, and CHIP providers specialize in treating children; CHIP is needed to assist low-income families in states that have not expanded Medicaid; CHIP is more affordable than many plans offered through state exchanges; and an estimated 2 million children would live in families who are not eligible for subsidies to purchase insurance through an exchange due to the "family glitch," which considers the cost of coverage for individual workers, not families, when assessing affordability (MACPAC, 2017; Vestal, 2014). The uncertainty surrounding the future of the ACA, the extent of Medicaid expansion, and the viability of the exchanges means the reasons CHIP was created in the first place—to provide insurance to uninsured low- to moderate-income children—continues today.

▶ Medicare

Medicare is the federally funded health insurance program for older adults and some persons with disabilities. As a completely federally funded program with uniform national guidelines, Medicare's administration and financing is quite different from that found in Medicaid and CHIP. This section reviews who Medicare serves, what benefits the program provides, how Medicare is financed, and how Medicare providers are reimbursed. As with Medicaid and CHIP, the ACA included several provisions relating to Medicare. These changes include new coverage for preventive services, bonus payments for primary care services, and assistance in paying for prescription drugs. At the same time, a number of changes will result in reduced reimbursement for providers. When the ACA was passed, its Medicare-related provisions were projected to result in $533 billion in savings and $105 billion in new Medicare spending, for a net

reduction of $428 billion in Medicare spending over 10 years (KFF, 2010).

Medicare Eligibility

Medicare covers two main groups of people—older adults and the disabled. In 2017, there were 58 million enrollees, including 49 million older adults and 9 million persons with disabilities, end-stage renal disease (ESRD), or amyotrophic lateral sclerosis (ALS, also called Lou Gehrig disease) enrolled in Medicare (HHS, 2017). These figures are expected to grow dramatically in the next few decades, as the "baby boom" population will result in the share of people 65 years and older increasing from 16% of the population in 2018 to 22% in 2048 (CBO, 2018, p. 19). As shown in **FIGURE 11-6**, Medicare enrollment is projected to exceed 90 million people by 2050.

To qualify for Medicare under the elderly category, individuals must be at least 65 years old and a U.S. citizen or permanent legal resident with at least 5 years of continuous residency. To avoid paying premiums for

---

BOX 11-19 Discussion Questions

Although many Medicare beneficiaries are poor, there is no means test (income- or resource-specific eligibility level) to determine eligibility as there is with Medicaid and CHIP. Is there a good public policy reason for this difference? What would be the basis for making this distinction? Does the government have a different role to play in providing health care based on the population involved?

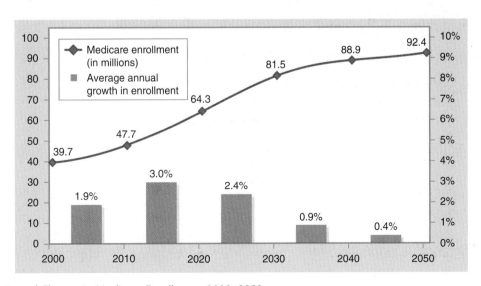

FIGURE 11-6 Projected Change in Medicare Enrollment, 2000–2050

Part A, older adults or their spouse must be eligible for Social Security payments by having worked and contributed to Social Security for at least 40 quarters (about 10 years). Individuals who are 65 years of age but do not meet the work requirements may become eligible for Medicare on the basis of their spouse's eligibility.

To qualify for Medicare as a person with disability, individuals must be totally and permanently disabled and receive Social Security Disability Insurance for at least 24 months, or have a diagnosis of either ESRD or ALS. There is no waiting period for individuals who qualify with an ALS or ESRD diagnosis. The disability categories do not have an age requirement, so these Medicare beneficiaries may be younger than 65 years, and Medicare beneficiaries younger than 65 years do not have to pay Part A premiums.

Unlike Medicaid and CHIP, Medicare eligibility is not based on an income or asset test; in other words, individuals of any income level are eligible for Medicare once they meet the eligibility requirements. Even though Medicare does not target low-income individuals, a significant portion of Medicare beneficiaries are indigent and in poor health (**FIGURE 11-7**). Half of Medicare beneficiaries are in families with annual incomes of $26,200 or less, and 34% had incomes under 200% FPL (KFF, 2016b). Among all Medicare beneficiaries, many have five or more chronic conditions, are in poor or fair health, or have a cognitive impairment (KFF, 2017a). In 2016, approximately 55% of beneficiaries were women (KFF, 2016c), 76% were white, 10% were African American, and 8% were Hispanic (KFF, 2016d). Women and racial and ethnic minorities are more likely to have lower income and fewer assets than their white, male counterparts.

In 2016, nearly 12 million low-income older adults were considered *dual eligibles*, meaning they were eligible for both Medicaid and Medicare (CMS.gov, 2018b). Dual-eligible beneficiaries receive most of their healthcare services through Medicare, but Medicaid is available to assist with Medicare's cost-sharing requirements and provide services not covered by Medicare, such as dental care and long-term services and supports. Not surprisingly, low-income beneficiaries tend to have significant healthcare needs. Medicare's dual eligibles are more likely than other beneficiaries to be in poor health, have several chronic conditions, and suffer from cognitive impairments (Musumeci, 2017) (**FIGURE 11-8**). Among dual eligibles, 41% have at least one mental health diagnosis, 68% have three or more chronic conditions, and half use long-term care support and services (CMS.gov, 2018b). Overall, 18% of dual-eligible enrollees report being in poor health

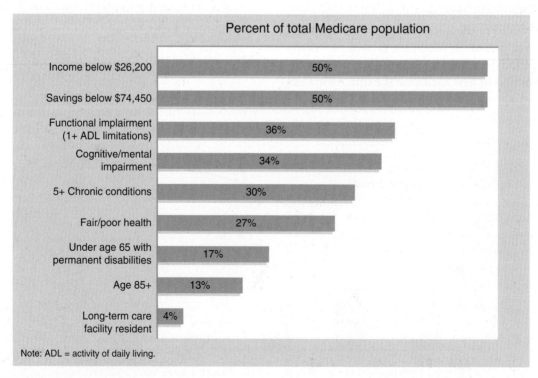

FIGURE 11-7 Characteristics of the Medicare Program

Source: Kaiser Family Foundation analysis of the Centers for Medicare & Medicaid Services Medicare Current Beneficiary 2013 Cost and Use file; Urban Institute/Kaiser Family Foundation analysis of DYNASIM data, 2017 (for income and savings). Retrieved from https://www.kff.org/medicare/issue-brief/an-overview-of-medicare/

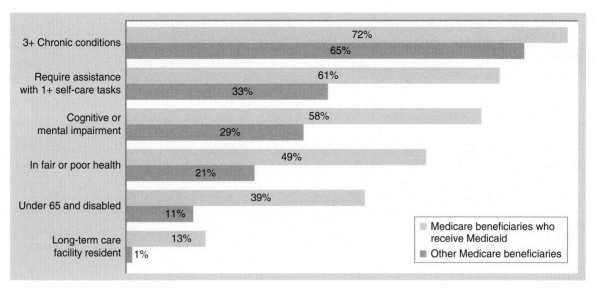

FIGURE 11-8 Health and Functioning of Medicare Beneficiaries Who Receive Medicaid Compared to Other Medicare Beneficiaries

Source: Kaiser Family Foundation analysis of CMS Medicarte Current Beneficiary Survey Cost & Use File, 2012.

as compared to 6% of other Medicare beneficiaries (CMS.gov, 2018b).

Given their frequent use of the healthcare system, dual eligibles consume a disproportionate share of resources. In 2012, this group constituted only 20% of Medicare beneficiaries but accounted for 34% of expenditures (CMS.gov, 2018b). Similarly, they made up 15% of the Medicaid population but were responsible for 33% of Medicaid spending (CMS.gov, 2018b). To assist with this high-need, high-cost population, the ACA created the Federal Coordinated Health Care Office (referred to as the Medicaid–Medicare Coordination Office) within CMS to improve the integration of services for dual eligibles (CMS.gov, 2018b).

Medicare Benefits

Medicare is split into several parts, each covering a specified set of services. Beneficiaries are automatically entitled to Part A, also known as Hospital Insurance (HI). Part B services, also known as Supplemental Medical Insurance (SMI), cover physician, outpatient, and preventive services. The ACA added coverage for certain preventive services without cost sharing, including an annual comprehensive risk assessment, provided without cost sharing when delivered in an outpatient setting. Part B is voluntary for enrollees, but 95% of Part A beneficiaries also opt to have Part B. Beneficiaries may choose to receive their benefits through Part C, Medicare Advantage (MA), which includes the Medicare managed care program and a few other types of plans. Part D is the new prescrip-

tion drug benefit. **TABLE 11-5** lists Medicare benefits by part, and **FIGURE 11-9** illustrates current spending on Medicare benefits. Significant growth is expected in spending on outpatient prescription drugs over the next 10 years. Although Medicare benefits are quite extensive, the list excludes services that one might expect to be covered in health insurance targeting older adults, such as nursing home care, routine eye care, dental care, and hearing exams and hearing aids (Cubanski et al., 2015).

There was rapid growth of Medicare managed care plans in the mid- to late 1990s, followed by a significant decline. Recently, enrollment has rebounded with 19 million enrollees (33% of Medicare beneficiaries) in 2017 (KFF, 2017a). However, as shown in **FIGURE 11-10**, enrollment is not spread evenly throughout the country; 40% of MA enrollees are in plans in 6 states (California, Florida, Hawaii, Minnesota, Oregon, Pennsylvania), while fewer than 20% are enrolled in plans in 13 states and the District of Columbia (Jacobson, Damico, Neuman, & Gold, 2017). In addition, many markets are highly concentrated. Insurance giants United and Humana signed 41% of all enrollees in 2017, and in 17 states one company accounted for at least half of enrollment (Jacobson et al., 2017).

Although HMOs have participated in Medicare since the 1970s, Part C has evolved over the last decade to include a number of new insurance options. In 1997, Congress added private FFS plans,[f] medical savings accounts coupled with high-deductible plans, county-based preferred provider organizations (PPOs), and point-of-service plans (Cubanski et al.,

TABLE 11-5 Medicare Benefits

Part	Services Covered
A	Inpatient hospital, 100 days at skilled nursing facility, limited home health following stay at a hospital or skilled nursing facility, and hospice care.
B	Physician, outpatient hospital, outpatient mental health, X-ray, laboratory, emergency department, and other ambulatory services; medical equipment; limited preventive services, including one preventive physical exam, mammography, pelvic exam, prostrate exam, colorectal cancer screening, glaucoma screening for high-risk patients, prostrate cancer screening, and cardiovascular screening blood test; diabetes screening and outpatient self-management; bone-mass measurement for high-risk patients; hepatitis B vaccine for high-risk patients; pap smear; and pneumococcal and flu vaccinations. New ACA benefits: cost sharing eliminated for select preventive services; coverage for personalized prevention plan, including comprehensive health assessment.
C	Managed care plans, private fee-for-service plans, special needs plans, and medical savings accounts. The plans provide all services in Part A and Part B and generally must offer additional benefits or services as well.
D	Prescription drug benefit.

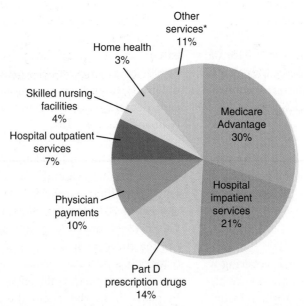

Total Medicare Benefit Payments, 2016: $675 billion

Note: *Consists of Medicare benefit spending on hospice, durable medical equipment, Part B drugs, outpatient dialysis, outpatient therapy, ambulance, lab, community mental health center, rural health clinic, federally qualified health center, and other Part B services.

FIGURE 11-9 Medicare Benefit Payments by Type of Service, 2016

Source: Congressional Budget Office, June 2017 Medicare Baseline.

2015). As part of the Medicare Prescription Drug Improvement and Modernization Act of 2003 (MMA), Congress added regional PPOs and "special needs plans" for the institutionalized and for beneficiaries with severe and disabling conditions (Cubanski et al., 2015). Most enrollees chose HMOs (11.9 million) or local PPOs (4.9 million) in 2017, with much smaller enrollment in the other types of plans (Jacobson et al., 2017). MA plans must cover all Part A and B services, and many offer additional services such as eyeglasses, hearing exams, and gym memberships as an inducement to enroll (Cubanski et al., 2015). Recent policy

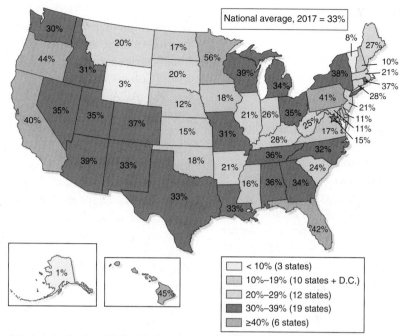

Share of Medicare Beneficiaries Enrolled in Medicare Private Health Plans, by State, 2017

National average, 2017 = 33%

< 10% (3 states)
10%–19% (10 states + D.C.)
20%–29% (12 states)
30%–39% (19 states)
≥40% (6 states)

Note: Includes Medicare Medical Savings Accounts (MSAs) cost plans and demonstrations. Includes special needs plans as well asother Medicare Advantage plans. Excludes beneficiaries with unknown county addresses and beneficiaries in territories other than Puerto Rico.

FIGURE 11-10 Enrollment in Medicare Advantage Plans Varies Across States

Source: Reproduced from Jacobson, G., Damico, A., Neuman, T., & Gold, M. (2017, June 6). Medicare Advantage 2017 spotlight: Enrollment market update. Retrieved from https://www.kff.org/medicare/issue-brief/medicare-advantage-2017-spotlight-enrollment-market-update/

changes allow MA plans to provide more supplemental benefits (e.g., portable wheelchair ramps, non-skilled in-home workers) to targeted beneficiaries, including chronically ill enrollees (Wynne & Horowitz, 2018).

The MMA also created Part D, Medicare's prescription drug benefit. The drug benefit was made available to recipients beginning in 2006, and 43 million beneficiaries were enrolled in Part D in 2018 (Cubanksi, Damico, & Neuman, 2018). In 2018, Medicare contracted with 782 private drug insurance plans (PDPs) in each of 34 regions (KFF, 2017b). Most Part D enrollees (58%) are in PDPs, with 42% in MA plans (Cubanski et al., 2018). Three firms—Humana, UnitedHealth, and CVS Health—have signed up over half of all Part D enrollees (Cubanski et al., 2018). Part D plans have flexibility to determine their formulary (beyond the federally required minimum), formulary tiering, cost sharing, and utilization management options (Cubanski et al., 2015). If at least two plans are not available in a region, the government contracts with a fallback plan (a private plan that is not an insurer) to serve that area. All plans must cover at least two drugs in each therapeutic class or category of Part D drugs. PDPs must maintain a medical loss ratio of at least 85%, meaning no more than 15% of revenue may be spent on administrative expenses or profits (Cubanski et al.,

2015). Dual eligibles (individuals enrolled in both Medicaid and Medicare) may no longer obtain prescription drug coverage under Medicaid; they must receive their prescription drug benefit through Medicare. In addition, low-income subsidies are available to those who need assistance paying for Part D. In 2018, 12 million enrollees received these subsidies (Cubanski et al., 2018).

To obtain prescription drugs through Medicare, beneficiaries have the choice of remaining in traditional FFS Medicare under Parts A and B and enrolling in a separate private prescription drug plan, or enrolling in a Part C plan through MA that includes prescription drug coverage. MA plans are required to offer basic prescription drug benefits and may offer supplemental prescription drug benefits for an additional premium. Some beneficiaries may also have access to employer-sponsored health insurance that includes prescription drug benefits. These beneficiaries may keep their employer coverage only, keep their employer coverage and enroll in Part D, or drop their employer coverage. Finally, beneficiaries may also choose not to obtain any prescription drug coverage. However, in certain circumstances, beneficiaries who decline to enroll in Part D during the allotted enrollment period and do not have other comparable prescription drug coverage will be charged a penalty of

1% of the national average premium for every month they do not enroll (KFF, 2017b).

Medicare Spending

Medicare expenditures reached almost $702 billion in 2017, which accounted for 15% of the total federal budget and 20% of total personal health expenditures (Cubanski & Neuman, 2018). Medicare spending is projected to increase to $1.3 trillion in 2028, with an aggregate growth rate of 7.3%. In 2017, Medicare spent a greater share of its funds on services under Parts B and D than in prior years, with a reduced share going toward Part A services (**FIGURE 11-11**). In addition, payments to MA plans for Parts A and B services almost doubled from 18% of benefit payments in 2007 to 30% in 2017 (Cubanski & Neuman, 2018). Spending levels would be even higher without savings created by the ACA. The growth in Medicare spending is expected to be slower in the next decade as compared to historical data, but spending rates are expected to rise in the long term due to increased use of services based on increased severity of illness, the aging population, and growth of healthcare costs (Cubanski & Neuman, 2018).

Not all Medicare beneficiaries cost the same amount to care for because of the disparities in the amount and type of services they require. As shown in Figure 11-9, 21% of Medicare's expenditures pay for hospital services, while physician and outpatient ser-

vices combined account for another 17% of Medicare payments. As with Medicaid and private insurance, a relatively small group of beneficiaries use a high proportion of these and other services. In 2010, 10% of all beneficiaries accounted for 58% of Medicare expenditures (Cubanksi et al., 2015).

The ACA established an Independent Payment Advisory Board, which has the task of submitting proposals to reduce the rate of Medicare spending if Medicare exceeds specified targets. The Secretary of Health and Human Services was required to implement proposals submitted by the board unless Congress enacts alternative proposals that achieve the same level of savings. Congress limited the board's options by prohibiting consideration of proposals that ration care, increase revenue, change benefits, change eligibility, or change cost sharing. This board, which was never constituted and was derided by policymakers and politicians from both sides of the aisle, was repealed as part of a budget bill in 2018.

Medicare Financing

Medicare is a federally funded program. Unlike Medicaid and CHIP, state governments do not generally contribute to Medicare spending, and therefore a matching system is not required. Although Medicare financing is simpler than Medicaid financing in many respects, each Medicare part has its own financing rules, adding some complexity to the program (**FIGURE 11-12**). In addition, beneficiary contributions in the form of premiums, deductibles, and co-payments contribute to financing Medicare expenditures.

Part A (HI) benefits are paid from the HI Trust Fund, funded through a mandatory payroll tax. Employers and employees each pay a tax of 1.45% of a worker's earnings (self-employed persons pay both shares, for a total tax of 2.9%), which is set aside for the Trust Fund. The ACA increases this rate for higher-income tax payers. Individuals who earn over $200,000 and couples who earn over $250,000 now pay a tax of 2.35% on their earnings (Cubanski & Neuman, 2018). In addition, beneficiaries pay a deductible for each inpatient hospital episode, and co-insurance for hospital care beyond 60 days, skilled nursing care beyond 20 days, outpatient drugs, and inpatient respite care (Cubanksi et al., 2015).

By relying on payroll taxes, Medicare Part A uses current workers and employers to pay for health benefits for the disabled and those older than 65 years, many of whom are already retired. This formula is problematic in the face of the looming retirement of those from the baby boom generation; while the number of enrollees is expected to grow to more than

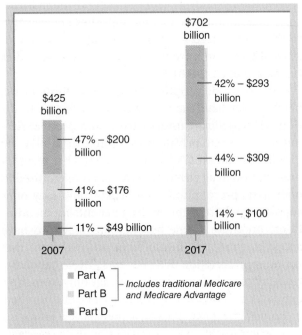

FIGURE 11-11 Medicare Payments for Parts A, B, and D, 2007–2017

Source: KFF Analysis of Medicare spending data from 2008 and 2018 Annual Report of the Board of Trustees of the Federal Hospital Insurance and Federal Supplementary Medical Insurance Trust Funds. Table II.B1.

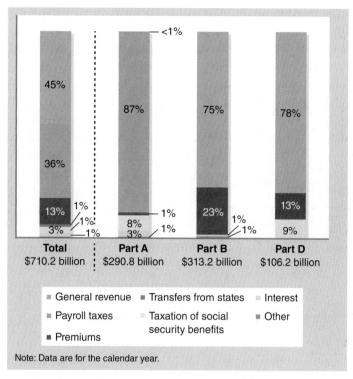

FIGURE 11-12 Sources of Medicare Revenue, 2016

BOX 11-20 Discussion Questions

Lawmakers were concerned that adding a prescription drug benefit to Medicare would encourage employers to drop prescription drug coverage to the beneficiaries who receive prescription drugs through retiree health plans. In an effort to avoid a shift in older people who rely on public insurance instead of private insurance for their prescription drug coverage, Congress included in the MMA a tax-free subsidy to encourage employers to maintain prescription drug coverage. While the ACA eliminates the tax deduction, the subsidy remains in place. The amount of the subsidy is based on the prescription drug costs of individuals who remain with the employer's plan and do not enroll in Part D. In 2017, approximately 2 million beneficiaries purchased coverage through employer retiree plans and employers received a subsidy of 28% of their costs between $405 and $8,350 per retiree (KFF, 2017b).

Is this subsidy a good idea? Is the proper role of government to pay private companies to maintain insurance coverage? If so, should it occur for other benefits? Do you have a preference regarding giving incentives for private entities to provide insurance coverage versus the government financing the coverage directly?

90 million by 2050, the country will not experience a similar growth in workers to support those enrollees. As shown in **FIGURE 11-13**, from 2010 to 2050, the number of workers supporting each enrollee is expected to decline from 3.4 to 2.3. Because of this and for other reasons, the 2014 Medicare Board of Trustees estimated that the Part A HI Trust Fund would be exhausted by 2026 (Cubanski & Neuman, 2018).

Part B (SMI) is financed through general federal tax revenues and monthly premiums, deductibles, and cost sharing paid by beneficiaries. Beneficiaries with incomes over $85,000 (or $170,000 for a couple) will pay a higher income-related monthly premium than other beneficiaries. Instead of increasing each year, this income threshold was frozen from 2009 to 2019 as part of the ACA, meaning more beneficiaries will be subject to the higher premium during those years. In addition to the monthly premium, beneficiaries pay an annual deductible for physician and medical services and have co-insurance requirements for outpatient hospital care, ambulatory surgical care, clinical diagnostic services, outpatient mental health services, and most preventive services.

Despite the federal government's and beneficiaries' investment in Medicare benefits, beneficiaries still face out-of-pocket expenses due to cost-sharing and service-related costs. In 2013, beneficiaries in traditional

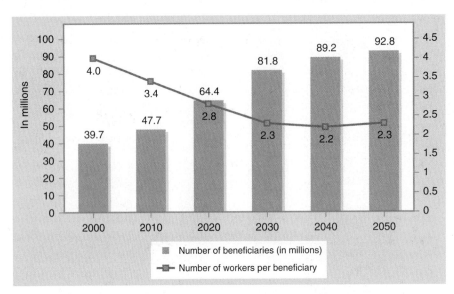

FIGURE 11-13 Number of Medicare Beneficiaries and Number of Workers per Beneficiary, 2000–2050

Source: Kaiser Family Foundation based on the 2014 Annual Report of the Boards of Trustees of the Federal Hospital Insurance and Federal Supplementary Medical Insurance Trust Funds.

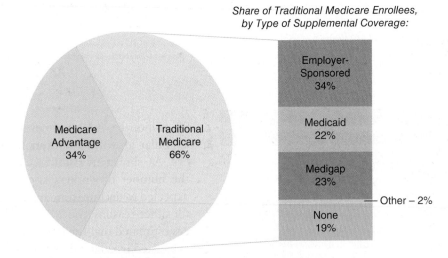

FIGURE 11-14 Distribution of Medicare Advantage and Traditional Medicare Enrollment and Types of Supplemental Coverage Among Medicare Beneficiaries, 2013

Source: Kaiser Family Foundation. (2017a). An overview of Medicare. Retrieved on July 25, 2018 from https://www.kff.org/medicare/issue-brief/an-overview-of-medicare/

Medicare paid just over $6,000 on average for out-of-pocket Part A and B services. Enrollees in MA plans may pay up to $6,700 in out-of-pocket costs (KFF, 2017a). As a result, many beneficiaries have some type of supplemental insurance. These "Medigap" policies, as they are known, are sold by private insurers and are intended to cover the cost of payments required by Medicare, such as premiums and co-payments. In addition, some Medigap policies offer benefits that are not covered by Medicare. **FIGURE 11-14** illustrates the most common type of supplemental options, and **FIGURE 11-15** shows that the highest proportion of out-of-pocket spending

was attributed to long-term care services. Older, sicker, and female Medicare beneficiaries experience the highest out-of-pocket costs (KFF, 2017a).

Part C MA plans provide services from Parts A and B and receive their funding from the sources described above. The federal government contracts with private plans and pays them a capitated rate to provide Medicare benefits to program participants. The plans charge beneficiaries varying premiums and co-payments. In addition, enrollees pay their regular Part B premiums. Most enrollees (81%) have a choice of a zero-premium plan, but only half choose to enroll in such plans, indicating

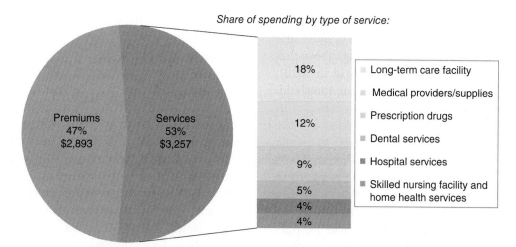

Average Total Out-of-Pocket Spending on Services and Premiums, 2013: $6,150

Note: Analysis excludes beneficiaries enrolled in Medicare Advantage plans those enrolled in Part A or Part B only.

FIGURE 11-15 Average Out-of-Pocket Spending on Services and Premiums by Medicare Beneficiaries, 2013

Source: Kaiser Family Foundation. (2017a). An overview of Medicare. Retrieved on July 25, 2018 from https://www.kff.org/medicare/issue-brief/an-overview-of-medicare/

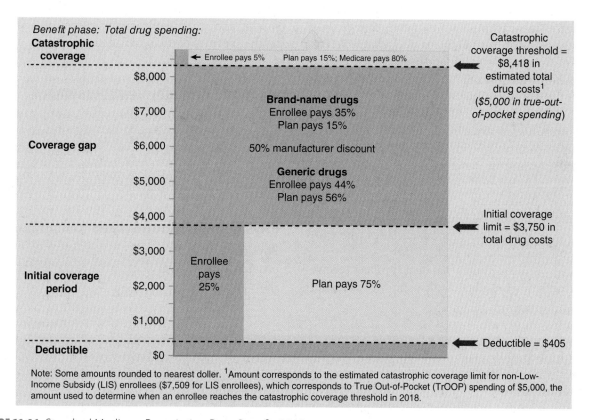

FIGURE 11-16 Standard Medicare Prescription Drug Benefit, 2018

Source: Kaiser Family Foundation. (2017b). The Medicare Part D prescription drug benefit. Retrieved from https://www.kff.org/medicare/fact-sheet/the-medicare-prescription-drug-benefit-fact-sheet/

other features are also important to enrollees (e.g., provider network, extra services) (Jacobson et al., 2017).

Part D, Medicare's prescription drug benefit, is financed through an annual deductible, monthly premiums, general revenues, and state payments for dual enrollees. Generally, premiums are set to cover 25.5% of Part D costs. As with Part B, enrollees pay a tiered pre-

mium based on their income. Individuals with incomes over $85,000 and couples with incomes over $170,000 pay a surcharge that ranges from 35% to 80% of Part D, depending on their income. Just over 3 million enrollees are expected to pay this surcharge in 2017 (KFF, 2017b). As shown in **FIGURE 11-16**, beneficiaries pay an annual deductible ($405 in 2018), 25% of the cost of drugs up to a set amount ($3,750 in 2018) during the initial coverage period, 35% of the cost of brand-name drugs and 44% of the costs of generic drugs above that amount to a catastrophic threshold ($8,418 in 2018), and 5% of the cost above the catastrophic threshold. When Part D was first created, the coverage gap in Medicare between the initial coverage period and the catastrophic coverage period was referred to as the *doughnut hole* because beneficiaries had to pay 100% of the costs of drugs. The ACA included provisions to close the doughnut hole such that beneficiaries will pay only 25% cost sharing in that range of drug spending by 2020. Beneficiaries received a $250 rebate for purchases made in the doughnut hole in 2010. To close the coverage gap, beneficiaries will receive a phased-in discount for generic and brand-name drugs purchased in the doughnut hole going forward. In addition, the amount of out-of-pocket spending needed to reach the catastrophic level was reduced from 2014 to 2019, but will revert back to its original level in 2020 without further congressional action (Cubanski et al., 2015).

In 2018, most Part D plans will charge a co-payment, often varied by drug, and over 60% will charge a deductible. In addition, 65% of plans do not offer coverage in the gap beyond what is required by the ACA (KFF, 2017b). Under Part D, deductibles, premiums, benefit limits, and catastrophic thresholds are not fixed, but indexed to increase with the growth in per-capita Medicare spending for Part D. To offset these charges, the MMA included provisions to assist low-income beneficiaries by reducing or eliminating cost-sharing requirements and the doughnut hole. There are three low-income assistance tiers for beneficiaries who earn up to 150% FPL (Cubanski et al., 2015).

The MMA also requires that dual enrollees receive their prescription drug benefit through Medicare, not Medicaid. Under the MMA, states are now required to help fund Medicare's prescription drug benefit for dual enrollees through a MOE or "clawback" provision. This provision requires states to pay the federal government a share of expenditures the states would have made to provide prescription drug coverage to dual enrollees. The state share begins at 90% in 2006 and tapers down to 75% in 2015 and beyond. Many states are resisting these requirements, and some are threatening not to pay their share. To the extent states adhere to the clawback provision, it represents the first time that states are assisting with Medicare financing. If states choose to provide dual enrollees with prescription drug coverage through Medicaid, states must use 100% of their own dollars to finance the coverage, even if the beneficiary does not enroll in Part D.

TABLE 11-6 provides a summary of Medicare financing provisions. Because Part C is financed by parts A and B and is an alternative to A and B, it is not included in the table. Whether beneficiaries have cost sharing and other requirements under Part C depends on the specifics of each managed care plan.

Medicare Provider Reimbursement

Medicare's reimbursement rules vary by provider type and by whether care is provided through an FFS arrangement or an MA (i.e., managed care) plan. This section reviews physician and hospital reimbursement methodologies under both payment systems.

Physician Reimbursement

Physicians who are paid by a managed care plan to provide Medicare services to beneficiaries follow the same general rules for managed care reimbursement.

TABLE 11-6 Medicare Financing by Part				
Medicare Part	**Government Financing Scheme**	**Annual Deductible**	**Monthly Premium**	**Cost Sharing**
A	Trust fund through mandated employer and employee payroll taxes	Yes	No, if Social Security work requirements are met	Yes
B	General federal tax revenue	Yes	Yes—tiered by income	Yes
D	General federal tax revenue and state clawback payments for dual enrollees	Yes—except some low-income beneficiaries	Yes—tiered by income (some low-income beneficiaries do not pay premiums)	Yes—except some low-income beneficiaries

However, physicians providing care on an FFS basis are paid according to the Medicare fee schedule, although the ACA included a 10% bonus payment from 2011 to 2015 for primary care providers who operated in Health Professional Shortage Areas. The fee schedule assigns a relative weight to every service to reflect the resources needed to provide the service. These weights are adjusted for geographic differences in costs and multiplied by a conversion factor (a way to convert the relative value that defines all medical services on the fee schedule into a dollar amount) to determine the final payment amount. Payment rates are changed through upward or downward shifts in the conversion factor. Although the ratio of Medicare physician fees to private insurance varies considerably by location, overall, Medicare physician fees are about 75% of those provided by private insurers (Medicare Payment Advisory Commission [MedPAC], 2018, p. 95), but about 44% higher than reimbursement rates provided by Medicaid (CBO, 2015).

In 1997 Congress established a formula for reimbursing physicians, referred to as the Sustainable Growth Rate (SGR), as a way to control spending on physician services. The formula set an overall target amount for spending on physician services (and related services such as laboratory tests) in Part B. Payment rates were adjusted to reflect actual spending as compared to the target level—if actual spending was higher than the target level, payment rates were cut, but if actual spending was lower than the target level, payment rates were raised. From 1997 to 2001, physician spending was slightly below the target (MedPAC, 2015). Since 2003, however, spending has exceeded the target level. Congress has not had the political will to impose reimbursement cuts called for by the formula. Since 2003, Congress suspended the formula annually because it would have resulted in rate reductions, and instead legislated rate increases for physicians. Deferring reimbursement cuts year after year has led to an untenable situation. If the SGR formula had been followed in 2015, physician fees would have been cut 21% that year (CBO, 2015).

In March 2015, Congress passed and President Obama signed into law the Medicare Access and CHIP Reauthorization Act of 2015 (MACRA). This bipartisan bill scrapped the SGR formula, provided physicians additional reimbursement, and created a new payment structure tying reimbursement to quality. MACRA includes a 0.5% annual update for physician reimbursement from 2015 to 2019 and then maintains level reimbursement from 2019 to 2025. In addition, physicians will be given the opportunity to supplement their reimbursement if they participate in a new Merit-Based Incentive Payment System (MIPS) or alternative payment model (APM) (e.g., bundled payments or accountable care organizations) (National Law Review, 2015). After 2026, physicians participating in an APM will receive a 1% reimbursement update, instead of a 0.5% increase for nonparticipants.

The MIPS program is an attempt to streamline three existing programs that tie physician reimbursement to improved quality and use of electronic health records: the Physician Quality Reporting System, the Value-Based Modifier, and the Promoting Interoperability (originally named Meaningful Use) program for electronic records (National Law Review, 2015). Based on their scores, physicians can receive cuts or additions to their reimbursement updates, up to a capped amount. As of 2018, physician cost is included in the MIPS score (Wilensky, 2018). Physicians who choose not to participate in MIPS must pay a penalty. It is estimated that 3% of physicians were penalized for the 2017 reporting year (Wilensky, 2018). Many interested stakeholders believe MIPS is not working as intended. In its 2017 report, the Medicare Payment Advisory Commission proposed scrapping MIPS for a new system because MIPS was not helping beneficiaries choose physicians, was not helping physicians improve their quality of care, and was not helping CMS identify and reward physicians who provide

BOX 11-21 Discussion Questions

The clawback provision is controversial and highlights some of the tensions about state flexibility and national uniformity that policymakers face when designing public programs. The clawback seems to contradict the prior decision to provide states with flexibility and program design responsibilities under Medicaid. In addition, it changes the decision to use only federal funds to pay for Medicare. Given decisions made by states prior to the MMA, there are many variations among state prescription drug benefits that will be "frozen" in place with the clawback provision. At the same time, the MMA creates a uniform rule about how all states finance prescription drug funding in the future, which could impact state-level decisions about dual enrollee coverage.

Is the clawback provision a good idea? Should states help pay for federal prescription drug coverage? Is there a better design? Should states or the federal government control Medicaid prescription drug coverage that is provided to dual enrollees? Should dual enrollees be treated differently than other Medicaid beneficiaries?

high-value care (Wilensky, 2018). Medical associations and the American Hospital Association agree MIPS is not working well but prefer that CMS fix the program instead of replace it (Wilensky, 2018).

CMS released its final rule implementing MACRA in November 2016. These rules included a transition period in 2017 that gave providers more flexibility and fewer reporting requirements in the MIPS program, additional models to qualify as an APM, and eligibility thresholds that may exempt more physicians (Patel, Darling, & Ginsberg, 2016). CMS estimated that over half of physicians would be exempt from MIPS because they do not have patient contact, they have low Medicare revenue or patient volume, they are new Medicare providers, or they participate in an APM (Patel et al., 2016). Under MACRA, physicians who participate in and receive a significant amount of their revenue through APMs that include the risk of financial loss and a quality improvement component will receive a 5% bonus from 2019 to 2024. In addition, participation in an APM releases physicians from the requirement to participate in MIPS and most Promoting Interoperability programs (National Law Review, 2015). CMS continues to explore APM structures, including creating the Bundled Payments for Care Improvement Advanced model that pays a retrospective amount for services over a 90-day period (Geilfuss & Romano, 2018) and allowing MA providers to qualify as APMs (Dickson, 2018).

BOX 11-22 Discussion Questions

Controlling Medicare spending is a difficult task. Even if provider reimbursement rates are reduced, physicians and hospitals may increase volume and intensity of services to make up for lost revenue. The ACA included a number of pilot programs and demonstration projects to experiment with reforming the way health care is financed and delivered, and MACRA increased the incentives for physicians to participate in these experiments. Some of these projects include bundling payment for acute care services; using value-based purchasing, which ties payments to quality outcomes; and creating accountable care organizations that bring together providers across the healthcare spectrum and reward organizations with better outcomes. The ACA created the CMS Innovation Center to oversee these and other reform projects.

What approach to reducing costs and improving quality do you prefer? What are the advantages and disadvantages of these ideas?

Hospital Reimbursement

Hospitals are paid for acute inpatient services on a prospective basis using diagnostic-related groups (DRGs). DRGs sort patients into more than 500 groups based on their diagnoses. Various diagnoses are grouped together if they have similar clinical profiles and costs. Each DRG is assigned a relative weight based on charges for cases in that group as compared to the national average for all groups. In addition, the part of the DRG covering hospitals' cost of labor is adjusted by a wage index to account for different geographic costs (MedPAC, 2005, p. 43). Hospitals may also receive additional payments for providing high-cost outlier cases; incurring costs associated with use of new technology; incurring indirect medical education costs; serving a high proportion of low-income patients; or being a qualified sole community provider, a rural referral center, a small Medicare-dependent hospital, a rural hospital treating fewer than 200 admissions, or a critical access hospital (a qualified rural hospital that provides critical care services) (MedPAC, 2005, pp. 43–44).

For outpatient care, hospitals are reimbursed by Medicare using a different prospective system. Each outpatient service is assigned to one of about 800 ambulatory payment classification (APC) groups. APCs have a relative weight based on the median cost of the service as compared to the national average. Again, a conversion factor is used to calculate the specific dollar amount per APC, and the labor cost portion is adjusted based on a hospital wage index to account for geographic cost differences. APC payments may be adjusted when hospitals use new technologies or biologics and when they treat unusually high-cost patients (MedPAC, 2005, p. 44).

The ACA included a number of provisions that reduced reimbursement for hospitals and other Medicare providers, including skilled nursing facilities and hospices. These rate reductions include "market basket" updates, which set the prices for a mix of goods and services, and a lowering of DSH payments, which are given to hospitals that provide services to a relatively high proportion of Medicaid and uninsured patients. In addition, hospitals will receive reduced payments for services connected to preventable readmissions and hospital-acquired conditions.

MA Reimbursement

MA plans are paid a capitated rate by the federal government to provide Parts A, B, and D benefits to each enrollee in their plan. Plans submit a bid to the federal government that estimates their cost per enrollee, and these bids are compared to benchmarks established by statute and that vary by county. The benchmark is the maximum Medicare will pay for Part A and B services in that county. If the bid is below the benchmark, Medicare and the plan split the difference and the portion returned to the plan is referred to as a rebate and must be used to provide additional benefits to enrollees (Cubanski et al., 2015). Once a bid is accepted, a contract between plans and the federal government details the services the plan will provide and the premiums, deductibles, and cost sharing it will charge beneficiaries.

The ACA includes significant reductions in MA payments. On average, MA plans had become 14% more expensive than FFS providers for comparable services (Cubanski et al., 2015). The ACA phases in reduced payments that bring MA plans closer to the benchmark payment for traditional Medicare services in their county. Additional reductions will occur due to changes in the risk-adjustment formula. On the other hand, plans that provide high-quality care may be eligible for additional payments under the new law (Cubanski et al., 2015). MA plans are also required to follow the 85% medical loss ratio rule, limiting the amount of revenues that can be used for profits and administration.

The Future of Medicare

While the Republican leadership in Congress included Medicare reform in its agenda for overall entitlement reform and reduced federal government spending, serious Medicare reform efforts have yet to materialize. The focus of its efforts to date has been to repeal and replace the ACA and to reform Medicaid. While there is broad agreement across the political spectrum that Medicare's financing is unsustainable going forward, there is less accord about how to address that problem. If Medicare is altered dramatically, one of the options frequently discussed is turning it into a premium support program. In this type of program, the federal government provides beneficiaries with a set amount of funds to purchase health insurance, with the beneficiary making up the difference between the allotment and the cost of the premium (Glied, 2018). Of course, both the amount of savings for the federal government and the burden on beneficiaries would depend on the size of the premium support provided to beneficiaries.

In any case, by shifting from an entitlement program to a specific allotment, much of the financial risk of rising healthcare costs would fall on beneficiaries, not the federal government (Glied, 2018). While it is doubtful that a significant restructuring will happen anytime soon, other policy changes—such as simplifying the program structure, increasing future beneficiaries' share of costs, increasing the eligibility age, and encouraging the use of private plans through competition—are more likely to become part of the debate over Medicare's future.

▶ Conclusion

This chapter provided you with an overview of the three main public programs that provide health insurance coverage to millions of people in the United States and raised a series of policy questions for your consideration. Based on the size of the programs, their costs to the federal and state governments, and their importance to millions of (often low-income) individuals, the role and structure of Medicaid, CHIP, and Medicare are constantly being debated. Some people would like to see coverage expanded to ensure that everyone has adequate access to health insurance, others would like to dismantle the programs in the interest of eliminating government-funded entitlements, and still others suggest incremental changes to the programs. The debate continues even with the passage of the ACA. Some want to repeal the law, while others are discussing cuts to entitlement programs as a way to reduce the federal deficit. Each of these decisions, and many others, reflect the recurring themes that have been discussed throughout this chapter: choosing between state flexibility and national uniformity; determining the appropriate role for government, the private sector, and individuals in healthcare financing and delivery; defining a primary decision-making goal (e.g., fiscal restraint, equity/social justice, improved health outcomes, uniformity); and settling on the appropriate scope of coverage to offer beneficiaries. Given these programs' expected increase in beneficiaries and the complementary increase in their cost, it is likely that the debates over Medicaid, CHIP, and Medicare will continue vigorously in the foreseeable future.

References

Accius, J., Flowers, L., & Flinn, B. (2017, March). *Low-income Medicare beneficiaries rely on Medicaid for critical help.* Retrieved from https://www.aarp.org/content/dam/aarp/ppi /2017-01/low-income-medicare-beneficiaries-rely-on-medicaid -for-critial-help.pdf

Advisory Board. (2018, June 8). *Where states stand on Medicaid expansion.* Retrieved from https://www.advisory.com/Daily -Briefing/Resources/Primers/MedicaidMap

American Association for Long-Term Care Insurance. (n.d.). *Long term care insurance partnership plans.* Retrieved from http://www.aaltci.org/long-term-care-insurance/learning-center/long-term-care-insurance-partnership-plans.php

Armstrong v. Exceptional Child Center, U.S., No. 14-15 (2015, March 31).

Bipartisan Budget Act of 2018, Pub. L. No. 115-123, 132 Stat. 64 (2018).

Blumberg, L., Holahan, J., Karpman, M., & Elmendorf, C. (2018, July). *Characteristics of the remaining uninsured: An update.* Retrieved from https://www.urban.org/sites/default/files/publication/98764/2001914-characteristics-of-the-remaining-uninsured-an-update_0.pdf

Brooks, T., Wagnerman, K., Artiga, S., Cornachione, E., & Ubri, P. (2017, January 12). *Medicaid and CHIP eligibility, enrollment, renewal, and cost sharing policies as of January 2017: Findings from a 50-state survey.* Retrieved from https://www.kff.org/report-section/medicaid-and-chip-eligibility-enrollment-renewal-and-cost-sharing-policies-as-of-january-2017-medicaid-and-chip-eligibility/

Center on Budget and Policy Priorities. (2016). *Policy basics: Introduction to Medicaid.* Retrieved from https://www.cbpp.org/research/health/policy-basics-introduction-to-medicaid

Children's Health Insurance Program Reauthorization Act of 2009, Pub. L. No. 111-3, 48 Stat. 998 (2009).

CMS.gov. (2016). *2016 actuarial report on the financial outlook for Medicaid.* Retrieved from https://www.cms.gov/Research-Statistics-Data-and-Systems/Research/ActuarialStudies/Downloads/MedicaidReport2016.pdf

CMS.gov. (2018a, April 17). *NHE fact sheet.* Retrieved from https://www.cms.gov/research-statistics-data-and-systems/statistics-trends-and-reports/nationalhealthexpenddata/nhe-fact-sheet.html

CMS.gov. (2018b, February). *People enrolled in Medicaid and Medicare.* Retrieved from https://www.cms.gov/Medicare-Medicaid-Coordination/Medicare-and-Medicaid-Coordination/Medicare-Medicaid-Coordination-Office/Downloads/MMCO_Factsheet.pdf

CMS.gov. (2018c, May 11). *Report on state section 1937 benchmark plans.* Retrieved from https://www.cms.gov/Regulations-and-Guidance/Legislation/DeficitReductionAct/index.html

Congressional Budget Office. (2015). *Medicare's payment to physicians: The budgetary effects of alternative policies relative to CBO's January 2015 Baseline.* Retrieved from https://www.cbo.gov/publication/49923

Congressional Budget Office. (2018). *The 2018 long-term budget outlook.* Retrieved from https://www.cbo.gov/system/files?file=2018-06/53919-2018ltbo.pdf

Cubanski, J., Damico, A., & Neuman, T. (2018, May 17). *Medicare Part D in 2018: The latest on enrollment, premiums, and cost sharing.* Retrieved from https://www.kff.org/medicare/issue-brief/medicare-part-d-in-2018-the-latest-on-enrollment-premiums-and-cost-sharing/

Cubanski, J., & Neuman, T. (2018, June 22). *The facts on Medicare spending and financing.* Retrieved from https://www.kff.org/medicare/issue-brief/the-facts-on-medicare-spending-and-financing/

Cubanski, J., Swoope, C., Bocutti, C., Jacobson, G., Casillas, G., Griffen, S., & Neuman, T. (2015, March 20). *A primer on Medicare: Key facts about the Medicare program and the people it covers.* Retrieved from https://www.kff.org/medicare/report/a-primer-on-medicare-key-facts-about-the-medicare-program-and-the-people-it-covers/

Cunningham, P., Rudowitz, R., Young, K., Garfield, R., & Foutz, J. (2016, January 9). *Understanding Medicaid hospital payments and the impact of recent policy changes.* Retrieved from https://www.kff.org/report-section/understanding-medicaid-hospital-payments-and-the-impact-of-recent-policy-changes-issue-brief/

Decker, S. L. (2012). In 2011, nearly one-third of physicians said they would not accept new Medicaid patients, but raising fees may help. *Health Affairs, 31*(8), 1673–1679. doi:10.1377/hlthaff.2012.0294

Decker, S. L. (2018). No association found between the Medicaid primary care fee bump and physician-reported participation in Medicaid. *Health Affairs, 37*(7), 1092–1098. doi:10.1377/hlthaff.2018.0078

Deficit Reduction Act of 2005, Pub. L. No. 109-362, 107 Stat. 312 through 685 Stat. 1025 (2006).

Department of Health and Human Services. (2017, January 26). *HHS 2017 budget in brief—CMS—Medicare.* Retrieved from https://www.hhs.gov/about/budget/fy2017/budget-in-brief/cms/medicare/index.html

Department of Labor. (2018). *Premium assistance under Medicaid and the Children's Health Insurance Plan (CHIP).* Retrieved from https://www.dol.gov/sites/default/files/ebsa/laws-and-regulations/laws/chipra/model-notice.pdf

Dickson, V. (2018, June 29). *CMS to test Medicare Advantage as alternative payment model under MACRA.* Retrieved from https://www.carevalue.com/cms-to-test-medicare-advantage-as-alternative-payment-model-under-macra/

Dranove, D., Garthwaite, C., & Ody, C. (2017, May 3). *The impact of the ACA's Medicaid expansion on hospitals' uncompensated care burden and the potential effects of repeal.* Retrieved from https://www.commonwealthfund.org/publications/issue-briefs/2017/may/impact-acas-medicaid-expansion-hospitals-uncompensated-care

Fremstad, S., & Cox, L. (2004, November). *Covering new Americans: A review of federal and state policies related to immigrants' eligibility and access to publicly funded health insurance.* Retrieved from https://kaiserfamilyfoundation.files.wordpress.com/2013/01/covering-new-americans-a-review-of-federal-and-state-policies-related-to-immigrants-eligibility-and-access-to-publicly-funded-health-insurance-report.pdf

Garfield, R., Damico, A., & Orgera, K. (2018, June 12). *The coverage gap: Uninsured poor adults in states that do no expand Medicaid.* Retrieved from https://www.kff.org/medicaid/issue-brief/the-coverage-gap-uninsured-poor-adults-in-states-that-do-not-expand-medicaid/

Geilfuss, C. F., II, & Romano, D. H. (2018, January 12). *CMS announces advanced alternative payment model—BPCI advanced.* Retrieved from https://www.healthcarelawtoday.com/2018/01/12/cms-announces-an-advanced-alternative-payment-model-bpci-advanced/

Georgetown University Health Policy Institute. (2017, February 6). *The Children's Health Insurance Program.* Retrieved from https://ccf.georgetown.edu/2017/02/06/about-chip/

Glied, S. (2018). Financing Medicare into the future: Premium support fails the risk-bearing test. *Health Affairs, 37*(7), 1073–1078. doi:0.1377/hlthaff.2018.0008

Grants to States for Medical Assistance Programs, 53 Fed. Reg. 36571 (September, 1988) (codified in 42 C.F.R. pts. 430-498).

HEALTHY KIDS (Helping Ensure Access for Little Ones, Toddlers, and Hopeful Youth by Keeping Insurance Delivery Stable) Act of 2018, Pub. L. No. 115-120, 132 Stat. 28 (2018).

Hing, E., Decker, S. L., Jamoom, E. (2015). *Acceptance of new patients with public and private insurance by office-based physicians: United States, 2013.* Retrieved from https://www .cdc.gov/nchs/data/databriefs/db195.pdf

Jacobson, G., Damico, A., Neuman, T., & Gold, M. (2017, June 6). *Medicare Advantage 2017 spotlight: Enrollment market update.* Retrieved from https://www.kff.org/medicare/issue-brief /medicare-advantage-2017-spotlight-enrollment-market -update/

Kaiser Family Foundation. (2010). *Summary of key changes to Medicare in the 2010 health reform law.* Retrieved from https:// www.kff.org/health-reform/issue-brief/summary-of-key -changes-to-medicare-in/

Kaiser Family Foundation. (2012a). *State adoption of coverage and enrollment options in the Children's Health Insurance Reauthorization Act of 2009.* Retrieved from https://www.kff .org/medicaid/fact-sheet/state-adoption-of-coverage-and -enrollment-options/

Kaiser Family Foundation. (2012b). *The Medicaid medically needy program: Spending and enrollment update.* Retrieved from https://kaiserfamilyfoundation.files.wordpress.com/2013 /01/4096.pdf

Kaiser Family Foundation. (2013). *Premium assistance in Medicaid and CHIP: An overview of current options and implications of the Affordable Care Act.* Retrieved from https://www.kff.org /medicaid/issue-brief/premium-assistance-in-medicaid-and -chip-an-overview-of-current-options-and-implications-of -the-affordable-care-act/

Kaiser Family Foundation. (2016a). *Distribution of Medicaid spending by service.* Retrieved from https://www.kff.org /medicaid/state-indicator/distribution-of-medicaid -spending-by-service/?dataView=1&currentTimeframe=0&s ortModel=%7B%22colId%22:%22Location%22,%22sort%22: %22asc%22%7D

Kaiser Family Foundation. (2016b). *Distribution of Medicare beneficiaries by federal poverty level.* Retrieved from https:// www.kff.org/medicare/state-indicator/medicare-beneficiaries -by-fpl/?currentTimeframe=0&sortModel=%7B%22colId%22 :%22Location%22,%22sort%22:%22asc%22%7D

Kaiser Family Foundation. (2016c). *Distribution of Medicare beneficiaries by gender.* Retrieved from https://www.kff.org /medicare/state-indicator/medicare-beneficiaries-by-gender/? currentTimeframe=0&sortModel=%7B%22colId%22:%22Loc ation%22,%22sort%22:%22asc%22%7D

Kaiser Family Foundation. (2016d). *Distribution of Medicare beneficiaries by race/ethnicity.* Retrieved from https://www.kff .org/medicare/state-indicator/medicare-beneficiaries-by-race ethnicity/?currentTimeframe=0&sortModel=%7B%22colId% 22:%22Location%22,%22sort%22:%22asc%22%7D

Kaiser Family Foundation. (2016e). *Distribution of the non-elderly with Medicaid by Race/Ethnicity, 2016.* Retrieved from https://www.kff.org/medicaid/state-indicator/distribution -by-raceethnicity-4/?currentTimeframe=0&selected Distributions=white--black--hispanic--other&selectedRows =%7B%22wrapups%22:%7B%22united-states%22:%7B%7D %7D%7D&sortModel=%7B%22colId%22:%22Location%22, %22sort%22:%22asc%22%7D

Kaiser Family Foundation. (2016f). *Federal and state share of Medicaid spending.* Retrieved from https://www.kff.org /medicaid/state-indicator/federalstate-share-of-spending/?cu rrentTimeframe=0&sortModel=%7B%22colId%22:%22Locati on%22,%22sort%22:%22asc%22%7D

Kaiser Family Foundation. (2016g). *Total Medicaid spending.* Retrieved from https://www.kff.org/medicaid/state-indicator /total-medicaid-spending/?currentTimeframe=0&selectedDis

tributions=total-medicaid-spending&sortModel=%7B%22col Id%22:%22Location%22,%22sort%22:%22asc%22%7D

Kaiser Family Foundation. (2017a). *An overview of Medicare.* Retrieved from https://www.kff.org/medicare/issue-brief/an -overview-of-medicare/

Kaiser Family Foundation. (2017b). *The Medicare Part D prescription drug benefit.* Retrieved from https://www.kff.org /medicare/fact-sheet/the-medicare-prescription-drug -benefit-fact-sheet/

Kaiser Family Foundation. (2018a). *Medicaid/CHIP coverage of lawfully-residing immigrant children and pregnant women.* Retrieved from https://www.kff.org/health-reform/state -indicator/medicaid-chip-coverage-of-lawfully-residing -immigrant-children-and-pregnant-women/?currentTimefra me=0&sortModel=%7B%22colId%22:%22Location%22,%22s ort%22:%22asc%22%7D

Kaiser Family Foundation. (2018b, July 26). *Medicaid waiver tracker: Which states have approved and pending section 1115 Medicaid waivers?* Retrieved from https://www.kff .org/medicaid/issue-brief/which-states-have-approved-and -pending-section-1115-medicaid-waivers/

Kardish, C. (2015, April 17). *Medicare deal delays but deepens hospital cuts.* Retrieved from http://www.governing.com /topics/health-human-services/gov-medicare-deal-delays -hospital-cuts.html

Medicaid.gov. (n.d.a.). *About section 1115 demonstrations.* Retrieved from https://www.medicaid.gov/medicaid/section -1115-demo/about-1115/index.html

Medicaid.gov. (n.d.b). *Alternative benefit plan coverage.* Retrieved from https://www.medicaid.gov/medicaid/benefits/abp/index .html

Medicaid.gov. (n.d.c). *April 2018 Medicaid and CHIP enrollment data highlights.* Retrieved from https://www.medicaid .gov/medicaid/program-information/medicaid-and-chip -enrollment-data/report-highlights/index.html

Medicaid.gov. (n.d.d). *Cost sharing out of pocket costs.* Retrieved from https://www.medicaid.gov/medicaid/cost-sharing/out -of-pocket-costs/index.html

Medicaid.gov. (n.d.e). *Federal policy guidance.* Retrieved from https://www.medicaid.gov/federal-policy-Guidance/index .html

Medicaid.gov. (2018). *Medicaid managed care enrollment and program characteristics, 2016.* Retrieved from https:// www.medicaid.gov/medicaid/managed-care/downloads /enrollment/2016-medicaid-managed-care-enrollment -report.pdf

Medicaid and CHIP Payment and Access Commission. (n.d.a). *Medicaid enrollment changes following the ACA.* Retrieved from https://www.macpac.gov/subtopic/medicaid-enrollment -changes-following-the-aca/

Medicaid and CHIP Payment and Access Commission. (n.d.b). *Medically needy thresholds as percent of FPL.* Retrieved from https://www.macpac.gov/medically-needy-program -thresholds/

Medicaid and CHIP Payment and Access Commission. (2011). *Federal CHIP financing.* Retrieved from https://www.gpo.gov /fdsys/pkg/GPO-MACPAC-MACBasics-CHIP-2011-09/pdf /GPO-MACPAC-MACBasics-CHIP-2011-09.pdf

Medicaid and CHIP Payment and Access Commission. (2017). *Recommendations for the future of CHIP and children's coverage.* Retrieved from https://www.macpac.gov/wp-content /uploads/2017/01/Recommendations-for-the-Future-of -CHIP-and-Childrens-Coverage.pdf

Medicaid and CHIP Payment and Access Commission. (2018). *State Children's Health Insurance Program (CHIP)*. Retrieved from https://www.macpac.gov/wp-content/uploads/2015/03/State-Childrens-Health-Insurance-Program-Fact-Sheet.pdf

Medicare Access and CHIP Reauthorization Act of 2015, Pub. L. No.114-10, 129 Stat. 87 (2015).

Medicare Payment Advisory Commission. (2005, March). *Report to the Congress: Medicare payment policy*. Retrieved from http://medpac.gov/docs/default-source/reports/Mar05_EntireReport.pdf?sfvrsn=0

Medicare Payment Advisory Commission. (2015, June). *Report to the Congress: Medicare and the health care delivery system*. Retrieved from http://medpac.gov/docs/default-source/reports/june-2015-report-to-the-congress-medicare-and-the-health-care-delivery-system.pdf?sfvrsn=0

Medicare Payment Advisory Commission. (2018, March). *Report to the Congress: Medicare payment policy*. Retrieved from http://medpac.gov/docs/default-source/reports/mar18_medpac_entirereport_sec_rev_0518.pdf?sfvrsn=0

Medicare Prescription Drug Improvement and Modernization Act of 2003, Pub. L No. 108-173, 117 Stat. 2066 (2003).

Musumeci, M. (2017, February 16). *Medicaid's role for Medicare beneficiaries*. Retrieved from https://www.kff.org/medicaid/issue-brief/medicaids-role-for-medicare-beneficiaries/

Musumeci, M. (2018, July 2). *Explaining* Stewart v. Azar: *Implications of the court's decision on Kentucky's Medicaid waiver*. Retrieved from https://www.kff.org/medicaid/issue-brief/explaining-stewart-v-azar-implications-of-the-courts-decision-on-kentuckys-medicaid-waiver/

National Federation of Independent Business v. Sebelius, 132 S. Ct. 2566 (2012).

National Law Review. (2015, April 20). *With SGR repealed, replacement policy creates new priorities—Sustainable growth rate*. Retrieved from https://www.natlawreview.com/article/sgr-repealed-replacement-policy-creates-new-priorities-sustainable-growth-rate

Neprash, H. T., Zink, A., Gray, J., & Hempstead, K. (2018). Physician participation in Medicaid increased only slightly following expansion. *Health Affairs, 37*(7), 1087–1091. doi:10.1377/hlthaff.2017.1085

Paradise, J. (2015, March 9). *Medicaid moving forward*. Retrieved from https://www.kff.org/health-reform/issue-brief/medicaid-moving-forward/

Paradise, J., Lyons, B., & Rowland, D. (2015, May 6). *Medicaid at 50*. Retrieved from https://www.kff.org/medicaid/report/medicaid-at-50/

Paradise, J., & Musumeci, M. (2016, June 9). *CMS' final rule on Medicaid managed care: A summary of major provisions*. Retrieved from https://www.kff.org/medicaid/issue-brief/cmss-final-rule-on-medicaid-managed-care-a-summary-of-major-provisions/

Passel, J. (2005, June 14). *Unauthorized migrants: Numbers and characteristics*. Retrieved from http://www.pewhispanic.org/2005/06/14/unauthorized-migrants/

Patel, K., Darling, M., & Ginsberg, P. (2016, December 15). *Key takeaways from the final MACRA rule, plus remaining challenges*. Retrieved from https://www.brookings.edu/blog/usc-brookings-schaeffer-on-health-policy/2016/12/15/key-takeaways-from-the-final-macra-rule-plus-remaining-challenges/

Personal Responsibility and Work Opportunity Reconciliation Act of 1996, Pub. L. No. 104-193, 100 Stat. 2105 (1996).

Rosenbaum, S. (2002). Medicaid. *New England Journal of Medicine, 346*(8), 635–640. doi:10.1056/NEJM200202213460825

Rosenbaum, S. (2014). Medicaid payments and access to care. *New England Journal of Medicine, 371*, 2345–2347. doi:10.1056/NEJMp1412488

Rosenbaum, S., Mehta, D., Dorley, M., Hurt, C., Rothenberg, S., & Lopez, N. (2015, May 11). *Medicaid benefit design for newly eligible adults: State approaches*. Retrieved from http://www.commonwealthfund.org/publications/issue-briefs/2015/may/medicaid-benefit-designs-newly-eligible-adults-state-approaches?redirect_source=/publications/issue-briefs/2015/may/medicaid-benefit-designs-for-newly-eligible-adults

Rudowitz, R., & Garfield, R. (2018, April 12). *Ten things to know about Medicaid: Setting the facts straight*. Retrieved from https://www.kff.org/medicaid/issue-brief/10-things-to-know-about-medicaid-setting-the-facts-straight/

Ryan, J. (2009). *The Children's Health Insurance Program (CHIP): The Fundamentals*. Retrieved from https://www.nhpf.org/library/background-papers/BP68_CHIPFundamentals_04-23-09.pdf

Social Security Act of 1935, Title XIX , 42 U.S.C. §§ 1308 & 1396 (1965).

Solomon, J., & Schubel, J. (2017, August 29). *Medicaid waivers should further program objectives, not impose barriers to coverage and care*. Retrieved from https://www.cbpp.org/research/health/medicaid-waivers-should-further-program-objectives-not-impose-barriers-to-coverage#_ftn7

Stewart v. Azar. 313 F.Supp.3d 237 (2018).

U.S. Census Bureau. (2017). *Health insurance coverage in the United States: 2016* (Current Population Reports, P60-260). Washington, DC: U.S. Government Printing Office.

Vestal, C. (2014). *Children's health program faces cloudy future under ACA*. Retrieved from http://www.pewtrusts.org/en/research-and-analysis/blogs/stateline/2014/12/4/childrens-health-program-faces-cloudy-future-under-aca

Wilensky, G. (2018, April 5). Will MACRA improve physician reimbursement? *New England Journal of Medicine, 378*, 1269–1271. doi:10.1056/NEJMp1801673

Wynne, B., & Horowitz, M. (2018, June 7). *With great power comes great responsibility: Medicare Advantage's newfound supplemental benefit flexibility*. Retrieved from https://www.commonwealthfund.org/blog/2018/great-power-comes-great-responsibility-medicare-advantages-newfound-supplemental-benefit

▶ Endnotes

a. Puerto Rico, the U.S. Virgin Islands, Guam, Northern Mariana Islands, and American Samoa participate in Medicaid. However, financing rules are different in these territories than in the 50 states. Federal spending is capped and appropriated by Congress annually.

b. A special 5% adjustment allowed by law effectively brings the eligibility rate to 138% FPL.

c. Community health centers have their own per-visit prospective payment system for reimbursement under Medicaid.

d. Although federal law does not elaborate on the specifics of section 1115 waivers, other federal guidance does. In 1994, HHS prepared a non-binding notice, "Demonstration Proposal Pursuant to Section 1115(a) of the Social Security Act," 59 Fed. Reg. 49249 (1994), and then the Health Care Financing Administration (now CMS) published "Review Guide for Section 1115 Research and Demonstration Waiver Proposals for State Health Care Reform." The *State Medicaid Manual* also contains information relating to Section 1115 waivers.

e. Because New Jersey and New York had already expanded coverage to children beyond 300% FPL prior to CHIPRA, those states are allowed to use their enhanced CHIP match up to their capped allotment.

f. Private FFS plans, usually offered at the county level, provide the standard Medicare coverage, but beneficiaries may see only physicians who participate in the plan and must pay premiums and co-payments or co-insurance to the private plan instead of to individual providers. In return, the private plan may offer additional services not covered by Medicare.

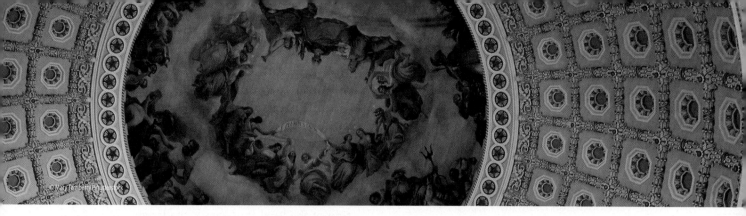

CHAPTER 12

Healthcare Quality Policy and Law

LEARNING OBJECTIVES

By the end of this chapter you will be able to:

- Discuss licensure and accreditation in the context of healthcare quality
- Describe the scope and causes of medical errors
- Describe the meaning and evolution of the medical professional standard of care
- Identify and explain certain state-level legal theories under which healthcare professionals and entities can be held liable for medical negligence
- Explain how federal employee benefits law often preempts medical negligence lawsuits against insurers and managed care organizations
- Describe efforts to measure and incentivize high-quality health care

▶ Introduction

This chapter steps away from the topics of healthcare access and coverage to focus on healthcare quality. As with access and coverage, healthcare quality has various dimensions, and the topic of healthcare quality has increasingly been a focal point of researchers, analysts, health professionals, and consumers. For instance, in the span of only a couple of years, the influential Institute of Medicine (IOM, which is now called the National Academy of Medicine) released two major reports pertaining to healthcare quality: *To Err Is Human: Building a Safer Health System* (Kohn, Corrigan, & Donaldson, 2000), which focused on the specific quality concern of patient safety, and *Crossing the Quality Chasm: A New Health System for the 21st Century* (Committee on Quality of Health Care in America, 2001), which described how the healthcare delivery system should be overhauled to improve care.

Like healthcare access and coverage issues, healthcare quality is a key concern in health policy and law. For example, long-standing problems related to the administration of health care—like racial and ethnic health disparities, and the geographic variation in the amount or type of care provided to patients—have drawn responses from policymakers and the legal system. Furthermore, policy and legal responses are often needed as healthcare quality is affected by changes in the marketplace or by advances in medical technology. For instance, institutional payers for healthcare services—traditional insurers, employers, and managed care

Michelina Bauman was born on May 16, 1995, in New Jersey. The managed care organization (MCO) through which her parents received healthcare coverage had precertified coverage for 1 day in the hospital postbirth, and both Michelina and her mother were discharged from the hospital 24 hours after Michelina was born. The day after the discharge, Michelina became ill. Her parents telephoned the MCO, but they were neither advised to take Michelina back to the hospital nor provided an in-home visit by a pediatric nurse as promised under the MCO's "L'il Appleseed" infant care program. Michelina died that same day from meningitis stemming from an undiagnosed strep infection.

companies—are more involved in healthcare practice now than was the case historically (Furrow, Greaney, Johnson, Jost, & Schwartz, 2001, p. 26), a fact that spurred policymakers and courts to reconsider traditional notions of healthcare quality and liability.

The role of law as a monitor of the quality of health care was on display in the context of the no-duty-to-treat principle and the case of *Hurley v. Eddingfield* (1901). Indiana's physician licensure law was described as a filter to weed out individuals without the requisite skills to safely and adequately practice medicine. Licensure, in theory, permits a second healthcare quality function as well: it allows state regulators to monitor the conduct of medical practitioners even after they have been licensed—although, as discussed later, this function has not been performed with much vigor over the years.

Holding healthcare professionals and entities liable for substandard care is another (and perhaps the most well-known) legal tool used to promote quality in health care. Physicians have no legal duty to accept a patient into their practice or to provide care upon request, except in limited circumstances. However, a doctor's decision to treat a patient establishes a legally significant physician–patient relationship, under which the physician owes the patient a reasonable duty of care. Failure to meet what is termed the *professional standard of care*—the legal standard used in medical negligence cases to determine whether health professionals and entities have adequately discharged their responsibility to provide reasonable care to their patients—can result in legal liability for reasonably foreseeable injuries.[a]

As you will soon discover, the laws and legal principles that define the circumstances under which aggrieved individuals can successfully sue an MCO for substandard care or coverage determinations are complex. This complexity stems from multiple facts. First, the legal framework applied to medical negligence cases was developed long before the advent of managed care. Second, the hybrid nature of managed care (combining as it does the financing and delivery of care) defies easy categorization and makes application of the legal framework challenging. And third, a federal law (the Employee Retirement Income Security Act, or ERISA) pertaining to employee benefit plans preempts (i.e., precludes) many typical state-level legal claims against MCOs.

The next section of this chapter provides a brief overview of healthcare licensure and accreditation in the context of healthcare quality. The chapter then turns to an overview of errors in health care. Although medical errors are only one small component of the broad subject of healthcare quality, they are commonly included in the quality discussion and serve as a jumping-off point for a discussion of healthcare liability. The chapter then turns to a full discussion of the professional standard of care and its evolution, followed by a description of some of the state legal theories under which hospitals, traditional insurers, and MCOs can be held liable for substandard medical professional conduct. It then explores the complex area of how ERISA preempts lawsuits premised on these same legal theories. Finally, the chapter describes the concepts of measuring and incentivizing healthcare quality.

▶ Quality Control Through Licensure and Accreditation

The licensing of healthcare professionals and institutions is an important function of state law. As noted previously, healthcare licensure is centrally about filtering out those who may not have the requisite knowledge or skills to practice medicine; in other words, states exercise their police powers when applying licensure laws in order to protect residents from being subjected to substandard health care. State licensure laws both define the qualifications required to become licensed and the standards that must be met for purposes of maintaining and renewing licenses (Rosenbaum, Frankford, Law, & Rosenblatt, 2012).

As important as the licensing function is, however, historically it has been used in the promotion of healthcare quality in only the bluntest sense. This stems from the fact that in most states, the only method by which to promote quality through licensure is, simply, the granting or denial of the license to practice medicine. In other words, there exists no middle ground between being granted a license and not being granted (or renewed for) a license, no ongoing monitoring or application of standards intended to promote quality and ensure competence in the face of evolving medical care practices. In designing licensing laws, most state legislatures assume that medical professional trade associations (e.g., the American Medical Association) and/or accrediting bodies have sufficient ethical and practice standards to effectively regulate healthcare practitioners and that the purpose of licensure as a quality control measure is to identify and deal with a relatively small number of cases of individual provider deviation from those standards (Rosenbaum et al., 2012). This assumption is correct, to a point; private professional and industry standards do indeed exist, though their effect on day-to-day quality is debatable. Some commentators maintain that accreditation amounts to little more than self-serving indicia of individual or institutional exceptionalism, while others argue that accreditation plays an important and useful role alongside licensure. There are many examples of healthcare accreditation bodies: The Joint Commission (formerly the Joint Commission on Accreditation of Healthcare Organizations), which may be best known for its review and accreditation of hospitals; the National Committee for Quality Assurance, which accredits MCOs; the Healthcare Facilities Accreditation Program; the Commission on Accreditation of Rehabilitation Facilities; the Community Health Accreditation Program; the Utilization Review Accreditation Commission; and others.

A second historical fact related to licensure's effect (or lack thereof) on healthcare quality—one that plays into detractors' claims about the self-serving nature of today's industry-designed accreditation processes—is that state licensing schemes were designed not with healthcare quality, per se, in mind, but rather with an eye toward protecting the medical professions from unscrupulous or incompetent providers and bad publicity. Thus, the laws tended to focus on preventing relatively rare instances of grossly poor-quality care, rather than on long-term promotion of high-quality care.

One final topic pertaining to licensure that bears mentioning is the immensely important role it plays in defining the permissible "scope of practice" of the various types of healthcare providers. It is one thing for state legislators to define the meaning of practice for various broad medical fields (e.g., there is not so

much overlap between, say, medicine and dentistry as to cause a huge number of policy and legal disputes), but quite another for legislators to define the lawful activities of doctors as compared to physician assistants as compared to nurses, and even more specifically of advanced practice nurses as compared to licensed practical nurses as compared to registered nurses. It is in delineating permissible scopes of practice within fields and subspecialties that fierce policy disputes take place.

Yet, it is not surprising that these disputes take place. Licensure laws define who has the power to engage in medical practice, who gets to practice specific types of health care, and how and when professional standards of conduct are enforced. In short, licensure laws have the power to determine who is in, as they say, and who is out. Some states are relatively more inclusive in their approach to the licensing of healthcare professionals, while others hew closely to a more traditional approach in which physicians are granted broad scope of practice powers while other professionals (e.g., nurses) have far less ability to diagnose and treat patients. The latter approach is being hotly contested, as nurses and other nonphysician healthcare professionals decry their inability to practice to their full education and training, particularly in light of the healthcare workforce shortages that plague the nation (Iglehart, 2013) and the large number of individuals who were newly able to access health insurance (and thus more likely to seek care) under the Affordable Care Act (ACA).

▶ Medical Errors as a Public Health Concern

Notwithstanding licensure laws and accreditation standards, medical errors are bound to, and often do, occur. And while medical errors are obviously not a new problem, framing the issue as a public health problem is a relatively new phenomenon, and healthcare providers, public health professionals, and policymakers have in recent years committed increased attention to the problem of medical errors.

The regularity with which medical errors occur and the resulting extent of adverse health outcomes and mortalities indicate that the problem is not confined to one ethnic or racial population, socioeconomic group, or geographic area. One study indicates that medical errors in hospitals and other healthcare facilities may now be the *third-leading* cause of death in the United States (Makary & Daniel, 2016), behind only heart disease and cancer. This prevalence suggests that factors such as unskilled or poorly trained doctors and poor communication systems within facilities contribute to more deaths annually than do respiratory disease, accidents, strokes, Alzheimer disease, diabetes, flu and pneumonia, kidney diseases, and suicide, which round out the top 11 causes of death (Makary & Daniel, 2016). The negative effects of medical errors on individual patients and on society as a whole—including associated reductions in work productivity, lost income, and the costs associated with correcting injuries resulting from errors—support the conclusion that medical errors are properly classified as a public health problem requiring a strong response from policymakers and the legal system.

There are various causes of medical errors. Some causes are, relatively speaking, concrete—such as failure to complete an intended medical course of action, implementation of the wrong course of action, use of faulty equipment or products in effecting a course of action, failure to stay abreast of one's field of medical practice, or health professional inattentiveness. For example, according to the previously mentioned IOM reports, errors in the prescribing, administering, and dispensing of medications result in at least 1.5 million injuries or deaths annually in the United States (Kaufman, 2006). Furthermore, "mistakes in giving drugs are so prevalent in hospitals that, on average, a patient will be subjected to a medication error each day he or she occupies a hospital bed" (Kaufman, 2006). Yet according to the IOM reports, "at least a quarter of the injuries caused by drug errors are clearly preventable" (Kaufman, 2006). Some of the errors are spawned by something as simple as name confusion among pharmaceuticals; for example, it is easy to see how physicians, nurses, and pharmacists could easily confuse the arthritis drug Celebrex, the anticonvulsant drug Cerebyx, and the antidepressant drug Celexa when prescribing, administering, and filling medications (Nordenberg, 2000).

There are more abstract causes of medical errors, as well. For example, they can result from the fact that "much of medical treatment is still primitive: the etiologies and optimal treatments for many illnesses are not known [and] many treatment techniques, such as cancer chemotherapy, create substantial side effects" (Furrow et al., 2001, p. 30). Also, many people argue that the culture of medicine—including its history of elitism, its focus on memorization in both diagnosing and treating illness, and its dedication to secrecy when adverse medical outcomes occur—helps to explain the extent of medical errors.

Just as there are multiple causes of medical errors, so are there various strategies—some broad and systemic, others more incremental—for preventing and reducing their occurrence. For instance, hospitals usually employ two vehicles to minimize medical errors and assure quality care for patients: risk management programs and peer review processes. Risk management programs monitor risks associated with nonphysician personnel and with facilities under the direct control of hospital administrators; peer review processes entail a secretive evaluation of hospital-based physician practices by physicians themselves. Most physicians encounter the peer review process when they apply for "staff privileges" at a hospital, which grant doctors the ability to use the hospital for their own private practice, including the ability to admit patients and use the hospital's resources in treating patients. Once a doctor is granted such privileges, he or she is subject to ongoing peer review. Many analysts maintain that the secretive manner in which the peer review process is conducted stifles meaningful improvements to patient safety and that it is too reactive, responding to errors only after they have occurred.

Recently, public and private policymakers have begun shifting their attention to medical error reforms that are less reactive and more centered on error prevention and patient safety improvements. There are two primary objectives of these reforms: to redesign healthcare delivery methods and structures to limit the likelihood of human error and to prepare in advance for the inevitable errors that will occur in healthcare delivery regardless of the amount and types of precautions taken. Medical error reform could entail various approaches, including improving standardization of medical procedures, enforcing mandatory reporting of medical errors, reducing reliance on memory in medical care, increasing and improving medical information technology systems, encouraging patients to be more participatory in their own medical care, and establishing a national focus on the topic of patient safety (Furrow et al., 2001, pp. 43–64). For example, the federal Patient Safety and Quality Improvement Act (PSQIA) was signed into law in 2005 in response to the *To Err Is Human* report. PSQIA created a system for use by healthcare providers to anonymously report medical error data for systematic analysis. The hope is that by aggregating, analyzing, and disseminating the data analyses to healthcare providers nationwide, healthcare professionals and entities will increase their knowledge about what leads to adverse medical outcomes and alter their practice methods accordingly.

BOX 12-2 Discussion Questions

What do you think of the term *medical error* as a descriptor of adverse medical outcomes? After all, there are many medical procedures (e.g., invasive surgeries) and treatments (e.g., chemotherapy) that not only are inherently risky, but also cause painful and dangerous (and often unpreventable) side effects (i.e., that lead to "adverse" medical results). Given this fact, is it conceivable that the healthcare delivery system could ever operate free of "error"? Can you think of other terms that better (or more fairly) convey the range of adverse outcomes attending healthcare practice?

Promoting Healthcare Quality Through the Standard of Care

Not all medical errors rise to the level of being contrary to law. This section details the measure used by the legal system to determine which errors trigger legal protections: the professional standard of care. The standard of care is key both to the provision of high-quality health care and to legal claims that a health professional's, hospital's, or MCO's negligence in rendering medical care resulted in injury or death. This type of liability falls under the law of *torts*, a term that derives from the Latin word for "twisted" and that applies to situations where the actions of an individual or entity "twist away" from being reasonable and result in harm to others. Generally speaking, proving tort liability is not easy, and this task is no less difficult in the specific context of medical care. A patient seeking to hold a health professional or entity responsible for substandard care or treatment must demonstrate the appropriate standard of care, a breach of that standard by the defendant, measurable damages (e.g., physical pain or emotional suffering), and a causal link between the defendant's breach and the patient's injury.[b]

The Origins of the Standard of Care

The professional standard of care has its origins in 18th-century English common law. Courts in England had established that a patient looking to hold a physician legally accountable for substandard care had to prove that the doctor violated the *customs of his own profession*, as determined by *other professionals within the profession*. In other words, no objective standard was used by courts to measure the adequacy of physician practice.[c] Furthermore, courts were not in the

habit of making searching analyses of whether the customs and standards proffered by the profession as defensible were at all reasonable. This type of physician deference was incorporated into America's legal fabric, as policymakers and courts delegated key decisions about medical practice—including determinations as to whether a specific practice undertaken in the treatment of a particular patient was acceptable or negligent—to the medical profession itself.

The law's reliance on health professionals to determine the appropriate standard of medical care was not without its problems. In effect, this laissez-faire approach made it virtually impossible for an injured patient to successfully recover monetary damages from a negligent doctor, because the patient was required to find another health professional willing to testify that the doctor's treatment violated the customary standard of care. (This type of testimony was certainly uncommon, as health professionals rarely openly questioned the practices of other members of the profession.) Moreover, using professional custom as the touchstone for determining legal liability had the effect of thwarting the modernization of medical care, because practicing physicians knew they would be judged, in essence, based on how other physicians customarily practiced.

Furthermore, establishing a violation of professional custom was not the only hurdle injured patients had to clear in their effort to hold their physicians legally accountable for substandard care. English courts also developed what became known as the "locality rule," which held that testimony provided on behalf of a patient as to whether a physician's actions met the standard of care could come only from physicians who practiced *within the same or similar locality* as the physician on trial. Thus, not only did aggrieved patients need to find a physician willing to testify that a fellow member of the profession violated customary practice, they needed to find this expert witness within the (or a similar) locality in which the defendant-doctor actually practiced. As they did with the professional custom rule, U.S. courts gradually adopted the English locality rule. For example, the Supreme Judicial Court of Massachusetts ruled that a small-town physician was bound to possess only the skill that physicians and surgeons of ordinary ability and skill, practicing in similar localities with opportunities for no larger experience, ordinarily possess, and that he was not bound to possess the high degree of art and skill possessed by eminent surgeons practicing in larger cities and making a specialty of the practice of surgery (*Small v. Howard*, 1880).

Courts' application of the locality rule severely limited patients' ability to bring medical malpractice actions against their physicians. Indeed, some injured patients were prevented from even initially mounting a case, because they were unable to convince a "geographic colleague" of their own physician to serve as an expert witness. (This problem was particularly acute in rural communities where there were fewer doctors to begin with, and where collegiality was the norm.) Furthermore, the locality rule likely resulted in at least a few local medical standards that were set by doctors who were less than completely skilled. The rule had another effect, as well: it led to a gulf among localities and cities in the standard of medical care practiced, and thus to different standards of care for similarly situated patients. Imagine, for example (notwithstanding the fact that the professional custom rule generally discouraged advancements in the standard of medical care), that physicians in a large town or city upgraded their practice techniques to reflect new medical technologies. Small-town practitioners had little incentive to model their big-city colleagues in the improvement of their own practice techniques, because the locality rule limited testimony as to the reasonableness of a physician's care to practitioners in the same or similar locality as the doctor on trial and their own actions would never be measured against the elevated techniques of their big-city counterparts.

By the 1950s, policymakers and courts grew wary of a healthcare system effectively in charge of policing itself; not surprisingly, this view was reflective of society more broadly, which during the civil rights era adopted a set of values heavily influenced by social justice and circumspect of concentrated institutional power. It also reflected the fact that no matter how chilling the effects of the professional custom and locality rules, the practice of medicine—particularly the dissemination of medical research findings—had obviously evolved from the 1800s. These facts both vastly altered the law's approach to measuring physician care and promoted higher-quality health care (Rosenbaum et al., 2012).

The Evolution of the Standard of Care

Under the law's modernized approach to the standard of care, both legal pillars of the physician autonomy era—the professional custom rule and the locality rule—were more or less razed.

The Professional Custom Rule

Courts no longer defer to professional custom as solely determinative of whether a physician's actions reached the accepted standard of care. Instead, courts now analyze whether the custom itself is reasonable in light of existing medical knowledge and technology.[d] Although evidence of professional custom remains probative in determining whether the standard of care has been met, courts consider a range of other relevant evidence as well. Thus, the benchmark courts employ today to determine whether a health professional's treatment of a particular patient rose to the standard of care is whether it was *reasonable given the "totality of circumstances."*

Furthermore, it is no longer the case that evidence as to what is and is not customary medical practice is limited to what medical professionals themselves testify. Although evidence as to medical custom may still be introduced by medical professionals, objective clinical and scientific evidence—such as scientific research and clinical trial results—are now considered relevant in determining medical negligence. For example, the well-known case of *Helling v. Carey* (1974) shows how advances in medical knowledge can obliterate long-standing medical customs and replace them with new requirements. In *Helling*, a 32-year-old woman sought treatment from a series of ophthalmologists for glaucoma-type symptoms. The ophthalmologists, however, refrained from screening the patient for glaucoma, on the ground that professional custom called for the screen only in patients beyond the age of 40 years because the incidence of glaucoma in younger people was low. The State of Washington's Supreme Court ruled that notwithstanding the fact that the ophthalmologists had properly adhered to accepted custom, the *custom itself* was outdated based on current medical knowledge and was therefore unreasonable. The court effectively determined that a new treatment standard was required of the ophthalmology profession and held that the defendant-physicians were liable for the patient's blindness.

The key legal principle at work in *Helling* is that courts can (and do, in rare circumstances) determine for an entire industry (medical or otherwise) what is legally required of them, despite long-standing industry practices. This principle is premised on the famous case of *T. J. Hooper v. Northern Barge Corp.* (1932), in which the U.S. Second Circuit Court of Appeals held that a tugboat company was liable for damages to cargo it was shipping because the company failed to maintain radio-receiving equipment that could have warned the crew of a storm that battered the boat. The company argued that it should not be liable for the damage because at the time it was not typical practice in the tugboat industry to carry radio equipment. In response, the court wrote the following:

> There are, no doubt, cases where courts seem to make the general practice of the calling the

standard of proper diligence.... Indeed in most cases reasonable prudence is in fact common prudence; but strictly it is never its measure; *a whole calling may have unduly lagged in the adoption of new and available devices.* It never may set its own tests, however persuasive be its usages. *Courts must in the end say what is required;* there are precautions so imperative that even their universal disregard will not excuse their omission. (*T. J. Hooper v. Northern Barge Corp.*, 1932)

Essentially, the court determined that the tugboat company was not acting reasonably under the circumstances, but was instead hewing too closely (and foolishly) to what should have been considered an outmoded industry practice. This same view appeared to drive the court in *Helling v. Carey.* Indeed, the idea that the quality of health care provided by a health professional should be measured by an objective standard based on reasonableness under the circumstances—rather than by other professionals cloaked in the protections of outright autonomy—is today considered the norm. Furthermore, this view extends to big cities and small towns alike, and to both well-off and indigent patients.

The Locality Rule

Just as professional custom was transformed by the courts from being conclusive evidence of proper medical practice to being merely one piece of the evidentiary puzzle, so too was the locality rule mostly undone by more modern judicial thinking. Based in part on the fact that medical education and hospital-based care were becoming increasingly standardized under national accreditation efforts, courts stopped restricting evidence regarding the appropriate standard of care to the locality in which a physician practiced. Instead, most states have adopted what could be termed the "reasonably competent physician" standard, described as

> that degree of care and skill which is expected of a reasonably competent practitioner in the same class to which he belongs, acting in the same or similar circumstances. Under this standard, advances in the profession, availability of facilities, specialization or general practice, proximity of specialists and special facilities, together with all relevant considerations, are to be taken into account. (*Shilkret v. Annapolis Emergency Hospital Ass'n*, 1975)

Under this revised standard, the practice of medicine nationally is key, because for purposes of determining medical liability, a physician's actions are now measured objectively against those of a reasonably prudent and competent practitioner under similar circumstances, not against the actions of physicians who practice within a particular defendant's locality. Thus, in the eyes of most state laws, local medical practice customs have properly given way to higher expectations where health quality is concerned.

At the same time, some states still retain the locality rule as the appropriate standard for the admissibility of medical evidence, and some states use a modified rule that takes into account local resources and other factors in determining whether a defendant-doctor was able to meet the standard of care. For an example of the latter point, see *Hall v. Hilbun* (1985), in which the Mississippi Supreme Court determined that the locality rule still had relevance to the extent that a physician's imperfect care resulted not from his substandard medical knowledge and skills, but from the fact that he did not have access to needed resources and equipment. In this type of situation, the court reasoned, health professionals who genuinely attempt to meet the requisite standard of care should not be held legally responsible when factors outside their control prevent them from doing so. The court in *Hall* went on to explain that under these circumstances, a physician is required to be aware of extant limitations and to actively demonstrate an effort to assist patients as best he can by, for example, referring them to doctors and facilities better able to care for them.

For purposes of determining legal liability for substandard treatment, the notion of distinguishing between medical knowledge and skills on the one hand and medical resources and outside factors on the other has particular relevance when the treatment involves an indigent patient whose care implicates broad contextual problems, such as poor living conditions or insufficient access to providers. Here, again, many courts look to see whether the treating physician's actions demonstrate an understanding of the proper level of care and a sincere effort to reach that level. However, do not confuse the fact that the law does not generally hold physicians liable for the consequences of resource problems attending the healthcare system, or of poverty, with the idea that different standards of care exist for the well-off and for the poor. As far as the law is concerned, there is a unitary standard of care to be applied regardless of a patient's socioeconomic status, and physicians can certainly be held legally responsible for mistreating an indigent patient.

Together, the revamped legal rules pertaining to medical custom and local practice were combined to create what is called the *national standard of care.*

> ### BOX 12-3 Discussion Questions
>
> Give some thought to the term *national standard of care*. What do you think it means, from both a healthcare quality and legal (i.e., evidentiary) perspective? Are you aware of any national body—governmental or otherwise—that determines the efficacy of new diagnostic protocols or treatment modalities? In the absence of such an entity, how are health professionals put on notice that a new medical care standard for a particular procedure or treatment has emerged?

We turn now to a discussion of how this standard is applied to healthcare institutions and insurers.

▶ Tort Liability of Hospitals, Insurers, and MCOs

Just as physicians are now held to a national standard of care in cases challenging the quality of their care and treatment, so too have courts moved to apply this same standard to hospitals, traditional health insurers, and MCOs. The following sections consider each party's liability considerations in turn.

Hospital Liability

By the early 1900s, the healthcare industry began to rely much more heavily than had been the case previously on hospitals (as opposed to physicians' offices or patients' homes) as a focus of patient care. As with all healthcare settings, hospital-based medical practice created circumstances that led patients to challenge the quality of care provided. Out of necessity, the legal system (specifically, state-level courts) responded to these challenges by applying theories of liability—premised on the national standard of care—meant to hold hospitals accountable for negligence that occurred within their walls. Two theories—one premised on hospitals' relationship with doctors and one based on the actions and decisions of hospitals themselves—dominate the field of hospital liability. The former theory is called vicarious liability; the latter is termed corporate liability.

Vicarious Liability

The concept of vicarious liability, which maintains that one party can be held legally accountable for the actions of another party based solely on the type of relationship existing between the two parties, is premised on the long-standing principles of "agency" law. Under this field of law, where one party to a relationship effectively serves (or is held out to society) as an agent of another party, a court can assign legal responsibility to the other party where the agent's actions negligently result in injury to a person or damage to property. For example, vicarious liability allows a hospital to be held responsible in some situations for the negligent acts of the doctors that practice medicine under its roof—not because the hospital itself somehow acted negligently, but rather because the doctor is (or is viewed as by the law) an agent of the hospital.

One relatively easy way for a plaintiff to win a lawsuit premised on vicarious liability is to establish through evidence that the two parties at issue are engaged in an employer–employee relationship, and that the employee (i.e., the agent) was acting within the normal scope of her professional duties when the act of negligence occurred. In these instances, courts frequently look to the employer to adequately supervise the employee while on the job and hold the employer responsible when an employee's negligent acts occur within the parameters of the employee's job responsibilities.

However, many "agents" of the companies they are hired to work for are not formal employees; rather, they are hired as independent contractors. Indeed, this is true of most hospital–physician relationships. Historically, agency law respected hiring entities' decisions to hire individuals as independent contractors rather than as employees, and the general legal rule is that employers are not accountable for the illegal actions of these contractors. Nonetheless, there are exceptions to this rule, and courts have developed theories of vicarious liability—such as *actual agency*, *apparent agency*, and *nondelegable duty*—that are more concerned with the scope of an employer–independent contractor relationship than with the formal characterization of the relationship as determined by the parties themselves. In other words, employers cannot avoid legal liability simply by labeling a hired worker as an independent contractor, because courts will analyze the relationship to determine whether it operates at the end of the day like a typical employer–employee relationship.

Actual agency exists—and the negligence of an independent contractor can be imputed to his employer—when the employer exercises de facto supervision and control over the contractor. Thus, for example, agency can be shown to exist between a healthcare corporation and a health professional when the particular facts pertaining to the relationship reveal that the corporation actually exercises control over the professional, even though the professional is not technically an employee. Similarly, the doctrine of apparent agency (also called ostensible agency) is another exception to the general rule that employers should not be legally exposed for the negligence of their independent contractors. In the context of health care, this type of agency exists, for example, when a patient seeks care from a hospital emergency department (rather than from any particular physician working in that department) and the hospital has led patients to believe that physicians are employees of the hospital, such as via a billboard extolling the skills of the physicians who practice in its emergency department (*Mehlman v. Powell*, 1977). Finally, courts have also associated the doctrine of vicarious liability with certain duties considered so important to society as to be legally "nondelegable." For example, the importance of a hospital's obligation to maintain control over the care provided in its emergency department led one court to rule that it would be improper for the hospital to claim immunity from vicarious liability when its independent contractor furnished substandard medical care (*Jackson v. Power*, 1987).

Corporate Liability

As opposed to vicarious hospital liability, which is predicated on the negligence of individual health professionals, corporate liability holds hospitals accountable for their own "institutional" acts or omissions. In other words, a hospital can also be held liable when its own negligent acts as a corporation cause or contribute to a patient's injury. Several general areas give rise to litigation around hospitals' direct quality of care duties to patients: failure to screen out incompetent providers (i.e., negligence in the hiring of clinicians), failure to maintain high-quality practice standards, failure to take adequate action against clinicians whose practices fall below accepted standards, and failure to maintain proper equipment and supplies (Rosenbaum et al., 2012).

The most famous hospital corporate liability case is *Darling v. Charleston Community Memorial Hospital* (1965). In *Darling*, the Illinois Supreme Court found Memorial Hospital liable for negligent treatment provided to plaintiff Dorrence Darling, an 18-year-old who suffered a broken leg while playing in a college football game. The poor treatment Darling received by the hospital's emergency department staff—his leg cast was not properly constructed and its application cut off blood circulation—ultimately resulted in amputation of Darling's leg below the knee. The court held the hospital liable not for the actions of the emergency department staff, but for *its own* negligence: according to the court, Memorial Hospital did not maintain

a sufficient number of qualified nurses for post–emergency department bedside care (when Darling's leg became gangrenous), and it neither reviewed the care provided by the treating physician nor required the physician to consult with other members of the hospital staff.

Insurer Liability

Like hospitals, conventional (i.e., indemnity) health insurers historically were not susceptible to being sued under tort principles; rather, they were subject mainly to breach of contract lawsuits when they failed to reimburse medical claims for services covered under beneficiaries' health insurance policies. This protection from tort liability stemmed from two related facts: first, normative insurer practice was to leave medical judgments and treatment decisions in the hands of doctors, meaning it was rare for an insurer-related action to lead to the type of injury covered by tort law; second, to the extent that an insurer did deny a beneficiary's claim for insurance coverage, it did so retrospectively—in other words, *after* the beneficiary received needed diagnostic tests, treatments, medications, and so on. This effectively meant that when beneficiaries sued their health insurer, they did so not because they had been physically or emotionally injured by the insurer's decision to deny an insurance claim, but because there was a dispute as to whether the insurer was going to pay for the already-received medical care.[e] Thus, although coverage denials had potentially enormous economic implications for affected beneficiaries, they did not tend to raise healthcare access or quality issues.

In the years following the *Darling* decision, however, courts began to apply tort liability principles to traditional indemnity insurers when their coverage decisions were at least partially responsible for an individual's injury or death,[f] which had the effect of opening insurers to a fuller range of potential damages (e.g., pain and suffering) than had been the case previously (when, under breach of contract principles, insurers were liable only for the actual cost of care they had initially declined to cover). This increased exposure to liability grew out of the fact that insurers were becoming more aggressive in their use of *prospective* coverage decisions, and courts were aware of how these types of coverage determinations could impact access to and the quality of health care. The advent of managed care as the primary mechanism for delivering and financing health care only magnified this concern, given managed care's use of techniques such as utilization review, and opened the door to one of the most contentious aspects of health services quality today: the extent to which patients can sue MCOs for negligent coverage or treatment decisions.

Managed Care Liability

Just as state courts were important in the extension of tort principles to health professionals, hospitals, and insurers, so too did they inaugurate application of these principles to MCOs. Modern MCOs are complex structures that heavily regulate the practices of their network physicians. Indeed, perhaps the most defining aspect of managed care is its oversight of physician medical judgment through various mechanisms—utilization review, practice guidelines, physician payment incentives, and so on.

A function of managed care's oversight of physician practice is that there is no longer any doubt that application of the professional standard of care for the purpose of determining negligence extends beyond the literal quality of health care delivered and reaches the very *coverage* of that care. This is because managed care has so altered coverage decision-making practices to focus on prospective decisions; where this type of coverage determination used to be the exception, it is now the rule. Instead of coverage denials leading to disputes over who was going to pay for an already-received medical service, prospective managed care coverage decisions more or less determine whether an individual receives treatment at all (Rosenbaum, Frankford, Moore, Borzi, 1999).

Needless to say, the negative impact of prospective coverage decisions on individuals' ability to access necessary, high-quality care is no small policy matter. At the same time, in one critical legal sense it does not particularly matter whether a dispute between an MCO and one of its beneficiaries is framed as one of negligence in healthcare *quality* or healthcare *coverage*; either way, the key issue is whether the medical judgment exercised by the MCO met the professional standard of care. In applying this standard, courts have had little trouble finding MCOs liable under state law both for the negligence of their network physicians and for their own direct negligence. (However, as discussed in the next section, these court decisions presume the nonapplicability of ERISA, a federal law that often precludes individuals from suing their managed care company under state tort laws.)

There have been a number of cases in which courts have determined that MCOs can be held vicariously liable for the negligent actions of their network physicians where a patient can prove an agency relationship under one of the theories (actual agency, apparent agency, or nondelegable duty) described

previously. In these cases, courts perform an exhaustive examination of the facts to determine the specific relationship between the treating physician and the MCO or the ways in which the MCO portrays and obligates itself to its beneficiaries. For example, in the case of *Boyd v. Albert Einstein Medical Center* (1988), a Pennsylvania court closely analyzed the literature of a health maintenance organization (HMO) for evidence of a contractual relationship to its beneficiaries to determine whether the HMO could be held vicariously liable under a theory of apparent agency for the treatment of a woman who died after physicians negligently treated her for a lump in her breast. Among other things, the court noted that the HMO's contract with its beneficiaries agreed to "provide healthcare services and benefits to members in order to protect and promote their health" and that the patients' contractual relationship was with the HMO, not with any individual physician in the HMO's network. In the end, the court determined that because the patient looked to the HMO itself for care and the HMO held itself out as providing care through its network physicians, the HMO was vicariously liable for the patient's negligent treatment.

Similarly, courts have applied the doctrine of corporate liability to MCOs. Courts have given various reasons for subjecting MCOs to this type of liability: at least in their role as arrangers or providers of health care, MCOs are much like hospitals; MCOs have the resources to monitor and improve the quality of healthcare delivery; and MCOs maintain tremendous authority over the makeup of their physician networks. The case of *Jones v. Chicago HMO Ltd. of Illinois* (2000) is a good example of the application of corporate liability principles to managed care. In *Jones*, the plaintiff called her MCO-appointed physician (Dr. Jordan) after her 3-month-old daughter (Shawndale) fell ill with constipation, fever, and other problems. Both an assistant to Dr. Jordan and, eventually, Dr. Jordan himself explained that Shawndale should not be brought to the physician's office but should instead be treated at home with castor oil. A day later, Shawndale was still sick and her mother took her to a hospital emergency department, where she was diagnosed with bacterial meningitis secondary to an ear infection. Shawndale was permanently disabled as a result of the meningitis. It emerged through pretrial testimony that the defendant MCO had assigned 4,500 to 6,000 patients to Dr. Jordan, far more than its own medical director deemed acceptable under the professional standard of care. The Illinois Supreme Court agreed, ruling that MCOs breach a legal duty as a corporate entity by assigning an excessive number of patients to any

What do you think about the role and success of tort law in promoting high-quality health care? Does it help to deter errors? If not, why?

single network physician, because doing so can affect the quality of care provided to beneficiaries.

This section reviewed generally the application of the professional standard of care to hospitals, insurers, and MCOs and described certain state-level theories of liability that are implicated when patients claim that the care they received fell short of this standard. However, as alluded to earlier, ERISA often preempts (i.e., supersedes) these kinds of state law liability claims against insurers and MCOs. This chapter now turns to a discussion of ERISA and its preemptive force.

▶ Federal Preemption of State Liability Laws Under ERISA

Generally speaking, ERISA prohibits individuals from recovering damages for death and injuries caused by substandard medical professional conduct to the extent that the individual receives her health coverage through a *private employer–sponsored* benefit plan. (Among others, individuals who work for federal, state, and local public employers are not covered by ERISA's rules.) Because approximately 150 million workers and their families in the United States receive this type of health coverage, and because managed care represents the dominant structure of healthcare delivery, the issue of whether individuals with private employer–sponsored managed care coverage can recover damages for substandard medical professional conduct is paramount.

Overview of ERISA

One of the most complex areas of federal civil law, ERISA[g] was established in 1974 mainly to protect the employee pension system from employer fraud. However, the law was drafted in such a way as to extend to all benefits offered by ERISA-covered employers, including health benefits. Because ERISA does not distinguish among employers based on size, essentially all employees in this country who receive health and other benefits through a private employer can be said to work for an "ERISA-covered" employer.

ERISA employs two main devices to protect employee pensions and other benefits. First, it imposes "fiduciary" responsibilities on those individuals or entities that administer various types of employer-sponsored benefit plans (in the case of health benefits, these are often conventional insurers or MCOs, or the employers themselves). A person or entity with fiduciary responsibilities is analogous to a trustee, who is expected to act primarily for another's benefit in carrying out his or her duties. Put differently, a fiduciary is one who manages money or property (like a pension fund or healthcare benefit) for another person and who is expected to act in good faith in that management. One critical fiduciary responsibility is to act with an eye toward the best interests of the person who has placed his or her trust in the fiduciary, rather than seeking personal enrichment through trustee activities.

The second tool used by Congress in ERISA to regulate employee benefits is a set of uniform, nationwide rules for the administration of employee benefits. However, although ERISA closely regulates the structure and operation of pension plans, the law includes few substantive standards governing the design or administration of health (or other) employee benefits. This stems mainly from the fact that Congress's main purpose in passing ERISA was to confront the employer fraud and underfunding evident in the pension system in the early 1970s (after all, the title of the law hints that its purpose is to specifically protect employee *retirement income*), not to regulate all employee benefit plans. However, the language used by ERISA's drafters is both broad and ambiguous, and courts have interpreted the statute as applying well beyond the field of pensions (Rosenbaum et al., 2012). As a result of the dearth of substantive standards pertaining to employee health benefits, employers enjoy discretion under ERISA to decide whether to offer health benefits at all and, if they do, to offer a benefit package of their choosing. This discretion allows the employer to design the benefit plan itself or buy an "off the shelf" insurance policy from a health insurer. If the employer chooses the latter, it also must decide whether to use a conventional insurer or a managed care company; if using a managed care company, it must decide whether to include physician incentive schemes in its benefit plan.

ERISA's lack of substantive health benefit regulations is compounded by the fact that the law contains few avenues for employees to remedy negligent benefit plan administration, including substandard conduct in the administration of health plan benefits. As mentioned, ERISA precludes the recovery of monetary damages under state law theories of liability when employer-sponsored benefits are improperly denied; Congress was of the opinion in fashioning ERISA that payment of these types of damages would drain employer benefit plans of needed resources. However, one might assume that when Congress broadly displaces state laws aimed at remedying negligence (as it did with ERISA), it would put in place meaningful enforcement provisions in the federal law. Yet the remedies available under ERISA are dramatically more limited than those available under state law. Under ERISA (1974), employees and their beneficiaries are effectively limited to suing to prospectively force a plan administrator to grant a covered benefit, to recover payment retrospectively when a covered benefit was improperly denied, and to enforce a plan administrator's fiduciary responsibilities. The upshot of these rights is that they allow an employee injured by an action or decision of his benefit plan to recover *nothing beyond the actual cost of the benefit due in any event*.

Furthermore, in *Pilot Life Insur. Co. v. Dedeaux* (1987), the U.S. Supreme Court held that ERISA's enforcement provision constituted not merely *a* remedy for negligent administration of an employee benefit plan, but rather the *exclusive* remedy. This means that all other state remedies generally available to individuals to remedy corporate negligence are preempted (and thus not available) to employees whose health benefits are provided through an ERISA-covered plan.

ERISA Preemption

To ensure the uniform regulation and administration of employee pension plans (and, as it turned out, other employee benefits) across the nation, Congress included in ERISA one of the most sweeping preemption provisions ever enacted under federal law. The uniqueness of the scope of ERISA's preemptive force is underscored by the fact that the states in America's governmental structure maintain broad authority to regulate many fields (including the fields of health care and health insurance) as they see fit, and federal law generally supplements, but does not replace, state law.

Furthermore, ERISA actually implicates two different types of preemption. The first, known as "conflict preemption," occurs when specific provisions of state law clearly conflict with federal law, in which case the state law is superseded. The second form of preemption triggered by ERISA is "field preemption," which the courts employ when they interpret federal law to occupy an entire field of law (e.g., employee benefit law), irrespective of whether there are any conflicting state law provisions (this is the type of

preemption at work in ERISA's remedial provisions, described earlier). The practical import of this second type of preemption is that a wide range of state laws are preempted by ERISA even though they do not directly conflict with it. All in all, it is little wonder that ERISA is considered to function as a "regulatory vacuum."

The length of ERISA's conflict preemption provision belies its preemptive scope, and its wording belies the enormous amount of litigation it has engendered. The substantive entirety of the preemption clause reads: "[ERISA] shall supersede any and all State laws insofar as they may now or hereafter relate to any employee benefit plan." Courts have grappled with the meaning of this language for decades. For example, the term *relate to* has been interpreted by the U.S. Supreme Court to include any state law that has "a connection with or reference to" an employee benefit plan (*Shaw v. Delta Air Lines, Inc.*, 1983), but not those that have only a "remote and tenuous" relationship to benefit plans (*New York State Conference of Blue Cross & Blue Shield Plans v. Travelers Insur. Co.*, 1995). Thus, the former types of state laws are preempted, while the latter are not. The Supreme Court has also weighed in on the meaning of "employee benefit plan" (*Fort Halifax Packing Co. v. Coyne*, 1987).

In addition to the preemption clause itself, however, there are two additional pieces to the ERISA conflict preemption puzzle that only add to the law's complexity. The second piece is referred to as the "insurance savings" clause, which says that the preemption clause shall not "be construed to exempt or relieve any person from any law of any State which regulates insurance." This essentially means that even where a state law relates to an employee benefit plan, it is saved from preemption if it regulates insurance (*Metropolitan Life Insur. Co. v. Massachusetts*, 1985). The Supreme Court has interpreted this provision to mean a state law is saved from preemption if it is specifically directed toward entities engaged in insurance and substantially affects the risk-pooling arrangement between an insurer and its beneficiaries (*Kentucky Ass'n of Health Plans, Inc. v. Miller*, 2003). The practical effect of the savings clause, then, is to narrow the reach of the preemption clause, because state laws that meet the "regulates insurance" test fall outside the scope of ERISA preemption.

The final element of ERISA conflict preemption is the "deemer" clause, which addresses the distinction between fully insured and self-insured employee health benefit plans. A fully insured health plan (sometimes referred to simply as an insured plan) is one in which an employer purchases health insurance coverage (i.e., pays premiums) to a conventional insurance company or MCO, and in return the insurance company or MCO accepts the financial risk of paying claims for covered benefits. A self-insured health plan (also called a self-funded plan) exists when an employer retains some or all of the financial risk for its employees' claims for covered benefits. Nearly one-half of all U.S. employers self-insure their health benefit plans.

ERISA's deemer clause reads in pertinent part: "An employee benefit plan shall [not] be deemed to be an insurance company or other insurer, ... or to be engaged in the business of insurance ... for purposes of any law of any State purporting to regulate insurance companies." The purpose of this clause is to prohibit states from deeming employee benefit plans as the functional equivalent of health insurers, and its practical effect is critical for the tens of millions of employees who receive their health benefits under self-insured plans: the deemer clause prevents state laws that meet the "regulates insurance" test from applying to self-insured employee health benefit plans (*Metropolitan Life Insur. Co. v. Massachusetts*, 1985). In other words, even state laws "saved" from preemption do not apply to self-insured plans because under ERISA these types of plans are "deemed" not to be insurance companies. The ultimate result of the deemer clause's application is to *exempt completely* self-funded employee benefit plans from state insurance law. This exemption allows sponsors of self-funded plans enormous discretion to design the plans as they choose.

The Intersection of ERISA Preemption and Managed Care Professional Medical Liability

The final matter to discuss in the context of ERISA preemption has been one of the most unstable over the past several years: the extent to which ERISA preempts state tort law claims by individuals against managed care companies for negligent coverage decisions and substandard provision of care. This issue has played out over a series of federal court decisions attempting to define with some precision ERISA's application in the context of employer-sponsored managed care plans.

In the 1992 case of *Corcoran v. United HealthCare, Inc.*, the Fifth Circuit Court of Appeals ruled that Florence Corcoran's state law claim against United HealthCare for the wrongful death of her fetus had to be dismissed under ERISA, regardless of any medical negligence on the part of the MCO. The court held that even if the company improperly denied coverage of preterm labor management services for Mrs. Corcoran, her state lawsuit seeking damages for a negligent coverage decision was preempted because the company's determination was, in the language of ERISA, sufficiently "related to" Mrs. Corcoran's employee benefit plan.

Three years later, the Third Circuit Court of Appeals ruled in *Dukes v. U.S. Healthcare, Inc.* (1995) that although individuals in ERISA-covered health benefit plans may not be able to sue under state law for an MCO's negligent coverage denial (i.e., for a company's decision as to the *quantity* of care covered under the plan), they can seek state law damages where a managed care company's negligence is connected to the *quality* of care actually provided. The Third Circuit essentially ruled that Congress did not intend in passing ERISA to supersede state laws aimed at the regulation of healthcare quality, historically a subject area under the states' purview. Instead, according to the court, federal policymakers enacted ERISA to alleviate national companies' concerns over abiding by many different state pension and employee benefit laws and to instead subject them to a uniform set of funding and administration rules. Whatever Congress meant by a "state law that relates to an employee benefit plan," the *Dukes* court did not interpret ERISA's preemption provision to sweep in laws pertaining to the quality of medical care provided to beneficiaries of employer-sponsored health benefit plans.

In the 5 years after *Dukes* was decided, federal court decisions applying ERISA to managed care plans more or less subscribed to this quantity/quality distinction. However, the Supreme Court stepped into the fray in 2000 in the case of *Pegram v. Herdrich*, seemingly altering the approach lower courts had been taking when analyzing ERISA preemption of state law negligence claims against MCOs. The main issue in *Pegram* was whether physician incentive arrangements were violative of the fiduciary responsibility rules contained in ERISA (incidentally, the court ruled they were not). However, the court included several paragraphs in its decision about the role of the treating physician in the case, who also happened to be one of the owners of the managed care company being sued for negligently failing to order a diagnostic test. In so doing, the court described two different kinds of decisions made by MCOs:

> What we will call pure "eligibility decisions" turn on the plan's coverage of a particular condition or medical procedure for its treatment. "Treatment decisions," by contrast, are choices about how to go about diagnosing and treating a patient's condition: given a patient's constellation of symptoms, what is the appropriate medical response? *These decisions are often*

practically inextricable from one another... . This is so not merely because ... treatment and eligibility decisions are made by the same person, the treating physician. It is so because a great many *and possibly most* coverage questions are not simple yes-or-no questions, like whether appendicitis is a covered condition (when there is no dispute that a patient has appendicitis), or whether acupuncture is a covered procedure for pain relief (when the claim of pain is unchallenged). The more common coverage question is a when-and-how question. Although coverage for many conditions will be clear and various treatment options will be indisputably compensable, physicians still must decide what to do in particular cases.... In practical terms, these eligibility decisions cannot be untangled from physicians' judgments about reasonable medical treatment. (*Pegram v. Herdrich*, 2000)

Importantly, the court went on to suggest that these intertwined decisions fall beyond ERISA's reach and that state laws implicated when these decisions are negligently made are not preempted, though the court provided no clear guidance as to when managed care decisions tipped sufficiently toward coverage or care to pull them out of the realm of being "mixed." Following the decision, many federal courts faced with ERISA's application to claims by managed care beneficiaries adopted *Pegram*'s approach over the one developed in *Dukes*. Courts favored *Pegram*'s approach because it opened the door to state law remedies for individuals (like Florence Corcoran) who were injured as a result of managed care negligence but who otherwise had no way to recover for their loss.

In the 2004 case of *Aetna Health, Inc. v. Davila*, however, the Supreme Court appeared to close the door it seemed to open in *Pegram*, suggesting that lawsuits premised on the intertwined or "mixed" decisions made daily by MCOs escape ERISA's preemptive force only when the decisions include actual treatment by an MCO medical employee. The *Davila* decision actually represented a pair of cases (the other one originally called *Cigna v. Calad*) consolidated by the court due to the similarity of the respective plaintiffs' claims. Both Juan Davila and Ruby Calad were members of ERISA-covered employee health benefit plans. Davila was injured when Aetna chose to substitute a less expensive medication for the one he normally took to control his arthritis pain; Calad suffered complications after being prematurely discharged from the hospital subsequent to Cigna's decision to cover just 1 day of hospitalization postsurgery. Rather

BOX 12-5 Discussion Questions

The critical intersection between health care and health insurance as exemplified by the *Davila* decision leads to an important question: is it reasonable to treat a healthcare coverage decision as having nothing to do with health care itself? Put another way, given the expense of health care today, do you believe that individuals and families can afford necessary health care if there is no third party responsible for covering at least some of the cost?

than filing appeals directly with their insurance companies, Davila and Calad sued under a state law called the Texas Health Care Liability Act. They argued that their respective insurer's decision breached a duty under the Texas law to exercise reasonable care in healthcare decision making and that the breach caused their injuries.

In rejecting both plaintiffs' claims, the Supreme Court ruled that ERISA preempts lawsuits for damages against ERISA-covered plans for negligent healthcare coverage decisions, even when the coverage decision was predicated on flawed medical judgment. Thus, *Davila* makes clear that when an individual covered by an ERISA plan complains only of negligent coverage decision making (including the wrongful denial of a benefit) on the part of an MCO, ERISA shields the MCO from liability beyond the actual value of the benefit itself.[h] However, the Supreme Court in *Davila* also explained that notwithstanding ERISA, MCOs remain liable under state tort laws for negligence when acting in their capacity as providers or arrangers of health care. Although this ruling sustains the general distinction made by the federal court of appeals in the *Dukes* decision, its effect on the legal remedies available to injured patients is likely to be limited, given that policymakers and courts still view coverage decision making, rather than the provision of health care, as the primary aim of MCOs.

▶ Measuring and Incentivizing Healthcare Quality[i]

We turn now to the final topics in this chapter: what exactly is meant by healthcare "quality," how is it measured, and how should policy be designed in order to encourage and reward it? Given the explosive growth in healthcare costs in the United States over the past few decades, combined with evidence from leading researchers and experts[j] that collectively points to the disconnect between high spending and healthcare quality and to serious deficiencies in healthcare quality overall, these are important questions.

To analyze these questions, focusing on the Medicare program is particularly instructive. As the single largest payer (in terms of dollars spent) in the U.S. health system, Medicare is a major national driver of policy in other markets (both public and private). Therefore, how the Medicare program addresses issues pertaining to quality is not only important to Medicare beneficiaries and providers but also to other purchasers and stakeholders whose policies and procedures are often driven, or at least influenced, by Medicare policy. The remainder of this section will focus on how the Medicare program, as authorized by federal legislation, is working to improve the quality and lower the cost of healthcare delivery. It also addresses similar efforts of other payers and stakeholders, including the role of health information technology in facilitating quality improvement.

Traditionally, the Medicare program has paid for healthcare services on a fee-for-service (FFS) basis, with the exception of inpatient hospital services, which are paid based on diagnosis-related groups under the prospective payment system (PPS), and the Medicare Advantage and Prescription Drug plans, which are paid on a capitated basis. All payment systems (public and private) tend to incentivize something; in the case of FFS, it is indiscriminate increases in the volume of treatments and services, while in case-based or capitation systems, it is indiscriminate reductions in volume. Whatever the payment arrangement, the challenge is to promote both quality and value while also apportioning financial risk appropriately. However, because Medicare has historically lacked a programwide and deliberate approach to promoting quality and value, and because it has relied principally on an FFS approach to payment for physician and other services, the program has experienced incredible growth in the volume of services for which it pays.

Over the years, Congress has passed a series of laws designed to move both the Medicare and Medicaid programs from passive purchasers of volume-based health care to active purchasers of high-quality, high-value health care based in large part on successful demonstration projects. For example, as authorized under the Medicare Prescription Drug and Modernization Act of 2003 (MMA) and extended by the Deficit Reduction Act of 2005 (DRA), hospitals that reported on specific quality measures receive the full annual payment update, while failure to participate resulted in a decrease in the annual payment update. Similarly, as authorized by the Tax Relief and Health Care Act of 2006 (TRHCA) and extended by the Medicare, Medicaid, and SCHIP Extension Act of 2007 (MMSEA), and made permanent by the Medicare Improvements for Patients and Providers Act of 2008 (MIPPA), the Physician Quality Reporting System (PQRS) offered bonus payments to Medicare physicians who reported on specific quality measures. The Health Information Technology for Economic and Clinical Health Act (HITECH), enacted as part of the American Recovery and Reinvestment Act of 2009 (ARRA), provided significant financial incentives to Medicare and Medicaid providers for "meaningfully using" electronic health records to improve the quality of care delivery.

Incentives to improve the quality of Medicare-covered care were also a focus of the ACA. The ACA set forth a broad vision for quality measurement, reporting, and financial incentives in Medicare, including quality measure development, quality measurement (including payment incentives), public reporting, and value-based purchasing. The ACA also called for other payers and stakeholders to align their efforts with federal efforts. In short, the ACA greatly expanded the existing efforts noted previously while introducing new tools for the Medicare program to identify, measure, and pay for high-quality care, while encouraging other payers and stakeholders to do the same. The ACA also moved the country toward implementing a "national quality strategy" that would work to align quality improvement and value-based purchasing initiatives among and across payers, both public and private.

Since passage of the ACA, several other pieces of healthcare-related legislation have extended and refined its quality improvement initiatives. The American Taxpayer Relief Act of 2012 (ATRA) made several changes to quality and utilization-based payment adjustments created or modified by the ACA, revised reporting requirements under the PQRS, and established a commission to develop a plan for delivering high-quality long-term care services. The Improving Medicare Post-Acute Care Transformation Act of 2014 (the IMPACT Act) required that long-term care hospitals, skilled nursing facilities, home health agencies, and inpatient rehabilitation facilities report specific, standardized data on quality and resource-use measures. Most notably, the Medicare Access and CHIP Reauthorization Act of 2015 (MACRA) established a new payment methodology to reward physicians either for quality improvement or the adoption of an alternative value-based payment model, provided additional funding for quality measure development, and expanded the availability of Medicare data to support public and private quality improvement efforts.

Quality Measure Development

Residing at the core of public and private efforts to improve the quality of care in the United States are measures used to evaluate the quality of providers' clinical care. But what constitutes quality clinical care? The answer to this question varies by stakeholder. A patient is likely focused on a good outcome and good relationship with his or her provider. A health plan is likely focused on whether the provider achieved a good outcome at the lowest cost (based on time and resources used). A provider is likely focused on whether the desired outcome was achieved and payment was made. Given the diversity of stakeholders involved in healthcare delivery, there is great variation in the definition of quality, even between and among different types of providers (e.g., primary care physicians and specialists).

To address the varying perspectives on quality, the U.S. Department of Health and Human Services (HHS) uses a multistakeholder approach to design and approve quality measures that are specific to provider types (e.g., hospital-specific measures). This approach, mandated by the ACA and MACRA, requires that HHS select an organization (currently the National Quality Forum, or NQF) to convene multistakeholder groups to provide consensus-based input on quality measures. HHS considers the measures endorsed by the NQF when selecting quality and efficiency measures for use in public reporting, performance-based payment, and other programs applicable to Medicare and Medicaid providers. Most public and private quality improvement efforts also use the measures that are approved by the NQF. Specialty groups representing specific types of providers and other stakeholders develop and endorse quality and performance measures applicable to their members prior to NQF review; these include the Ambulatory Quality Alliance (AQA), Pharmacy Quality Alliance (PQA), National Committee for Quality Assurance (NCQA; health plan measures), and Hospital Quality Alliance (HQA).

The ACA also provided some clarification for defining quality measures. It defines a "quality measure" as a "standard for measuring the performance and improvement of population health or of health plans, providers of services, and other clinicians in the delivery of healthcare services." The HHS Secretary, acting through its Centers for Medicare and Medicaid Services (CMS), is required to identify gaps where no quality measures exist and any existing quality measures that need to be improved, updated, or expanded

for use in federal healthcare programs (including Medicare, Medicaid, and CHIP). Identified gaps are reported on a publicly available website, and the HHS Secretary provides grants to organizations to develop, update, or expand quality measures. Priorities for new measures include those that assess outcomes, functional status, care coordination across episodes, shared decision making, use of health information technology, efficiency, safety, timeliness, equity, and patient experience. The Secretary also develops (and updates) outcome measures for acute and chronic diseases and primary and preventive care for hospitals and physicians.

Quality Measurement

The ACA reauthorized and developed quality measurement programs for multiple types of providers participating in the Medicare program. For example, the ACA reauthorized incentive payments under the PQRS through 2014 and instituted a penalty for physicians who do not report PQRS measures beginning in 2015. The PQRS (along with other performance-related programs) was replaced under MACRA's Quality Payment Program (QPP) Merit-Based Incentive Payment System (MIPS) track as of January 2017. Physicians participating in MIPS are evaluated on their performance across four categories, including quality (the category that replaced the PRQS), and receive a reduction or a bonus beginning in the 2019 payment year. MACRA provides funding for development and selection of MIPS quality measures and requires that selected measures address several quality domains (clinical care, safety, care coordination, patient and caregiver experience, and population health and prevention), with priority given to outcome, patient experience, care coordination, and resource utilization measures, emphasizing outcome measures where feasible. The ACA required the HHS Secretary to provide feedback to eligible professionals on their performance on reported quality measures under PQRS, and MACRA similarly requires the Secretary to provide feedback on performance related to selected quality measures and resource utilization.

Public Reporting

In addition to informing providers about the quality of care they deliver, quality information enables consumers to make more informed provider choices. The CMS currently posts a significant amount of quality and cost of care information on their suite of *Compare* websites (e.g., Hospital Compare[k]). The ACA also expanded required public reporting to Medicare physicians and several other provider types, including long-term care hospitals, inpatient rehabilitation hospitals, psychiatric hospitals, hospice programs, and non-PPS cancer hospitals. Information reported must include the quality measures as well as assessments of patient health outcomes, risk-adjusted resource use, efficiency, patient experience, and other relevant information deemed appropriate by the HHS Secretary. Beginning in 2013, CMS also made several changes to their data release policy, publishing data sets containing physician-identifiable information on utilization and payment in the Medicare Part B and Part D programs. As of early 2018, CMS further enhanced transparency by providing Medicare Part C program claims data to researchers upon request and announced plans to release Medicaid and CHIP encounter data.

Value-Based Purchasing

The voluntary quality improvement programs described previously focused on developing provider-specific quality measures and incentivizing providers to report specific quality information. Typically, the programs began with providers collecting and reporting information to CMS and then transitioned to linking incentive payments to the reporting. While these "pay for reporting" programs have been successful in encouraging providers to assess the quality of care they are delivering through the reporting mechanisms, they do not take into account individual patient outcomes or population health outcomes (i.e., they do not "pay for *performance*"). However, CMS's End-Stage Renal Disease Quality Incentive Program (QIP) began reducing payments to facilities that do not meet or exceed certain performance benchmarks in 2012. In addition, as authorized by the DRA, CMS has implemented a similar type of payment program that reduces payments to hospitals that have the highest rates of certain hospital-acquired conditions (HACs). (HACs stand in contrast to conditions that were present on admission.) It is worth noting that these programs are not unique to the Medicare program; many state Medicaid programs and private payers have also developed and implemented similar programs.[1]

Until passage of the ACA, CMS was not able to move beyond "pay for reporting" programs or the HAC Reduction Program because it did not have the necessary legal authority to vary payments based on actual provider performance. Specifically, the ACA required the implementation of Medicare value-based purchasing programs for most hospitals subject to the inpatient PPS. Value-based purchasing programs for home health agencies and skilled nursing facilities were respectively implemented in 2016 and 2018, and,

as required by the ACA, a program for ambulatory surgical centers is in development. These value-based programs require the Medicare program to financially reward and penalize providers based on their performance on specified quality measures and other indicators, such as rates of readmission and HACs. For example, through the hospital value-based purchasing program, eligible hospitals began receiving incentive payments for discharges after October 1, 2012, that met certain performance standards. Quality domains on which hospital performance is evaluated include patient- and caregiver-centered experience (based on the hospital's HCAHPS score, which stands for Hospital Consumer Assessment of Healthcare Providers and Systems), clinical process of care, patient safety (measured by rates of certain healthcare-associated infections), and efficiency and cost reduction (based on spending per Medicare beneficiary). Information regarding the performance of individual hospitals under the program is available online through the Hospital Compare website.

The ACA authorized a physician and physician practice group value-based purchasing program that provided differential payments to physicians and physician practice groups under the fee schedule based on the quality of care furnished compared to cost. MACRA's Quality Payment Program replaced the ACA's value-based payment modifier for physicians participating in the MIPS track with the "cost" performance category beginning in 2018. The MIPS cost category evaluates physician performance on cost of care and resource utilization measures relevant to specific episodes of care.

In early 2015, HHS announced its goals of making 30% of FFS Medicare payments to alternative payment models, such as accountable care organizations (ACOs) or bundled payment arrangements, and of tying 85% of FFS payments to quality or value through programs such as hospital value-based purchasing and hospital readmissions reduction by the end of 2016. It achieved both goals ahead of schedule in early 2016 and announced its intention to make 50% of payments to alternative payment models and to tie 90% of payments to quality or value by the end of 2018. These new goals were halted in early 2018 to allow the new administration time to review the impact of these new payment models and programs, though HHS remains publicly committed toward value-based payment reform. Similarly, MACRA's Quality Payment Program includes the Alternative Payment Model participation track, which offers an incentive payment to physicians participating in certain alternative payment models who meet volume-based thresholds.

National Quality Strategy

To better align quality improvement initiatives across payers, the ACA also required the development of a national quality strategy to improve the delivery of healthcare services, patient health outcomes, and population health. HHS released its initial report to Congress, titled "National Strategy for Quality Improvement in Health Care," in March of 2011, outlining aims and priorities for quality improvement. The Strategy was updated in 2014 with levers representing core business functions, resources, and/or actions that stakeholders could use to align to the Strategy. What follows is a summary of the updated Strategy (Agency for Healthcare Research and Quality, 2016):

- **Adopting national aims:** The National Quality Strategy will pursue three broad aims that will be used to guide and assess local, state, and national efforts to improve healthcare quality. These aims include the following:
  - Better care: Represents efforts to improve the overall quality of health care by making care more patient centered, reliable, accessible, and safe.
  - Healthy People/Healthy Communities: Encompasses efforts to improve the health of the population by supporting interventions that address behavioral, social, and environmental determinants of health.
  - Affordable care: Seeks to reduce the cost of quality health care for individuals, families, employers, and government.
- **Setting priorities:** To advance these three aims, the strategy focuses on six priorities:
  - Making care safer by reducing harm caused in the delivery of care.
  - Ensuring that each person and family is engaged as partners in his or her care.
  - Promoting effective communication and coordination of care.
  - Promoting the most effective prevention and treatment practices for the leading causes of mortality, starting with cardiovascular disease.
  - Working with communities to promote wide use of best practices to enable healthy living.
  - Making quality care more affordable for individuals, families, employers, and governments by developing and spreading new healthcare delivery models.
- **Using levers to achieve improved health and health care:** In addition to adopting one or more of these aims and priorities, stakeholders can align

to the National Quality Strategy using any of the following nine levers:
- Payment: Payment arrangements should reward and incentivize high-quality, patient-centered care.
- Public reporting: Public reporting initiatives compare costs, treatment outcomes, and patient experience for consumers.
- Technical assistance: These efforts foster learning environments that offer training, resources, tools, and guidance to help organizations achieve quality improvement goals.
- Certification, accreditation, and regulation: These activities ensure that providers adopt or adhere to approaches to meet safety and quality standards.
- Consumer incentives and benefit designs: These are designed to help consumers adopt healthy behaviors and make informed decisions.
- Measurement and feedback: These activities provide performance feedback to plans and providers to improve care.
- Health information technology: These tools improve communication, transparency, and efficiency for better coordinated health and health care.
- Workforce development: These activities involve investing in people to prepare the next generation of healthcare professionals and support lifelong learning for providers.
- Innovation and diffusion: This lever aims to foster innovation in health care, in quality improvement, and within and across organizations and communities.

Annual reports have provided an update on quality improvement in the national tracking measures and highlighted public and private accomplishments in the six priority areas at the federal, state, and local levels. For the Strategy's fifth anniversary update in 2016, the annual report was combined with the annual National Healthcare Quality and Disparities Report to describe the nation's progress toward improving healthcare access, quality, and disparities. The report found that while quality had continued to improve since adoption of the National Quality Strategy, wide variation existed across its six priorities (the annual reports are available on the AHRQ website). In addition to the National Quality Strategy, multiple HHS agencies, as well as several state health departments, have their own quality strategies, many of which use the National Quality Strategy as their foundation.

Private Payer Efforts

While the federal government drives much of the quality improvement activity in the United States, private payers also make significant contributions to quality measurement and improvement and to related payment initiatives. For example, payers have created set payments for care during specific periods (i.e., a modified global payment arrangement) that connect payments to quality goals and provide bonuses to participants that meet or exceed set benchmarks. Others use NQF, NCQA, and similar measures to assess providers' performance and resource consumption; providers achieving set thresholds in both metrics are designated as high-quality performers online, for consideration by beneficiaries and other stakeholders. These are not unique examples; most payers post quality information about their network providers to enable their enrollees to make more informed decisions. Other efforts focus on incentives to ensure patient satisfaction, such as offering refunds to any patient who reports a negative healthcare encounter, or aim to achieve compliance with best practice guidelines, such as agreeing to bear the costs of any care associated with complications arising after a procedure. Organizations develop, implement, refine, and expand on these innovative approaches, which can encourage others to adapt and adopt successful models and methods of quality improvement.

It is important for private payers to be involved in quality improvement initiatives. Absent common standards across payers for provider quality and value, systemwide delivery and payment reform will be hampered. Because providers typically contract with federal payers (e.g., Medicare) as well as multiple private payers, they will likely be subject to different definitions of quality and different requirements for demonstrating value. This makes it a challenge for providers to align their quality improvement efforts. Multipayer efforts enable more efficient quality measurement and validate the importance of systemwide quality improvement.

Underscoring the importance of multi-stakeholder involvement, HHS established the Health Care Payment Learning and Action Network in 2015. This network virtually convenes thousands of stakeholders (including payers, providers, employers, patients, states, and consumer groups) to set goals related to payment reform, share best practices, and decrease variation in payment methodologies. Interested individuals and organizations can register to participate in the network via the CMS Innovation Center's website.

In addition, across the country, multi-stakeholder collaboratives and community groups are partnering with employers, payers, providers, and consumers to further public/private efforts to improve quality. For example, Aligning Forces for Quality, a signature Robert Wood Johnson Foundation initiative from 2007 to 2015, established alliances in 16 communities across the United States. These multi-stakeholder alliances collected and reported provider performance data, tested new care delivery and payment reform models, and disseminated best practices. Providers used the information provided by the alliances to improve quality of care for the nearly 40 million residents of those 16 communities, demonstrating the value of multi-stakeholder partnerships in healthcare delivery transformation.

Role of Health Information Technology

Health information technology, or health IT, provides critical support for quality improvement and payment reform. Health IT includes electronic features that facilitate care delivery, such as decision support tools, electronic health records, and electronic prescribing functions. Health IT enables instant sharing of health information throughout a facility, among providers in different locations, and with the patient. Health IT can prevent clinical errors that may have dire consequences, such as by alerting providers of potential adverse drug interactions or treatment contraindications. These features facilitate quality improvement across clinical settings. Beyond clinical functions, health IT can also facilitate quality improvement efforts by collecting and analyzing data related to outcomes and process measures for use by a provider in required reporting or conducting quality improvement initiatives. However, connecting health IT systems and allowing providers to communicate across different health IT systems remains a challenge. HHS's Office of the National Coordinator for Health Information Technology is working with other stakeholders to foster a health IT environment where patient information can be shared electronically across the entire care spectrum, regardless of the technology used.

The value of health IT is demonstrated through federal efforts to encourage its adoption. For example, the meaningful use program, created in 2009 by the HITECH Act, established incentives for providers and hospitals to adopt electronic health records. The Center for Medicare and Medicaid Innovation, established by the ACA, tests new payment and delivery models and must consider whether a model uses technology in making its selections. MACRA's Quality Payment

Program phased out the meaningful use program and replaced it with the Promoting Interoperability (formerly Advancing Care Information) performance category for MIPS-participating physicians beginning in 2017. This dimension's name change was designed to emphasize the importance of improving interoperability, flexibility, and patient access to information. This new category requires use of certified electronic health record technology (CEHRT); incentive payments for this category are calculated based on performance in measures related to use of CEHRT to engage patients and exchange health information.

▸ Conclusion

This chapter introduced the concept of healthcare quality generally, briefly described the concepts of licensure and accreditation, discussed the specific quality concern of medical errors, detailed the topic of legal liability for substandard healthcare provision and decision making, and covered measurement of healthcare quality. While the majority of the chapter was dedicated to legal accountability for negligence in healthcare delivery, this is of course just one method used to promote high-quality care. Policymakers, health services researchers, the health professions themselves, and others have proposed or implemented several additional strategies (e.g., related to the healthcare system's organizational structure, or to evidence-based medicine, or to information technology) aimed at remedying existing quality concerns and improving the quality of care going forward, some of which are reflected in federal legislation. Many of these strategies have yet to take hold on a national scale, however, and finding effective ways to mesh them with existing legal rules—and navigating the legal system's responses to them—are issues with which the country will continue to grapple.

References

Aetna Health, Inc. v. Davila, 542 U.S. 200 (2004).

Agency for Healthcare Research and Quality. (2016). *National Strategy for Quality Improvement in Health Care*. Retrieved from https://www.ahrq.gov/workingforquality/about/agency -specific-quality-strategic-plans/nqs3.html

Boyd v. Albert Einstein Med. Ctr., 547 A. 2d 1229 (Pa. Super., 1988).

Canterbury v. Spence, 464 F.2d 772 (D.C. Cir. 1972).

Committee on Quality of Health Care in America. (2001). *Crossing the quality chasm: A new health system for the 21st century*. Washington, DC: National Academy Press.

Corcoran v. United Healthcare Inc., 965 F.2d 1321 (5th Cir. 1992).

Darling v. Charleston Cmty. Mem. Hosp., 211 N.E.2d 253 (Ill. 1965).

Dukes v. U.S. Healthcare, Inc., 57 F. 3d 350 (3d Cir. 1995).

Employee Retirement Income Security Act of 1974, 29 U.S.C. §§ 1132, 1144(a)-(b)(2)(A) & (B) (1974).

Fisher, E. S., Wennberg, D. E., Stukel, T. A., Gottlieb, D. J., Lucas, F. L., & Oinder, E. L. (2003). The implications of regional variations in Medicare spending. Part 1: the content, quality, and accessibility of care. *Annals of Internal Medicine, 138*, 273–287.

Fisher, E., Goodman, D., Skinner, J., & Bronner, K. (2009). *Health care spending, quality and outcomes: More isn't always better*. Retrieved from http://www.dartmouthatlas.org/downloads /reports/Spending_Brief_022709.pdf

Fort Halifax Packing Co. v. Coyne, 482 U.S. 1 (1987).

Furrow, B. R., Greaney, T. L., Johnson, S. H., Jost, T. S., & Schwartz, R. L. (2001). *Health law: Cases, materials and problems*. St. Paul, MN: West Group.

Gruenberg v. Aetna Insur. Co., 510 P. 2d 1032 (Cal. 1973).

Hall v. Hilbun, 466 So.2d 856 (Miss. 1985).

Helling v. Carey, 519 P.2d 981 (Wash. 1974).

Hurley v. Eddingfield, 59 N.E. 1058 (Ind. 1901).

Iglehart, J. K. (2013). Expanding the role of advanced nurse practitioners: Risks and rewards. *New England Journal of Medicine, 368*, 1935–1941.

Integrated Healthcare Association. (n.d.). *AMP commercial HMO*. Retrieved from https://www.iha.org/our-work/accountability /value-based-p4p

Jackson v. Power, 743 P. 2d 1376 (Alaska, 1987).

Jones v. Chicago HMO Ltd. of Illinois, 730 N.E. 2d 1119 (2000).

Kaufman, M. (2006, July 21). Medication errors harming millions, report says. *Washington Post*. Retrieved from http://www .washingtonpost.com/wp-dyn/content/article/2006/07/20 /AR2006072000754.html

Kentucky Ass'n of Health Plans, Inc. v. Miller, 538 U.S. 329 (2003).

Kohn, L. T., Corrigan, J. M., & Donaldson, M. S. (Eds.). (2000). *To err is human: Building a safer health system*. Washington, DC: National Academy Press.

Kuhmerker, K., & Hartman, T. (2007). *Pay-for-performance in state Medicaid programs: A survey of state Medicaid directors and programs*. Retrieved from https://www.commonwealthfund .org/publications/fund-reports/2007/apr/pay-performance -state-medicaid-programs-survey-state-medicaid

Makary, M. A., & Daniel, M. (2016). Medical error—The third leading cause of death in the U.S. *The BMJ*. Retrieved from https://www.bmj.com/content/353/bmj.i2139

McGlynn, E. A., Asch, S. M., Adams, J., Keesey, J., Hicks, J., DeCristofaro, A., & Kerr, E. (2003). The quality of health care delivered to adults in the United States. *New England Journal of Medicine, 348*, 2635–2645.

Mehlman v. Powell, 378 A. 2d 1121 (Md. 1977).

Metropolitan Life Insur. Co. v. Massachusetts, 471 U.S. 724 (1985).

New York State Conference of Blue Cross & Blue Shield Plans v. Travelers Insur. Co., 514 U.S. 645 (1995).

Nordenberg, T. (2000). *Make no mistake: Medical errors can be deadly serious*. Retrieved from https://permanent.access.gpo .gov/lps1609/www.fda.gov/fdac/features/2000/500_err.html

Patient Protection and Affordable Care Act (Pub. L. 111-148) § 3013 (2010), adding Public Health Service Act § 931.

Patient Safety and Quality Improvement Act of 2005, 42 U.S.C. § 299 et seq. (2005).

Pegram v. Herdrich, 530 U.S. 211 (2000).

Pilot Life Insur. Co. v. Dedeaux, 481 U.S. 41 (1987).

Rosenbaum, S., Frankford, D. M., Law, S. A., & Rosenblatt, R. E. (2012). *Law and the American health care system* (2nd ed.). Westbury, CT: The Foundation Press.

Rosenbaum, S., Frankford, D. M., Moore, B., & Borzi, P. (1999). Who should determine when health care is medically necessary? *New England Journal of Medicine, 340*(3), 229–233.

Shaw v. Delta Air Lines, Inc., 463 U.S. 85 (1983).

Shilkret v. Annapolis Emergency Hospital Ass'n, 349 A. 2d 245, 253 (Md. 1975).

Slater v. Baker and Stapleton, 95 Eng. Rep. 860, 862 (King's Bench 1767).

Small v. Howard, 128 Mass. 131 (1880).

T. J. Hooper v. Northern Barge Corp., 60 F.2d 737 (2d Cir. 1932).

Van Vector v. Blue Cross Ass'n, 365 N.E. 2d 638 (Ill. App. Ct., 1977).

Wennberg, J. (Ed.) (1996). *The Dartmouth atlas of health care in the United States 1996.* Hanover, NH: American Hospital Publishing, Inc.

Wennberg J. E., Fisher, E. S., & Skinner, J. S. (2002). Geography and the debate over Medicare reform. *Health Affairs,* (suppl.), W96–W114.

▶ Endnotes

a. For example, in the lawsuit stemming from the facts described at the outset of this chapter, the parents of the infant who died alleged that their MCO's decision to precertify only 24 hours of hospital care coverage did not meet the requisite standard of care in several healthcare quality respects: it was not medically appropriate and was motivated by financial profit, not Michelina's health and well-being; it forced Michelina's premature discharge from the hospital; it was made despite the MCO's knowledge that newborns are particularly at risk for developing illnesses; and it discouraged physicians participating in the MCO's provider network from readmitting infants to the hospital when problems arose after discharge.

b. Because the law's evolving view of the standard of care closely mirrors its view of the medical profession more generally, it is worth pausing for a moment to reflect on the health policy and law conceptual framework that is focused on historical, social, political, and economic views. This framework includes three perspectives: professional autonomy, social contract, and free market. The first perspective, dominant from about 1880 to 1960, argues that physicians' scientific and medical expertise leaves them in the best position to determine whether care rendered to patients is of adequate quality, and thus that legal oversight of the medical profession should be driven by the profession itself. The second perspective guided policymaking and legal principles for roughly 20 years beginning around 1960 and maintains that healthcare delivery and financing should be governed by enforcement of a "social contract" that generally elevates patient rights and societal values over physician autonomy and control. The free market perspective—dominant since the 1990s—contends that healthcare services are most efficiently delivered in a deregulated marketplace controlled by commercial competition. Bear in mind the first two perspectives specifically as you read this section.

c. One of the most commonly cited English cases for this rule is *Slater v. Baker and Stapleton* (1976), in which the court ruled that the appropriate legal standard for determining a surgeon's liability was "the usage and law of surgeons … the rule of the profession" as testified to by practicing surgeons.

d. An example of this shift can be seen in the case of *Canterbury v. Spence* (1972), which is often discussed in the context of a patient's right to make informed healthcare decisions. The *Canterbury* court ruled that a professional-oriented standard for measuring the legality of a physician's disclosure of information to a patient should be replaced by an objective standard predicated on what a reasonable patient would need to be told to effect the aforementioned right.

e. For example, see *Van Vector v. Blue Cross Ass'n* (1977).

f. For example, see *Gruenberg v. Aetna Insur. Co.* (1973).

g. Even citations to ERISA are complicated, because the law's section numbers in the U.S. Code (where much of ERISA can be found under Title 29) do not always correspond to the section numbering in the original act as written by Congress. For a helpful website effectively decoding where ERISA provisions are located in the U.S. Code, go to http://benefitslink.com/erisa/crossreference.html.

h. Note how this outcome can reasonably be viewed as incentivizing ERISA plans to arbitrarily deny patients' claims for healthcare coverage, because even in the event that plans are found to have acted negligently, they are responsible for paying only the cost of the denied benefit, but nothing more.

i. We are deeply grateful to professors Jane Thorpe and Elizabeth Gray, our colleagues in the Department of Health Policy and Management and experts in healthcare quality promotion, for the drafting of this section.

j. There is extensive literature on this topic. See, for example, Fisher, Goodman, Skinner, & Bronner, 2009; Fisher et al., 2003; McGlynn et al., 2003; Wennberg, 1996; Wennberg, Fisher, & Skinner, 2002.

k. Go to www.medicare.gov/hospitalcompare /search.html? to see the hospital comparisons, and to www.medicare.gov/ to access other Compare websites.

l. See, for example, Integrated Healthcare Association, n.d.; Kuhmerker & Hartman, 2007.

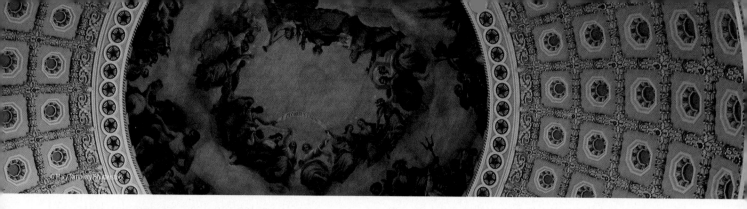

CHAPTER 13

Public Health Preparedness Policy

Rebecca Katz and Claire Standley

LEARNING OBJECTIVES

By the end of this chapter you will be able to:

- Describe what public health preparedness is and understand the scope of events that can lead to a public health emergency
- Understand the threats from and history of the use of weapons of mass destruction
- Define public health threats from biologic agents and naturally occurring diseases
- Describe key policies and laws that support public health preparedness and the infrastructure that has been built to support preparedness activities at the federal, state, and local levels

▶ Introduction

The last 15 years have seen many changes in terms of how the United States views homeland security and the role of the public health community in maintaining that security. There is an ever-evolving threat of the terrorist use of weapons of mass destruction (WMDs)—including the use of a biologic weapon—against the population. Infectious diseases continue to emerge and reemerge around the world, and the globalization of our food supply and the speed and volume of international travel make us all vulnerable to the emergence of a new agent anywhere in the world. Media reports include constant reminders of the devastating effects of natural disasters—such as hurricanes, fires, and earthquakes—and the lack of infrastructure and resources in many parts of the world leave many regions particularly vulnerable to natural disasters and epidemics.

All of these factors—and mounting evidence that large-scale catastrophes and epidemics can dramatically affect the economic, social, and security foundations of a nation—have led to the rapid emergence at the federal, state, and local levels of a new subdiscipline within public health: public health preparedness. Public health preparedness refers to the ways in which nations, states, and communities identify, prepare for, respond to, contain, and recover from emergencies. When this approach is applied around the world, it is often referred to as "global health security." It is imperative that public health students and professionals develop an awareness of the threats to population health and to the stability of societies, and the activities and frameworks developed to address these threats. Public health students must also be able to identify and work with other sectors with relevant responsibilities, as effective coordination among multiple sectors is essential to true public health preparedness.

The goal of this chapter is to introduce readers to the field of public health preparedness by providing an overview of the complex issues that must be considered by public health professionals in designing preparedness and response plans, policies, and laws. This chapter begins by defining public health preparedness and examining the types of threats that can lead to public health emergencies. It then describes possible policy responses to public health threats and emergencies, including a discussion of preparedness infrastructure, engagement, guidance documents, and some key pieces of U.S. legislation. The chapter closes by explaining the multitude of actors—from local to international—involved in public health preparedness and global health security.

▶ Defining Public Health Preparedness

Public health preparedness is a term that represents concerns and actions that have occurred throughout history. The term itself, however, and the field devoted to thinking about, preparing for, and mobilizing resources to respond to public health emergencies are relatively new.

The Association of Schools and Programs of Public Health (2012) defines public health preparedness as "a combination of comprehensive planning, infrastructure building, capacity building, communication, training, and evaluation that increase public health response effectiveness and efficiency in response to infectious disease outbreaks, bioterrorism, and emerging health threats." A group at the RAND Corporation, however, proposed a definition in 2007 that is a broader and better characterization of the field:

> Public health emergency preparedness . . . is the capability of the public health and health care systems, communities, and individuals, to prevent, protect against, quickly respond to, and recover from health emergencies, particularly those whose scale, timing, or unpredictability threatens to overwhelm routine capabilities. Preparedness involves a coordinated and continuous process of planning and implementation that relies on measuring performance and taking corrective action. (Nelson, Lurie, Wasserman, & Zakowski, 2007)

This definition raises the question, what exactly is a public health emergency? According to the RAND definition, it is an event "whose scale, timing, or unpredictability threatens to overwhelm routine capabilities." These types of events fit into four basic categories:

1. The intentional or accidental release of a chemical, biologic, radiologic, or nuclear (CBRN) agent
2. Natural epidemics or pandemics, which may involve a novel, emerging infectious disease, a reemerging agent, or a previously controlled disease, or that may occur in areas with limited infrastructure or resources
3. Natural disasters, such as hurricanes, earthquakes, floods, or fires
4. Man-made environmental disasters, such as large-scale oil spills

For any of these categories of events to be classified as a public health emergency, it is not just enough for the event to occur, but it also must pose a high probability of large-scale morbidity or mortality, or a risk of future harm.

According to the health policy organization Trust for America's Health, public health preparedness requires the basic functions of a public health system, such as epidemiology, laboratory capacity, and event-based surveillance capacity (Levi, Segal, Lieberman, May, & Laurent, 2014). These core functions need to be supplemented by specialized training, procedures, laws, regulations, and planning so that all relevant sectors can operate effectively and in a coordinated fashion during a crisis. Preparedness also requires the development of systems for surge capacity and distribution of medical countermeasures, with the goal of promptly detecting a crisis and managing a response to rapidly mitigate the consequences of the crisis and move toward recovery.

At the global level, the World Health Organization's (WHO's) Revised International Health Regulations, adopted in 2005, define a public health emergency of international concern as "an extraordinary event which is determined . . . to constitute a public health risk to other States through the international spread of disease and to potentially require a coordinated international response" (WHO, 2016). Such an emergency can involve any of the above four types of public health events, as long as it is unusual, is unexpected, and has the potential to cross international borders.

Some public health issues that have been called "emergencies" do not meet the criteria of any of the previous definitions. Public health preparedness refers to planning for and responding to acute events, as opposed to chronic conditions that evolve over time. The prevalence of breast cancer, for example, may be a "public health crisis," but it is not considered an emergency within the purview of public health preparedness (Harford, Azavedo, Fischietto, & Breast Health Global Initiative Healthcare Systems Panel, 2008).

Effective public health preparedness spans a wide range of activities. This chapter focuses primarily on the policy and legal actions to support preparedness, and application of the principals of emergency management to public health operations, but a "prepared community" also entails the ability to do the following (Nelson et al., 2007):

- Perform health risk assessments.
- Establish an incident command system or related structure.
- Actively engage and communicate effectively with the public.
- Have functional epidemiologic and laboratory capacity to perform surveillance, detect emerging events, and appropriately diagnose patients.
- Deploy rapid response teams to investigate outbreaks.
- Develop, stockpile, and distribute medical countermeasures (e.g., drugs and vaccines).
- Have "surge capacity" within the medical system to provide care for large populations during an emergency.
- Maintain appropriate workforces, financial resources, communication systems, and logistics to detect, respond to, and recover from events.

The responsibility of the public health community to prepare for and address acute health emergencies is thus extensive and can be a challenge, particularly in environments where the public health system is under-resourced.

▶ Threats to Public Health

As noted previously, there are four main categories of threats the public health community must be prepared to address. The first is the intentional or accidental release of a CBRN agent, followed by naturally occurring infectious diseases, natural disasters, and finally man-made environmental disasters with serious public health consequences. This section provides a brief overview of each of these threats.

CBRN Threats

The release of chemical, biologic, radiologic, or nuclear agents into a population center can have devastating consequences to the public's health. These agents may be released intentionally through an act of warfare or terrorism or unintentionally through human or mechanical error. For example, an explosion at a nuclear plant may not be intentional, yet it obviously can still expose workers or nearby populations to harmful radiation (Cerezo, 2011). An improperly disposed-of piece of medical equipment may be found by children, passed around a neighborhood, and result in multiple deaths from radiation sickness (WHO, 2007). A train carrying industrial chemical agents may derail, subjecting local communities to lethal doses of agents (Wenck et al., 2007). A laboratory worker may discover that a protocol intended to kill anthrax spores prior to transfer to a lower-level biosafety laboratory was not successful, potentially exposing dozens of staff to the agent (Centers for Disease Control and Prevention [CDC], 2014a). What leads a CBRN agent to be released into a population varies greatly, but the consequences of fear, disruption, sickness, and death result regardless. Public health preparedness plays an essential role in mitigating the consequences of CBRN events.

Chemical Threats

There is a wide variety of chemical agents and toxins capable of causing injury or death to humans, ranging from chemicals found in cleaning supplies purchased at a local drug store to carefully developed weapons designed to incapacitate and kill (**BOXES 13-2** and **13-3**). Toxins are nonliving poisons produced by living entities, such as plants, fungi, insects, and animals. Because they are chemical by-products of biologic agents, they occupy a conceptual gray area between chemical and biologic weapons, and countries do not always agree on how toxins should be categorized for the purposes of arms control and legal international obligations, although they are covered under the Biological and Toxin Weapons Convention. Chemical agents may be highly toxic and can enter the body through inhalation or through the skin. Adding to the complexity of treatment of a chemical agent injury is the fact that illness or death can come within minutes

---

BOX 13-2 Types of Chemical Agents

- **Nerve agents** primarily act on the nervous system, causing seizures and death. Examples of this category include sarin, VX, tabun, and soman. This category also includes fourth-generation chemical weapons, known as novichok agents, which are thought to be much more lethal than VX.
- **Blister agents or vesicants** primarily cause irritation of the skin and mucous membrane. Examples of this category include mustard gas and arsenical lewisite.
- **Choking agents or pulmonary toxicants** primarily cause damage to the lungs, including pulmonary edema and hemorrhage. Examples include phosgene, diphosgene, and chlorine.
- **Blood agents** primarily cause seizures and respiratory and cardiac failure in high doses. Examples include hydrogen cyanide and cyanogen cyanide.
- **Riot control agents** cause incapacitation due to irritation of eyes and respiratory system. Examples include CN, CS, PS, and CR.
- **Psychotomimetic agents**, in low doses, cause psychiatric effects. An example is lysergic acid diethylamide (LSD).
- **Toxins** cause symptoms that range from death to incapacitation, depending on the agent. Examples include ricin and saxitoxin.

Source: Ganesan et al. (2010).

BOX 13-3 Examples of Chemical Agents Impacting Public Health

Khan al-Assal Chemical Attack, Syria

On March 19, 2013, a rocket landed in the village of Khan al-Assal, in the Aleppo region of Syria. Upon impact, a gas was released, ultimately leading to over 20 fatalities and wounding many dozens more. Samples analyzed by both Russia and the United States identified the agent as sarin. The Syrian government and the opposition faction were quick to trade accusations of responsibility, and the Syrian government requested that the United Nations investigate the incident further. After lengthy delays due to a lack of access and disagreement over the scope of the investigation, a United Nations team finally arrived in August 2013, only to have their mandate quickly overshadowed by a second sarin attack at Ghouda. The team eventually concluded that the perpetrators "likely" had access to the Syrian military's chemical weapons stockpile but the "evidentiary threshold" for assigning responsibility was not met. At the time of the attack, Syria was not a signatory to the Chemical Weapons Convention. This example demonstrates the challenges of preparing for, responding to, and attributing responsibility for chemical incidents in the midst of a conflict situation.

Salisbury Novichok Poisonings, 2018

On March 4, 2018, Sergei Skripal, a former Russian military intelligence officer and double agent for the United Kingdom, and his daughter Yulia collapsed while sitting on a public bench in Salisbury, England. It was quickly determined by the local hospital that they had been poisoned by a toxic agent. Testing at the United Kingdom's Defence Science and Technology Laboratory at Porton Down identified the cause as a novichok nerve agent, a potent organophosphate believed to have been developed by the Soviet Union during the Cold War. This finding was further confirmed by the Organization for the Prohibition of Chemical Weapons. A police officer involved in the initial response on March 4 was also exposed and required hospitalization. All three victims eventually recovered fully. After trace elements of the agent were found at public sites visited by the Skripals earlier in the day, Public Health England was forced to reassure the public of the "very low risk" of exposure and restricted access to nine locations for decontamination. On April 13, the United Kingdom's National Security Advisor, Sir Mark Sedwill, stated the government's assertion that only Russia possessed the technical and operational means, as well as motive, to carry out the attack. On June 30, a British couple without known links to the Skripals fell ill at their house and were also determined to have been exposed to novichok. Police believed they had possibly handled a contaminated item, highlighting the challenges of controlling even a small, likely targeted, poisoning attack with a lethal nerve agent.

Sources: BBC (2018a, 2018b), Brunning (2018), Holmes and Solomon (2013), United Nations (2013), Vale, Mars, and Maynard (2018).

---

of exposure, or take as long as several hours (Ganesan, Raza, & Vijayaraghavan, 2010).

There are several main categories of chemical warfare agents: blister (e.g., mustard gas), blood (e.g., cyanide), choking (e.g., chlorine), and nerve (e.g., sarin).

Toxins are also a major category of agents, as are psychotomimetic agents, which can alter mental status. In addition, there is a class termed riot control agents, which produce temporary, usually nonfatal irritation of the skin, eyes, and respiratory tract. Riot control agents, often known as "tear gas," include chloroacetophenone (CN), chlorobenzylidenemalononitrile (CS), chloropicrin (PS), and dibenzoxazepine (CR). The Chemical Weapons Convention and the U.S. government do not consider this class of agents to be chemical weapons. Other nations, however, disagree (Hu et al., 1989).

The public health response to chemical events will range depending on the event itself, its origin, and the location. Possible activities may include the following (Melnikova, Wu, & Orr, 2015):

- Issuing shelter-in-place orders
- Evacuating populations
- Organizing decontamination efforts
- Restricting entry to particular areas
- Ensuring food and water are safe for consumption
- Monitoring both immediate and long-term health effects

Nuclear Threats

A nuclear weapon that involves fission (the splitting of atoms)—such as the bomb that the United States dropped on Hiroshima, Japan, during World War II, or the weapons created and stockpiled by a small number of nations since—leaves a limited role for the public health community. Such weapons, if released, would instantly destroy people, buildings, and anything else in the vicinity. There would be no need for a public health response, because the chances of survival would be minimal. The explosion, however, would leave behind large amounts of radioactivity, a threat to which we now turn.

Radiologic Threats

A radiologic event is an explosion or other release of radioactivity. Such an event might be caused by any of the following: a simple, nonexplosive radiologic device, an improvised nuclear device designed to release large amounts of radiation with a large blast radius (such as a "suitcase bomb"), a dispersal device that combines explosive materials and radioactive material (such as a "dirty bomb"), or damage to a nuclear reactor that results in the release of radiation (Durham, 2002).

Even a small dose of radiation can cause some detectable changes in blood. Large doses of radiation can lead to acute radiation syndrome (ARS). First signs of ARS are typically nausea, vomiting, headache, diarrhea, and some loss of white blood cells. These signs are followed by hair loss, damage to nerve cells and to cells that line the digestive tract, and severe loss of white blood cells. The higher the dose of radiation, the less likely the person will survive. Those who do survive may take several weeks to 2 years to recover,

and survivors may suffer from leukemia or other cancers (CDC, 2017).

The public health implications of radiologic exposure can be significant. In addition to all other functions, the public health community will be responsible for the following (CDC, 2014c):

- Participating in shelter-in-place or evacuation decisions
- Identifying exposed populations through surveillance activities
- Conducting or assisting with environmental decontamination
- Determining safety requirements for working in or near the site of the incident
- Conducting near- and long-term follow-up with exposed populations

Biologic Threats

Biologic warfare is the military use of a biologic agent to cause death or harm to humans, animals, or plants. In warfare, the targets of biologic agents are typically governments, armed forces, or resources that might affect the ability of a nation to attack or defend itself. Similarly, bioterrorism is the threat or use of a biologic agent to harm or kill humans, plants, or animals. Unlike biologic warfare, though, the target of bioterrorism is typically the civilian population or resources that might affect the civilian economy. Agroterrorism refers to the knowing or malicious use of biologic agents to affect the agricultural industry or food supply (Monke, 2004).

For a biologic agent to be an effective weapon, it should ideally (from the perpetrator's perspective) have high toxicity; be fast acting; be predictable in its impact; have a capacity for survival outside the host for enough time to infect a victim; be relatively indestructible by air, water, or food purification; and be susceptible to medical countermeasures available to the attacker, but not the intended victim(s). Of the many biologic agents that exist in nature (including parasites, fungi and yeasts, bacteria, *Rickettsia*, viruses, prions, and toxins), most effort is directed at a small group of bacteria, viruses, and toxins as the primary source of potential biologic weapons (**BOXES 13-4** and **13-5**).

BOX 13-4 Biologic Agents in Nature

Bacteria Free-living unicellular organisms
Viruses Core of DNA or RNA surrounded by a coat of protein; require host cell in order to replicate; much smaller than bacteria
Toxins Toxic substances produced by living organisms

BOX 13-5 Major Biologic Threat Agents

Anthrax (*Bacillus anthracis*)
Botulism (*Clostridium botulinum* toxin)
Brucellosis (*Brucella* species)
Food safety threats (e.g., *Salmonella* species, *Escherichia coli* O157:H7, *Shigella*)
Glanders (*Burkholderia mallei*)
Melioidosis (*Burkholderia pseudomallei*)
Plague (*Yersinia pestis*)
Psittacosis (*Chlamydia psittaci*)
Q fever (*Coxiella burnetii*)
Ricin toxin
Smallpox (*Variola major*)
Staphylococcal enterotoxin B
Tularemia (*Francisella tularensis*)
Typhoid fever (*Salmonella Typhi*)
Typhus fever (*Rickettsia prowazekii*)
Viral encephalitis (alphaviruses [e.g., Venezuelan equine encephalitis, eastern equine encephalitis, western equine encephalitis])
Viral hemorrhagic fevers (filoviruses [e.g., Ebola, Marburg] and arenaviruses [e.g., Lassa, Machupo])
Water safety threats (e.g., cholera [*Vibrio cholera*], *Cryptosporidium parvum*)
Emerging infectious diseases such as Zika virus, Nipah virus, and hantaviruses

Source: CDC (2018a).

There have been a series of attempts to classify and characterize biologic threat agents over the past 15 years. Here we present two of the major classifications, as well as a list of major biologic threats.

This first classification was used primarily by policy planners at the federal level between 2005 and 2010 (The White House, 2007). It looks at the spectrum of agents and defines them as follows:

- **Traditional:** These are naturally occurring microorganisms or toxins that have long been connected with bioterrorism or biologic warfare, either because they have been used in the past or they have been studied for use. There are a finite number of agents that are relatively well understood. The policy and public health community has devised specific plans to address the potential use of these agents. Examples include smallpox and anthrax.
- **Enhanced:** Enhanced agents are traditional biologic agents that have been altered to circumvent medical countermeasures. This group includes agents that are resistant to antibiotics.
- **Emerging:** This category includes any naturally occurring emerging organism or emerging

infectious disease. Examples include severe acute respiratory syndrome, H5N1, and novel H1N1.
- **Advanced:** The final category on the spectrum of biologic threats encompasses novel pathogens and other artificial agents that are engineered in laboratories. It is virtually impossible to plan for the specific threats posed by this category of agents, thus forcing policymakers to address biologic threats with a much broader strategic approach.

The second classification method for biologic threat agents is the Category A, B, and C list. This categorization originated with a 1999 CDC Strategic Planning Workgroup, which looked at the public health impacts of biologic agents, the potential of those agents to be effective weapons, public perception, and fear and preparedness requirements. The Workgroup also examined existing lists, including the Select Agent Rule list, the Australia Group list for export control, and the WHO list of biologic weapons (Elrod, 2011).

The resulting list begins with Category A, which includes the highest-priority pathogens with the perceived highest threat. They can cause large-scale morbidity and mortality and often require specific preparedness plans on the part of the public health community. Category B includes the second-highest threat group. Most of the agents in this category are waterborne or foodborne. These agents have been used intentionally in the past or were part of offensive research programs. The morbidity and mortality from these agents are not as significant as from Category A agents, but they are still considerable and they require enhanced surveillance and diagnostic capacity. The last group is Category C, which encompasses emerging pathogens or agents that have become resistant to medical countermeasures. These agents may cause high morbidity and mortality, and may be easily produced and transmitted (CDC, 2018a).

There is a long history of the intentional use of biologic agents. One regularly cited example derives from the 1346–1347 siege of the city of Kaffa (now Feodosija), Ukraine, by the Mongols. The Mongols reportedly catapulted corpses contaminated with plague over the walls of the city, causing an outbreak of *Yersinia pestis* (Wheelis, 2002). Another historical example comes from 1767, when British troops gave smallpox-infested blankets to Native Americans, which may have directly led to a massive outbreak of smallpox among this immunologically naïve population (Ranlet, 2000).

The most well-known bioterrorism event in the United States occurred in the fall of 2001, just weeks after the World Trade Center attacks. That event, eventually named "Amerithrax" by the Federal Bureau of

Investigation (FBI), targeted political figures and media outlets through the use of finely milled anthrax (*Bacillus anthracis*) that was sent through the mail. Twenty-two people became ill, and five died. Thousands of post office workers, congressional staff, and other potentially exposed individuals received prophylactic antibiotics and were offered vaccines.

The total disruption caused by what was, in the end, the equivalent of about a sugar packet amount of anthrax demonstrates how destructive and disruptive biologic weapons can be. In fact, they have been called "weapons of mass disruption." Vast infrastructure and funding came in response to the Amerithrax attack.

Public health preparedness against biologic weapons threats spans a wide range of activities. These activities include pre-event surveillance and detection, research and development of medical countermeasures, preparedness planning, and community engagement. Post-event, the public health community's responsibilities include mitigating the event's consequences through containment of the agent (using pharmaceutical and nonpharmaceutical interventions), delivering medical countermeasures in a timely manner, providing mass-casualty care, performing environmental decontamination, issuing messages to the public, and ensuring community resilience.

Naturally Occurring Disease Threats

Naturally occurring diseases can have both direct and indirect impacts on national security and require the same attention in terms of public health preparedness as CBRN agents (**BOX 13-6**). The direct impact of disease on national security arises from the potential proliferation or use of a biologic weapon, or the intentional spread of disease within specific populations. In addition, the impact of disease on the armed forces directly affects security because morbidity and mortality affect "readiness"—the ability of the nation to defend itself militarily and to engage in armed battles around the world. Until World War II, more soldiers died from infectious diseases than from direct combat injuries (Murray, Hinkle, & Yun, 2008). Disease altered the outcomes of conflicts and affected the balance of power among states. Even today, troop exposure to diseases affects morbidity and mortality, which then impacts overall military readiness. Hospital admissions from disease continue to outnumber injuries and wounds during U.S. military deployments. As a result, the military has invested significant resources in infectious disease research, building diagnostic laboratory capacity around the world, disease surveillance infrastructure, and vaccine development (Global Emerging Infections Surveillance, 2018; Murray et al.,

---

BOX 13-6 U.S. Biosafety Incidents in 2014

Over the summer of 2014, three significant biosafety incidents occurred involving U.S. government facilities. The first incident took place in early June at the Centers for Disease Control and Prevention's (CDC's) Roybal Campus in Atlanta. On June 5, a laboratory worker used an improper method to deactivate anthrax spores that were being transferred to several lower biocontainment laboratories on the same campus. The mistake was discovered over a week later, when culture plates left in the original laboratory showed signs of bacterial growth. Thirty-five staff and 67 visitors were considered at risk of exposure to anthrax as a result of the error.

The second incident also involved the CDC. On July 9, it was discovered that a sample of low-pathogenic avian influenza shipped to the U.S. Department of Agriculture from the CDC was contaminated with highly pathogenic H5N1. Because the sample was assumed to be of low risk, safety and security precautions required for shipping of select agents were not carried out. All handling of the sample at both institutions took place under BSL-3 conditions, minimizing the risk of accidental exposure. The contamination was determined to have taken place at the CDC influenza laboratory, and the discovery was made by the USDA on May 23. However, the incident was not reported for another 6 weeks.

The third incident occurred in mid-July, when several vials labeled as smallpox were discovered on the National Institutes of Health (NIH) campus in Bethesda, Maryland. The vials dated from the 1950s, when smallpox was still widespread, and are believed to have been part of a previous Food and Drug Administration (FDA) facility on the site. While some of the viral contents were shown to still be viable, the vials were well sealed and the risk of exposure was deemed to be very low.

While no casualties resulted from any of these incidents, they highlight the potential risks of accidental exposure to dangerous biologic agents as a result of poor bio-risk management practices. In January 2016 an expert review, commissioned by the CDC, found that while the agency had made some progress, "considerable work" remained to be done to achieve a culture of safety.

Sources: CDC (2014a, 2014b, 2014d), Kaiser (2014), Maron (2014), Sun (2014).

2008; Walter Reed Army Institute of Research, 2018; Writer, DeFraites, & Keep, 2000).

Indirectly, disease affects security because it can create large-scale morbidity and mortality, leading to massive loss of life and affecting all sectors of society. Such morbidity and mortality could result in economic loss and even long-term deterioration of economic viability. Fear of disease, in addition to disease itself, can lead to societal disruption, which can lead to civil disorder, political unrest, and, ultimately, destabilization. Chronic diseases, now the leading cause of morbidity and mortality around the world, already have a substantial global economic impact, with lower- and middle-income countries, already more vulnerable to financial shocks, increasingly heavily impacted (Abegunde, Mathers, Adam, Ortegon, & Strong, 2007).

Globalization; movement of people, animals, and goods; rapid urbanization; and changing human behaviors and land use all create opportunities for the emergence of infectious diseases. These diseases emerge from every corner of the world and, because of rapid transportation networks, can spread from international airports around the world in 24 to 48 hours. Pathogens with differing routes of exposure will spread at varying rates, but it has been estimated that a respiratory virus could spread globally and kill as many as 30 million people in a single year (Gates, 2018).

While disease can emerge anywhere and spread everywhere, it tends to adversely affect regions and countries that are least able to address the threat (WHO, 2007). Over the past four decades, there has been a fourfold increase in the number of emerging infectious diseases, and these diseases continue to emerge in all corners of the world (Doucleff & Greenhalgh, 2017; Fauci, 2017). Additionally, researchers have conducted "hot spot analyses" to identify conditions such as the presence of vectors, land use, and climate characteristics to identify where particular types of disease (like ones that are mosquito-borne) are likely to occur (Allen et al., 2017).

The regions where public health emergencies are most likely to emerge are the same regions experiencing critical shortages of healthcare personnel and that tend to have the least developed healthcare infrastructure (National Intelligence Council, 2008; WHO, 2007). On top of this problem, many of the current and developing megacities (cities with a population of 10 million people or more) can be found in the same regions that have poor healthcare infrastructure, understaffed healthcare workforces, and the most public health emergencies (National Intelligence Council, 2008). These conditions mean it is possible that a public health emergency will emerge in a place that is understaffed, under-resourced, and overpopulated—all conditions that may contribute to the spread of disease.

Public health preparedness for naturally occurring diseases must focus on basic scientific research

> **BOX 13-7** Discussion Question
>
> How can a naturally occurring disease event lead to a public health emergency? Describe how disease can impact national, regional, or international security.

to better understand the threats and work to design effective drugs, vaccines, and other therapeutics, and ensure the existence of sufficient production capacity for these tools. Effective, comprehensive, global surveillance systems are essential for early detection of disease to enable rapid response and containment efforts. Medical, community, and public sector coordination are necessary for distribution of countermeasures, surge capacity for mass care, mortuary services when necessary, and nonpharmaceutical interventions, including isolation and quarantine. Public health officials are also responsible for ensuring that a sufficient workforce is available to detect, report on, and respond to emergencies and to help bring about a recovery as quickly as possible.

Natural Disasters

It is an absolute certainty that natural disasters will occur all over the world: hurricanes will form, earthquakes will occur near fault lines, active volcanoes will erupt, tornadoes will sweep through regions, snow will fall, fire will spread, and low-lying regions will flood (**BOX 13-8**). Public health emergency preparedness is as much about planning for and responding to these types of disasters as it is about responding to terrorist events. In fact, the public health community is much more likely to engage in a response to a natural disaster than to an intentional or accidental one, based on probability of events.

Natural disasters have the potential to impact very large populations. They can lead to morbidity and mortality, disrupt basic services, pose environmental challenges, and completely unhinge a community. **TABLE 13-1** illustrates the magnitude, as measured in mortality, of major natural disasters.

Public health professionals have long been engaged in disaster response; as long as there have been emergencies, there have been medical personnel attending to the needs of populations. The CDC started responding officially to disasters in the 1960s, when an Epidemic Intelligence Service team traveled to Nigeria to help maintain public health programs in the midst of a civil war. Over the decades, the CDC has developed public health and epidemiologic tools to address the realities of disaster situations and

BOX 13-8 Recent U.S. Response to Hurricanes

Hurricane Katrina and the Public Health Response

On August 29, 2005, Hurricane Katrina landed on the Gulf Coast of the United States, reaching Mississippi, Louisiana, and Alabama. It came ashore with winds of 115 to 130 miles per hour and brought with it a water surge that in some locations rose as high as 27 feet. The surge pushed 6–12 miles inland and flooded approximately 80% of the city of New Orleans. Some 93,000 square miles were affected, resulting in 1,300 fatalities, 2 million displaced persons, 300,000 destroyed homes, and almost $100 billion in property damage.

Katrina was the worst domestic natural disaster in recent history, but the consequences of the event were made worse by a faltering levee system designed by the U.S. Army Corps of Engineers and a failure of government at all levels to properly prepare for and respond to the disaster. First, long-term warnings went unheeded. It was clear that a hurricane of this type would eventually hit the region, yet local and state officials, even after running exercises based on such a scenario, failed to properly prepare. Local and state officials were unable to evacuate all of the citizens, struggled with logistics, and did not make proper preparations for dealing with vulnerable populations, including nursing home residents. The federal government failed to adequately anticipate the needs of the state and local authorities, and the insufficient coordination resulted in a lack of resources and a too-slow response.

The public health and medical response coordinated by the federal government followed the traditional response to a flood or hurricane: focus on sanitation and hygiene, water safety, surveillance and infection control, environmental health, and access to care. Katrina, though, also presented unique challenges, such as the inability of displaced persons to manage chronic disease conditions and access medications, death and illness from dehydration, and mental health problems, all associated with the widespread devastation among those affected.

Almost all offices and branches of the federal Department of Health and Human Services (of which the CDC is a part) eventually became involved in the response to Katrina. The CDC sent staff to the affected areas, deployed the Strategic National Stockpile to provide drugs and medical supplies, and developed public health and occupational health guidance. The FDA issued recommendations for handling drugs that might have been affected by the flood. The NIH set up a phone-based medical consultation service for providers in the region. The Substance Abuse and Mental Health Services Administration set up crisis counseling assistance and provided emergency response grants.

In addition, the National Disaster Medical System deployed 50 Disaster Medical Assistance Teams to try to accommodate and treat hurricane victims. Disaster Mortuary Operational Response Teams also deployed to help process bodies. The Department of Defense set up field hospitals at the New Orleans International Airport and aboard naval vessels. The Department of Veterans Affairs evacuated both of its local hospitals—one prior to the storm, one afterward.

The 2017 Atlantic Hurricane Season: The Response to Hurricanes Harvey, Irma, and Maria

A combination of climatic conditions, including warmer-than-usual sea temperatures in the tropical Atlantic, led the 2017 Atlantic hurricane season to be the most devastating since 2005, and the fifth most active since recordkeeping began in the 1930s. In particular, three storms—Hurricanes Harvey, Irma, and Maria—had a substantial impact on the U.S. mainland and Puerto Rico. Along the Gulf Coast of Texas, Louisiana, and Florida, Hurricanes Harvey and Irma hit within 2 weeks of each other, causing an estimated $175 billion of damage. Ten days later, Hurricane Maria slammed directly into Puerto Rico, which had already been heavily impacted by Irma. The federal response was rapid, with President Trump immediately approving disaster declarations for all three storms.

However, there were significant differences between the impact of the three storms, as well as the federal responses. The Federal Emergency Management Agency (FEMA) already had supplies and personnel stationed in Texas before Hurricane Harvey made landfall, and leveraged existing memoranda of understanding with local and state authorities, as well as the National Guard, to coordinate response efforts closely. Local and federal responders had even previously trained together, under the $2 billion invested by FEMA in training of local authorities since 2005. Similarly, within 4 days of Hurricane Irma's landfall in Florida, FEMA had deployed more than 2,650 staff (out of a total of more than 40,000 federal response personnel) to support response efforts.

In contrast, the federal response to Hurricane Maria in Puerto Rico was criticized by the United Nations and other observers for being sluggish and inadequate. Already stretched thin by the Harvey and Irma responses, only 10,000 federal response personnel were initially deployed, many of whom were trainees or lacked previous response experience. Few supplies were in place ahead of time, and being an island, FEMA faced considerable logistical challenges in sending provisions, tarpaulins, and other key supplies to Puerto Rico, leading to major shortages of food and shelter, particularly as Maria had destroyed more than one-third of homes on the island. The Army Corps of Engineers, deployed to help repair homes destroyed by the hurricane, managed to put up just over 400 roofs in the month following the storm, whereas they had repaired more than 10 times that many in Florida in the same time frame after Irma. The hurricane also crippled Puerto Rico's electricity grid; as late as May 2018, over 100,000 residents were still without power, highlighting the slow recovery faced by the island.

Sources: Barron (2017), Einbinder (2018), Greenough and Kirsch (2005), Greshko (2017), Lister (2005), Philipps (2017), The White House (2006).

BOX 13-9 Discussion Questions

How did the public health community respond to Hurricane Katrina? What lessons can be learned to better prepare for future response efforts?

   To what extent did the response to the 2017 hurricane season reveal improvements to public health preparedness for natural disasters, versus gaps still remaining?

TABLE 13-1 Major Natural Disasters, 1900 to Present

Date	Event	Location	Approximate Death Toll
June–November, 2017	Hurricanes	Caribbean Basin	Up to 8,750
April 25, 2015	Earthquake	Gorkha, Nepal	9,000
March 11, 2011	Earthquake/tsunami	Tohoku, Japan	15,800–18,500
January 12, 2010	Earthquake	Port-au-Prince, Haiti	170,000–230,000
May 2, 2008	Cyclone	Myanmar	138,000
December 26, 2004	Tsunami (Indian Ocean)	Indonesia, Thailand, Sri Lanka, India, and more	220,000 (+)
July 28, 1976	Earthquake	Tangshan, China	242,000–655,000
November 13, 1970	Cyclone	Bangladesh	500,000
May–August 1931	Yellow River and Yangtze River floods	China	1–3.7 million
May 22, 1927	Earthquake	Xining, China	200,000
September 1, 1923	Earthquake and fires	Tokyo, Japan	143,000
December 16, 1920	Earthquake	Haiyuan, China	200,000

Sources: Associated Press (2010), CBC News (2010), Kishore et al., (2018), Noji (1997), Office of U.S. Foreign Disaster Assistance (1993), U.S. Geological Survey (2004).

displaced populations. The public health community enters a disaster situation and establishes prevention and control measures, collects critical data to support response, and works to meet the short- and long-term needs of the population (Gregg, 1989; Noji, 1997). Often, the most experienced public health and medical professionals on the ground during an emergency come from the nongovernmental organization (NGO) community, which has decades of experience responding to and helping populations recover from disasters. In fact, the American Red Cross, an NGO, has a federal charter to engage in disaster relief, and

has specific responsibilities outlined in the National Response Framework based on its recognized expertise in this area (Department of Homeland Security [DHS], 2013). In addition, military assets are used during emergencies to get qualified personnel to the event site quickly and, most importantly, provide logistical support, because some disasters require resources only the militaries of the world possess (e.g., the ability to reach isolated populations, bring supplies to remote regions, and establish care and living centers in harsh environments) (VanRooyen & Leaning, 2005; Wiharta, Ahman, Halne, Löfgren, & Randall, 2008).

Man-Made Environmental Disasters

The fourth category of public health emergencies is man-made environmental disasters. These are events where human intervention, accident, or other engagement leads to an environmental disaster with direct implications for population health (**BOX 13-10**). Long-term human conduct that degrades the environment could conceivably fall into this category, but for purposes of studying public health preparedness, the more important concern is with acute events, such as the 2010 oil spill disaster in the Gulf of Mexico, primarily affecting the Gulf Coast, which resulted from an explosion on an oil rig. This and similar disasters required the public health community to team with a variety of sectors at the local, state, and federal levels, understand the consequences to human health, and take actions to mitigate the consequences and address the health concerns of the community.

BOX 13-10 Fukushima Nuclear Disaster

The most serious radiation accidents have been associated with nuclear power plants. While the total number of accidents occurring at nuclear power plants is a matter of debate, at least 33 significant accidents are believed to have taken place since the 1950s. The most recent serious incident occurred at Fukushima Nuclear Power Plant in Japan, starting on March 11, 2011. The incident began when the facility was struck by a tsunami, itself caused by the magnitude 9.0 Tohoku earthquake. Seawater flooding the nuclear facility caused the plant's power (including backup generators) to fail. With no mechanism for continued cooling, the reactors began to heat up; eventually, three out of the facility's six nuclear reactors melted, resulting in a massive release of radioactive material, and the largest nuclear incident since Chernobyl in 1986. Investigations into the Fukushima disaster concluded the catastrophe must be considered "man-made": the findings of a 2008 tsunami risk assessment had been ignored by the facility's management; there was institutionalized "corruption, collusion, and nepotism" between the nuclear industry and regulatory authorities; and the Japanese government's eventual response to the disaster was thoroughly criticized for its poor crisis command, inadequate legal structure for nuclear crisis management, and lack of communication and transparency. While there were no immediate casualties from the incident, more than 100,000 people were evacuated from their homes and an estimated 1,000 died as a result of maintaining the evacuation. Concerns over the long-term impact of radiation exposure remain.

Sources: Kaufmann and Penciakova (2011), Secretariat of the Investigation Committee on the Accidents at the Fukushima Nuclear Power Station (2012), Tanter (2013), Wheatley, Sovacool, and Sornette (2017).

▶ Public Health Preparedness Policy

While government officials have long been aware of public health emergencies and the need for coordinated action to detect, report, and respond appropriately, the U.S. preparedness infrastructure did not truly take shape until after the attacks on U.S. soil on September 11, 2001 (commonly referred to as 9/11). Almost immediately after the World Trade Center, Pentagon, and subsequent anthrax letter attacks, the United States embarked on a series of changes that resulted in the most massive reorganization of the federal government since World War II. The first significant organizational change was announced on October 8, 2001, when Executive Order 12338 established both the federal Office of Homeland Security and the Homeland Security Council within the White House. This was followed by the Homeland Security Act of 2002, which created the Department of Homeland Security (DHS) by reorganizing multiple existing agencies under a single department and creating new responsibilities around homeland security and preparedness.

Within DHS, the main office created to address public health preparedness is the Office of Health Affairs. This office has several divisions. The Health Threats Resilience Division oversees biodefense activities, including Project BioWatch, the National Biosurveillance Integration Center, and state and local initiatives. The Workforce Health and Medical Support Division works to strengthen national medical emergency response capacity (DHS, n.d.). Importantly, FEMA, responsible for much of the emergency disaster response activities at the federal level, is also part of DHS.

In addition to the creation of DHS, in the wake of the 9/11 attacks, Congress passed new statutes and many existing government departments and agencies established new regulations, directives, and offices, expanded existing offices, and redirected resources toward preparedness and homeland security. The following agencies and offices are most directly linked to public health preparedness policy at the federal level.

Federal Response Agencies and Offices

Department of Health and Human Services (HHS)

HHS is the primary federal agency charged with ensuring the health of Americans. It comprises several offices that are key to U.S. health policy, public health, and healthcare provision.

Office of the Assistant Secretary for Preparedness and Response (ASPR). The Office of the Assistant Secretary for Preparedness and Response was created by the Pandemic and All-Hazards Preparedness Act of 2006 and replaced the office previously known as the Office of Public Health Emergency Preparedness. ASPR is composed of multiple components, including the Biomedical Advanced Research and Development Authority (BARDA), the Office of Emergency Management, and the Office of Policy and Planning (HHS, 2014). ASPR is responsible for leading the nation's "medical and public health preparedness for, response to, and recovery from disasters and public health emergencies" (HHS, 2018a). In addition to policy development, the office supports state and local capacity during emergencies by providing federal support. This support includes deployment of clinicians through the National Disaster Medical System. ASPR also hosts a series of preparedness programs, including the Hospital Preparedness Program (HHS, 2018b). As of July 2018, the Trump administration planned to transfer oversight of the Strategic National Stockpile to ASPR, with it having previously been managed by the CDC (Sun, 2018).

Centers for Disease Control and Prevention (CDC). The CDC has a vast array of offices and subject-matter expertise that would be used during a public health emergency. Many of the preparedness and response activities are consolidated in the Office of Public Health Preparedness and Response. This office coordinates and responds to public health threats through a multitude of programs, including an emergency operations division that constantly maintains situational awareness of potential threats; a division dedicated to supporting preparedness at the state, local, tribal, and territorial level through cooperative agreements providing funding to state and local entities for preparedness for all-hazard threats; and a division devoted to regulating the federal Select Agent program (CDC, 2018b).

National Institutes of Health (NIH). The NIH is engaged in public health preparedness through a variety of offices. The Office of Science Policy houses the National Science Advisory Board for Biosecurity, which is a committee of experts focused on advancing biotechnology. The National Institute of Allergy and Infectious Diseases hosts a robust research agenda, both intramural and in support of extramural programs, that supports the research and development of medical countermeasures against radiologic, nuclear, and chemical threats, and supports biodefense

activities (NIH, 2015). Additionally, divisions across NIH support research programs that might focus on special-population or clinical outcomes from public health emergencies, such as mental health, children's health, or disease mapping for preparedness.

The Food and Drug Administration (FDA). The FDA has multiple offices that focus on emergency preparedness and response. These offices are responsible for ensuring regulatory oversight, monitoring infrastructure, and facilitating the delivery of appropriate countermeasures. Specifically, the Office of Crisis Management coordinates emergency and crisis response, as related to FDA-regulated products. The Center for Biologics Evaluation and Research oversees safety and effectiveness of biologic products, including CBRN medical countermeasures. The Office of Counterterrorism and Emerging Threats works on policies, strategies, and interagency communication relating to counterterrorism. It also oversees Emergency Use Authorization for medical countermeasures (FDA, 2018a).

Department of Agriculture (USDA)

The Animal and Plant Health Inspection Service (APHIS) at USDA has a broad mission to protect and promote U.S. agricultural health. APHIS also works with DHS and FEMA to provide assistance and coordination during emergencies. This assistance ranges from containing disease in poultry, such as in cases of avian influenza, to protecting the health of livestock and crops from foreign disease. The Agricultural Research Service provides research support that can be essential during an emergency (USDA, n.d.).

Federal Bureau of Investigation (FBI)

The FBI, which operates under the Department of Justice, created a new WMD Directorate in 2006. This Directorate works in several areas, including countermeasures and preparedness, investigations and operations, and intelligence analysis. The investigative component directs the WMD threat credibility assessments and manages all WMD criminal investigations. On preparedness, the FBI works with field components, as well as with other agencies. In particular, the FBI works closely with the CDC using the "Crim-Epi" model, in which law enforcement and epidemiologists cooperate in the investigation of potential WMD events in a way that enables the FBI to collect information that will lead to a prosecution, but that also enables epidemiologists to investigate, treat, and minimize morbidity and mortality (FBI, n.d.).

Department of Defense (DoD)

The DoD has a massive infrastructure designed to address threats of any nature, including public health emergencies. The military is trained in emergency response and preparedness as critical components of an effective armed forces. While most DoD programs focus on protecting the war fighter, several also have implications for the broader civilian population. There is an active chemical and biologic defense program that involves research, development, and testing defense systems and equipment, including medical countermeasures. The Cooperative Threat Reduction programs work to reduce the threat of WMDs around the world, while building global capacity for detection and response to biologic threats. There is a large-scale laboratory network both in the United States and abroad engaged in basic scientific research for infectious diseases, as well as epidemiologic response to public health emergencies. There is also a robust surveillance and response program for naturally occurring diseases (Sandor, 2011).

Preparedness Statutes, Regulations, and Policy Guidance

Statutes, regulations, and policy guidance documents form the foundation of public health preparedness. In the always-evolving, operations-based field of public health preparedness, the legal and regulatory framework creates the baseline from which all policymaking, planning, and action is taken. As this is a relatively new discipline, the statutes, regulations, and policy guidance are also relatively new, changing to meet evolving threats, incorporating lessons from previous experiences, and adapting to feedback from those directly involved with implementing the relevant policies and laws. The following is a brief description of the key laws (both statutory and regulatory) and policy documents that currently guide preparedness efforts.

Public Health Improvement Act of 2000 (Public Law 106-505)

The Public Health Improvement Act of 2000 has 10 titles, or sections, 9 of which address traditional public health interests such as sexually transmitted diseases, Alzheimer disease research, organ donation, clinical research, and laboratory infrastructure. Title 1, however, addresses emerging threats to the public's health. This section authorizes the Secretary of HHS to take appropriate response actions during a public health emergency, including investigations, treatment, and prevention. The act established the Public Health

Emergency Fund to support response activities and directed the HHS Secretary to establish a working group to focus on the medical and public health effects of a bioterrorist attack.

USA PATRIOT Act of 2001 (Public Law 107-56)

The Uniting and Strengthening America by Providing Appropriate Tools Required to Intercept and Obstruct Terrorism (USA PATRIOT) Act was passed by Congress and signed into law in October 2001 immediately following the 9/11 attacks, and during the height of the anthrax letters scare. This law includes a multitude of terrorism-related policies. Among them are provisions related to acquiring, handling, and transporting particularly dangerous pathogens; assistance to first responders; and funding for substantial new investments in bioterrorism preparedness and response.

Public Health Security and Bioterrorism Preparedness and Response Act of 2002 (Public Law 107-188)

Signed into law in June 2002, the Bioterrorism Act (as it is known) was the first major piece of legislation dedicated entirely to public health preparedness. The act has five titles:

1. **National Preparedness for Bioterrorism and Other Public Health Emergencies:** Addresses national preparedness and response planning by calling for the development and maintenance of medical countermeasures, creation of a national disaster medical system, support for communications and surveillance among all levels of public health officials, creation of a core academic curriculum concerning bioweapons and other public health emergencies, improvements to hospital preparedness, and measures to address workforce shortages for public health emergencies. Also codifies what had already been established—a strategic national stockpile of medical countermeasures.
2. **Enhancing Controls on Dangerous Biological Agents and Toxins:** Addresses the control over select agents.
3. **Protecting Safety and Security of Food and Drug Supply:** Addresses bioterrorist threats to the food supply, and what the FDA is permitted to do to address this threat. It also touches on the importance of

ensuring the safety of drugs imported into the United States.

4. **Drinking Water Security and Safety:** Directs communities to do a full assessment of the vulnerabilities of the water supply to terrorist attacks.

5. **Additional Provisions:** Addresses miscellaneous provisions, including some focused on prescription drug user fees and Medicare plans.

Smallpox Emergency Personnel Protection Act of 2003 (Public Law 108-20)

In December 2002, the Bush administration announced a program to vaccinate both military personnel and civilian emergency health workers against smallpox. The vaccine program for the military was obligatory, while the civilian vaccination program was voluntary. The Smallpox Emergency Personnel Protection Act, which became law nearly 3 months after the vaccination program started, focuses on compensation related to medical care, lost income, or death resulting from receipt of the smallpox vaccine.

The Project Bioshield Act of 2004 (Public Law 108-276)

While the Bioterrorism Act of 2002 codified into law the requirement for a Strategic National Stockpile, there remained in practice a problem: because of the vast costs involved with producing and no guaranteed market in which to sell CBRN medical countermeasures (drugs and vaccines), pharmaceutical companies were reluctant to develop and bring to market these countermeasures. As a result, the National Stockpile remained under-resourced. The Bioshield Act of 2004 aimed to create a guaranteed government-funded market for medical countermeasures, and included funding to purchase the products while they are still in the final stages of development. The act also allowed HHS to expedite spending to procure products, hire experts, and award research grants pertaining to CBRN, and to allow for emergency use of countermeasures even if they lacked final FDA approval. However, most of the funds were used to target only three pathogens—anthrax, smallpox, and botulism—which led some to criticize the Obama administration for diverting funds that could have been used to develop therapeutics against other biologic agents, such as the Ebola virus. (For more about this act, see Box 13-13 at the end of the chapter.)

Public Readiness and Emergency Preparedness Act of 2005 (Division C of the Department of Defense Emergency Supplemental Appropriations; Public Law 109-148)

Because the Project Bioshield Act allowed the Secretary of HHS to force the use of medical countermeasures for emergency purposes without final FDA approval, manufacturers, distributors, program administrators, prescribers, and dispensers expressed concern to policymakers that they could be held liable for any negative consequences associated with the use of unapproved countermeasures. In response, Congress and the Bush administration passed the Public Readiness and Emergency Preparedness Act (PREP Act), which limits liability associated with public health countermeasures used on an emergency basis. The only exception is in the event of "willful misconduct."

Pandemic and All-Hazards Preparedness Act of 2006 (Public Law 109-417)

The Pandemic and All-Hazards Preparedness Act, known as PAHPA, reauthorized the Bioterrorism Act of 2002 and added broad provisions aimed at preparing for and responding to public health and medical emergencies, regardless of origin. PAHPA is organized into the following four main titles:

1. **National Preparedness and Response, Leadership, Organization, and Planning:** This title makes the HHS Secretary the lead person for all public health and medical responses to emergencies covered by the National Response Framework (the act actually refers to the National Response Plan, which was later updated and renamed the National Response Framework). It also established the position of Assistant Secretary for Preparedness and Response at HHS and required HHS to create a National Health Security Strategy.

2. **Public Health Security Preparedness:** This section of the act focuses on developing preparedness infrastructure, primarily at the state and local level, to include pandemic plans, interoperable networks for data sharing, and telehealth capabilities. It also addresses laboratory security and the need to ensure readiness of the Commissioned Corps of the Public Health Service to respond to public health emergencies.

3. **All-Hazards Medical Surge Capacity:** This title has several key provisions, including the transfer of the National Disaster Medical System (NDMS) back to HHS from DHS. Thus, HHS is responsible for evaluating capacity for a medical patient surge during a public health emergency and is required to establish a Medical Reserve Corps of volunteers to assist during such emergencies. Title III also requires HHS to develop public health preparedness curricula and establish centers for preparedness at schools of public health.

4. **Pandemic and Biodefense Vaccine and Drug Development:** The final title of PAHPA builds on the Bioshield Act of 2004 by requiring the establishment of BARDA within HHS to coordinate countermeasure research and development. Although the Bioshield Act enticed manufacturers to develop countermeasures, it did not do enough to assist companies during the expensive years of product research and development. Through payment structure reform, Title IV permits BARDA to better enable countermeasure development and production.

Pandemic and All-Hazards Preparedness Reauthorization Act of 2013 (Public Law 113-5)

The PAHPA was reauthorized in 2013 as the Pandemic and All-Hazards Preparedness Reauthorization Act (PAHPRA). PAHPRA is organized into the following four main titles:

1. Strengthening National Preparedness and Response for Public Health Emergencies
2. Optimizing State and Local All-Hazards Preparedness and Response
3. Enhancing Medical Countermeasures Review
4. Accelerating Medical Countermeasure Advanced Research and Development

At the time of this writing, a bill has been introduced to reauthorize PAHPA until 2023, but has not yet been passed into law.

Implementing Recommendations of the 9/11 Commission Act of 2007 (Public Law 110-53)

In August 2007, Congress passed the Implementing Recommendations of the 9/11 Commission Act,

which, as the title suggests, focuses on implementing the recommendations from the 9/11 Commission Report. The act includes numerous specific provisions pertaining to preparedness, such as preparedness grants to state and local entities, improving the incident command system, improving the sharing of intelligence information across the federal government, enhancing efforts to prevent terrorists from gaining entry into the United States, increasing the safety of transportation, and improving generally the preparedness infrastructure. It also includes sections on diplomatic engagement and advancing democratic values abroad. Specific to public health, Title XI of the act addresses enhanced defenses against WMDs, particularly the need to maintain a National Biosurveillance Integration Center that reports to Congress on the "state of … biosurveillance efforts."

National Defense Authorization Act of Fiscal Year 2017 (Public Law 114-328)

In December 2016, Congress passed the National Defense Authorization Act for Fiscal Year 2017. Title X of the act (subtitle G, section 1086) calls for the Secretaries of Defense, HHS, DHS, and USDA to jointly develop a national biodefense strategy and an associated implementation plan, including a review of all biodefense policies, practices, programs, and initiatives. The strategy was to be submitted to Congress no later than 275 days after December 23, 2016, and then revised biennially. As of this writing, the biodefense strategy has been drafted, but not yet submitted to Congress.

Presidential Directives

Biodefense for the 21st Century: National Security Presidential Directive 33/ Homeland Security Presidential Directive 10, April 2004

In 2004 the Bush administration released Homeland Security Presidential Directive (HSPD) 10, which provided a strategic overview of the biologic weapons

> **BOX 13-11** Discussion Questions
>
> The PAHPRA of 2013 included changes to each of the four main titles of the previous PAHPA law. Looking back at PAHPA (2006), how significant do you think these changes were, and what might have been the rationale behind the revisions? How does this act compare to the current reauthorization?

threat and the administration's approach to framing biodefense initiatives. The directive described four essential pillars of the national biodefense program: threat awareness, prevention and protection, surveillance and detection, and response and recovery. This document remained the primary policy directive concerning biodefense until the National Strategy for Countering Biological Threats was released in late 2009.

Public Health and Medical Preparedness: Homeland Security Presidential Directive 21, October 2007

Building upon HSPD 10, and in accordance with HSPD 18 (released early in 2007, it pertained to the development of medical countermeasures, led by HHS but with DoD retaining control over development specific to the armed forces), HSPD 21 was released in the fall of 2007 and defines four critical components of public health and medical preparedness. The four components are a robust and integrated biosurveillance system, the ability to stockpile and distribute medical countermeasures, the capacity to engage in mass-casualty care in emergency situations, and resilient communities at the state and local levels. The directive also mandates the creation of task forces, studies, and plans to meet public health and medical preparedness needs.

Establishing Federal Capability for the Timely Provision of Medical Countermeasures Following a Biological Attack, Executive Order 13527, December 2009

In the last days of 2009, President Obama released Executive Order 13527, establishing a policy of timely provision of medical countermeasures in the event of a biologic attack and tasking the federal government with assisting state and local entities in this endeavor. The order also spells out the role of the U.S. Postal Service in the delivery of medical countermeasures and calls on HHS to develop continuity of operations plans in the event of a large-scale biologic attack.

National Strategy for Countering Biological Threats, Presidential Policy Directive 2, November 2009

The National Strategy for Countering Biological Threats was released in time for Undersecretary of State Ellen Tauscher to share it with the international community at the December 2009 Meeting of States Parties of the Biological Weapons Convention. The strategy, the first major policy statement by the Obama administration on the topic of biologic threats, spells out seven major objectives:

- **Promote** global health security.
- **Reinforce** norms of safe and responsible conduct.
- **Obtain** timely and accurate insight on current and emerging risks.
- **Take** reasonable steps to reduce the potential for exploitation.
- **Expand** our capability to prevent, attribute, and apprehend.
- **Communicate** effectively with all stakeholders.
- **Transform** the international dialogue on biologic threats.

While many of the Bush administration directives focused on policies for responding to a biologic threat, the Obama strategy directive placed more emphasis on prevention, with particular stress on the importance of working with international partners, reinforcing norms of responsible scientific conduct, and engaging scientists so that they can continue beneficial work in the life sciences (National Security Council, 2009).

National Preparedness Presidential Policy Directive 8, March 2011

In early 2011, the Obama administration released Presidential Policy Directive (PPD) 8, replacing HSPD 8. The PPD required the development of a national preparedness goal (as did HSPD 8) and the creation of a National Preparedness System to integrate guidance, programs, and processes to build and sustain capabilities essential for preparedness. PPD 8 takes an "all-of-nation" approach, identifying the importance of collaboration between governments at all levels and the private and not-for-profit sectors as well as the public in order to enhance resilience.

International Agreements

In addition to domestic statutes, regulations, and formal policy guidance documents, there are a host of formal international agreements that attempt to coordinate global efforts to respond to the threats posed to populations by WMDs and infectious diseases. These international agreements include a series of arms control treaties, including the Geneva Protocol, the Biological and Toxin Weapons Convention, the Chemical Weapons Convention, and the Nuclear Nonproliferation Treaty. In addition, United Nations Security Council Resolution 1540 obligates Member States of the United Nations (including the United States) to ensure they do not support nonstate actors in their efforts to develop, acquire, possess, or use nuclear, chemical, or biologic weapons.

As mentioned previously, the WHO's World Health Assembly adopted the International Health Regulations in 2005. This agreement recognizes the threat of emerging infectious diseases, the globalization of society, and the need for improved surveillance, response, communication, and coordination to effectively detect and respond to public health threats. A primary purpose of the regulations is to improve global health security through international collaboration and communication by detecting and containing public health emergencies at the source.

Explicitly linking public health objectives with the security implications of international disease threats, the Global Health Security Agenda (GHSA) was launched in 2014 as an effort to elevate and accelerate progress toward a world free from infectious disease threats. While focused on preventing, detecting, and responding to epidemics—rather than all public health emergencies—the GHSA encourages the development of many of the same preparedness and response capacities that would be needed to address any manner of

public health hazard. Depending on the type of public health emergency, there are a range of global actors that become involved to aid, augment, or help govern national response efforts. These actors range from Interpol, to WHO, to the Food and Agriculture Organization, to organizations connected to arms control efforts, such as the Organization for the Prohibition of Chemical Weapons and the International Association for Atomic Energy. In addition, there are networks of laboratories, regional cooperation organizations, and a vast conglomeration of nongovernmental organizations that may become involved in the detection of, response to, and recovery from global public health emergencies.

BOX 13-12 Discussion Questions

Describe the federal preparedness infrastructure that evolved after 9/11. Are there things about the departments, agencies, and offices that to you represent improvements over the pre-9/11 infrastructure? Are there aspects that seem redundant or misplaced?

BOX 13-13 Policy Case Study: Domestic Response to the 2014–2016 Ebola Outbreak

Several of the federal preparedness laws and regulations of the early 2000s focused on the need to develop and stockpile a ready supply of medical countermeasures to be deployed in the event of a public health emergency. However, many pathogens of concern are relatively rare, or occur endemically only in lower-income or resource-constrained countries. As such, there was reluctance from the pharmaceutical and drug manufacturing industries to commit significant research and development dollars to products that might not have a commercially viable market. The Project Bioshield Act of 2004 sought to change that by establishing a government-funded market for such countermeasures, and thus incentivize the development of vaccines and therapeutics that would not otherwise be cost-effective. Subsequent legislation changed how the development of medical countermeasures were funded to better incentivize private sector companies to remain committed and financially viable during the lengthy process between initial development of a product and final approval by the FDA.

Given the length of time required for a product to come to market, the Project Bioshield Act also allowed for HHS to authorize the emergency use of countermeasures even if they had not yet been approved by the FDA. Of course, FDA approval processes are critical for determining safety and efficacy, so the concern was raised about liability in the event that a non-FDA-approved countermeasure, used for a legitimate public health emergency, produced a severe side effect or failed as a treatment. Manufacturers feared that liability in these situations would fall on them, leading to a reticence to even engage in the development of the product. In response, Congress passed the PREP Act, which provides immunity from liability for any claims resulting from the use of a medical countermeasure approved for use during a public health emergency. There have been eight PREP Act Declarations since its inception, addressing countermeasures for smallpox, pandemic influenza, botulinum toxin, and anthrax, as well as for nonbiologic threats such as radiation.

Starting in late 2013, erupting in 2014, and continuing into 2015 and 2016, Ebola virus disease spread through Guinea, Sierra Leone, and Liberia, infecting and killing thousands more people than any previous Ebola outbreak. The virus spread to countries outside of West Africa, including the United States, through global travel and the return of infected medical volunteers. The scale of the outbreak prompted several pharmaceutical companies to accelerate research and development of Ebola vaccines and therapeutics; despite such products being incentivized under the

(continues)

Project Bioshield Act, virtually no companies had focused on Ebola virus, and few countermeasures were at an advanced stage of testing. There was tremendous public fear and pressure mounted on public health and medical officials to ensure that U.S. patients with Ebola were given every available treatment, even if experimental. In August 2014, the media widely reported on the remarkable recovery of two American Ebola patients in Liberia, who had been given doses of an experimental drug called ZMapp. It is not clear if and what liability protections were waived for the initial use of this and other experimental Ebola therapeutics on U.S. patients, though the provision of these treatments were sanctioned under the auspices of the FDA's "compassionate use exemption" whereby a patient may receive unapproved treatment outside of already-approved clinical trials. However, HHS subsequently issued a PREP Act declaration providing immunity from liability for the manufacturing, administration, and use of Ebola-related vaccines, including several Ebola vaccines under development, and later issued a declaration for therapeutics such as ZMapp.

This example demonstrates the importance of establishing a legal framework for preparedness to ensure the appropriate and timely use of medical countermeasures in the event of a public health emergency. Having a process in place to protect manufacturers allowed them to move forward with getting potentially lifesaving products to a frightened, at-risk population.

Sources: FDA (2018b), HHS (2017), Health Resources and Services Administration (2017), Kadlec (2013), Monahan and Halabi (2015).

▶ Conclusion

The United States has made great strides in public health preparedness in the past decade. This success was due in no small part to a massive influx of funding to support federal, state, and local entities in building capacity, planning, and response efforts. Between 2003 and 2007, DHS alone awarded over $27 billion in preparedness grants to state and local governments, although this represents only a small fraction of total state and local preparedness expenditures (Schnirring, 2011).

However, budgets steadily decreased from highs in 2002–2003, and after the financial crisis of 2008, preparedness budgets were reduced further as the nation and its individual states grappled with debt, deficits, and reduced revenues (Murthy, Molinari, LeBlanc, Vagi, & Avchen, 2017; Watson, Watson, & Sell, 2017). For example, funding for CDC's domestic Centers for Public Health Preparedness program dropped from an average of over $25 million per year between 2004 and 2007 to less than $15 million for 2008 and 2009 (Richmond, Hostler, Leeman, & King, 2010). Reduced funding means that policymakers and program managers have to make difficult decisions about how best to allocate and plan for preparedness activities in a resource-constrained environment. High-profile public health incidents, including the 2009 H1N1 pandemic, the handful of Ebola cases identified in 2014, and the identification of domestic transmission of Zika virus during the 2015–2016 global outbreak have thus far resulted in only one-off appropriations of funding, rather than substantial long-term investments. Yet even these allocations may prove transient. In fiscal year 2015, the CDC received $1.77 billion earmarked for Ebola preparedness and response, including more than $500 million for domestic preparedness and response activities (CDC, 2015); in 2016, however, facing congressional deadlock over allocation of new funds to fight the emerging Zika epidemic, the Obama administration diverted over $500 million of Ebola funds toward Zika research, prevention, and control efforts (McNeil, 2016).

Assuming sufficient funding, there are several areas of public health preparedness that should be targeted for further development, both domestically and internationally. These include the following:

- **Comprehensive disease surveillance:** The development of a fully integrated, national disease surveillance system capable of early detection of events should be supported. This may involve integration of electronic health records and exploration of other information and technology opportunities.
- **Workforce:** The public health workforce, particularly epidemiologists and laboratory workers, and encompassing both human and animal health, must be developed and sustained.
- **Resilience and community planning:** The public health community must continue to engage community members and work with local entities to develop recovery and resilience plans.
- **Countermeasures:** Continued investment must be made in the basic research and development of medical countermeasures, as well as in exploring ways to store and disperse such countermeasures during a public health emergency.

- **Chemical and radiologic preparedness:** Public health professionals must continue to conduct research and better understand chemical and radiologic threats to further develop plans to address such events.
- **Public and private partnerships:** Local, state, and federal entities must continue to explore partnerships with the private sector to enhance preparedness efforts, improve coordination, and decrease costs.

Finally, the public health community must continue to develop opportunities and curricula to train the next generation of public health professionals.

BOX 13-14 Discussion Question

What are the distinct roles of local, state, federal, and international governments and organizations in managing a public health emergency of international concern?

Understanding threats; planning effectively to detect, respond to, and recover from emergencies; and appropriately engaging with counterparts across communities, governments, and nations are essential to future public health practice and policy.

References

Abegunde, D. O., Mathers, C. D., Adam, T., Ortegon, M., & Strong, K. (2007). The burden and costs of chronic diseases in low-income and middle-income countries. *The Lancet, 370*(9603), 1929–1938. https://doi.org/10.1016/S0140-6736(07)61696-1

Allen, T., Murray, K. A., Zambrana-Torrelio, C., Morse, S. S., Rondinini, C., Di Marco, M., . . . Daszak, P. (2017). Global hotspots and correlates of emerging zoonotic diseases. *Nature Communications, 8*(1), 1124. https://doi.org/10.1038/s41467-017-00923-8

Associated Press. (2010, February 11). Haiti earthquake: Conflicting death tolls lead to confusion. Retrieved from https://www.theguardian.com/world/2010/feb/11/haiti-earthquake-conflicting-death-tolls

Association of Schools and Programs of Public Health. (2012). *Practical Implications, Approaches, Opportunities and Challenges of a Preparedness Core Curricula in Accredited Schools of Public Health.* Washington, DC: Author.

Barron, L. (2017). U.S. emergency response efforts in Puerto Rico aren't good enough, U.N. experts say. *Time.* Retrieved from http://time.com/5003470/united-nations-puerto-rico-hurricane-response/

British Broadcasting Corporation. (2018a, August 2). Amesbury Novichok poisoning: What we know so far. *BBC News.* Retrieved from https://www.bbc.com/news/uk-44721558

British Broadcasting Corporation. (2018b, April 20). Skripal poisoning: Salisbury toxic hotspots clean-up begins. *BBC News.* Retrieved from https://www.bbc.com/news/uk-43833582

Brunning, A. (2018). What we do (and don't) know about novichok agents. *American Scientist, 106*(3), 139. https://doi.org/10.1511/2018.106.3.139

CBC News. (2010). The world's worst natural disasters. Retrieved from https://www.cbc.ca/news/world/the-world-s-worst-natural-disasters-1.743208

Centers for Disease Control and Prevention. (2014a). *CDC lab incident: anthrax, June 2014.* Retrieved from https://www.cdc.gov/anthrax/news-multimedia/lab-incident/index.html

Centers for Disease Control and Prevention. (2014b). *CDC media statement on newly discovered smallpox specimens.* Retrieved from https://www.cdc.gov/media/releases/2014/s0708-NIH.html

Centers for Disease Control and Prevention. (2014c). *Radiation emergencies: Information for public health professionals.* Retrieved from https://emergency.cdc.gov/radiation/publichealth.asp

Centers for Disease Control and Prevention. (2014d). Report on the potential exposure to anthrax Centers for Disease Control and Prevention. *International Microbiology, 17*(2), 119–127.

Centers for Disease Control and Prevention. (2015). *FY 2015–2019 Ebola response funding.* Retrieved from https://www.cdc.gov/budget/ebola/index.html

Centers for Disease Control and Prevention. (2017). *Acute radiation syndrome: A fact sheet for physicians.* Retrieved from https://emergency.cdc.gov/radiation/arsphysicianfactsheet.asp

Centers for Disease Control and Prevention. (2018a). *Bioterrorism agents/diseases, A–Z.* Retrieved from https://emergency.cdc.gov/agent/agentlist.asp

Centers for Disease Control and Prevention. (2018b). *Office of Public Health Preparedness and Response.* Retrieved from https://www.cdc.gov/phpr/index.htm

Cerezo, L. (2011). Radiation accidents and incidents. What do we know about the medical management of acute radiation syndrome? *Reports of Practical Oncology and Radiotherapy: Journal of Greatpoland Cancer Center in Poznan and Polish Society of Radiation Oncology, 16*(4), 119–122. https://doi.org/10.1016/j.rpor.2011.06.002

Department of Health and Human Services. (2014). *ASPR organization chart.* Retrieved from https://www.hhs.gov/about/agencies/orgchart/aspr/index.html

Department of Health and Human Services. (2017). *HHS accelerates development of first Ebola vaccines and drugs.* Retrieved from https://www.hhs.gov/about/news/2017/09/29/hhs-accelerates-development-first-ebola-vaccines-and-drugs.html

Department of Health and Human Services. (2018a). *HHS Office of the Assistant Secretary for Preparedness and Response.* Retrieved from https://www.phe.gov/about/aspr/Pages/default.aspx

Department of Health and Human Services. (2018b). *Hospital Preparedness Program (HPP).* Retrieved from https://www.phe.gov/Preparedness/planning/hpp/Pages/default.aspx

Department of Homeland Security. (n.d.). *Workforce Health and Medical Support Division.* Retrieved from https://www.dhs.gov/workforce-health-and-medical-support-division

Department of Homeland Security. (2013). *National Response Framework, Second Edition.* Retrieved from https://www.fema.gov/media-library-data/20130726-1914-25045-1246/final_national_response_framework_20130501.pdf

Doucleff, M., & Greenhalgh, J. (2017, February 14). Why killer viruses are on the rise. *National Public Radio*. Retrieved from https://www.npr.org/sections/goatsandsoda/2017/02/14/511227050/why-killer-viruses-are-on-the-rise

Durham, B. (2002). The background and history of manmade disasters. *Advanced Emergency Nursing Journal, 24*(2), 1–14.

Einbinder, N. (2018, May 1). How the response to Hurricane Maria compared to Harvey and Irma. *Frontline*. Retrieved from https://www.pbs.org/wgbh/frontline/article/how-the-response-to-hurricane-maria-compared-to-harvey-and-irma/

Elrod, S. (2011). Category A–C agents. In R. Katz & R. Zilinskas (Eds.), *Encyclopedia of Bioterrorism Defense* (2nd ed.). Hoboken, NJ: Wiley and Sons.

Fauci, A. S. (2017). Pandemic preparedness in the next administration: Keynote address by Anthony S. Fauci. *YouTube*. Retrieved from https://www.youtube.com/watch?v=DNXGAxGJgQI

Federal Bureau of Investigation. (n.d.). Homepage. Retrieved from https://www.fbi.gov/

Food and Drug Administration. (2018a). *Counterterrorism and emerging threats*. Retrieved from https://www.fda.gov/emergencypreparedness/counterterrorism/default.htm

Food and Drug Administration. (2018b). *Expanded access: Information for patients*. Retrieved from https://www.fda.gov/NewsEvents/PublicHealthFocus/ExpandedAccessCompassionateUse/ucm20041768.htm

Ganesan, K., Raza, S. K., & Vijayaraghavan, R. (2010). Chemical warfare agents. *Journal of Pharmacy and Bioallied Sciences, 2*(3), 166–178. https://doi.org/10.4103/0975-7406.68498

Gates, B. (2018). *Speech by Bill Gates*. Retrieved from https://www.securityconference.de/de/aktivitaeten/munich-security-conference/munich-security-conference/msc-2017/reden/speech-by-bill-gates/

Global Emerging Infections Surveillance. (2018). Homepage. Retrieved from https://www.health.mil/Military-Health-Topics/Health-Readiness/Armed-Forces-Health-Surveillance-Branch/Global-Emerging-Infections-Surveillance-and-Response

Greenough, P. G., & Kirsch, T. D. (2005). Public Health response—Assessing needs. *New England Journal of Medicine, 353*(15), 1544–1546. https://doi.org/10.1056/NEJMp058238

Gregg, M. (1989). *The public health consequences of disasters*. Atlanta, GA: Centers for Disease Control and Prevention.

Greshko, M. (2017). *Why this hurricane season has been so catastrophic*. Retrieved from https://news.nationalgeographic.com/2017/09/hurricane-irma-harvey-season-climate-change-weather/

Harford, J., Azavedo, E., Fischietto, M., & Breast Health Global Initiative Healthcare Systems Panel. (2008). Guideline implementation for breast healthcare in low- and middle-income countries. *Cancer, 113*(S8), 2282–2296. https://doi.org/10.1002/cncr.23841

Health Resources and Services Administration. (2017). PREP Act declarations. Retrieved from https://www.hrsa.gov/get-health-care/conditions/counter-measures-comp/declarations.html

Holmes, O., & Solomon, E. (2013). Alleged chemical attack kills 25 in northern Syria. *Reuters*. Retrieved from https://www.reuters.com/article/us-syria-crisis-chemical-idUSBRE92I0A220130319

Hu, H., Fine, J., Epstein, P., Kelsey, K., Reynolds, P., & Walker, B. (1989). Tear gas—harassing agent or toxic chemical weapon? *JAMA, 262*(5), 660–663.

Kadlec, R. (2013). *Renewing the Project BioShield Act: What has it bought and wrought?* Retrieved from https://www.bio.org/sites/default/files/CNAS_RenewingTheProjectBioShieldAct_Kadlec.pdf

Kaiser, J. (2014, July 11). Lab incidents lead to safety crackdown at CDC. *Science*. Retrieved from http://www.sciencemag.org/news/2014/07/lab-incidents-lead-safety-crackdown-cdc

Kaufmann, D., & Penciakova, V. (2011, March). Japan's triple disaster: Governance and the earthquake, tsunami and nuclear crises. *Brookings Institution*. Retrieved from https://www.brookings.edu/opinions/japans-triple-disaster-governance-and-the-earthquake-tsunami-and-nuclear-crises/

Kishore, N., Marqués, D., Mahmud, A., Kiang, M. V., Rodriguez, I., Fuller, A., . . . Buckee, C. O. (2018). Mortality in Puerto Rico after Hurricane Maria. *New England Journal of Medicine*, NEJMsa1803972. https://doi.org/10.1056/NEJMsa1803972

Levi, J., Segal, L. M., Lieberman, D. A., May, K., & Laurent, R. S. (2014). Outbreaks: Protecting Americans from infectious diseases. *Trust for America's Health*. Retrieved https://www.tfah.org/releases/outbreaks2013/

Lister, S. A. (2005). *Hurricane Katrina: The public health and medical response*. Retrieved from http://www.au.af.mil/au/awc/awcgate/crs/rl33096.pdf

Maron, D. F. (2014). CDC botched handling of deadly flu virus. Retrieved from https://www.scientificamerican.com/article/cdc-botched-handling-of-deadly-flu-virus/

McNeil, D. G. (2016). Obama administration to transfer Ebola funds to Zika fight. Retrieved from https://www.nytimes.com/2016/04/07/health/zika-virus-budget-ebola.html

Melnikova, N., Wu, J., & Orr, M. F. (2015). Public health response to acute chemical incidents—Hazardous substances emergency events surveillance, nine states, 1999–2008. *Morbidity and Mortality Weekly Report, 64*(SS02), 25–31.

Monahan, J., & Halabi, S. (2015). Legal preparedness and Ebola vaccines. *Lancet (London, England), 386*(9991), 338–339. https://doi.org/10.1016/S0140-6736(15)61408-8

Monke, J. (2004). *CRS report for Congress: Agroterrorism; Threats and preparedness*. Retrieved from https://fas.org/irp/crs/RL32521.pdf

Murray, C. K., Hinkle, M. K., & Yun, H. C. (2008). History of infections associated with combat-related injuries. *The Journal of Trauma: Injury, Infection, and Critical Care, 64*(Suppl), S221–S231. https://doi.org/10.1097/TA.0b013e318163c40b

Murthy, B. P., Molinari, N.-A. M., LeBlanc, T. T., Vagi, S. J., & Avchen, R. N. (2017). Progress in public health emergency preparedness—United States, 2001–2016. *American Journal of Public Health, 107*(S2), S180–S185. https://doi.org/10.2105/AJPH.2017.304038

National Institutes of Health. (2015). *NIAID organization*. Retrieved from https://www.niaid.nih.gov/about/niaid-organization

National Intelligence Council. (2008). *Global trends 2025: A transformed world*. Retrieved from https://www.dni.gov/files/documents/Newsroom/Reports and Pubs/2025_Global_Trends_Final_Report.pdf

National Security Council. (2009). *National strategy for countering biological threats*. Retrieved from https://www.hsdl.org/?view&did=31404

Nelson, C., Lurie, N., Wasserman, J., & Zakowski, S. (2007). Conceptualizing and defining public health emergency preparedness. *American Journal of Public Health, 97*(Suppl 1), S9–S11. https://doi.org/10.2105/AJPH.2007.114496

Noji, E. K. (1997). The public health consequences of disasters. *Prehospital and Disaster Medicine, 15*(4), 147–157.

Office of U.S. Foreign Disaster Assistance. (1993). *Disaster history: Significant data on major disasters worldwide, 1900–present.* Retrieved from https://pdf.usaid.gov/pdf_docs/PNABP986.pdf

Philipps, D. (2017). Seven hard lessons federal responders to Harvey learned from Katrina. Retrieved from https://www.nytimes.com/2017/09/07/us/hurricane-harvey-katrina-federal-responders.html

Ranlet, P. (2000). The British, the Indians, and Smallpox: What actually happened at Fort Pitt in 1763? *Pennsylvania History: A Journal of Mid-Atlantic Studies.* University Park, PA: Penn State University Press.

Richmond, A., Hostler, L., Leeman, G., & King, W. (2010). A brief history and overview of CDC's Centers for Public Health Preparedness Cooperative Agreement Program. *Public Health Reports (Washington, DC: 1974), 125* (Suppl 5), 8–14. https://doi.org/10.1177/00333549101250S503

Sandor, K. (2011). Department of Defense. In R. Katz & R. A. Zilinskas (Eds.), *Encyclopedia of bioterrorism defense* (pp. 1–8). Hoboken, NJ: John Wiley & Sons.

Schnirring, L. (2011). Public health groups sound warning about preparedness cuts. Retrieved from http://www.cidrap.umn.edu/news-perspective/2011/05/public-health-groups-sound-warning-about-preparedness-cuts

Secretariat of the Investigation Committee on the Accidents at the Fukushima Nuclear Power Station. (2012). *Investigation Committee on the Accident at the Fukushima Nuclear Power Stations of Tokyo Electric Power Company.* Retrieved from http://www.cas.go.jp/jp/seisaku/icanps/eng/

Sun, L. H. (2014). Expert panel finds CDC remains weak on lab safety despite some progress. *The Washington Post.* Retrieved from https://www.washingtonpost.com/national/health-science/expert-panel-finds-cdc-remains-weak-on-lab-safety-despite-some-progress/2016/01/04/8df100bc-b298-11e5-9388-466021d971de_story.html?noredirect=on&utm_term=.de3474cc6d7b

Sun, L. H. (2018, April 24). Inside the secret U.S. stockpile meant to save us all in a bioterror attack. *Washington Post.* Retrieved from https://www.washingtonpost.com/news/to-your-health/wp/2018/04/24/inside-the-secret-u-s-stockpile-meant-to-save-us-all-in-a-bioterror-attack/?utm_term=.c788e89b8469

Tanter, R. (2013). After Fukushima: A survey of corruption in the global nuclear power industry. *Asian Perspective, 37*(4), 475–500.

The White House. (2006). *The federal response to Hurricane Katrina: Lessons learned.* Retrieved from http://library.stmarytx.edu/acadlib/edocs/katrinawh.pdf

The White House. (2007). *Homeland Security Presidential Directive/HSPD-18: Medical Countermeasures Against Weapons of Mass Destruction.* Retrieved from https://fas.org/irp/offdocs/nspd/hspd-18.html

United Nations. (2013). *United Nations mission to investigate allegations of the use of chemical weapons in the Syrian Arab Republic.* Retrieved from https://unoda-web.s3.amazonaws.com/wp-content/uploads/2013/12/report.pdf

U.S. Department of Agriculture. (n.d.). *About the U.S. Department of Agriculture.* Retrieved from https://www.usda.gov/our-agency/about-usda

U.S. Geological Survey. (2004). *M 9.1—Off the west coast of northern Sumatra.* Retrieved from https://earthquake.usgs.gov/earthquakes/eventpage/official20041226005853450_30#executive

Vale, J. A., Marrs, T. C., & Maynard, R. L. (2018). Novichok: A murderous nerve agent attack in the UK. *Clinical Toxicology,* 1–5. https://doi.org/10.1080/15563650.2018.1469759

VanRooyen, M., & Leaning, J. (2005). After the tsunami— Facing the public health challenges. *New England Journal of Medicine, 352*(5), 435–438. https://doi.org/10.1056/NEJMp058013

Watson, C. R., Watson, M., & Sell, T. K. (2017). Public health preparedness funding: Key programs and trends from 2001 to 2017. *American Journal of Public Health, 107*(S2), S165–S167. https://doi.org/10.2105/AJPH.2017.303963

Wenck, M. A., Van Sickle, D., Drociuk, D., Belflower, A., Youngblood, C., Whisnant, M. D., . . . Gibson, J. J. (2007). Rapid assessment of exposure to chlorine released from a train derailment and resulting health impact. *Public Health Reports (Washington, DC: 1974), 122*(6), 784–792. https://doi.org/10.1177/003335490712200610

Wheatley, S., Sovacool, B., & Sornette, D. (2017). Of disasters and dragon kings: A statistical analysis of nuclear power incidents and accidents. *Risk Analysis, 37*(1), 99–115. https://doi.org/10.1111/risa.12587

Wheelis, M. (2002). Biological warfare at the 1346 Siege of Caffa. *Emerging Infectious Diseases, 8*(9), 971–975. https://doi.org/10.3201/eid0809.010536

Wiharta, S., Ahman, H., Halne, J.-Y., Löfgren, J., & Randall, T. (2008). *The effectiveness of foreign military assets in natural disaster response.* Stockholm International Peace Research Institute. Retrieved from https://www.sipri.org/publications/2008/effectiveness-foreign-military-assets-natural-disaster-response

World Health Organization. (2007). *The world health report 2007—A safer future: Global public health security in the 21st century.* Retrieved from http://www.who.int/whr/2007/en/

World Health Organization. (2016). *International Health Regulations (2005)* (3rd ed.). Geneva, Switzerland: World Health Organization.

Walter Reed Army Institute of Research. (2018). Homepage. Retrieved from http://www.wrair.army.mil/

Writer, J. V., DeFraites, R. F., & Keep, L. W. (2000). Non-battle injury casualties during the Persian Gulf War and other deployments. *American Journal of Preventive Medicine, 18* (Suppl 3), 64–70. Retrieved from http://www.ncbi.nlm.nih.gov/pubmed/10736542

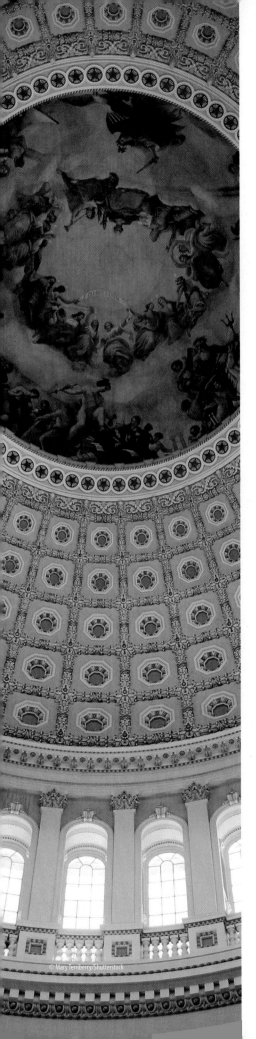
© Mary Terriberry/Shutterstock

PART III

Basic Skills in Health Policy Analysis

Parts I and II covered fundamental concepts of health policy and law and engaged in a substantive discussion of essential issues in health policy. This analysis of the *content* of health policy and law is paired in Part III with a tutorial covering one of the most important *skills* in the field of health policy: writing a health policy analysis.

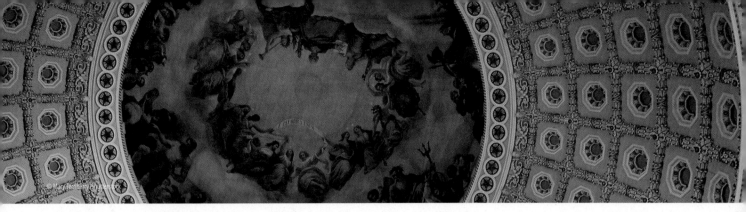

CHAPTER 14

The Art of Structuring and Writing a Health Policy Analysis

LEARNING OBJECTIVES

By the end of this chapter you will be able to:

- Understand the concept of policy analysis
- Analyze a health policy issue
- Write a health policy analysis
- Develop descriptive and analytic side-by-side tables

▶ Introduction

Imagine you work for the governor of a state that recently received a large sum of federal money for antibioterrorism efforts and your boss asks you how it should be spent. How will you respond? Or, assume you are an assistant to the director of a state nutrition program for low-income children and the program's budget was slashed by the legislature. The program's director needs to reduce costs and turns to you for help. How will you approach this problem? Finally, pretend you work in the White House as a domestic policy advisor and the president is considering revising the administration's methane emissions guidelines. What guidance will you offer?

While the *substance* of health policy and law has been discussed in detail up to this point, this chapter teaches you what policy analysis is and the *skill* of addressing complex health policy questions through a written policy analysis.

We use the following definition to describe a policy analysis: *an analysis that provides informed advice to a client that relates to a public policy decision, includes a recommended course of action/inaction, and is framed by the client's powers and values.* We briefly review each element of this definition in this chapter.

▶ Policy Analysis Overview

In this section we define policy analysis and review the purposes for developing one. In the following section, we provide a step-by-step process detailing how to create a written health policy analysis.

Client-Oriented Advice

The client is the particular stakeholder that requests the policy analysis, and the analysis must be developed to suit the client's needs. (The client, for example, could be a policymaker who hires you, a fictional policy-maker in an exercise developed by your professor, or an employer who asks you to analyze a problem.) In general, a stakeholder refers to an individual or a group that has an interest in the issue at hand. There may be many stakeholders related to a particular policy issue. Of course, the client requesting an analysis is also a stakeholder because that person or entity has an interest in the issue. However, to avoid confusion, we refer to the person or group that requests the analysis as the client, and the other interested parties as stakeholders.

Informed Advice

Providing informed advice means the analysis is based on thorough and well-rounded information. The information included in the analysis must convey all sides of an issue, not just the facts and theories supporting a particular perspective. If a decision maker is presented with evidence supporting only one course of action or one side of a debate, it will be impossible for the client to make a well-informed decision. In addition, to be effective in persuading others to favor the recommended policy, your client must be able to understand and, when necessary, refute alternative solutions to the problem.

Public Policy Decision

Policy analyses involve public policy decisions. A public policy problem goes beyond the individual sphere and affects the greater community.

Providing Options and a Recommendation

A key component of any policy analysis is providing the client with several options to consider, analyzing those options, and settling on one recommendation. In other words, a policy analysis is not simply a background report that identifies a variety of issues relating to a particular problem; instead, it gives the client ideas about what steps to take to address the problem and concludes by recommending a specific course of action.

Your Client's Power and Values

Finally, the analysis should be framed by the client's power and values. Framing the analysis based on the client's *power* is fairly straightforward and uncontroversial: the options presented and the recommendation made must be within the power of the client to accomplish. On the other hand, the notion of framing an analysis according to the client's *values* is more

controversial. In most conceptualizations of policy analysis, including the one discussed later in this chapter, the process is roughly the same: define the problem and provide information about it, analyze a set of alternatives to solve the problem, and implement the best solution based on the analysis (Patton & Sawicki, 1993, p. 3). As new information is uncovered or the problem is reformulated, analysts may move back and forth among these steps in an iterative process (Stone, 2002, p. 47). However, although there is general agreement that politics and values play a role in policy analysis, there is disagreement over at which stage of the analysis they come into play.

To understand this controversy, it is necessary to discuss two models of policy analysis: the rational model and the political model. The rational model was developed in an attempt to base policy decisions on reason and science rather than the vagaries of politics (Stone, 2002, p. 7). In the traditional rational model, the analyst does not consider politics and values. Instead, he or she should recommend the "rational, logical, and technically desirable policy" (Stone, 2002, p. 51). According to the rational model, the *decision maker* infuses the analysis with politics and values once the analyst's work is complete.

Professor John Kingdon and others have moved away from the rational model and toward a political model. Kingdon suggests that policy analysis occurs through the development of three streams: problems, policies, and politics (Kingdon, 1995). The problem stream is where problems are defined and noticed by decision makers. The policy stream is where solutions are proposed. These proposals may be solutions to identified problems, but they are often favored projects of policymakers or advocates that exist separate from specific problems that have garnered attention. Finally, the political stream refers to the ever-changing political mood. As a general matter, these streams develop separately, only coming together at critical junctures when the problem reaches the top of the agenda, the solutions to that problem are viable, and the political atmosphere makes the time right for change (Weissert & Weisser, 2002, p. 87).

Kingdon's approach discusses occurrences the rational model does not consider, such as why some problems are addressed and others are not, why some solutions are favored even if they are not technically the best approach, and why action is taken at some junctures but not at others (Kingdon, 1995). In addition, the rational model refers to only one cycle of problems. As Kingdon and others have noted, solutions to one problem often lead to unintended consequences that create other problems to be addressed, resulting in an ongoing policy analysis cycle instead of an event with a start and a finish (Weissert & Weissert, 2002, p. 260).

Professor Deborah Stone also focuses on the role of politics and values in analysis (Stone, 2002, pp. 1–4). She argues that the idea of the rational policy analysis model misses the point because "analysis itself is a creature of politics" (Stone, 2002, p. 8). According to Stone, every choice, from defining a problem, to selecting analytic criteria, to choosing which options to evaluate, to making a recommendation, is political and value-laden. As she states, "Rational policy analysis can begin only after the relevant values have been identified and … these values change over time as a result of the policymaking process" (Stone, 2002, p. 32). She contends that policy analysis should do the very things that the rational model does not permit—allow for changing objectives, permit contradictory goals, and turn apparent losses into political gains (Stone, 2002, p. 9). The goal of the rational model founders—to divorce analysis from the vagaries of politics—is simply not possible in Stone's view.

Having differentiated these models, we now return to our definition of policy analysis: *an analysis that provides informed advice to a client that relates to a public policy decision, includes a recommended course of action/inaction, and is framed by the client's powers and values.* You can see that this definition follows Stone's political model of policy analysis, requiring the analysis to be developed with a particular client's values in mind. After reviewing the numerous examples provided in the following section, it will be evident that client values permeate all aspects of a policy analysis. Only after you take into account your client's values, combine it with the information you have gathered, place it in the prevailing political context, and understand your client's powers, can you make an appropriate policy recommendation.

Multiple Purposes

The ultimate product of a policy analysis is a recommendation to a specific client about how to address a problem. However, a policy analysis has several other purposes as well. It provides general information necessary to understand the problem at hand and may be an important tool to inform stakeholders about a policy problem. In addition, the analysis may be a vehicle for widespread dissemination of ideas and arguments. Although your analysis is targeted to the client requesting advisement, it may also be used to inform and persuade other supporters, opponents, the media, the general public, and others. Finally, it

will help you, the policy analyst, learn how to think through problems and develop solutions in an organized, concise, and useful way.

Policy analyses can take many forms—a memorandum, an oral briefing, a report, and so on—and, correspondingly, have varying degrees of formality. This chapter explains how to construct a *short, written* analysis because it is a commonly used, highly effective, and often practical way to provide a policy analysis to your client. In addition, the principles embedded in a policy analysis can then be used in whatever other format(s) your client prefers. Whether you are aiding a governor, the director of a state program, the CEO of a private business, or any other decision maker, you often will not have the opportunity to discuss issues in person or for a significant length of time. Furthermore, given time pressures, the demands on high-level policymakers, the need for rapid decision making, and the variety of issues most policymakers deal with, many clients will not read a lengthy analysis. That is why it is essential for anyone who wants to influence policy to be able to craft a clear and concise written analysis.

▶ Structuring a Policy Analysis

We now turn to a five-step method for writing a thorough yet concise policy analysis. Regardless of the subject matter, you can use this structure to analyze the question your client is considering. As you review each part of the analysis, notice the various disciplines and tools that may be part of writing an effective policy analysis. Analysts draw from a variety of disciplines—law, economics, political science, sociology, history, and others—and use a number of quantitative and qualitative tools when explaining issues, analyzing options, and making recommendations.

Although policy analyses come in various formats and use different terminology, they will all contain these essential elements:

- **Problem identification:** Defines the problem addressed in the analysis
- **Background:** Provides factual information needed to understand the problem
- **Landscape:** Reviews the various stakeholders and their concerns
- **Options:** Describe and analyze several options to address the problem
- **Recommendation:** Offers one option as the best action to pursue

The following sections discuss each of these elements in detail.

Problem Identification

Define the Problem

The first step in writing a policy analysis is to clearly define the problem you are analyzing. A problem identification should be succinct and written in the form of a question that identifies the problem addressed in the analysis. It usually consists of a single sentence, though it may be two sentences if you are analyzing a particularly complex issue. Although a problem identification is simple to define, it is often one of the most difficult parts of the analysis to do well. It is also one of the most important.

The problem identification is the key to your analysis because it frames the problem at hand. Indeed, some policy battles are won or lost simply by how the problem identification is crafted. For example, consider the different questions asked in these problem identifications:

Problem identification 1:

What type of tax credit, if any, should the president include in the next budget proposal?

Problem identification 2:

What type and size of health insurance tax credit should the president include in the next budget proposal?

The first problem identification asks what type of tax credit, if any, should be considered. One possible answer to that question is that no tax credit of any kind should be considered. Another answer could involve a tax credit, but not one related to health insurance. The second problem identification suggests that the option of not proposing a health insurance tax credit is unacceptable. Instead, the second problem identification lends itself to an analysis of identifying the pros and cons of various health insurance tax credit options. In other words, one option that may be considered based on the first problem identification (no tax credit) is excluded based on the second problem identification.

Consider another example:

Problem identification 1:

Which health issue should be the governor's top priority?

Problem identification 2:

Should the governor's priority of reducing the number of obese residents be accomplished by relying on currently existing programs?

Again, the first problem identification asks an open-ended question about identifying the governor's top

priority. The answer may be obesity, but it may be any other health issue as well. The second problem identification starts with the governor committed to reducing the obesity rate and asks how to best accomplish that goal. Again, these problem identification lead to very different analyses and (most likely) different recommendations.

It is possible that your client's values will be evident from the way the problem identification is phrased. For instance, in the second example, the second policy statement clearly reflects the governor's desire to reduce the obesity rate. Consider another example. You have been asked to write a policy analysis about the merits of importing low-cost prescription drugs from Canada. How might the problem identification differ if your client is a pharmaceutical lobbying group versus if your client is an elder rights association? Here are two possible problem identifications.

An acceptable way to identify the problem for the pharmaceutical lobbying firm:

How can this firm help improve medical care quality in the United States by reducing the importation of dangerous prescription drugs from Canada?

An acceptable way to identify the problem for the elder rights association:

How can this association help seniors obtain low-priced prescription drugs from Canada?

The vast differences in these problem identifications reflect differing viewpoints regarding the importation of prescription drugs. A pharmaceutical lobbying firm is more likely to be concerned about reduced profits for its drug company clients and therefore would want to deter or restrict importation, which could lead to more competition in the market. One way to accomplish that goal is to phrase the issue as a safety/quality-of-care concern. An elder rights association is more likely to be concerned with high-priced prescription drugs in the United States and would therefore want to promote drug importation (assuming, of course, there is no actual safety concern with the drugs). One way to accomplish that goal is to phrase the issue as one of cost reduction.

It is also possible to identify the problem in a neutral manner. From the immediately previous example, analysts for both groups could use the following phrasing.

Neutral problem identification:

What action should [the client] take in response to recent congressional proposals relating to importing prescription drugs from Canada?

Neutral wording is not necessarily better or worse than value-driven phrasing. The value-driven phrase provides additional information about the direction of the policy analysis and clearly limits some of the options that might otherwise be considered. Neutral wording is often broader, leaving more options on the table at the outset. Yet, even if neutral phrasing is used, the options the analyst considers and the recommendation the analyst makes will still be constrained by the client's values and needs.

Because it is possible to identify problems numerous ways for any issue, how do you develop the best one? In general, you want to use the one that provides the best fit for your analysis. If you decide to focus on all safety-related concerns, for example, the pharmaceutical lobbying firm example would be a good fit. If, however, the firm chose to have one safety-related option, one state government-focused option, and one convenience-centered option, then you would want a broader problem identification that allows for all types of options. For example, "How can this firm help improve consumers' experience purchasing prescription drugs?" would allow for various types of options. In addition, you want to make sure your problem identification is analytically manageable and does not include your recommendation.

Make the Problem Identification Analytically Manageable

Acceptable phrasing can be broad or narrow. One is not better than the other; they suit different purposes. Policy analyses with broad problem identifications may require more diverse information in terms of background and may consider a wider range of issues in the paper's landscape section. Also, the recommendations may promote "big picture" changes instead of specific and tailored ideas. Narrower wording may require less extensive background and landscape information, but they may not capture big picture, systemic concerns relating to the problem under consideration.

Reflect on the following examples. They both may be acceptable problem identifications, depending on the needs of your client.

A broad problem identification:

What action should the U.S. Department of Health and Human Services take to avoid another flu vaccine shortage?

A narrow problem identification:

How can the U.S. Department of Health and Human Services create incentives for additional manufacturers to supply flu vaccine to the United States?

The first one could result in a variety of recommendations, such as improving surveillance to lower the incidence of flu in the future, developing new vaccines that have longer-lasting immunity, or finding ways to entice additional manufacturers to provide supplies to the United States. It is a broad problem identification that will lead to an analysis that could recommend a wide variety of actions. The second one focuses on one particular way to decrease a flu vaccine shortage—increasing the number of suppliers. Although the analysis will also provide a number of options, all of the options will address the specific issue of increasing suppliers. Again, there is no single right or wrong way to phrase a problem. Whether it is more useful to have a broad or narrow problem will depend on the needs and concerns of your client.

However, it is possible to make a problem identification so vague that it will be impossible to write a sound policy analysis. Unfortunately, there is no easy way to differentiate an acceptably broad problem phrasing from an unmanageably vague one when you begin your analysis. You will know your wording is too vague, however, if you find it impossible to write a *complete and concise* policy analysis and you can think of too many diverse options to include (if you can think of 5 to 10 possible options your statement is probably workable; if you can think of 15 or more options, your statement is probably too broad). Your paper will require too much information in the background and landscape sections if you draft an overly vague problem identification. In addition, you will find that you cannot devise a coherent series of options addressing the problem because the problem identification is too broadly defined. Instead of a concise and useful policy analysis, you will end up with a lengthy and unfocused paper.

If you believe your problem identification may be so vague that it is analytically unmanageable, ask yourself if you are addressing one specific problem that may be countered with a few specific options. If you are having trouble narrowing your problem identification, you can try including limitations based on geography (e.g., refer to a particular state or city), time (e.g., focus on the next year or over the next 5 years), or numerical boundaries (e.g., use a goal of reducing a figure by a certain percentage or a budget by a specific dollar amount). Consider this example:

An unmanageably vague problem identification:

What is the best use of the Centers for Disease Control and Prevention's resources to improve the health status of our citizens?

This phrasing is not analytically manageable. It is extremely broad and unfocused. Using this problem identification, your analysis could address any health issue, such as access to care problems, the need to improve vaccination rates, racial disparities in health care, or many others. The list is endless and your policy analysis will be as well.

A manageable problem identification:

What preventive health issue should be the top priority for the Centers for Disease Control and Prevention next year?

This one is analytically manageable. It is focused on preventive measures specifically and is limited to determining the top priority. In addition, the problem is focused on what can be done in the upcoming year. This second problem identification allows for a much more concise and directed policy analysis.

Do Not Include the Recommendation in Your Problem Identification

Another pitfall when identifying problems is crafting a problem in a way that suggests a particular solution to the issue. A problem identification should define a specific problem; it should not indicate how that problem should be solved. If the answer is preordained, why bother with the analysis? When phrasing your problem , ask yourself if you can imagine four, five, or six potentially viable options to address the problem. If you cannot, then you have not defined the problem well.

For example, assume you've been asked to address how to reduce medical malpractice insurance premiums. Here is a problem identification that leads the reader to one conclusion:

A leading problem identification:

To what extent should jury awards be limited in malpractice cases in order to reduce malpractice premiums?

This phrasing leads to one very specific solution (limiting jury awards) as a way to counter a broad problem (reducing malpractice premiums). The only question presented by this problem identification is what the award limit should be. It does not provide a range of options for reducing malpractice premiums (one of which may be limiting jury awards) for your client to consider. (Of course, if you were specifically asked to address how to limit jury awards in malpractice cases, this would be an appropriate problem identification.) A better way to word the problem would be, "What action should be taken to stem the rise in malpractice premiums nationwide?"

This problem identification lends itself to an analysis that considers several options. Possible alternatives include limiting jury awards, enacting regulations that limit the amount insurance companies can increase premiums each year, and a host of other options. This wording also narrows the focus of the analysis to national solutions.

Once you have written your concise and precise problem identification, you have set the framework for your analysis. Every other section of the analysis should relate directly to the problem you identified. Remember that writing a policy analysis is an iterative process; you must review, revise, and tighten the information and arguments throughout the writing process. As you review the other components of your policy analysis, it may become evident that what you thought was the best way to describe the problems can be further improved. There is nothing wrong with revising your wording as you craft your analysis, as long as you remain true to your client's values and power.

The Background Section

The first substantive information your analysis provides is in the background section. The background informs the reader why the particular problem has been chosen for analysis. This section should make clear why the issue is important and needs to be addressed now. In addition to providing general information about the topic, your background and landscape (discussed next) sections provide the information necessary to assess the options you lay out.

Much of the information in the background will be relevant regardless of who assigned the analysis. However, because the background provides information necessary to understand the problem, it is essential to understand the knowledge level of your client when constructing the background. For example, assume you are writing an analysis relating to state preparedness planning for smallpox vaccination in the event of a bioterror attack. Regardless of your client, your background would likely include information about why a smallpox attack is a threat, including (but not limited to) the following:

- Reference to the September 11, 2001, attacks on the World Trade Center and subsequent events
- The belief that although smallpox has been eradicated as a natural disease, it is likely that samples of the virus still exist
- Reference to any information provided by the federal government or other sources relating to the possibility of a bioterror attack

If your client does not have knowledge relating to smallpox, you would also include details about smallpox transmission, the effects of the disease, the vaccination procedure, and the risks associated with vaccination.

In addition, your background should include whatever factual information is necessary to fully assess the options discussed. Remember, your client needs a complete picture, not just the information that supports the recommended action or your client's viewpoint. By the time the reader reaches your paper's options section, all of the information necessary to evaluate the options should have been presented in your background or landscape.

For example, assume one of your options for the smallpox vaccination state preparedness analysis is immediate compulsory vaccination of all first responders and establishment of a protocol for vaccinating the remaining population if there is a smallpox outbreak. In that case, your background (and possibly the landscape) should provide information regarding who first responders are, where they are located, how many there are, legal issues relating to compulsory vaccination, and so on.

Because the background section is an informational—not analytical—part of the analysis, the material provided in it should be mostly factual. The tone of the background is not partisan or argumentative. It should simply state the necessary information.

The Landscape Section

Together, the background and landscape sections frame the context of the analysis for your client. Whereas the background provides factual information to assist the client in understanding what the problem is and why it is being addressed, the landscape provides the overall context for the analysis by identifying key stakeholders and the factors that must be considered when analyzing the problem. In the following discussion, you will read about numerous types of people, groups, and issues that might be included in a landscape. These examples are meant to provide suggestions and provoke thought about what should be included in an analysis. It would be impossible to include everything discussed here in any single landscape section. It is the job of the policy analyst to choose among these options—to be able to identify whose views and which factors are the most salient ones in creating a complete landscape.

Identifying Key Stakeholders

Up to this point, the policy analysis discussion has focused on just one stakeholder: the client who asked for the policy analysis. The landscape brings in other stakeholders who have an interest in the issue. Although it is often impossible to include every possible stakeholder in a single analysis, it is necessary to identify the key stakeholders whose positions and concerns must be understood before a well-informed decision can be made.

How do you identify the key stakeholders particular to your issue? Unfortunately, there is no magic formula. The best approach is through research and thinking. Also, bear in mind that the stakeholders and issues discussed in the landscape must relate to your overall policy analysis. Your options must address the problem identified initially, and all of the information necessary to assess the options must be presented in the background and landscape. As you learn about the problem to be analyzed and think about options for addressing the problem, it should become apparent which stakeholders have a significant interest in the issue.

For example, assume your analysis relates to proposed legislation regulating pharmacists and pharmaceuticals. Who are possible key stakeholders regarding this issue? They may include several parties:

- Democratic and Republican politicians (you might need to distinguish among those in Congress, state legislatures, and governors)
- Pharmaceutical industry
- Health insurance industry
- AARP and other elder rights groups
- Advocacy groups for the disabled
- Pharmacists' lobby
- Foreign pharmaceutical companies
- Internet-based pharmaceutical companies

Can you think of others?

Deciding which stakeholders *must* be included in an analysis depends on the exact problem being analyzed and which options are included in the analysis. For example, assume you are writing an analysis about requirements relating to how pharmacists inform consumers about their medications. If your problem deals with face-to-face encounters only, Internet-based pharmaceutical companies would not be a key stakeholder. Alternatively, if the problem definition deals with purchasing limitations over the Internet, Internet-based pharmaceutical companies must be included in the analysis. If one of your options focuses on comprehension among older adults, elder rights groups should be included in the analysis. If your client is someone running for public office in a county where the health insurance industry is a major employer, the views of those companies would be essential to include. In other words, although it is possible to make a generic list of the types of individuals and groups that could be included, the specific list for any policy analysis will depend on the client for whom the analysis is being written, the specific problem being addressed, and the options being considered.

Identifying Key Factors

Once you have settled on a list of key stakeholders, it is necessary to analyze their position on the issue at the center of the analysis. Earlier, we described the landscape as the portion of the analysis that provides the overall context of the issue. The "overall context" refers to the mix of factors that are relevant when any decision is being made. These factors are used to analyze stakeholder positions. Although there is not one comprehensive list of context factors and not all factors are relevant to all analyses, the list in **BOX 14-1** includes some common factors that could be discussed.

BOX 14-1 Possible Factors to Include in a Landscape Section

Political Factors

What is the political salience of the issue?
Is this a front-burner issue?
Is this a controversial issue?
Are your client, legislators, and the general public interested in addressing this issue?
Has this or a similar healthcare issue been addressed recently?
Do key constituents, opponents, interest groups, or other stakeholders have an opinion about the issue? Who is likely to support or oppose change?
Is there bipartisan support for the issue?
Is there a reason to act now?
Is there a reason to delay action?

Social Factors

Who is affected by this problem?
According to the client who assigned the analysis, are influential or valued people or groups affected by this problem?
Is there a fairness concern relating to this issue?
Is there a stigma associated with this issue?

Economic Factors

What is the economic impact of addressing this problem? Of not addressing it?
Are various people or groups impacted differently?
Are there competing demands for resources that relate to this issue?
What is the economic situation of the state or nation? How does this affect the politics relating to this issue?
How will addressing this issue affect healthcare costs/healthcare spending?

Practical Factors

Is it realistic to try to solve this problem?
Do others need to be involved to be able to solve this problem?
Is the technology available to solve this problem?
Would it be more practical to solve this problem later?
Are other people in a better position to solve this problem?
What do we know about solutions that do or do not work?
If this problem cannot be solved, is it still necessary (politically, socially) to act in some way to address the problem?
Is evidence available to support potential solutions?

Legal Factors

Are there legal restrictions affecting this problem?
Is there a need to balance public health concerns and individual legal rights?
Are there legal requirements that impact the analysis?
Is new legislative authority necessary to solve the problem?
Is there legal uncertainty relating to this problem?
Is future litigation a concern if action is taken?

Quality-of-Care Factors

Does this problem address quality-of-care issues?

Do some solutions focus on quality of care more than others?

Do quality-of-care concerns vary based on which provider is involved?

Is evidence available about the best ways to improve quality of care?

Has the client already taken any actions to improve quality of care?

The list of factors in Box 14-1 is by no means exhaustive, but rather is intended to provide a sense of the types of questions that are often relevant to understanding the context of a problem. Just as it would be impossible to discuss every stakeholder who might be connected to the problem, it would be impossible to include in a concise analysis of all the issues raised by the five factors listed in Box 14-1. It is the policy analyst's job to identify not only which key stakeholders must be included, but also which key factors must be discussed.

Consider again the example relating to limiting prescription drug purchases made over the Internet. The following key factors would likely be included:

- **Political factor:** Who supports or opposes the limitation and how influential are they?
- **Economic factor:** Would it be costly to implement this limitation or costly to key constituents who may need more prescription drugs than are allowed by the limit? Would it provide an economic benefit to some stakeholders?
- **Practical factor:** Is it possible to implement and enforce a restricted purchasing system over the Internet?
- **Legal factor:** Are there legal barriers to limiting Internet prescription drug purchases?

For each factor, the analysis should discuss relevant views of the stakeholders you included in your analysis. For example, when discussing economic factors, the analysis might explain that Internet-based pharmaceutical companies would experience a loss of revenue, some consumers would pay more for prescription drugs if they needed more than the limited amount, and storefront pharmaceutical companies would make money because consumers probably would have to fill more of their orders in person. Depending on the political situation, the analysis might explain that the client's most influential constituents are older adults who use many prescription drugs and are likely to oppose any restriction, or that storefront pharmaceutical companies are large campaign contributors and would support a restriction.

Structuring the Landscape Section

The landscape may be organized by stakeholder or by factor. In other words, it is acceptable to identify stakeholder 1 and then describe that stakeholder's views based on various concerns, and then identify stakeholder 2 and describe that stakeholder's views, and so on. Alternatively, the landscape could be structured based on factors described in Box 14-1. Within that structure, the landscape would address one set of factors (e.g., economic), then another set (e.g., social), and so on. Some stakeholders may not have relevant views for all of the factors, but each stakeholder must be addressed as often as necessary to convey their policy position. For example, the economic factors section would identify various stakeholders and their views based on economic concerns. It would include information such as "Canadian companies would oppose regulating Internet pharmacies because it would increase the cost of doing business with Americans, while U.S. storefront pharmacists would support regulating Internet pharmacies because it may increase prices for their competitors' products."

When you discuss a particular view, it is important to identify which stakeholders hold that view. At the same time, do not insert opinions unattached to individuals or groups. For example, it would not be helpful to write, "Some oppose legislation regulating Internet pharmacies." Such a statement does not identify *who* opposes the legislation or *why* they oppose the legislation. If your client will be able to assess the political, practical, and ethical feasibility of taking a particular action, the client needs to understand where the various groups stand and why they hold those views. Thus, a more helpful sentence would be: "RxData, a large software company that assists Internet pharmacies and is a major employer in your congressional district, opposes legislation regulating Internet pharmacies because it will add costs to its business and may result in future employee layoffs." That sentence tells your client who is opposed to the legislation, why they are opposed to it, and why they are a key stakeholder.

The tone of the landscape should be neutral and objective. The landscape is not an argumentative section to persuade the reader that one view is better than another. Its purpose is to identify all of the key stakeholders and their concerns so the decision maker is well-informed before assessing options.

The Options Section

Once your client finishes reading the background and landscape sections, he or she should have a thorough understanding of the policy problem and the overall context in which a decision will be made. The time has come for him to consider what action to take. This is where your paper's options section comes in, providing three to five alternatives for your client to consider. This section is more than a recitation of various choices; it provides an analysis of each option by stating the positive and negative aspects of pursuing each path.

Identifying Options

The first step to writing your options section is to identify the various options you could analyze. Although you may develop a new option not previously considered by others, it is likely that you will find numerous possibilities that others have already suggested. Some places to find already-considered options include the following:

- Media
- Scholarly articles
- Interest group recommendations
- Think tanks/experts in the field
- Congressional testimony
- Legislation (passed or proposed)
- Agency reports

Another approach to developing options is to consider several major actions that policymakers often take to deal with a policy problem. For example, depending on the circumstances, the following actions could be added, eliminated, or altered by a policymaker in response to a policy problem:

- Taxes
- Subsidies
- Grants
- Laws
- Regulations
- Programs
- Government organizations
- Information
- Outreach

Once you have compiled a list of options, how do you choose the best three to five options to include in the analysis? As always, the guiding principle underlying your decision is to base your decision on your client's values and powers. You should not suggest an option that clearly violates your client's values because your client will not seriously consider that option. For example, if your client has rejected spending new state money to solve a problem, you should not include an option that would cost the state money (or if you do, you would need to be clear about how these funds would be offset). Also, it is important to remember the extent of your client's power. For example, on one hand, an analyst might recommend that a member of Congress introduce or sponsor a bill, or that an interest group submit a comment as part of the public notice and comment period before a regulation is finalized. On the other hand, an analyst should not recommend that a member of Congress force a state to pass a particular law, because that action is not within Congress's power (the responsibility of passing state laws falls to state legislatures). Similarly, an interest group cannot issue an executive order or force an administrative agency to craft a regulation in a particular way. In other words, any option you include must be within the ability of your client to undertake.

In addition, you will probably want to include in your analysis any major proposals that are currently being considered. You may also choose to include proposals backed by key allies and constituents. Even if your client does not act on these proposals, it is important to be able to explain why "mainstream" options are being rejected. Also, it may be appropriate to consider the status quo (the "do-nothing" approach) as an option. The status quo option works best when there is a specific reason for waiting to act; otherwise, it may appear to be an option because the analyst ran out of ideas. For example, if there is an evaluation under way of a key program, a valid status quo option would be to wait until the evaluation is complete and then reconsider the issue based on the findings. Simply suggesting to do nothing without a rationale is not acceptable. Even when considering the do-nothing tactic, it is necessary to evaluate the pros and cons of this option. In addition, your options should be different enough from one another to give your client a real choice. For example, if all of your options involved creating a big, new federal program and your client does not prefer that strategy, then the analysis is not useful. There is one final rule to follow: whichever alternative you ultimately recommend must be analyzed in the options section of your analysis.

All of the options included in the analysis must directly address the problem identified in your problem identification. For example, if your problem identification involved ways to reduce the number of uninsured individuals, an option that promotes increasing access to care for insured residents would be inappropriate because it does not directly address the problem. Indeed, everything in your analysis must flow from your problem identification, from what is included in the background and the issues discussed in your landscape, to the alternatives suggested in the options section, and (as discussed later) your final recommendation.

Assessing Your Options

Your options analysis must include a discussion of the pros (what is useful) and the cons (what is problematic) of each option. Although policymakers often seek a "silver bullet" that solves a problem without any negative effects, it is highly unlikely that such an option exists. As a result, an analysis must include the positive and negative aspects of an option. Also, all options must be analyzed equally. Do not provide more analysis for the option you decide to recommend even though it is your preferred option. Your client can make a fully informed decision only if you analyze what is both good and bad about each proposal.

To draft your pros and cons, you must identify the appropriate criteria for the analysis of the pros and cons and apply each criterion to all of the options. Many possible criteria could be used, so you must pick the ones that best fit your client's values and that address the key issues relating to the policy problem. Sometimes your client will provide you with criteria; other times you must deduce the correct criteria based on what you know about your client and the problem. Generally you should choose between three and five criteria for your evaluation of the pros and cons in this type of analysis. Typically, fewer than three will not allow for a full analysis, and more than five are difficult to assess in a relatively short analysis.

Your choice of criteria should reflect the concerns discussed in the landscape, where you identified the key factors relating to the problem. For example, if economic burden was an important aspect of the issue being considered, costs should be one of the criteria used to analyze the options. If the need for quick action was an important aspect of the issue, timeliness and administrative ease might be important criteria to consider. In general, cost and political feasibility are usually important criteria to include in your analysis. However, the specific criteria that are best for your analysis will depend on your client, the specific problem identification being addressed, and the landscape of the issue. **BOX 14-2** provides some criteria that could be considered when analyzing options. Can you think of others?

BOX 14-2 Sample Options Criteria

Cost: How much does this option cost? (You may have to break this down: how much does it cost the federal government, state government, individuals, etc.?)

Cost–benefit: How much "bang for the buck" does this option provide? (This is a difficult criterion to assess in shorter, less complicated policy analyses because you often do not have the information necessary to make this determination.)

Political feasibility: Is this option politically viable? Is it likely to become law? Even if it is not likely to become law, is it likely to help your client politically?

Legality: Is this option legal? If so, are there any restrictions?

Administrative ease: Does this option have steep implementation hurdles?

Fairness: Are people affected by this option treated fairly/equally?

Timeliness: Can this option be implemented in an appropriate or useful amount of time?

Targeted impact: Does this option target the population/issue involved?

Effectiveness: How well does this option accomplish the goal set out in the problem identification?

Healthcare-specific criteria: Does this option improve quality of care, lower healthcare spending, reduce the incidence of a particular disease, etc.?

Structuring the Options Section

When structuring your options section, you may find it helpful to use headings or bullets delineating each option. Your headings should clearly label each option. Also, it is generally useful to separate out the options by paragraph instead of having a continuous page or two assessing all of the options. The first sentence or two of each options paragraph should be a clear description of that option so the client understands what is being proposed and exactly what action your client would be taking; then assess the pros and cons of the option based on the criteria you identified. You should explicitly state the criteria prior to your options description.

For example, assume you are writing a policy analysis for the Secretary of the Department of Health and Human Services about how to increase access to care for immigrants. After drafting the necessary background and landscape information, you decide to assess the following options: (1) creating a public education campaign, (2) providing grants to states, and (3) increasing funding to community health centers.

You decide the best criteria to use are cost to the federal government, political feasibility, and degree of increase in the number of immigrants who seek care. In your options section, you would have three different parts—one for each option—assessing the pros and cons based on the criteria you chose. Although the structure of the analysis may vary, you might have a paragraph looking something like this:

> **Option 1: Create a Public Education Campaign.** The Secretary of the Department of Health and Human Services should order the Centers for Disease Control and Prevention to create a public education campaign to alert immigrants to the various ways they can access health care in their area. The campaign will be delivered in English and the most common immigrant languages in the area and will occur on television, over the radio, and in public (e.g., billboards). In these difficult economic times, this is a relatively low-cost option (although if immigrants access more care, the cost of providing care will increase). In addition, the political feasibility is somewhat high because this option does not call for any policy changes, but rather merely alerting individuals to policies that already exist. On the other hand, the political feasibility is tempered because the option focuses on helping immigrants, a group that has been under attack politically in recent times. The most significant disadvantage of this option is that it may not be very effective in increasing the number of immigrants who access care because it does not increase access points, reduce the cost of care, or address concerns in the immigrant community about being deported if they participate in public programs.

You would write a similar analysis for each of the options under consideration.

Side-by-Side Tables

You may choose to assess your options with the help of a side-by-side table. This table may be descriptive or analytic. A descriptive table would provide a description of each option but not provide any analysis. An analytic table would assess the options based on the criteria chosen. In either case, the table should be appropriately labeled and easy to read. As a general matter, a side-by-side table should supplement, not replace, your textual analysis because it is difficult to provide sufficient information within the space provided by a table. However, a table is a useful visual aid that may enhance the reader's understanding of your options and overall analysis. **TABLES 14-1** and **14-2** provide examples of side-by-side tables.

As you can see from both tables, additional information is necessary for a complete analysis. In the text of your options section, you would need to provide a more complete explanation of each option. It is difficult (but not impossible) to provide sufficient depth of analysis in a chart without creating a busy, difficult-to-read table.

Although the second table uses the terms *low*, *medium*, and *high* to assess the options, other terms or symbols (e.g., +, −) may be used. In addition, you may choose to include phrases instead of single words or symbols. Whatever choice you make, be sure that it

TABLE 14-1 Descriptive Side-by-Side Table

Increasing Access to Care for Immigrants—Options Description			
	Public Education Campaign	**Grants to States**	**Health Center Funding**
General description	Campaign on radio, television, and public areas	Federal government provides funds to states to increase access to care for immigrants	Federal government provides funding to health centers for services
Populations affected	All will hear, focus on immigrants in community	Only immigrants in the state	All health center patients, including immigrants
Length of option	1 year	5 years, subject to annual appropriations	2 years
Payer	Federal	Federal	Federal

TABLE 14-2 Analytic Side-by-Side Table

Increasing Access to Care for Immigrants—Options Assessment

Options Criteria	Public Education Campaign	Grants to States	Health Center Funding
Cost to federal government	Low	Medium	High
Political feasibility	Medium	Low	High
Increase in access for immigrants	Low	High	Medium

BOX 14-3 Checklist for Writing a Policy Analysis

1. Problem Identification
Is my problem written as one sentence in the form of a question?
Can I identify the focus of my problem ?
Can I identify several options (but not *too* many) for solving the problem?

2. Background
Does my background include all necessary factual information?
Have I eliminated information that is not directly relevant to the analysis?
Is the tone of my background appropriate?

3. Landscape
Does the landscape identify all of the key stakeholders?
Are the stakeholders' views described clearly and accurately?
Is the structure of the landscape consistent and easy to follow?
Is the tone of the landscape appropriate?
Does the reader have all the information necessary to assess the options?

4. Options
Do my options directly address the issue identified in the problem identification?
Did I assess the pros and cons of each option?
Did I apply all of the criteria to each option's assessment?
Are the options sufficiently different from each other to give the client a real choice?
Are all of the options within the power of my client?

5. Recommendation
Is my recommendation one of the options assessed?
Did I recommend only one of my options?
Did I explain why this recommendation is the best option, despite its flaws?

is clear which assessment is positive and which is negative. When necessary, provide a legend explaining your terms. Also, some people prefer to use numerical assessments (e.g., 1 = low, 2 = medium, 3 = high). Although debates exist regarding the value of this type of quantitative assessment in a side-by-side chart, we strongly discourage it. Policy analysis is both an art and a science, and using a numerically based table can obscure that balance. An attempt to use quantitative measures may lead readers to assume a simple summation will suffice—just add up the columns and choose the best one. Overall, reducing the analysis to numerical labels hides the value judgments that are part of every analysis, fails to address whether certain criteria should be weighted more than others, and makes the optimal solution appear more certain than it probably is.

The Recommendation Section

The time has finally arrived in your policy analysis to make a recommendation. You should choose *one* of your options as your recommendation. Although it is possible to make more than one recommendation or a hybrid recommendation of multiple options, we discourage those approaches. Making multiple recommendations might make it necessary for your client to conduct further analysis to choose among the options, and making a hybrid recommendation (a combination of two or more options) is not appropriate unless the hybrid option was analyzed separately as a single option. In general, it is the analyst's job to organize and clarify the issues and place them in the context of the client's views and power. Ultimately, this approach should result in one path that you believe best suits your client.

The recommendation section should begin by clearly identifying which option is favored and why this option is preferred over the other ones. As mentioned in the options section, every alternative will have pros and cons. The recommendation section does not simply repeat the analysis in the options section. Instead, this portion of the analysis must explain why, despite the drawbacks, this is the best action to take based on your client's values and power. In addition, the recommendation section identifies what, if any, actions may be taken to mitigate or overcome the negative aspects of your recommendation.

▶ Conclusion

You now have a basic understanding of what policy analysis is and an introduction to the tools necessary to analyze a policy problem. Additionally, thinking through the process described in this chapter should train you to evaluate your options when *you* become the decision maker. The checklist in **BOX 14-3** provides examples of what should be included in each section of a written policy analysis.

References

Kingdon, J. (1995). *Agendas, alternatives, and public policies* (2nd ed.). New York, NY: Addison-Wesley Educational Publishers.

Patton C. V., & Sawicki, D. S. (1993). *Basic methods of policy analysis and planning* (2nd ed.). Englewood Cliffs, NJ: Prentice Hall.

Stone, D. (2002). *Policy paradox: The art of political decision making.* New York, NY: W. W. Norton.

Weissert, C. S., & Weissert, W. G. (2002). *Governing health: The politics of health policy* (2nd ed.). Baltimore, MD: Johns Hopkins University Press.

Glossary

accountable care organization (ACO) A group of healthcare providers that is collectively reimbursed for a single patient's care. This arrangement is meant to give providers an incentive to deliver high-quality, cost-effective care.

accreditation A process applied to healthcare institutions to ensure that all necessary and required processes, standards, competencies, ethics, and so on are up to par.

administrative law The body of law produced by executive (i.e., administrative) agencies of federal, state, and local governments.

Administrative Procedures Act A federal law that governs the way in which administrative agencies of the federal government may propose and establish regulations.

adverse selection A means of forming an insurance pool based on the idea that individuals with a higher-than-average risk of needing health care are more likely to seek health insurance coverage.

annual aggregate limit A cap imposed by health insurance companies on the amount a policy will pay during a single year.

bioterrorism The threat or use of a biologic agent, typically by a nonstate actor, to cause death or harm to humans, animals, or plants and specifically targeting civilian populations or resources.

block grant A large sum of money granted by the national government to a regional government with only general provisions as to how the money is to be spent.

bundling An arrangement by which providers are paid a predetermined amount for all services related to treating a specific condition, as opposed to compensating healthcare providers separately for every service performed. This arrangement is meant to give providers an incentive to deliver cost-effective care.

"Cadillac" healthcare plans Health insurance plans and other products whose value exceeds a stated annual dollar threshold.

cafeteria plans Employer-sponsored health benefit plans under which employees may set aside wages to be used for medical expenses not otherwise covered by their basic health insurance. Also referred to as flexible spending accounts (FSAs).

capitation A method of payment for health services in which a fixed amount is paid for each person served without regard to the actual number or nature of services provided.

catastrophic coverage A health insurance coverage option with limited benefits and a high deductible, intended to protect against medical bankruptcy due to an unforeseen illness or injury.

Centers for Disease Control and Prevention (CDC) The federal agency within the Department of Health and Human Services charged with disease prevention, education, and public health activities.

Centers for Medicare and Medicaid Services (CMS) The federal agency within the Department of Health and Human Services that administers the Medicare and Medicaid programs.

Children's Health Insurance Program (CHIP) A health insurance program targeted to low-income children, established in 1997 and reauthorized in 2009, that is administered by states and funded through a combination of federal and state payments.

COBRA The nickname for a law, enacted as part of the Consolidated Omnibus Budget Reconciliation Act of 1985, that allows individuals to continue to purchase employee health benefits for a period of 18 to 36 months following a "qualifying event" such as unemployment, death of a wage earner, divorce, or termination of minor dependent coverage.

co-insurance A form of beneficiary cost-sharing for covered health insurance benefits and services, expressed as a percentage of the approved payment amount for the benefit or service (e.g., 20% of the payable amount).

community health center A type of community clinic that provides a broad range of healthcare services and that charges on a sliding-scale fee basis. See also *federally qualified health center*.

community rating A method for setting a premium that requires health insurance providers to offer health insurance policies within a given territory at the same price to all persons without medical underwriting, regardless of individual health status.

comparative effectiveness research (CER) A type of health services research that compares different approaches to treating medical conditions in order to determine which methods are most likely to produce the best outcomes.

coordination of benefits A process by which health services are paid for by more than one health insurance plan. For example, if a child is insured through both parents, one insurer is generally considered the primary policy, and the secondary policy reimburses for services not covered under the primary policy.

co-payment A form of beneficiary cost-sharing for covered health insurance benefits and services, expressed as a flat dollar payment (e.g., $5.00 for a prescription drug).

cost-sharing A requirement that insured patients pay a portion of their medical costs, either as co-insurance or as a fixed co-payment.

culturally and linguistically appropriate care A federal standard designed to eliminate ethnic and racial disparities in health care.

deductible The amount patients must pay out of their own pocket before their health insurance policy begins contributing to the cost of their care.

Department of Defense (DoD) A federal agency that, among other functions, administers healthcare programs for active military and their dependents through a publicly funded and privately administered health program called TriCare.

Department of Health and Human Services (HHS) A federal agency that administers federal health and welfare programs and activities.

Department of Labor (DoL) A federal agency responsible for administration and enforcement of ERISA, a federal law that sets requirements for employer-provided health benefits that are not offered through state-licensed health insurance plans.

dependent coverage Health insurance coverage of a spouse, child, or domestic partner of an insured individual.

diagnostic-related group (DRG) A system used to classify patients (particularly under Medicare) for the purpose of reimbursing hospitals. Hospitals are paid a fixed fee for each case in a given category, regardless of the actual costs of providing care.

discrimination in health care Failure by providers to treat patients equitably for any of a number of reasons, including race, gender, age, ability to pay for care, or severity of illness. This term can also be used to describe the insurance company practice of medical underwriting and rating.

doughnut hole A gap in prescription drug coverage under Medicare Part D, for which beneficiaries pay 100% of their prescription drug costs after their total drug spending exceeds an initial coverage limit until they qualify for catastrophic coverage. The coverage gap will be gradually phased out under the Affordable Care Act by 2020.

dual eligibles Individuals who are eligible for both Medicaid and Medicare.

electronic medical record (EMR) An individual medical record that is stored electronically.

Employee Retirement Income Security Act (ERISA) A 1974 federal law that establishes standards governing both pension plans and "welfare benefit plans" (such as health benefits, dependent care benefits, and other types of benefits and services) and that is applicable to non-federal employers, multi-employer arrangements, and union plans.

employer responsibility A requirement that employers assist in covering workers and their dependents, either through the provision of a health plan or through a contribution toward coverage that may be expressed as payment of a flat dollar charge (e.g., $500 per worker), a percentage of payroll, a percentage of an annual insurance premium, or some other amount. Also referred to as an "employer mandate."

employer-sponsored insurance (ESI) A health benefit plan offered by an employer to its employees (and often to employee dependents). Some employers purchase plans from a traditional insurance company, while other (primarily large) employers may choose to directly insure their employees through their own plan.

entitlement program An insurance program that guarantees access to benefits or services based on established rights or by legislation (e.g., the Medicaid program).

epidemic A situation in which new cases of a certain disease, in a given human population during a given period, substantially exceed what is expected based on recent experience.

epidemiology The study of patterns of health and illness and associated factors at the population level.

essential benefits A list of core benefits established under the Affordable Care Act that must be included under any health insurance plan in order to meet minimum coverage requirements.

exchange-eligible employer An employer that is permitted to enroll in a health insurance exchange in order to offer health benefits to its employees.

exchange-eligible individual An individual who is permitted to obtain coverage through a health insurance exchange.

exchange-participating health benefit plan A health insurance plan offered to individuals and small employers through health insurance exchanges. They must meet federal insurance market and benefit requirements.

excise tax A tax on health insurance and health benefit plans whose annual dollar value exceeds a specified limit, as well as on the sale of specified healthcare items and services such as medical devices and equipment.

exclusion The practice by which an insurer or health benefit plan classifies certain otherwise-covered items and treatments as ineligible for coverage. Common exclusions include "experimental," "educational," and "cosmetic" treatments and services.

executive order A presidential directive, with the authority of a law, that directs and governs actions by executive officials and agencies.

fair marketing A term used to encompass a range of health insurance market reforms to protect consumers from medical underwriting and other practices designed to limit the amount an insurer pays for medical claims.

Federal Emergency Management Agency (FEMA) A federal agency responsible for responding to national emergencies, including natural disasters.

federalism A system of government in which sovereignty is constitutionally divided between a central governing authority and constituent political units (e.g., states), and in which the power to govern is shared between the national and state governments.

federally qualified health center (FQHC) A community health center that either receives funding under section 440 of the Public Health Service Act or has been certified as meeting the same criteria.

fee-for-service A method of paying for medical services under which doctors are paid for each service provided. Bills are paid by the patient, who then submits them to the insurance company for reimbursement.

fraud and abuse A range of wasteful healthcare activities, including billing for services not performed, billing for more expensive services than performed ("up-coding"), and performing inappropriate or unnecessary care.

gainsharing A system in which the government passes on savings from providing more-efficient care to insurers and providers.

guaranteed issue and renewal A rule that bars health insurers from denying or dropping an individual's coverage for any reason other than fraud or nonpayment of health insurance premiums. This rule is especially important to prevent insurance companies from denying coverage based on individuals' health status.

health disparity A situation in which one population group experiences a higher burden of disability or illness relative to another group.

health equity A situation in which everyone has the opportunity to attain his or her full health potential and no one is disadvantaged because of social conditions.

health information privacy and security Standards or procedures to ensure that personal health information is not compromised or disclosed in processing healthcare transactions.

health information technology (HIT) Technology that allows the comprehensive management of health information and enables its exchange among health professionals, healthcare providers, healthcare payers, and public health agencies.

health insurance exchanges Regulated marketplaces for the sale and purchase of health insurance established under federal law and operated in accordance with federal requirements.

health insurance exchange subsidies Federal subsidies made available on an income-related basis to exchange-eligible individuals for the purchase of health insurance coverage through health insurance exchanges.

health insurance issuers Entities that sell health insurance in the individual and employer-sponsored group markets.

Health Insurance Portability and Accountability Act (HIPAA) A federal law that regulates health insurers and health benefit plans in the group market and provides privacy protections for health information.

health maintenance organization (HMO) A type of health insurance plan that provides a coordinated array of preventive and treatment services for a fixed payment per month. Enrollees receive medically necessary services regardless of whether the cost of those services exceeds the premium paid on the enrollees' behalf.

health status All aspects of physical and mental health and their manifestations in daily living, including impairment, disability, and handicap.

health threat In the context of national or global security, an environmental, biologic, chemical, radiologic, or physical risk to public or community health.

healthcare/public health workforce A term used to define a range of health professionals in private and public practice who provide medical care and public health services such as primary care, disease diagnosis, and public education.

healthcare disparity A difference in access to healthcare services or to health insurance, or in the quality of care actually received.

high-risk insurance pool An insurance option for patients with existing medical conditions that make them expensive to insure.

homeland defense The protection of U.S. territory, populations, and infrastructure against external threats or aggression.

incidence The number of new cases of illness or disease during a specific period of time in a specific population.

Indian Health Care Improvement Act A federal law creating programs to strengthen healthcare options in Native American communities.

Indian Health Service A federal health program to provide health care to Native Americans and Alaska natives.

individual market The insurance market for individuals who are purchasing insurance for themselves and their families and are not part of a group plan, such as one offered by an employer. Also referred to as the nongroup market.

individual responsibility The requirement that all individuals must carry health insurance or pay a penalty. Also referred to as an "individual mandate."

insurance pool A group of individuals whose premiums are used to pay all covered medical costs of its members. Insurance companies may charge higher premiums to a pool whose members are older or less healthy than other pools in order to cover the risk that its members may submit more medical claims.

interest group An organization that uses various forms of advocacy to influence public opinion and/or policy. Groups vary considerably in size, influence, and purpose. Also referred to as special interest groups, advocacy groups, or lobby groups.

International Health Regulations A 2005 international treaty obligating all Member States of the World Health Organization to detect, report, and respond to potential public health emergencies of international concern. These regulations are aimed at improving global health security through international collaboration and communication.

large group market The market for health insurance or health benefit plans among employers whose employee numbers exceed a specified threshold size (e.g., 100 full-time workers).

lifetime aggregate limits Provisions included in health insurance contracts designed to limit the total amount the policy will pay out in claims and benefits over the lifetime of the policy.

long-term care A set of healthcare, personal care, and social services provided to persons who have lost, or never acquired, some degree of functional capacity (e.g., the chronically ill, aged, or disabled) in an institution or at home, on a long-term basis.

managed care Health insurance arrangements that integrate the financing and delivery of services to covered individuals.

market failure A concept within economic theory in which the allocation of goods and services by a free market is not efficient.

Medicaid A program established in 1965 to provide health insurance to low-income families and individuals with certain disabilities. It is administered by the states and funded jointly with the federal government.

medical home A clinic focused on primary care and preventive services that offers a range of coordinated treatment services.

medical-legal partnership An approach to health that integrates the expertise of healthcare, public health, and legal professionals and staff to address and prevent health-harming social and civil legal needs for patients and populations.

medical underwriting The insurance industry practice of assessing the medical condition of individuals at the time that insurance enrollment is sought in order to identify existing physical or mental health conditions that may affect an individual's or group's eligibility for enrollment, the application of preexisting condition exclusions or waiting periods, or the price to be charged for coverage.

Medicare A federal program enacted in 1965 that provides government-sponsored health insurance to individuals ages 65 years and older and certain individuals younger than 65 years with disabilities that meet federal requirements.

Medicare Advantage Optional private insurance plans in which Medicare beneficiaries may enroll to receive their federal benefits.

Medigap coverage Supplemental health insurance designed to cover all or most of the charges that are not covered by Medicare, including the 20% co-payment required for many outpatient services.

National Health Service Corps A commissioned corps of public health professionals employed by the federal Department of Health and Human Services. Members are assigned to settings that include clinics in underserved areas, state and local health departments, and federal agencies such as the Centers for Disease Control and Prevention.

National Institutes of Health A federal agency within the Department of Health and Human Services that is primarily responsible for conducting and supporting medical research.

notifiable disease A disease that, once diagnosed, must be reported under the law to a public health authority.

Office of the Inspector General (OIG) Located within the federal Department of Health and Human Services, this office is charged with protecting the integrity of programs administered by the Department, protecting the health and welfare of program beneficiaries, and reporting problems to the Department Secretary and to Congress.

pandemic An infectious disease that spreads through human populations across a large region, over multiple continents.

parity A term generally used to require that large group insurers or plans pay equivalent benefits for different kinds of services. For example, federal law requires "mental health parity," which means that for health plans that include mental health benefits as well as medical ones, the services must be covered with the same financial requirements and treatment limitations.

Patient Protection and Affordable Care Act Also known as the Affordable Care Act or ACA, a major federal health reform law enacted in March 2010.

patient protections Laws establishing protections for patients, such as the right to health information, to choice of providers, to access to care, to file a grievance, or to appeal a denied health benefit claim.

pay-for-performance (P4P) A healthcare payment system in which providers receive incentives for meeting quality and cost benchmarks (or, in some cases, penalties for not meeting established benchmarks).

performance measurement A set of recommendations, requirements, or data used to determine whether plans, providers, or programs meet or exceed a standard of care.

policy analysis An analysis that provides informed advice to a client that relates to a public policy decision, includes a recommended course of action/inaction, and is framed by the client's powers and values.

population health Health outcomes of a group of individuals, including the distribution of such outcomes within the group.

preexisting conditions Health conditions that exist prior to or at the time of enrollment into a health insurance or health benefit plan.

preferred provider organization (PPO) A health insurance plan in which providers agree to provide care to covered individuals at a negotiated price. Covered individuals receive all medically necessary services regardless of whether the cost of the services exceeds the premium paid, although members do have cost-sharing obligations.

premium The amount a business or individual pays regularly to maintain health insurance coverage.

premium rating An insurance industry practice determining health insurance premiums based on factors including age, health status, gender, industry, geography, or other factors.

prevalence The total number of cases of a disease or illness in the population at a given time.

preventive services Measures taken to prevent the development of disease or to treat illnesses early so that they do not become more acute and expensive to treat. Examples include vaccination, weight-loss programs, and mammograms.

primary care provider (PCP) A healthcare provider, such as a physician engaged in the practice of internal medicine, pediatric care, or geriatric care, or a nurse practitioner, who provides general medical care and coordinates treatment.

public health emergency An acute event capable of causing large-scale morbidity and mortality, either immediately or over time. These events have the ability to overwhelm normal public health and medical care capabilities.

public health insurance A health insurance plan that is administered by the government either directly or through the use of private contractors. Medicare, Medicaid, and CHIP all are considered forms of public health insurance.

public health preparedness The actions and policies associated with preventing, protecting against, responding to, and recovering from a major public health event.

quarantine The separation and restriction of movement of people or animals that may have been exposed to an infectious agent.

reinsurance A form of insurance that health insurers may purchase to protect themselves against losses that may occur should they underestimate how much they will pay out for medical claims in a year.

rescission A process by which an insurance company seeks to recover the amount paid out for covered services after discovering that information on a beneficiary's initial enrollment form was incomplete or incorrect.

retiree health benefits Health benefits provided by an employer to its retirees.

risk adjustment A tool for evaluating the relative risk of enrollees within insurance plans and providing for a financial transfer from plans with low-risk enrollees to plans with higher-risk enrollees.

safety net The collection of healthcare providers who serve patients regardless of patients' ability to pay for care. Providers include community health centers, public hospitals, local health departments, school- and church-based health clinics, and private physicians and nonprofit hospitals committed to serving uninsured and low-income, vulnerable patients.

skimming The insurance plan practice of enrolling predominantly healthy individuals in order to reduce the costs to the plan.

small group market The health insurance market for employers whose size is smaller than a specified threshold (e.g., 100 full-time workers).

social determinant of health (SDH) A factor outside of one's genetic predisposition that can cause or prevent poor health, as well as affect how disease can progress (or not) throughout one's lifetime. Examples include socioeconomic status, geographic birthplace, and housing quality.

stare decisis A Latin term that refers to the legal principle that prior case law decisions should be accorded great deference and should not be frequently overturned.

surge capacity The ability of clinical care facilities and laboratories to accommodate a sharp increase in patients and samples during a public health emergency.

telehealth The use of electronic information and telecommunications technologies to support long-distance clinical health care, patient and professional health-related education, public health, and health administration. Technologies may include videoconferencing, the Internet, store-and-forward imaging, streaming media, and terrestrial and wireless communications.

uncompensated care Services provided by physicians and hospitals for which no payment is received from the patient or from third-party payers.

underinsured Individuals with insurance policies that do not cover all necessary healthcare services, resulting in out-of-pocket expenses that exceed the ability to pay.

uninsured Individuals who lack public or private health insurance.

universal coverage The provision of at least basic or medically necessary health insurance for an entire population.

utilization review The examination, usually by an insurer or third-party administrator, of the necessity and/or appropriateness of healthcare services provided to a patient.

weapon of mass destruction (WMD) A weapon that causes large-scale destruction, generally through nuclear, radiologic, chemical, or biologic means.

wellness programs Special services and benefits offered by employers to employees in addition to health benefit plans, including nutrition classes, smoking-cessation programs, or gym memberships.

World Health Organization (WHO) The directing and coordinating authority for health within the United Nations system.

The following source was used, in part, in the compilation of this Glossary:

The Health Policy Institute of Ohio. (n.d.). *Glossary*. Retrieved from http://www.healthpolicyohio.org/tools/glossary/

Index

Page numbers followed by *f*, *t*, *b* and *n* indicate figures, tables, boxes and notes.

A